Laser Surface Treatment of Metals

NATO ASI Series

Advanced Science Institutes Series

A Series presenting the results of activities sponsored by the NATO Science Committee, which aims at the dissemination of advanced scientific and technological knowledge, with a view to strengthening links between scientific communities.

The Series is published by an international board of publishers in conjunction with the NATO Scientific Affairs Division

A	**Life Sciences**	Plenum Publishing Corporation
B	**Physics**	London and New York
C	**Mathematical and Physical Sciences**	D. Reidel Publishing Company Dordrecht and Boston
D	**Behavioural and Social Sciences**	Martinus Nijhoff Publishers Dordrecht/Boston/Lancaster
E	**Applied Sciences**	
F	**Computer and Systems Sciences**	Springer-Verlag Berlin/Heidelberg/New York
G	**Ecological Sciences**	

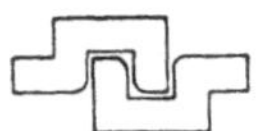

Series E: Applied Sciences – No. 115

Laser Surface Treatment of Metals

edited by

Clifton W. Draper

AT & T Engineering
Research Center
Princeton, NJ 08540
USA

and

Paolo Mazzoldi

Padova University
Department of Physics
Padova 35131
Italy

1986 **Martinus Nijhoff Publishers**
Dordrecht / Boston / Lancaster
Published in cooperation with NATO Scientific Affairs Division

Proceedings of the NATO Advanced Study Institute on Laser Surface Treatment of Metals, San Miniato, Italy, September 2-13, 1985

Library of Congress Cataloging in Publication Data

NATO Advanced Study Institute on Laser Surface Treatment of Metals (1985 : San Miniato, Italy)
Laser surface treatment of metals.

(NATO advanced science institutes series. Series E, Applied sciences ; 115)
Proceedings of the NATO Advanced Study Institute on Laser Surface Treatment of Metals, San Miniato, Italy, September 2-13, 1985"--P. iv.
Includes index.
1. Metals--Finishing--Equipment and supplies--Congresses. 2. Metallurgy--Laser use in--Congresses. Draper, Clifton W. II. Mazzoldi, Paolo. III. Title. IV. Series.
TS653.5.N37 1985 671'.7 86-21766

ISBN-13:978-94-010-8489-5 e-ISBN-13:978-94-009-4468-8
DOI:10.1007/978-94-009-4468-8

Distributors for the United States and Canada: Kluwer Academic Publishers, 101 Philip Drive, Assinippi Park, Norwell, MA 02061, USA

Distributors for the UK and Ireland: Kluwer Academic Publishers, MTP Press Ltd, Falcon House, Queen Square, Lancaster LA1 1RN, UK

Distributors for all other countries: Kluwer Academic Publishers Group, Distribution Center, P.O. Box 322, 3300 AH Dordrecht, The Netherlands

INTRODUCTION

This book contains the papers presented at a NATO Advanced Study Institute held at S. Miniato, Italy, from September 2 to 13, 1985, on the latest developments in the science and technology of modifications, in particular, of metallurgical surfaces due to laser treatment.

The objectives of the meeting were twofold. First, to inform participants of actual and developing technological applications of laser treatment in which fundamental science makes a strong contribution; second, to bring together scientists from widely different cultural backgrounds in material science and technology to promote mutual understanding and collaboration.

Laser surface processing comprises different operational regimes, depending on the interaction time and laser beam energy. By changing the characteristics of the laser-material interaction spectrum, a variety of modifications are possible, as transformation hardening, deep penetration welding, laser glazing, drilling, metastable alloys formation, and shock hardening.

The mechanism by which the laser light energy is absorbed by the material surface and the heat transfer models for evaluation of the melt depth and temperature obtained with different laser inputs are examined, in terms of technology applications, by many lecturers. The effectiveness of enhanced absorption techniques in the laser energy transfer to the metal surfaces has been analyzed in detail. The modification metallurgy and the variety of modifications which are possible have been investigated in the main part of the meeting, focusing on the performance of the modified surfaces.

In addition, some seminars have been devoted to laser annealing of semiconductors, the interaction of laser beams with living tissues, production of superconducting alloys by laser annealing and quenching, and laser preparation of metal surfaces for telecommunication needs.

An interesting comparison between different direct energy sources, as laser, electron or ion beams, has been presented by some lecturers.

The last session was devoted to development in laser material processing for the automotive industry with the contributions of experts from FIAT, General Motors and Rolls-Royce Industries.

The interdisciplinary nature of the meeting appears clearly in the wide range of interest in the material delivered by the lecturers.

Finally, probable directions for future research are discussed.

We thank all the chairmen, lecturers and participants who cooperated in the discussions and exchanges in different disciplines and between applied technologies and basic research.

We thank also all those organizations who generously supported the meeting:

- NATO, Scientific Affairs Division, provided the major balance of the funds under the framework of the NATO double-jump program for generating closer collaboration between industry and basic research organizations of the member countries.

- The industrial and national organizations below responded promptly, ensuring the remaining support:

Institute Co-Sponsors

American Society for Metals
Centro Informazioni Studi Esperienze
Cilas Alcatel
Coherent General
Consiglio Nazionale Delle Richerche
Ente Nazionale Energia Alternativa
European Research Office (USARDSG)
Ferranti, plc
FIAT
General Electric Company, plc
The Institute of Metals
International Society for Optical Engineering
The Laser Institute of America
Laser Optronix, srl
The Materials Research Society
The National Science Foundation
Newport Corporation
Padova University
Soitab
Valfivre

We are also very grateful to AT&T for assistance and support in the organization of the meeting and preparation of the book. In particular, Mary F. Edsall, whose skill at the word processor and editorial secretarial experience proved indispensable.

The support of these agencies, societies and companies made the attendance of 16 graduate students possible. These graduate students collectively wrote a meeting synopsis for their sponsors and we have decided to print it below as part of the book introduction.

EDITORS' INTRODUCTION - GRADUATE STUDENTS' REPORT

COMPILED BY DALE C. JACOBSON
Stevens Institute of Technology and AT&T Bell Laboratories

The NATO Material Science Panel has recognized for the past decade that laser treatment of surfaces is a field of enormous growth and that the technology developed by member countries should be shared. To this end NATO authorized an ADVANCED STUDY INSTITUTE, dedicated to LASER SURFACE TREATMENT OF METALS, under the direction of Dr. C. W. Draper of AT&T, USA, and Professor P. Mazzoldi of Padova University, Italy. The Institute took place in September, 1985, in San Miniato, Italy. The nine-day program included lectures, 90-minute talks, and contributed papers, 45 minutes in length. The Institute consisted of 18 lectures, 35 invited participants and 16 graduate students, for a total of 69 attendees.

Monday, September 2

Following a brief welcome and introduction by Clif Draper and Paolo Mazzoldi, the first session began with a talk by Prof. Walter Duley of York University in Canada. His presentation dealt with the quantity of energy deposited by a laser in the material being irradiated. Extensive studies have been performed to measure the reflection and transmission of laser irradiation which decrease the energy coupled to the material. The most striking result was the sensitivity of reflection to the cleanliness of the surface of the sample. If one is going to predict the reflectivity of a surface, that surface must be atomically clean. Wavelength and temperature dependence were also discussed.

Todd Rockstroh, a graduate student from the University of Illinois, presented a paper dealing with the production of plasmas by laser irradiation of metal surfaces. A two-dimensional model for the plasma temperature above the heat-affected zone was developed. Temperature measurements of the plasma were made using relative line intensity emission spectroscopy.

The afternoon session began with a presentation by Dr. Jean-Pierre Girardeau-Montaut, describing preliminary results of high-frequency, short-pulse laser irradiation of tungsten. A train 1 usec long of pulses 35 psec or less of UV or visible light was used to induce thermal and mechanical effects in the metal. It was shown that very rapid and periodic variations in temperature at the surface induce large stresses in the material.

Dr. Fritz Keilmann reported on a new mechanism of laser-material interaction. Stimulated scattering of laser light into surface electromagnetic waves which in turn are absorbed by the material. Surface rippling, a commonly observed phenomenon, can be explained by this model. It was shown the surface waves are strongly polarized.

The first session ended with a talk by Prof. Dona dalle Rose, where he showed the results of computer modeling of ultra rapid heat flow resulting from pulsed laser irradiation of metal surfaces. Diffusion of implanted impurities in the molten phase, segregation of these impurities upon recrystallization, and mixing of alternating layers as a result of laser irradiation of metals were discussed.

Tuesday, September 3

Dr. Frans Spaepen demonstrated melt quenching rates of 10^{12} K/sec for 30 ps pulsed laser radiation. The high rate promises the formation of new metastable/crystalline phases and metallic glasses. In particular, various Ni-Nb systems (23-81% Ni) were melted, with glasses forming far below the T_0 lines over the entire range of Ni.

Dr. Paul Peercy showed the results of laser melting of metallic (Al-Ni) systems with 10-100 ns pulses. The rapid solidification suppressed the formation of complex phases. Thus, a comparison of the laser-induced phases with ion implantation phases (currently under way) will permit the primary thermodynamic and kinetic processes to be evaluated.

It was shown by Steve Williamson, utilizing picosecond electron diffraction, that superheating can occur in 25 nm freestanding Al films. He attributes the onset of melting to the formation of defects.

Carolyn MacDonald utilized transient reflectance to measure melt lifetimes and melt/solid interface velocities in pure metals. It was shown that using a frequency doubled Nd-YAG 20 ps laser, interface velocities range from 60-100 meters/sec. This range of velocities implies a collision-limited regime.

Prof. Paolo Mazzoldi showed the surface peak formation resulting from laser-irradiated La- and Eu-implanted Ni systems. In a low-pressure oxygen or water vapor atmosphere, the effect is attributed to oxidation and solute trapping at the surface. A liquid phase diffusion analysis accounting for the two mechanisms reproduced the experimental results.

Joachim Fröhlingsdorf discussed the formation of amorphous Ga by irradiating a cryogenically cooled crystalline Ga substrate. An interesting feature was the repeatable switching of the substrate behavior between phases as the sample was heated a few degrees Kelvin and recooled.

Dale Jacobson demonstrated the laser melting of graphite (HOPG) at 4300 K at low ambient pressure and temperature. The results of TEM, and Rutherford backscattering and channeling implied that the liquid phase had indeed occurred. A free-electron gas model was shown to accurately predict the melt depth.

Aubrey Helms applied the techniques of Low-Energy Diffraction-Spot Profile Analysis (LEED-SPA) and RBS to the investigation of the structural reponse of single-crystal Mo and Bi samples to high-power laser pulses. The results indicate that the samples deform plastically in response to the high thermal stresses via the activation of dislocation sources lying on the major slip planes.

Wednesday, September 4

Dr. John Poate, Dr. Paul Peercy and Prof. Ugo Campisano presented three lectures on semiconductor-laser interactions. Intense interest in laser heating of semiconductors was generated a decade ago by the observation that ion implantation damage could be removed by laser melting. Defect-free crystals result from liquid phase epitaxy after pulsed laser irradiation yielding resolidification velocities up to 15 m/s with little segregaton of the implanted dopant. At higher velocities amorphous silicon is formed. Thermodynamic calculations give an estimate for the first-order melting temperature of amorphous Si 250 K below that of the crystalline material. This can be confirmed by calorimetry, transient conductance measurements, and observations of explosive crystallization. Lasers have proved unwieldy for bulk industrial application in silicon, but the understanding of the silicon regrowth processes led to the development of rapid thermal annealing furnaces and strip heaters. Models for describing solute trapping were presented by Dr. Michael Aziz and compared to data obtained from transient conductance measurements. Any description of the process requires deviation from local equilibrium; the most successful models also assume collision-limited growth.

Thursday, September 5

Prof. Jyotirmoy Mazumder lectured on creating a three-dimensional mathematical model for melting, mixing and resolidification as a result of cw laser irradiation. Mass and momentum transfer were included as well as heat conduction.

Dr. Gabriel Laufer presented a talk about the application of lasers in medicine - specifically, their use as a surgical cutting and cauterizing instrument. A thermodynamic model was developed to explain the damage to the surrounding tissue.

Dr. Michael Berry discussed the ablation of graphitic carbon and TaC as a result of higher power cw DF laser irradiation. He has measured the mass and energy distribution of the atoms that are removed from the surface as well as methods of protecting the surfaces against laser irradiation.

Dan Gnanamuthu presented a paper describing the problems one encounters when trying to apply laser technology to real industrial applications, such as beam shaping, polarization, energy coupling and heat transfer that affect solid phase transformations during surface modification. Mathematical models were presented that may be used to evaluate these parameters.

Paolo Gay talked about the work he has done with phosphate-based surface coating to increase the absorption of energy by the irradiated material. A two-dimensional model has been developed to explain the presented data.

Etienne Petit described how he had used AES and XPS to examine Al-Sb multilayered structures that had been prepared, laser irradiated and analyzed in UHV. Al-Sb alloy films are of interest in the field of optical data storage.

Ralf Koppmann described a technique in which Li and Al films were ablated by a Q-switched ruby laser. The energy and density distributions of the ablated particles were measured as a function of time by laser-induced fluorescence and mass spectroscopy. From this information plasma temperatures were calculated. This technique has a possible application of measuring very high temperatures, for example, in nuclear reactors.

Friday, September 6

The day began with a comprehensive account of the physico-chemical effects of laser-gas interaction as related to Laser Chemical Vapor Deposition (LCVD). Prof. Jean Tardieu de Maleissye lectured on laser chemistry and, in particular, surface and gaseous phase chemistry important in LCVD processes. Dr. Tom Jervis then presented results using a pulsed CO_2 laser to deposit metal films via LCVD. Depositions of Ni, Mo, and W have been produced and exhibit respectable conductivities. Interest in this cold deposition technique ranges from microelectronics to large-area coatings. The third talk by Dr. Jean-Pierre Celis described a technique that used a Nd:YAG laser to control the deposition rate in an electroplating process. Analysis of the thermal the electrochemical effects as well as optimal laser parameters of this technique were presented.

Finally, Prof. Lindsay Greer described the results of two separate experiments. The first showed rapid resolidification using picosecond laser pulses. The study of nucleation can benefit greatly from experiments performed on this fast time scale. Secondly, he presented the principles and applications of laser ionization mass analysis, citing the technique's importance as a versatile and most convenient first approach in microanalytic investigation.

Monday, September 9

The sixth day of lectures involved surface modifications to metallic substrates for engineering applications.

Dr. Hans Bergmann started the day with a comprenensive paper on continuous-wave CO_2 laser melting of cast irons. He described two approaches to this process: deep penetration surface melting and finish grinding, or precision casting (grinding if necessary) and surface melting. The hardnesses of the surface layers depended on the substrate material (ferritic, pearlitic, bainitric or austenitic) and graphite morphology (flaky or spheroid). Excellent wear properties in abrasive, adhesive and sliding/rolling tests were found, and these were borne out in actual component tests in a car engine. Push-pull and rotating bending tests showed a degradation in fatigue properties, but this was not thought to be critical when compared with the surface hardening and wear properties produced.

The second paper presented by Emmanuel Kerrand described the transformation hardening of 12% chromium steels by continuous-wave CO_2 lasers. The geometry and hardness of the treated zones with respect to different beam geometries was described and resultant residual stresses discussed. Graphite and black paint were used to improve coupling efficiencies, with black paint proving the better. Surface melting a chromium steel and low alloy steels was also carried out, along with cladding of a cobalt-based alloy.

Prof. Emilio Ramous described in the third paper the behavior of two absorbent coatings: DAG graphite and silica appliea in the form of water glass. The efficiency of the coatings was assessed by measuring the temperature at the rear of the specimens, with graphite proving the more efficient. The interaction between carbon and the substrate in both solid phase and surface melting treatments was reported.

Prof. Bill Steen started the afternoon session with a description of laser surface cladding. He discussed pre-placed powder beds, blown powder and particle injection techniques and concluded the blown powder technique was the easiest to use. With close control of powder feed rate and beam power, an absolute minimum of substrate is melted, resulting in minimum dilution of the clad layer. The optimum angle of incidence for blowing powder was discussed and the additional benefit of enhanced energy coupling by the powder noted. The relationships between treatment parameters and resultant microstructures were discussed.

Janet Folkes described the surface melting of titanium alloys and the resolidified microstructures, and went on to describe surface alloying with nickel pre-positioned by electroplating, platinum pre-positioned by ion-plating, and silver applied in a colloidal suspension. A problem with titanium and its alloys is its susceptibility to wear. A solution to this problem was suggested in the surface alloying with nitrogen to form a resolidified microstructure containing primary TiN. The structural features of the melt zone were reported and mechanisms for their formation discussed.

A second paper by Prof. Ramous reviewed the application of CO_2 laser surface melting to cast iron, steels and stellite alloys. It described the fine microstructures achieved in these materials, which included the complete solution of carbides in an alloy steel. Laser cladding with stellite resulted in higher hardnesses than the same clad with either the T.I.G. or acetylene process because of the finer microstructure.

The final paper of the day, presented by Charles Marsden, described laser carborizing of a martensitic stainless steel used in steam turbine blades, with an aim to overcome erosion problems. The carbon was applied in the form of colloidal graphite. A range of carbon content through hypoeutectic to hypereutectic compositions was obtained by increasing the number of repeated tracks. Large quantities of retained austenite were found and remained present even when quenched to liquid nitrogen temperatures.

Tuesday, September 10

Dr. Ed McCafferty described his work improving the corrosion properties of materials using lasers. He concentrated on the laser processing of various stainless steels and Al alloys. He discussed the "normalizing" of 304 stainless steel and its improvement to have properties similar to that of 316 stainless steel.

Prof. Jyotirmoy Mazumder presented a talk centering around the use of laser surface alloying and powder feed techniques for the development of corrosion and wear-resistant coatings. Several examples were given which included the formation of Fe-Cr-Ni alloys which mimic the corrosion properties of 304 stainless steel. Another example was the use of this technique to develop Fe-Cr-Mn-C alloys with good wear resistance.

Claude Chabrol reported investigations of the residual stresses induced in various steels after laser transformation. They studied the effect of a wide variety of parameters such as initial state laser power, interaction time and beam shape. Their analysis indicated compressive stresses within the treated region and tensile stresses in the transition zone.

Dr. Bernd Stritzker has been working to determine if pulsed laser quenching can be used to form new metastable materials with enhanced superconductivity properties. His talk centered around work done with anisotropic compounds. The conclusion was that there is hope that the laser may be used to quench new metastable materials, which will have the high T_c desired for superconducting materials.

Dr. Clif Draper outlined a number of uses of lasers in the telecommunications industry. Emphasis was made on why the laser had advantages in each of the applications reviewed. The laser has been used for surface treatment and surface alloying along with a vast array of other applications. The advantages and disadvantages of various types of lasers were discussed in relation to critical laser and materials parameters which are important in each application.

Dr. Carmen Afonso discussed the possibility of using the laser to develop new materials for optical storage. Much of the discussion concentrated on results of the Ge/Al system. She showed they could successfully produce amorphous Ge/Al films. They also observed mixing in both alloyed and eutectic films, with metastable phases being produced in the case of premixed systems.

Wednesday, September 11

The session started with a very informative talk on the development in laser material processing for the automotive industry, given by Dr. Aldo La Rocca. The talk concentrated on how the heat conduction equation can be solved given different boundary conditions and the diffusivity term. He correlated the physical parameters that were predicted with those that were measured. The model was then extended to more complex problems and used to understand practical problems in the auto industry, such as the cladding of valves.

Malcolm Macintyre from Rolls Royce discussed the use of lasers within their company. He said the use of electron beam welding was extensive in the production of modern engines and laser welding also had potential applications in many areas of the engine. Lasers were in production use for small hole drilling and laser cladding of turbine blades with cobalt-based alloys. Control of dilution to give optimum wear resistance and prevention of cracking in the heat-affected zone were important technical factors. In addition to substantial economic benefits in the use of lasers for this application, he emphasized in his talk the extensive testing needed before the introduction of new manufacturing techniques in order to meet the requirements of the Civil Aviation Authority.

The last speaker of the day was Dr. David Roessler of General Motors. He described the use of lasers at General Motors for cutting, welding, hardening, and cladding of parts and material. Laser alignment of parts and tools was discussed as well as the chemical analyzers of auto exhaust.

Thursday, September 12

Dr. Elton Kaufmann emphasized that in contradiction to pulsed laser irradiation, in the scanned laser cases the isotherm velocity increases as it approaches the surface, resulting in very different morphologies. His work described the behavior of $Fe_{40}Ni_{40}P_{14}B_6$ and a near eutectic composition of a Ta-Ir alloy. The above was used in order to explain the appearance of an amorphous overlayer above an initially polycrystalline regrown layer. The results were related to TTT curves.

Professor Barry Mordike suggested that gaseous laser surface alloying was dependent upon the equilibrium constant "K." He then went on to describe in considerable detail how gaseous nitriding, de-nitriding, carburizing and oxidizing of commercially pure titanium, IMI 318 and some iron-based alloys were related to K. Repeated cycles of treatment were also described. Methods of carbon and nitrogen detection were described as well as typical surface roughness. The effects of laser surface alloying on possivation currents, fatigue and tensile properties were also elucidated.

This NATO Study Institute certainly presented a broad scope of techniques and materials approached both from a science and engineering point of view. The interaction of scientists, engineers and graduate students was an excellent format for a cooperative learning experience.

This was especially true for the student attendees, who had an opportunity to see both the theory and application of laser solid interactions.

TABLE OF CONTENTS

CHAPTER 3. MODELING OF HEAT AND MASS TRANSFER

CHAPTER 6 - APPLICATION TO INDUSTRY

CHAPTER 7. LASER SURFACE CHEMISTRY

CHAPTER 8 - LASER ANNEALING OF SILICON

CHAPTER 1. INTERACTION AT METAL SURFACES

CHAPTER INTRODUCTION - W. W. DULEY

The interaction of high-power laser radiation with metals and other solids is capable of providing industry with a variety of novel and useful processing tools. However, the overall efficiency of this new technology is limited, in many instances, by the difficulty of obtaining effective coupling between incident laser radiation and the workpiece. High reflectivity, plasma shielding and gas absorption all conspire to reduce the overall coupling of laser radiation to solids and particularly to metals. At room temperature most elemental metals and alloys absorb less than 10% of incident radiation at 10.6 m, the wavelength of the CO_2 laser, so that some 90% of incident laser power is wasted unless steps are taken to artificially reduce sample reflectivity. During sample processing the ejection of material from the laser interaction region may create a plasma that can also absorb incident laser radiation.

This section contains several papers that describe these and other phenomena that are involved in the initial stages of the conversion of laser radiation to heat at the surface of a workpiece. Duley surveys experimental data relating to the absorptivity of metals at several laser wavelengths. These data are discussed in the context of current physical models and a comparison is made between the predictions of theory and these data. Despite the industrial importance of the CO_2 laser, little reliable experimental data on effective coupling coefficients are available, particularly at the elevated temperatures encountered during laser processing. Even less data is available at YAG and excimer wavelengths.

A variety of ways of increasing the absorptivity of metals are discussed by Duley. The simplest of these appears to be via the deposition of thin absorbing layers. Papers by Ramous, Gnanamuthu and Gay elsewhere in this conference have discussed the effect of absorbing surface layers in considerable detail.

A novel technique for increasing coupling efficiency via laser-induced periodic or grating structures is discussed in the paper by Keilmann. For some years such periodic structures have been observed on the surface of laser-irradiated solids. The work of Keilmann and others now shows that these structures arise as an interference effect between the incident laser beam and a propagating surface wave. The overall effect when the wavelength of the periodic structure is the same as that of the incident laser is to provide an enhancement of coupling efficiency. Industrial applications of this effect have yet to be developed.

A paper by Rockstroh and Mazumder describes some interesting preliminary data on the properties of the plasma produced over a metal surface. Photometry has been used to obtain two-dimensional maps of isophotes within such a plasma driven by a cw CO_2 laser at the 8500 W level.

Other papers in this section by Berry and co-workers and Koppmann et al. outline measurements related to the interaction of pulsed laser radiation with absorbing targets. The emission of atomic and molecular species during the ablation of a variety of target materials has been followed via time of flight (TOF) mass spectrometry and laser-induced fluorescence (LIF). The LIF-TOF combination promises to be a powerful diagnostic tool in the study of surface evaporation.

Overall, the papers presented here, as well as many others appearing elsewhere in the proceedings of this institute, show that while lasers are routinely used in a wide variety of processing applications, many interesting and important studies of the physical phenomena involved in such processes remain to be done. Hopefully, the work described here will point the way to such future studies.

LASER MATERIAL INTERACTIONS OF RELEVANCE TO METAL SURFACE TREATMENT

W. W. DULEY
York University, Toronto, Canada

Key Words: Reflectance, Drude, coupling

ABSTRACT

The physical processes involved in the initial stages of the coupling of laser radiation to metals are briefly reviewed. This is followed by an analysis of available theoretical descriptions of the absorptivity A and its temperature dependence. Experimental coupling coefficients for cw CO_2 laser radiation on metals over the range 20-1000°C are reported. The effect of oxidation on these coefficients is discussed. Finally, several methods of increasing A(T) are evaluated.

1. INTRODUCTION

The initial stage in all laser metal processing applications involves the coupling of laser radiation to electrons within the metal. This first occurs by the absorption of photons from the incident laser beam promoting electrons within the metal to states of higher energy. Electrons that have been excited electronically in this manner can divest themselves of their excess energy in a variety of ways. For example, if the photon energy is large enough, the excited electron can

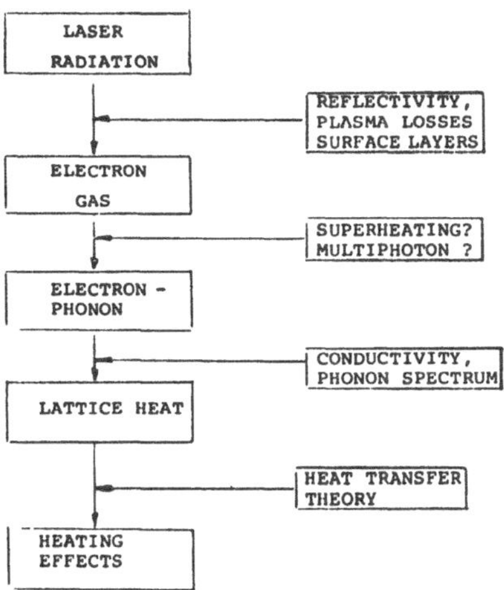

FIGURE 1. The stages in the conversion of photon energy to heat including the identification of relevant physical processes.

Draper, C.W. and Mazzoldi, P. (eds.), Laser Surface Treatment of Metals. ISBN 90-247-3405-3.

be removed entirely from the metal. This is the photoelectric effect and usually requires photon energies greater than several electron volts (eV).

Most laser processing applications, however, utilize lasers emitting photons with relatively low energy - the energy of CO_2 laser photons is only 0.12 eV while the photons obtained from the YAG laser have about 1.2 eV of energy. Electrons excited by absorption of CO_2 or YAG laser radiation do not therefore have enough energy to be ejected from the metal surface. Such electrons must, nevertheless, lose energy to return to an equilibrium state after photon excitation. This occurs when excited electrons are scattered by lattice defects. Such defects can be permanent structures such as dislocations, grain boundaries etc., or they may be evanescent structures such as the lattice deformation produced by photons. In either case, the overall effect is to convert electronic energy derived from the beam of incident photons into heat. It is this heat that is useful (indeed necessary!) in all surface treatment applications. The factors that influence the efficiency of the overall process (photon energy⟶heat energy) will be the subject of this paper. Figure 1 shows the dominant states in the conversion process from photon energy to heat energy in block diagram form.

2. REFLECTIVITY AND ABSORPTION

Reflection losses dominate many laser processing applications and are often the primary limiting factor to the overall efficiency of the conversion of laser radiation to heat in metallic systems. For normal incidence of radiation on a plane metal surface, the reflectivity can be written

$$R = \left|\frac{1 - Z}{1 + Z}\right|^2 \tag{1}$$

where Z is the surface impedance. Equation 1 is valid at all times. However, under conditions where the mean free path of excited electrons is less than or comparable to the skin depth, this expression for R may be written in terms of a complex refractive index $\tilde{n} = n - ik$

$$R = \frac{(n - 1)^2 + k^2}{(n + 1)^2 + k^2} \tag{2}$$

The absorptivity $A = 1 - R$ for an opaque solid becomes

$$A = \frac{4n}{(n + 1)^2 + k^2} \tag{3}$$

The latter expressions for R and A both assume that the field of the incident light wave decays exponentially as it penetrates into the metal.

If A is known, then the heating effect of a beam with intensity I_0 (watts m^{-2}) is simply AI_0. To get A, one can adopt three basic approaches. The first is to measure the refractive indices n and k at the particular wavelengths and sample temperatures required.

Such measurements are relatively straightforward (2), but in reality, little data at high temperature are available.

The second approach relies on theory to develop a way of relating n and k to other material properties such as electrical conductivity, effective electron mass, etc. Several of these theoretical models will be discussed below.

The third method gives perhaps the most reliable data. It involves the direct measurement of A during laser excitation. It has the advantage that any non-linearities that might not be predicted from theory will be immediately obvious.

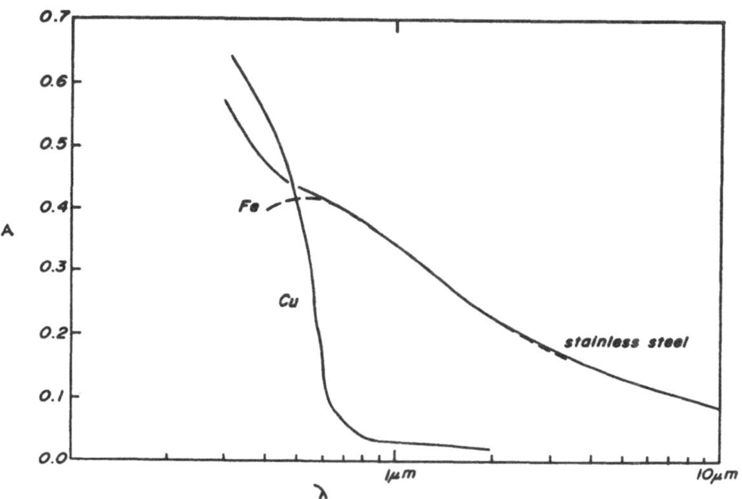

FIGURE 2. Wavelength dependence of absorptivity A for some metals.

Figure 2 shows the absorptivity A for iron and copper calculated from measured values of n and k (ref. 3,4) together with the measured A for a stainless steel as reported by Karlsson and Ribbing (5). It shows clearly the well-known decrease in A for metals in the infrared spectral region.

Figure 3 provides the solution to Eq.(3) in graphical form and shows curves of A vs. wavelength calculated using measured n,k values. It is apparent that both n and k are large in the IR. When both n and k are large and of comparable value, then A approaches the Hagen-Rubens result $A \sim 2/n$.

3. MODELING $A(\lambda)$

While the actual events occurring at an iradiated metal surface involve the absorption of photons, it is more convenient to adopt a wave approach. Here one imagines that the incident electromagnetic wave imposes an acceleration to conduction electrons within the metal. The equation of motion for these electrons is, as described by Drude (6),

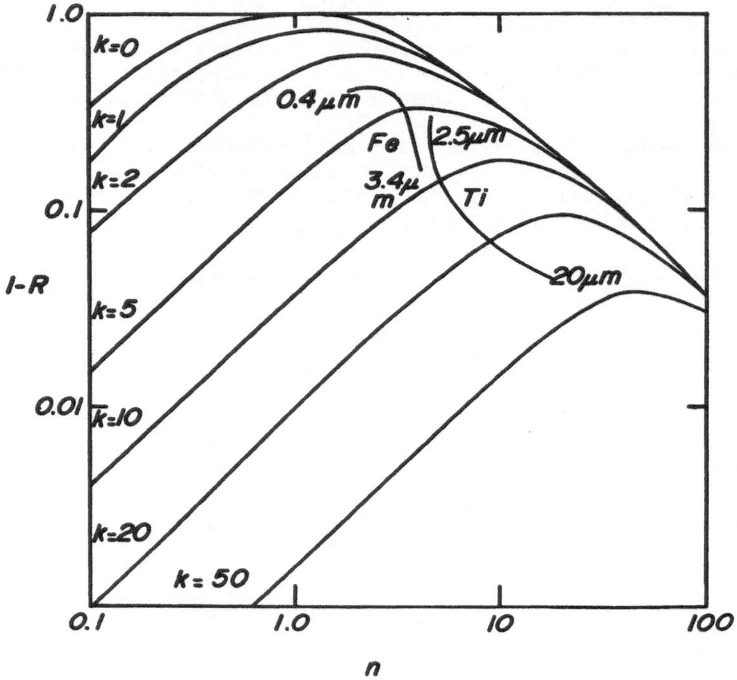

FIGURE 3. Solution to $A = 4n/[(n+1)^2 + k^2]$ in generalized form. $A(\lambda)$ calculated from measured n,k for Fe and Ti is also shown.

$$m \frac{dv_y}{dt} = -eE_y - \frac{m^* v_y}{\tau} \tag{4}$$

where the em wave is taken to be polarized with its E vector in the y direction. v_y is the y component of the electron speed while m^* = effective mass and τ = damping or relaxation time. The solution to Eq.(4) is

$$v_y = \frac{-e\tau E_y}{m^*(1 - i\omega\tau)} \tag{5}$$

where ω = angular frequency of em wave. The electron then moves under the influence of the applied field with an amplitude that is frequency dependent. This motion constitutes a current of density

$$J = \tilde{\sigma} E \tag{6}$$

where $\tilde{\sigma}$ is a complex electrical conductivity

$$\tilde{\sigma} = \sigma' + i\sigma'' \tag{7}$$

and

$$\sigma' = \frac{\sigma_0}{1 + (\omega\tau)^2} \quad ; \quad \sigma'' = \frac{\sigma_0 \omega\tau}{1 + (\omega\tau)^2} \tag{8}$$

where $\sigma_0 = Ne^2\tau/m^*$ is the dc electrical conductivity. σ' and σ'' can now be easily related to the dielectric constant $\tilde{\varepsilon} = \varepsilon_1 + i\varepsilon_2$. The components of $\tilde{\varepsilon}$ are

$$\begin{aligned} \varepsilon_1 &= 1 - \frac{\sigma''}{\omega\varepsilon_0} & \varepsilon_2 &= \frac{\sigma'}{\omega\varepsilon_0} \\ &= n^2 - k^2 & &= 2nk \end{aligned} \tag{9}$$

where $\varepsilon_0 = 8.85 \times 10^{-12}$ Coul/N-m^2. This is the Drude result. It is important to note, however, that quantum mechanical calculations yield the same result, but with a different interpretation for the parameters N, the electron concentration and τ the relaxation time (7,8).

In principle, then, the Drude theory, together with the input of data on the dc conductivity σ and τ, can be used to predict $A(\lambda)$ for metals. In practice the following limitations often occur:

(a) σ_0 required is often 5-10 times smaller than the dc value.
(b) Neither σ_0 nor τ are independent of wavelength.
(c) Excess absorption attributable to interband transmissions often occurs.

Limitations (a) and (b) are well illustrated by reference to Fig. 4, where σ_0 and τ, are derived from a fit between $A(\lambda)$ evaluated directly from Eq.(3) using measured n,k for Fe, and that calculated via the Drude theory. It can be seen that although the dc resistivity of Fe is $\sigma_0(\text{dc}) = 1.02 \times 10^7\ \Omega^{-1}\text{m}^{-1}$, σ_0 (Drude) is almost a factor of twenty times smaller. This can be attributed to the fact that optical radiation samples only the metal surface where defects, etc. may contribute to a lower effective conductivity.

τ is also seen to be a strong function of λ at 20°C but less so at 1400°C. The high temperature data show that the Drude theory may be most applicable at high temperature where relaxation times are short. A similar result is expected for alloys where defect scattering lowers τ.

Ujihara (7) has modified the Drude theory to incorporate a temperature-dependent τ. By doing an average over the photon frequency spectrum, he was able to show that $\tau \propto T^{-\chi}$ where χ is in the range 1-1.3 for metals such as Al, Cu, Au and Ag. Ujihara was successful in predicting R(T) for Cu at 1.06 μm, but several parameters in his model did not exhibit the correct temperature dependence (9).

For alloys, Weiting and Schriempf (10) show that the Drude theory is valid even at room temperature if the parameter N/m^* appearing in σ_0 is interpreted as a sum over individual groups of conduction electrons while τ was similarly weighted. They find that the temperature dependence of A (10.6 µm) for 304 stainless steel and a Ti-6Al-4V alloy are well predicted by such a modified Drude theory. Significant deviations between predicted and measured values of A for the same metals at 3.8 µm were, however, observed. This is as expected since interband transitions are most important at short wavelengths.

A summary of these and other data on A for various metals at CO_2, YAG and excimer laser wavelengths is given in Tables 1-3.

TABLE 1. Measured and calculated values of A at 10.6 µm.

Metal	Measured	Calculated	
		n,k	Drude
Fe	0.023		0.029
	0.053 (500°C)		0.053 (500°C)
Ti	0.23	0.074	0.08
Zr	0.15	0.053	
Cu		0.042	0.015
Al		0.075	0.019
Mo	0.05		0.027
Ta	0.1		0.044
304 SS	0.1		0.1
	0.14 (1000°C)		0.14 (1000°C)
Ti-6Al-4V	0.13		0.13
	0.14 (400°C)		0.14 (400°C)

TABLE 2. Measured and calculated values of A at 1.06 µm.

Metal	Measured	Calculated	
		Johnson, Christy	Gushkin et al.
Ti		0.39	
V		0.42	
Cr		0.42	
Mn		0.35	
Fe		0.39	0.36
			0.32 (1400°C)
Co		0.25	0.30
			0.30 (1400°C)
Ni		0.23	0.25
			0.27 (1400°C)
Cu	0.015	0.029	
	0.067 (liquid)	0.037 (150°C)	
Al	0.056		
	0.22 (liquid)		

TABLE 3. Values of A at 3.08 μm calculated from refractive indices.

Metal	Calculated	
	Johnson, Christy	Gushkin et al.*
Ti	0.47	
V	0.45	
Cr	0.51	
Mn	0.56	
Fe	0.59	0.40
		0.40 (1400°C)
Co	0.51	0.30
		0.36 (1400°C)
Ni	0.70	0.39
		0.44 (1400°C)
Cu	0.64	
	0.63 (150°C)	

* at 0.4 μm.

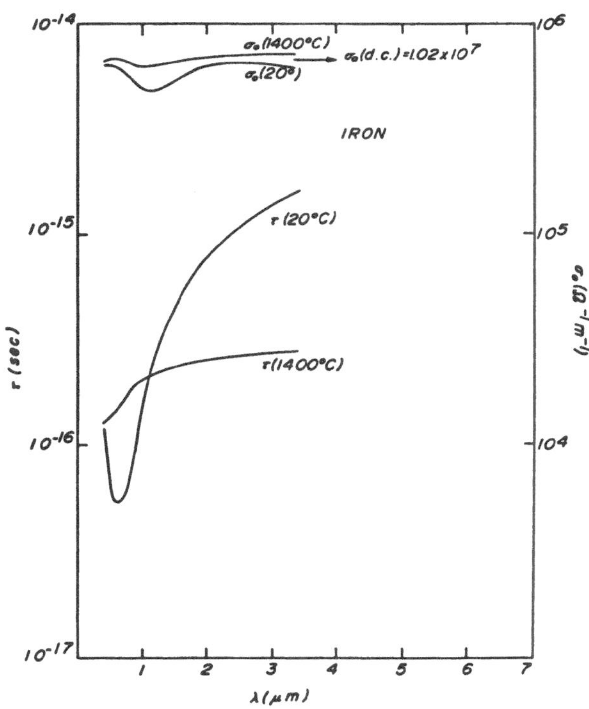

FIGURE 4. Wavelength dependence of σ_0 and τ derived from Drude model for Fe using n,k from Shvarev et al. (4).

4. EXPERIMENTAL VALUE FOR A (10.6 μm)

Figures 5-9 (at end of this manuscript) show some experimental data on the coupling coefficient (i.e., A) for 10.6 μm cw laser radiation on metals at temperatures in the range 20-1000°C. Experimental data were obtained using the technique developed by Duley et al. (11) for metals in vacuum. The simple temperature dependence exhibited by stainless steel (Fig. 9) is not apparent in the other data. Metals such as Ta and Ti actually show a decreasing coupling efficiency with increasing temperature while other metals such as Zr have a much more complex A(T) curve. Some of these effects may be attributable to the high-temperature annealing out of surface defects introduced during preparation of the metal sheets used. A similar effect has been noted by Weiting and de Rosa (12) in stainless steel.

The rapid increase in A(T) at temperatures approaching 1000°C in some samples may be due to the formation of oxide coatings since the residual pressure over the samples in the vacuum chamber used was $\sim 10^{-5}$-10^{-6} atmospheres.

5. EFFECT OF SURFACE LAYERS ON A

Thin refractory layers or coatings are occasionally used to enhance the coupling between laser radiation and metals for laser processing. In addition, many metals have thin oxide layers at their surface, or have surface layers whose composition is significantly different from that of the bulk metal. The change in reflectivity ΔR induced by such layers can be treated rigorously when optical constants are known (2). However, such calculations are often laborious. A simple approximation, valid when the film thickness $d << \lambda$, has been given by McIntyre and Aspnes (13). Their result is

$$\frac{\Delta R}{R} = -\frac{8\pi d}{\lambda} \, \mathrm{Im} \, \frac{1 - \tilde{\varepsilon}_2}{1 - \tilde{\varepsilon}_3} \tag{10}$$

where $\tilde{\varepsilon}_2$ = dielectric constant of film and $\tilde{\varepsilon}_3$ is that of the metal substrate. At a wavelength λ = 10.6 μm, a film with $d \sim 0.1$ μm can produce $\Delta R/R \sim 0.1$. Since $R \sim 1$ for metals at this wavelength, the absorptivity of the surface can be significantly increased even with a $\Delta R/R$ ratio as small as 0.1.

When $d \geq /2n_2$ where n_2 = real refractive index of coating, interference effects may become important. Here the net reflectivity may be a sensitive (and oscillatory) function of d. These effects have been modeled by Bunkin et al. (14) for YAG radiation incident on oxidized copper.

Duley et al. (11) have reported data on the effect of oxidation on the coupling coefficient for cw CO_2 laser radiation on several metals. These data were analyzed using the following simple approximation to Eq.(10).

$$\frac{\Delta R}{R} \sim -\frac{8\pi d k_2}{\lambda} \tag{11}$$

Assuming a parabolic rate law for oxidation, i.e., $d(t) \propto t^{1/2}$, then

$$A(t) = A(0) + C(T)R(T)t^{1/2} \quad (12)$$

where $A(t)$ = absorptivity after oxidation for time t at temperature T. $C(T)$ is a constant containing the parabolic rate constant, film density and $\alpha = 4\pi k_2/\lambda$ the film absorption coefficient. Data obtained for 304 stainless steel together with a theoretical fit using Eq.(12) are shown in Fig. 10.

6. METHODS OF INCREASING A

In this section I briefly discuss some methods that may be applied to increase the coupling of laser radiation to metallic surfaces.

6.1. Preheating

For many elemental metals and IR wavelengths $A(T)$ is well approximated by the linear relation

$$A(T) = A(20°C)[1 + B(T - 20°C)] \quad (13)$$

where B is constant. Typically $A(1000°C) \lesssim 5\ A(20°C)$ although deviations are commonly observed (cf. Figs. 5-9). Since A often increases with temperature, preheating using a conventional heat source may improve the efficiency of laser surface treatments. An estimate of the wavelength dependence of $\Delta R/R$ can be obtained from thermomodulation spectra (28).

6.2. Roughening

Surface roughening using sandblasting or rubbing with silicon carbide paper (12) has been shown to increase A at low temperatures. For stainless steel roughening with silicon carbide increased A by about 27%. However, this enhanced coupling was not maintained at temperatures in excess of 600°C. It was suggested that the effect of roughening was to introduce surface defects that were annealed out at elevated temperatures.

6.3. Surface Layers

From Eq.(10), it is evident that $\Delta R/R$ is maximized when $\tilde{\varepsilon}_2$ is large, i.e., n_2 and k_2 are as large as possible. Using the approximate result

$$\frac{\Delta R}{R} = -\frac{8\pi d k_2}{\lambda}$$

$$= -2dk\alpha \quad (14)$$

where α = absorption coefficient (cm^{-1}), one can see that $\Delta R/R$ is largest for strongly absorbing layers. At IR wavelengths oxide and other refractory films can have k_2 in the range 1-5 within lattice absorption bands (15,16). This yields $\alpha \leq 6 \times 10^4\ cm^{-1}$ at $10\ \mu m$ so that according to Eq.(11) a surface layer only some 100 nm thick can have a profound effect on reflectivity. However, such effects are localized over a relatively narrow spectral range (17).

In the visible and near ultraviolet α often rises to 5×10^5-10^6 cm^{-1} due to the excitation of electronic transitions.

6.4. Induced Grating Structures

Periodic surface structures (waves, "gratings") have been observed on many different types of solids during and after irradiation with laser radiation (18-20). Such structures are formed as the result of interference between the incident laser plane wave, $E_L \exp i(\omega t + k_L z)$ and a surface wave $E_{S\omega} \exp i(\omega t - k_{S\omega} y)$ generated by scattering from surface defects. The resultant surface standing wave intensity $I_0 + E_L E_{S\omega} \cos(k_S\, y)$ impresses a surface structure on the material with a period of $\Lambda \sim \lambda_{Laser}$.

When this occurs, the efficienty of coupling of incident laser radiation to the surface rises dramatically (21). This can be seen from the grating equation

$$\Lambda = \frac{m\lambda}{1 - \sin\phi} \qquad (15)$$

where ϕ is the angle that the incident laser beam makes with respect to the normal to the surface. m is the order of diffraction of radiation of wavelength λ by a grating with groove spacing Λ. When $\phi = 0$ (normal incidence), $\Lambda = m\lambda$ and incident radiation is diffracted strongly along the grating surface. This is the Woods anomaly and leads to an enhancement of energy absorption.

Large transient decreases in the reflectivity of metals during laser irradiation have been observed for some time (22,24). They have been variously attributed to a discontinuity in reflectivity at the solid-liquid transition (22) or to the onset of a metal-dielectric transition (25). Work on periodic structures now suggests an alternative explanation - that such decreases in R are due to the onset of laser-induced grating structures that greatly enhance coupling. Once this effect is better characterized, it is apparent that it may be useful in increasing the efficiency of laser-machining/heat-treating processes.

6.5. Electroreflectance

Since the reflectivity of metals depends on the concentration of electrical charge at the surface, reflectivity can be increased by application of an electrical field of the correct sign (26,27). In the infrared, the effect is small as can be seen from the following

$$A \sim \left[\frac{8}{\varepsilon_2}\right]^{1/2} \qquad (16)$$

where

$$\varepsilon_2 = \frac{\omega_p^2\, \omega_c}{\omega(\omega^2 + \omega_c^2)} = \frac{4\pi N e^2 \omega_c}{m^* \omega(\omega^2 + \omega_c^2)}$$

and ω_p = plasma frequency, ω_c = relaxation frequency. Thus

$A \propto N^{-1/2}$ and a decrease in N results in an increase in absorptivity. For $\omega << \omega_p$ significant variations in A (or R) can be induced by modest fields. For example, Garrigos et al. (26) have reported $\Delta R/R \sim 0.4$ at $\lambda = 0.04\,\mu m$ for copper. Possible laser machining implications of this technique have yet to be explored.

7. CONCLUSION

Despite the availability of a simple theory, the Drude formalism, the best way to obtain the absorptivity of a metal surface for laser radiation is to measure it experimentally. An alternative approach that yields satisfactory results involves the measurement of refractive indices n,k that are then used to calculate A. The Drude theory is capable of accurate prediction of A(T) at high temperatures and for disordered alloys. Drude predictions of the behavior of elemental metals, particularly at short wavelengths, are in most instances inaccurate. Modification of the Drude theory to take the temperature dependence of relaxation time into account yields an improved fit to experimental data. Little data on coupling coefficients are available at excimer wavelengths.

Several methods exist for increasing coupling of laser radiation during surface treatment. The most promising of these seems to be via induced grating structures.

REFERENCES

1. M. P. Givens, Solid State Physics 6, 313 (1958).
2. O. S. Heavens, Optical Properties of Thin Solid Films (Dover Publ., 1965).
3. P. B. Johnson and R. W. Christy, Phys. Rev. B 11, 1315 (1975).
4. K. M. Shvarev et al., High Temp. Res. 16, 441 (1978).
5. B. Karlsson and C. G. Ribbing, J. Appl. Phys. 53, 6340 (1982).
6. P. Drude, Ann. Physik 14, 677 (1904).
7. K. Ujihara, J. Appl. Phys. 43, 2376 (1972).
8. J. A. McKay and J. A. Rayne, Phys. Rev. B 13, 673 (1976).
9. W. T. Walter et al., in Lasers in Metallurgy, edited by K. Mukherjee and J. Mazumder, AIME 179 (1981).
10. T. J. Weiting and J. T. Schriempf, J. Appl. Phys. 47, 4009 (1976).
11. W. W. Duley, D. J. Semple, J.-P. Morency, and M. Gravel, Optics Laser Technology 11, 281 (1979).
12. T. J. Weiting and J. L. DeRosa, J. Appl. Phys. 50, 1071 (1979).
13. J. D. McIntyre and D. E. Aspnes, Surface Science 24, 417 (1971).
14. F. V. Bunkin et al., Sov. J. Quantum Electronics 10, 891 (1980).
15. F. Brehat et al., C. R. Acad. Sci. Paris B263, 1112 (1966).
16. A. Schlegel and P. Wachter, J. Physique 41, C5, 5 (1980).
17. M. Handke and C. Paulszkiewicz, Infrared Physics 24, 121 (1984).
18. M. Siegrist, G. Kaech, and F. K. Kneubuhl, Appl. Phys. 2, 45 (1973).
19. F. Keilmann, Phys. Rev. Lett. 51, 2097 (1983).
20. M. J. Soileau, IEEE J. Quantum Electron. QE-20, 464 (1984).
21. I. Ursu et al., Appl. Phys. Lett. 45, 365 (1984).
22. A. M. Bonch-Bruevich et al., Sov. Phys. Tech. Phys. 13, 640 (1968).
23. M. K. Chun and K. Rose, J. Appl. Phys. 41, 614 (1970).
24. C. T. Walters and A. H. Clauer, Appl. Phys. Lett. 33, 713 (1978).
25. A. M. Prokhorov et al., IEEE J. Quantum Electron. QE-9, 503 (1973).
26. R. Garrigos, R. Kofman and J. Richard, C. R. Acad. Sci. Paris 276, B55 (1973).
27. T. E. Furtak and D. W. Lynch, Il Nuovo Cimento 39B, 346 (1977).
28. R. Rosei and D. W. Lynch, Phys. Rev. B 5, 3883 (1972).

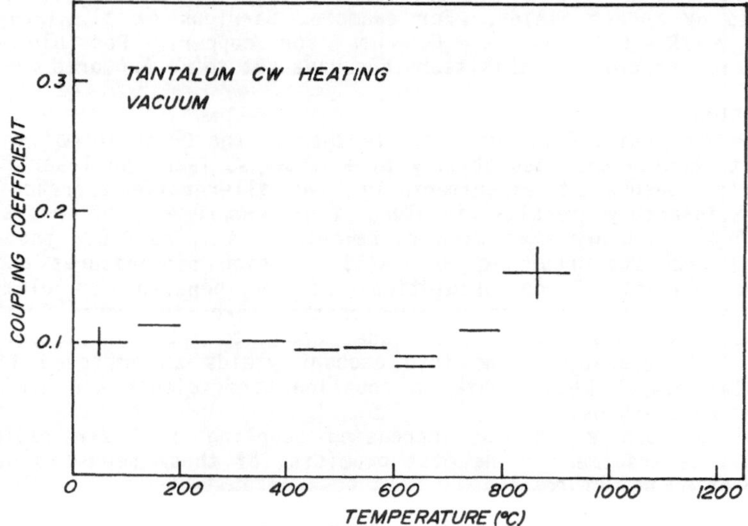

FIGURE 5. A (10.6 μm) vs. T for tantalum.

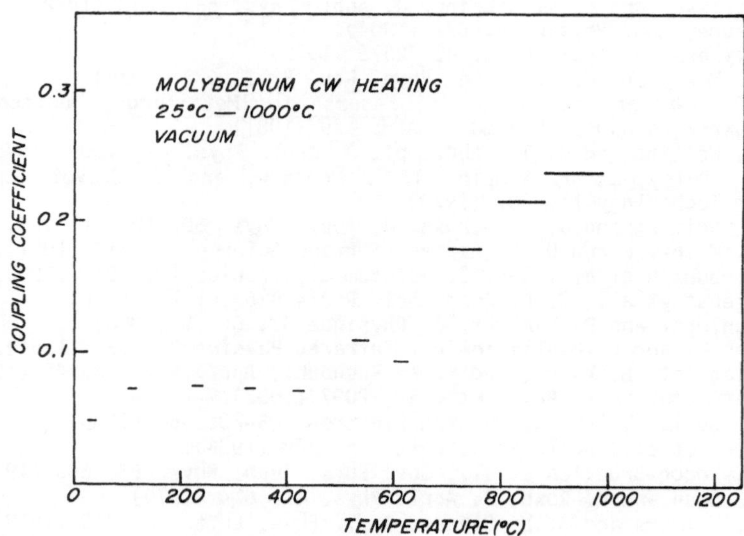

FIGURE 6. A (10.6 μm) vs. T for molybdenum.

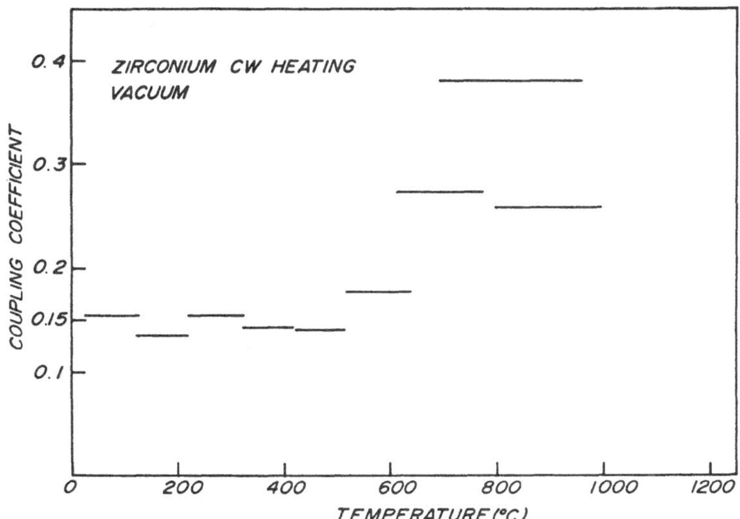

FIGURE 7. A (10.6 μm) vs. T for zirconium.

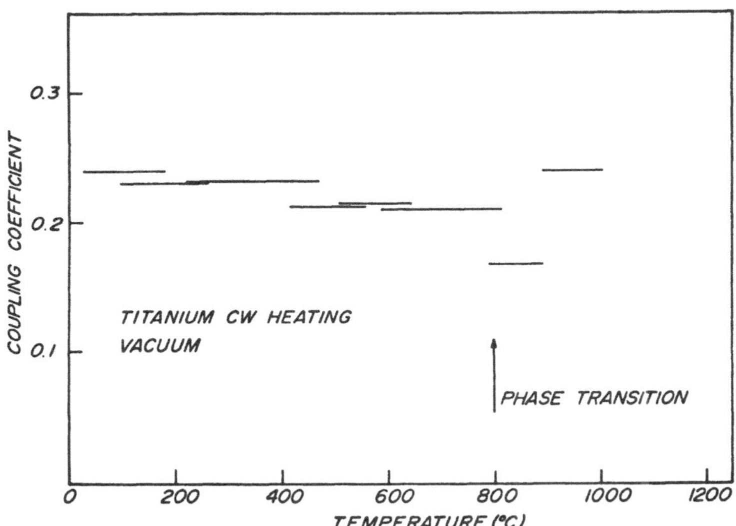

FIGURE 8. A (10.6 μm) vs. T for titanium.

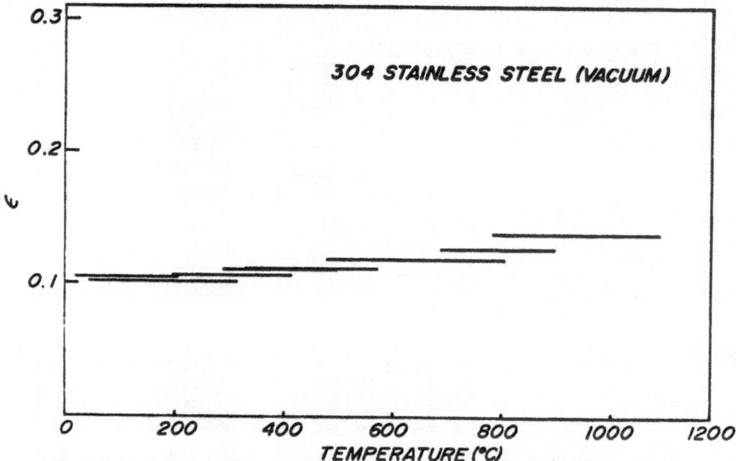

FIGURE 9. A (10.6 μm) vs. T for 304 stainless steel.

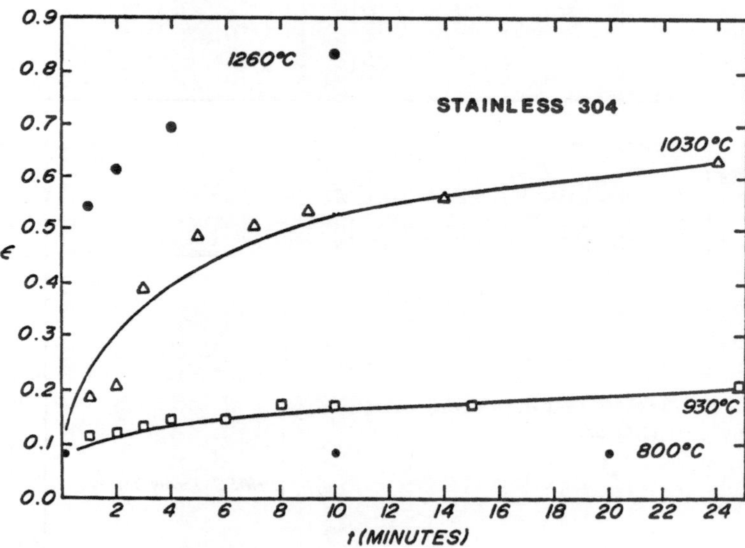

FIGURE 10. Coupling coefficient ε (≡A) for cw CO_2 radiation incident on 304 stainless steel oxidized for various times at indicated temperatures. A theoretical fit using Eq.(12) is shown for two data sets.

STIMULATED ABSORPTION OF CO_2 LASER LIGHT ON METALS

FRITZ KEILMANN
Max-Planck-Institut für Festkörperforschung, 7000 Stuttgart 80, FRG

Key Words: plasmons, periodic, ripples

ABSTRACT

A new mechanism has been identified for the interaction of high-power infrared radiation with metal surfaces. This mechanism is based on the occurrence of initial surface roughness, which by a stimulated process grows into a coherent periodic corrugation or "ripple" pattern, owing to a nonlinear interaction with surface plasmons. Once developed, this ripple pattern acts as an anti-reflective coating, enabling the full absorption of the incoming radiation on the metal surface. Evidence is given for the dynamics of this process in the case of CO_2 laser treatment of metals like Hg, In, Sn, Al and Pb.

1. INTRODUCTION

Twenty-five years after the invention of the laser, we see a strong penetration of laser machining tools into the industrial area of metal processing. This has occurred not as a result of increased understanding of the fundamental processes involved, but on a rather empirical basis. Now there is the demand from the applications side that calls for increased basic research. Looking closer to the laser-metal situation, the basic problem is all but trivial; the interaction involves a complicated connection of electrodynamics, thermodynamics, hydrodynamics and plasmadynamics.

I describe here a recently discovered connection between electrodynamics and hydrodynamics, mediated by surface electromagnetic waves (called surface plasmons on metals). This effect is important because it can strongly reduce the reflectivity of metals.

In laser metal processing the reflectivity of metals is a particularly awkward problem when using infrared radiation of the CO_2 laser, since on one hand the reflectivity is typically as high as 95% while the CO_2 laser is very attractive because of its high efficiency and low cost. Thanks to empirical studies, it was found that at some critical intensity near 10^7 watt/cm^2 the high reflectivity becomes fully depressed and thus the process becomes extremely effective. Why is this so?

Commonly one attributes the increased coupling to the gaseous plasma, which at high intensity, develops just above the surface. It is, however, not well understood how the plasma is initiated in the first place.

The possible role of some other not yet established mechanism enhancing the laser metal cutting process is indicated by a second observation: a distinct dependence on polarization of both the obtainable cut quality and cutting speed. Explanations put forward for this effect have been qualitative only. Altogether the situation remains unsatisfactory. The contribution of this paper is the explanation of a new mechanism which, if dominant at high intensity, inherently leads to both total absorption as well as strong polarization dependence.

2. SURFACE POLARITONS

It is known that there exist solutions of Maxwell's equations which describe electromagnetic waves bound to the surface of strongly conducting materials such as metals. These modes are called surface polaritons, or surface plasmons (3). They exist on metals at all frequencies in the optical and infrared range. Their characteristics are (i) a field maximum in the surface, (ii) an exponential decay of the field both into the metal and the air, and (iii) a strict TM polarization. Their phase velocity being somewhat slower than the free space velocity of light, these modes cannot be excited by a laser beam incident on an ideally flat surface. To accomplish excitation, it is necessary to have imperfections on the surface; an appropriate Fourier component of the surface structure has to contribute the missing momentum to phase-match the incoming laser to the surface wave.

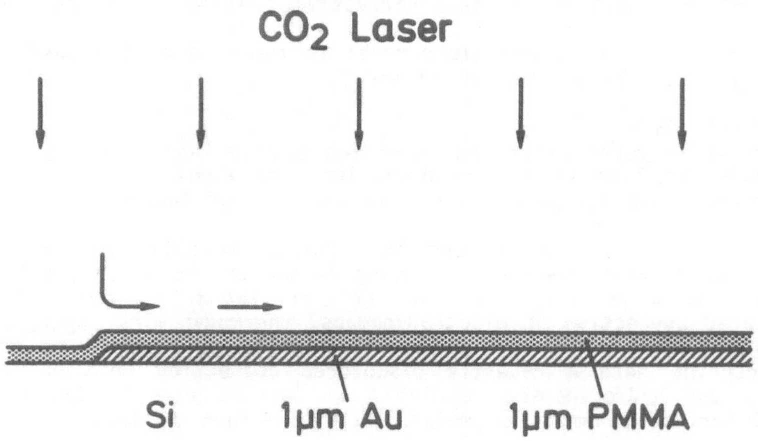

FIGURE 1. Schematic of the arrangement for the generation of surface plasmons on gold by irradiation with a CO_2 laser, and for photographing them in a thin plastic overcoat.

Let me illustrate this with an experiment (4), designed to photograph surface plasmons for the first time. A gold surface is prepared by vacuum deposition on a silicon substrate. A CO_2 laser beam incident normally (Fig. 1) is fully reflected from most of the surface and no plasmons are generated. It is only at the boundary (i.e., the discontinuity of dielectric constant of the surface) that surface plasmons can be generated (bent arrow). The surface plasmons are made visible by a holographic process where the incoming laser radiation serves as a reference wave; the resulting interference maxima and minima are permanently recorded by a thermoplastic deformation they produce in the PMMA layer (Fig. 2). The burn pattern in the plastic overcoat comes from the interference between the incoming laser wave and the surface wave. The

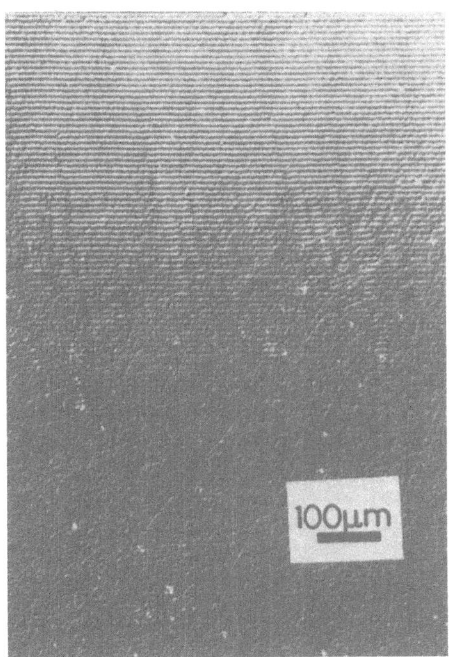

FIGURE 2. Microscope picture of the plate shown in Fig. 1, after exposure to CO_2 laser radiation.

period of the interference pattern equals the wavelength of the surface wave. Damping is clearly visible. Note that the surface wave is generated at one edge of the gold area only; generation at the other edge which runs parallel to the electric field is totally suppressed, demonstrating the distinctly polarized character of surface waves.

Two results of this experiment are of interest in our context. First, we observe a drastic polarization dependence of the excitation efficiency; surface waves are seen to be generated at one of the boundaries only, the one which is oriented perpendicularly to the laser polarization. Secondly, we observe a strong damping of the surface wave in a range of a few dozen wavetrains, documenting a strong attenuation in the metal.

This allows an important conclusion: If, somehow, all of the incoming laser radiation could be converted into surface plasmons, then all of it would end up absorbed in the metal.

3. STIMULATED SCATTERING INTO SURFACE PLASMONS

On a nearly smooth surface the scattering of incident light into surface plasmons is very small. If the surface is, however, deformable, the interference, as demonstrated in the photography experiment above, will lead to the appearance of a periodic deformation of the surface. In turn, such a periodic deformation can resonantly couple more incident light into the surface wave. This establishes a feedback situation: An instability results, which ends in a very deep periodic deformation of

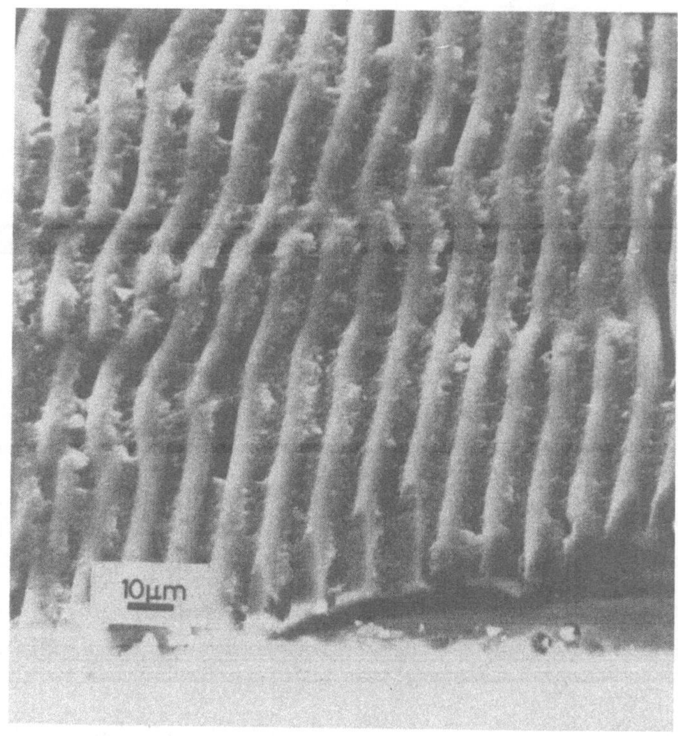

FIGURE 3. Electron micrographs of a glass surface damaged by a high-intensity CO_2 laser pulse, (a) view from above. The surface is periodically corrugated to a considerable depth of about 3 µm and period of 6 µm.

the surface, and a very efficient scattering of incident light into surface plasmons.

The existence of this process was first deduced from laser damage patterns we obtained on glass (1). Figure 3 shows such an example. The period, about 6 µm, equals the wavelength of the surface wave generated by the CO_2 laser light. We interpret this structure to be the remnant of a highly non-linear scattering process to be called "stimulated surface wave scattering." Evidence for the process to be present on metal surfaces was obtained in further experiments (2), designed to test the theoretical model.

Theoretically, the instability can be viewed as a parametric decay of the input laser wave into two other waves, the surface plasmon and the surface corrugation. Energy and momentum are conserved since the generated plasmon carries away the incoming photon energy, while the plasmon momentum is balanced by the "Umklapp" momentum of the corrugation grating. The theoretical treatment is therefore very similar to, e.g., stimulated Brilloin scattering, and thus can be named stimulated plasmon scattering.

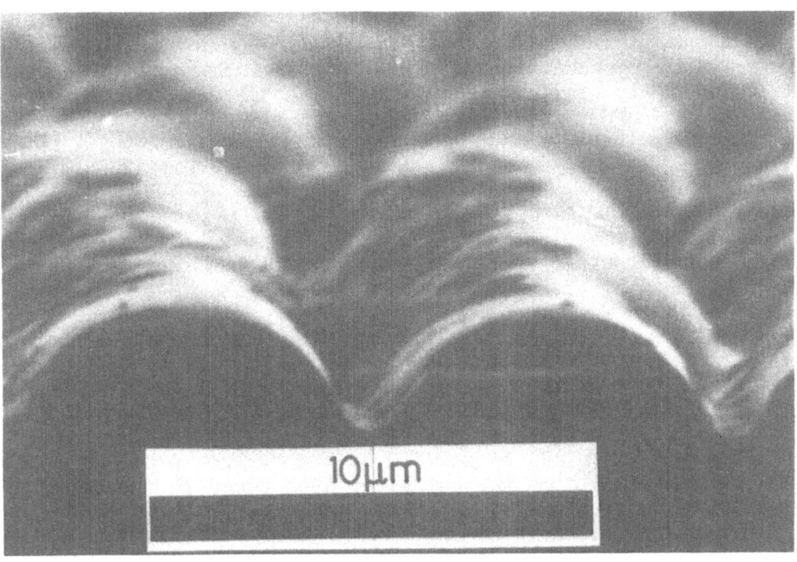

FIGURE 3. Electron micrographs of a glass surface damaged by a high-intensity CO_2 laser pulse, (b) view along the surface (1). The surface is periodically corrugated to a considerable depth of about 3 μm and period of 6 μm.

For a quantitative test of the model of stimulated plasmon scattering, I used liquid metal surfaces (2). With high-power CO_2 laser radiation at normal incidence, a periodic rippling of the surface was readily obtained. The experiment was performed with short pulses which allow an observation of both growth and decay phases. Visible laser light scattering was used to obtain quantitative data on the dynamics of the process.

During the application of the laser pulse I observed a time exponential growth of the corrugation depth. The corrugation grating constant equals very nearly the free space wavelength of the incident radiation, 10 μm. For Hg, I obtained an exponential time constant of $\tau = 45$ ns for an incident laser intensity of 3×10^7 W/cm^2. The final corrugation depth d produced depends on the applied fluence F, i.e., the product of intensity and irradiation time. For Hg, $d = 10$ nm with $F = 3.5$ J/cm^2, and $d = 100$ nm with $F = 5$ J/cm^2. At $F = 6.5$ J/cm^2, where we would expect $d = 1000$ nm, a radically different behavior is seen: The surface explodes and a strong plasma formation is seen. I interpret this by a transition of the absorptive property of the metal surface, from the Fresnel-type low absorption of a few percent as long as $d \ll 1$ μm to a total absorption when $d \sim 1$ μm. The latter critical depth can be deduced from the theory of grating efficiency, which predicts full coupling for a grating with a 5% depth-to-period ratio.

The experiment thus yields direct evidence that the initially highly reflective surface is transformed to a fully absorbing surface by being strongly rippled at the plasmon wavelength. Observations in the strongly absorbing phase are, however, extremely difficult because of the violent dynamics: At the critical point an increase in applied fluence of a few percent raises the power load absorbed into the material by a factor of 10 or 20. The strongly rippled phase can therefore be expected to be highly transient, since the enhanced power load is bound to trigger further instabilities, e.g., dielectric breakdown and plasma formation.

4. CONSEQUENCES FOR METAL PROCESSING

The stimulated surface plasmon scattering - or instability - has been found to be a general phenomenon. In laser metal processing it can initiate a highly absorbing phase. This transition takes place at intensities comparable to the magic intensities of 10^7 W/cm^2 used in laser processing of metals. The significance of this new process certainly deserves further experiments.

The potential importance, for metal processing, of the stimulated plasmon effect is further argumented by its ability to predict distinct polarization effects: When E is perpendicular to the cut direction, a part of the incoming light can be carried by the surface plasmons to the right and to the left, out of the cut line. The power in the center is thereby reduced. In the other case, when E is parallel to the cut direction, the surface waves propagate along the cut direction and thus deposit the energy along the cut line. In practice, one indeed observes a strong polarization dependence of the cut quality and speed, just in the manner predicted by the model. In general, one tries to have the polarization parallel to the cut line; where this is not practical (curved cuts), one has adapted to use circular polarization to obtain an isotropic cut quality.

5. CONCLUSIONS

Stimulated plasmon scattering is a new and seemingly general phenomenon in high-power laser-material interaction. Theory and experiments with 100 ns pulses give evidence of stimulated absorption to occur when CO_2 laser radiation of about 10^7 W/cm^2 hits even a highly reflecting metal. The resulting total absorption as well as the strong polarization dependence are of interest to laser metal processing.

REFERENCES

1. F. Keilmann and Y. H. Bai, Appl. Phys A 29, 9 (1982).
2. F. Keilmann, Phys. Rev. Lett. 51, 2097 (1983).
3. For a recent review, see A. A. Maradudin, in Festkörperprobleme, edited by J. Treusch (Vieweg, Braunschweig, 1981), Vol. 21, pp. 62-116.
4. F. Keilmann, unpublished.

CHARACTERIZATION OF LASER-INDUCED PLASMAS AND TEMPERATURE MEASUREMENT DURING LASER SURFACE TREATMENT

T. J. ROCKSTROH AND J. MAZUMDER
Department of Mechanical and Industrial Engineering, University of Illinois at Urbana-Champaign, 1206 West Green Street, Urbana, IL 61801

Key Words: plasma, thermography, emission spectroscopy

1. INTRODUCTION

The laser is a versatile tool for a number of surface treatment processes, which include solid state phase transformation as in surface hardening, melting and vaporization as in laser surface alloying. Due to short dwell times, high temperatures and steep gradients, it is difficult to measure surface temperatures during laser/target interaction. Processes involving vaporization are more complicated to monitor due to the resulting plasma formation. The plasma can attenuate the laser energy and affect the energy distribution transmitted to the surface. For proper process control and to understand the laser/plasma interaction mechanisms, an accurate estimate of plasma temperature and energy transport is needed. Infrared thermography and emission spectroscopy are the two techniques we have utilized to study the surface temperature and plasma temperature, respectively.

2. DIAGNOSTICS

2.1. IR Thermography

The application of remote temperature-sensing equipment, such as IR thermography, ultrasonics, and acoustic emission, has been limited to temperature profiling with little interest in absolute temperature measurement (1). By monitoring discontinuity and asymmetry in temperature profiles, faults and discontinuities in the heat treatment and joining processes can be isolated. Thermocouples and similar contact devices can be unwieldy due to the relatively slow response time and thermal intertia. By applying appropriate filtering techniques to an existing IR thermography system, a reproducible means of absolute temperature measurement in the 600-2000°C range has been developed (2).

The IR thermography system is an Inframetrics Model 525 thermal imaging system. The detector senses 3 to 12 μm radiation. The system is designed to operate in the -20-500°C range with an extended range of 1100°C. The non-linearity of the extended range reduces temperature resolution above 600°C. Pyrex was utilized as a filter due to its attenuation above 4 μm. Thus, by a combination of reduced detector response in the 3 to 4 μm range and attentuation above 4 μm, detector saturation is prevented. The system response was calculated by monitoring a blackbody temperature in a box oven. Subsequent measurements of a non-blackbody emitter and heating/cooling cycle of gray cast iron implied the accuracy to be $\pm$ 10%.

2.2. Spectroscopy

When sufficient laser energy is focused on a metallic workpiece, a plasma forms consisting of excited and ionized particles from the workpiece and ambient atmosphere. The absorption of laser radiation by the plasma is highly dependent on temperature and number density (pressure). The primary absorption mechanism is inverse Bremsstrahlung with contributions from photoionization. Figure 1 shows the basic laser-plasma interaction mechanisms for a flowing pure argon plasma. The mechanisms are similar for plasmas formed during laser processing of metals. The focused laser beam is absorbed by the metal which rapidly vaporizes. The high number density of free electrons in the metallic vapor is sufficient to initiate cascade breakdown in the ambient gas, forming the bulk of the plasma. The free electrons in the plasma core absorb the laser radiation via inverse Bremsstrahlung, a free-free mechanism. The electrons conduct energy to the heavier particles, but most of the energy is lost as line and continuum radiation. If the plasma temperature fields are measured, local and global laser radiation can be determined (3,4).

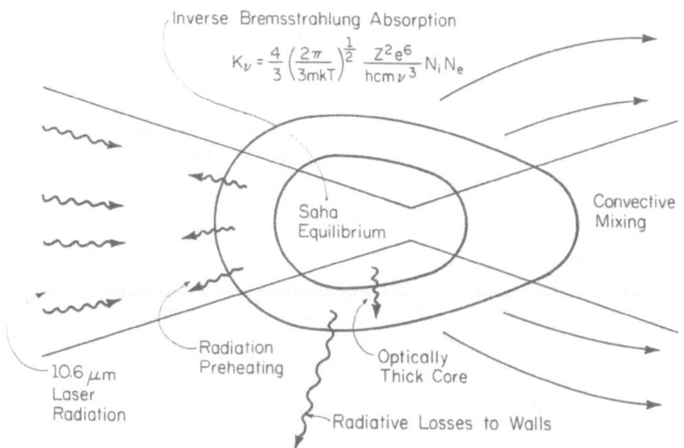

FIGURE 1. Laser-plasma interaction physics: flowing pure argon system.

The relatively high temperatures (> 8000°K) encountered in the plasma core render conventional temperature diagnostics impractical. Spectroscopic diagnostics have been adapted to the laboratory plasma via the assumption of local thermodynamic equilibrium (LTE). Two general techniques have been widely used to measure plasma temperatures, absolute and relative diagnostics.

Absolute techniques measure the intensity of a spectral line or narrow band of continuum radiation. The measured intensity is compared to a calibrated source such as a tungsten lamp. Henricksen (5) and Carlhoff (6) have utilized absolute measurements to map two-dimensional temperature profiles in laser-supported argon plasma. They found peak plasma temperatures on the order of 15,000°K. The equipment required to perform absolute measurements is relatively modest. System flexibility and calibration accuracy make error predictions questionable.

Relative techniques rely on the intensity ratio of two spectral events (line-to-continuum) from the same elemental plasma volume to determine temperature. Mills (7) and Key (8) have utilized relative techniques in atmospheric pressure argon arc plasmas with peak temperatures of 9000°K and 13,000°K, respectively. The temperature fields are reasonable, but both authors used ionic argon lines which at atmospheric pressure and the relatively low temperatures make the LTE assumption suspect. Tsao (9) used atomic argon lines and found peak temperatures of 8000°K. The low temperature may be explained by the small upper-level energy difference of atomic argon lines. The energy difference should be of the same order as the temperature to be resolved. Kobayashi (10) used an atomic and ionic line with peak temperatures of 18,000°K. The data is reasonable, but the different ionization stages introduce a more explicit dependence on LTE.

Based on the previous studies of laser- and arc-supported plasmas in argon, relative diagnostics have been chosen. The relative line-to-continuum method will be used initially in atmospheric plasmas at the low temperatures. If multiple lines and/or line pairs can be resolved, a self-consistency check on temperature and LTE can be performed.

3. EXPERIMENTAL RESULTS

3.1. Thermography

The IR thermography system was used to measure the surface temperature of a cylindrical gray cast-iron workpiece as it underwent laser surface heat treatment using an annular beam. The laser utilized in these experiments operates in the $TEM_{01}*$ mode. The laser energy is concentrated in an annulus with a mean radius of 2.3 inches (9 mm) with a Gaussian profile across the annulus. The axis of the cylindrical workpiece was placed along the centerline of the laser beam. A conical mirror section deflected the beam onto the workpiece, forming a circumferential heat treatment area as shown in Fig. 2. The measured temperatures were compared to the results of a mathematical model (11), both assuming an emissivity of 0.8. The model is a finite-difference simulation of the annular beam treating a cylindrical body. An energy balance including the radiation loss defines the cell temperature. Mass transfer in the form of carbon diffusion determines the interaction time once the laser parameters are fixed. Since the interaction time is a

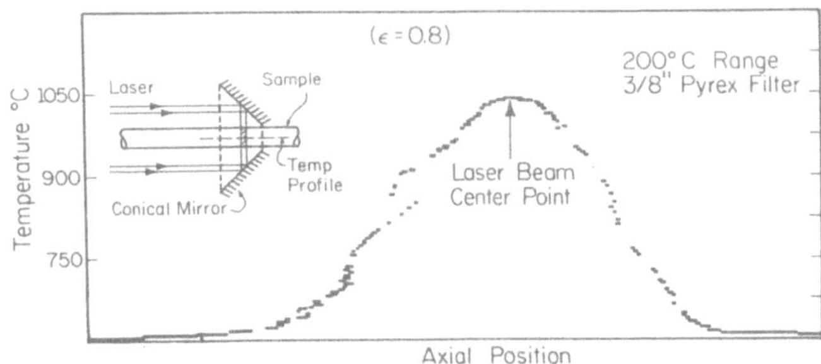

FIGURE 2. IR thermographic image of cylindrical gray cast iron: annular laser beam.

function of microstructure, a closed form solution of the fine pearlite carbon diffusion is coupled with the heat transfer equation to define a realistic interaction time. Figures 2 and 3 show the data and model, respectively, at 8.5 kW. The peak temperatures of the data and model were found to be within ± 7% at various power levels from 1 kW to 10 kW. Subsequent cross sectioning of the workpices verified the model accuracy of ± 10%, which further supports the ± 10% accuracy of the thermography system. Abscissa scaling was not performed in the series of experiments.

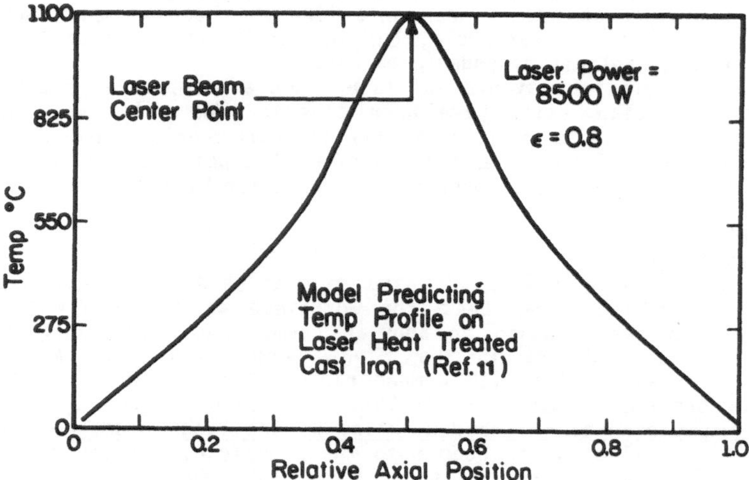

FIGURE 3. Results of mathematical model of cylindrical gray cast iron: annular laser beam.

More recently, the thermography system has been used to qualitatively map the behavior of pure argon plasmas under various flow conditions and laser power. Figure 4 shows the line of sight measured plasma intensity where the central regions are "hot." The round IR images contrast with the visible spectrum teardrop shape. The IR radiation is primarily Bremsstrahlung, which is proportional to the cube of the wavelength. Thus the cooler regions which do not radiate in the visible spectrum can contribute in the 3 to 4 μm range. Finally, quantitative measurements will be attempted when a calibration source such as the spectroscopic data can be directly compared to the thermography data.

3.2. Spectroscopy

Utilizing the relative line-to-continuum technique at the 415.86 nm argon line, peak electron temperatures of 17,000°K have been measured in laser-supported argon plasmas (3) as shown in Figure 5. The off-axis peak corresponds to the TEM01* laser beam peak. Figure 5 also shows the electron number density corresponding to the given temperature profile. The number density was calculated from the Saha equation based on LTE. The two figures demonstrate the relationship between temperature and number density which is necessary in the calculation of 10.6 μm

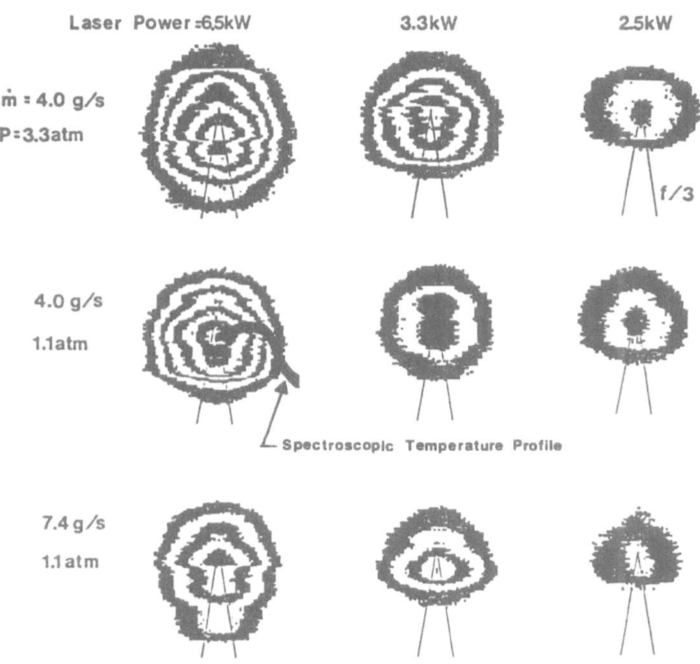

FIGURE 4. IR thermographic images of laser-sustained argon plasmas.

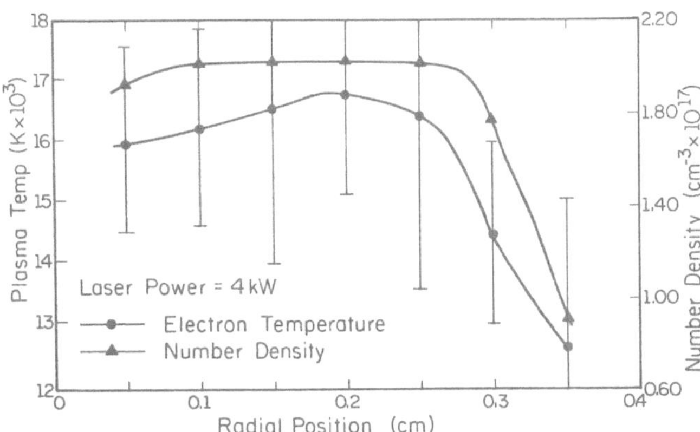

FIGURE 5. Radial temperature and number density profiles of laser-supported plasma in pure argon: core region.

radiation absorption in laser-supported plasma. Pure argon plasmas have been investigated initially to simplify the spectra and the diagnostic apparatus.

Figure 6 is a two-dimensional temperature mapping of a laser-supported argon plasma above 5054 aluminum plate. From the sequence of scans, a magnesium line was found in the region near the surface. This finding is in agreement with the various authors previously cited.

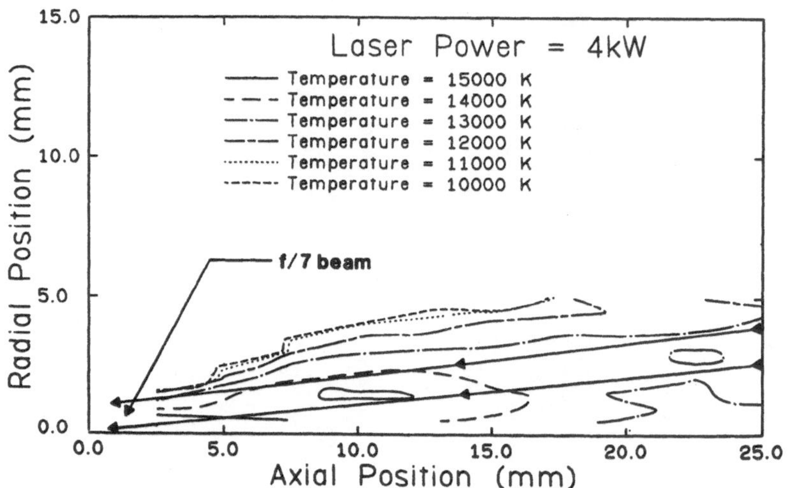

FIGURE 6. Two-dimensional temperature field of laser-supported plasma above 5054 aluminum plate: argon atmosphere.

From the temperature data of Figure 6, the inverse Bremsstrahlung absorption coefficient at 10.6 μm was calculated with a correction for photoionization absorption. The f/7-TEM01* beam was modeled using hermite polynomials. At each axial location, the Gaussian distribution was attenuated by the absorption coefficient and an energy balance performed to determine the energy transmitted to the next lower axial location. The net energy absorbed by the plasma of Figure 6 was determined to be 16% or 700 W, with 3.8 kW transmitted to the aluminum target.

The other effect of plasma absorption is that the Gaussian cross section is flattened, resulting in a "top hat" distribution at the workpiece. For the 1 mm spot size, the transmitted intensity is approximately 4.8×10^5 W/cm^2. Modeling the plasma as a 0.5 cm diameter disk, 2 mm above the workpiece, a calculation of the radiation from the plasma to the workpiece is roughly 10 watts. Thus our observations agree with the findings of previous authors reporting on pulsed laser interactions that plasma radiation alone cannot explain the enhanced coupling effect.

4. CONCLUSION

IR thermography has been adapted as a useful tool in temperature measurement during laser heat treatment. The accuracy of the system appears to be on the order of conventional temperature measurement devices. The system can be calibrated to higher temperatures approaching 4000°K. The system has been applied to qualitative measurements of laser-supported plasma behavior in pure argon. Eventually, the system may be used for quantitative measurements after calibration with spectroscopic data.

Relative line-to-continuum spectroscopy has been utilized to map the two-dimensional temperature of a cw laser sustained plasma above a metallic target. Heretofore, investigators have mapped arc-supported plasmas or pulsed events. The cw plasma above a metallic workpiece has been determined to absorb as much as 16% of the incident laser radiation. It was determined from a simple radiation model that radiation transport alone cannot explain the enhanced coupling effect. This conclusion agress with the various pulsed laser investigations. However, this result is highly dependent on laser parameters. In particular, pure argon plasmas have been shown experimentally to absorb more than 70% of the incident laser radiation (3).

REFERENCES

1. M. A. Khan, N. H. Madsen, and B. A. Chin, Proc. Soc. Photo-Opt. Instrum. Eng., 446 (1983).
2. T. J. Rockstroh and J. Mazumder, Appl. Opt. 24, 1343 (1985).
3. H. Krier et al., AIAA 18th Fluid Dynamics and Plasmadynamics and Lasers Conf., July 16-18, 1985, Cincinnati, Ohio, Paper No. AIAA-85-1551.
4. R. J. Glumb and H. Krier, ibid., Paper No. AIAA-85-1553.
5. B. B. Henriksen and D. R. Keefer, J. Appl. Phys. 46, 1080 (1975).
6. C. Carlhoff et al., Physica 103C, 439 (1981).
7. G. S. Mills, Welding Journal 56, 935 (1977).
8. J. F. Key, F. W. Chan, and M. E. McIllwain, Welding Journal 62 (1983).
9. K. C. Tsao and D. Pavelic, UK Welding Inst. Conf., (Welding Institute, UK, 1982), Paper No. 23.
10. M. Kobayashi and T. Suga, ibid., Paper No. 18.
11. L. C. Peterson, Jr., M.S. Thesis, University of Illinois at Urbana-Champaign (1984).

LASER/MATERIALS INTERACTIONS: CW DF LASER ABLATION OF CARBON*

RICHARD F. MENEFEE, BRENDAN D. KRENEK, AND MICHAEL J. BERRY
Houston Area Research Center, The Woodlands, TX 77380, and
Department of Chemistry, Rice University, Houston, TX 77251

Key Words: ablation, burnthrough, figure-of-merit

ABSTRACT

DF chemical laser interactions with isotropic (graphNOL) and anisotropic (pyrolytic graphite, diamond) carbons have been studied in order to analyze the intrinsic ablation performance of these materials and to measure their responses and properties under well-characterized laser irradiation conditions. Several hundred experiments were performed over a broad range of intensities in order to determine burnthrough times, reflectances at DF wavelengths, and front and back surface temperatures during irradiation. Burnthrough data were analyzed to provide Q* values (energies of ablation per gram of material) as a function of laser intensity and to understand energy and mass balances associated with laser-induced ablation. In addition, a laser probe absorption spectrometer was used to observe quantitative time-resolved spectra of carbon vapor species in laser-ablated plumes. All of the experiments are used to examine the physical and chemical processes that produce the phenomenology and effects characteristic of pure thermochemical ablation of materials by cw infrared lasers.

1. INTRODUCTION

The phenomenology of carbon ablation during radiative heating must be understood for aerospace applications. In addition, it is possible that surface metals and/or metal carbides can yield nonequilibrium distributions of carbon vapor species during laser ablation (1). In this work we set out to examine the interactions of cw infrared laser radiation with model isotropic and/or anisotropic carbons to determine fundamental aspects of laser/materials interactions and to explore possible nonequilibrium processes.

2. EXPERIMENTAL DETAILS

We used the Houston Area Research Center (HARC) Laser Test Resource to carry out experimental work on several types of pure carbon (including graphNOL, a nearly isotropic polycrystalline graphite, pyrolytic graphites, and diamond). The HARC Laser Test Resource includes a cw HF/DF chemical laser system, a test chamber, and beam and

---

* This work was supported by the Defense Advanced Research Projects Agency under Contract Number MDA903-82-C-0359 and Subcontract Number BDM-S309-0L7200 to the BDM Corporation and by the Robert A. Welch Foundation under Grants C-812 and K-099B.

sample diagnostic instrumentation. The facility has been used to study cw DF chemical laser interactions with more than 60 different materials in order to analyze their intrinsic ablation performance and to measure their time-resolved responses and properties under well-characterized laser irradiation conditions. Fundamental studies have been carried out to obtain a basic understanding of the chemical and physical processes that produce the phenomenology and effects associated with thermochemical ablation of carbon-based and other materials irradiated by cw infrared lasers at intensities up to 100 kW/cm^2.

Figure 1 shows a typical experimental configuration. The basic apparatus components are:

(1) A HF/DF cw chemical laser system (Helios Model CLIV) producing 100-200 W multiline output in the 2.6-3.0 μm (HF) and 3.7-4.1 μm (DF) spectral regions.
(2) An optical delivery system suitable for irradiating samples with excellent control of beam position, intensity, and time on target.
(3) Laser beam diagnostics to characterize wavelengths, short-term and long-term power levels, beam profiles, and intensity distributions on target.
(4) An evacuable sample chamber incorporating a carousel with 16 samples and accurate positioning controls; the chamber permits experiments in vacuum and in controlled atmospheres and has several viewing ports, together with an internally mounted integrating sphere reflectance measurement system.
(5) A laser probe absorption spectrometer for quantitative time-resolved measurements on plume species.
(6) Additional sample diagnostics instrumentation (optical pyrometers for front and back surface temperature measurements, a burnthrough detector, a microbalance for determination of mass losses, and a photomicrography system).
(7) A minicomputer system for experimental control and data acquisition (16 channels of information with a 40 kHz/channel acquisition rate).

The HARC Laser Test Resource was used to irradiate several hundred graphite samples at DF laser wavelengths within an intensity range of 10-50 kW/cm^2. These experiments were usually carried out in near vacuum (ca. 10 torr argon), but additional data were obtained at variable pressures of both air and argon.

Sample data obtained by irradiation of pyrolytic graphite are shown in Figure 2. For each data run, we obtain information on laser beam parameters (in order to specify laser intensities accurately) and sample responses. We also carry out postmortem inspections to determine mass losses and to record photomicrographs of selected samples.

3. RESULTS

Extensive experiments have been completed on graphNOL, a model form of graphite that is amenable to both detailed experimental and theoretical analyses. GraphNOL has isotropic and well-measured thermal properties; our measurements also provide time resolved optical properties which can be combined with all other required data as input for numerical computations of ablation behavior. The purpose of these experiments is to establish a complete understanding of physical and chemical phenomena on a quantitative level that permits us to develop energy and mass balances (including a determination of loss factors and scaling relations) for laser/materials interactions.

Figure 3 shows a set of data traces for graphNOL irradiated under similar conditions as used for the pyrolytic graphite run shown in Figure 2. Note that the sample reflectance is much lower and the back surface temperature rise is much faster for graphNOL compared to pyrolytic graphite. These different optical and thermal responses are directly related to the much faster ablation of graphNOL.

Figure 4 shows the results of numerous burnthrough measurements carried out on graphNOL samples of different thicknesses. In each plot of inverse burnthrough time vs. peak laser intensity, we obtain a linear least squares fit which yields burnthrough parameters I_t, the threshold intensity for ablation, and Q*, the effective figure-of-merit for ablation, which is equal to the effective enthalpy of ablation H_A divided by the energy coupling coefficient α. I_t is determined from the intercept ($t_{BT}^{-1} = 0$) and Q* from the slope of each linear fit using the relation: $Q^* = (\text{slope} \times \rho \times \ell)^{-1}$ where ρ and ℓ are the sample bulk density and thickness, respectively. Such linear plots are expected on the basis of surface energy balance considerations for the case of one-dimensional, quasi steady state thermochemical ablation of vaporizing materials (2).

Real systems exhibit two-dimensional effects due to radial conduction losses (3). Even in the flood loaded limit of laser irradiation by our Gaussian beams, part of the deposited laser energy is channeled into radial conduction losses that vary with sample diameter. In addition, conduction losses and radiative losses are expected to vary with sample thickness at a fixed sample diameter. Both sets of behavior are handled (in a phenomenological manner) by Klein's analysis (3) that develops scaling relations for the effective Q* as a function of a scaling parameter σ. Klein's procedure (3) yields nonlinear fits to burnthrough data which are also shown in Figure 4; these fits are entirely consistent with a model for thermochemical ablation of graphNOL, taking into account both radiative and nonradiative losses as well as our experimentally determined values of the energy coupling coefficients for DF laser absorption. Full analysis of our data to extract scaling relations and loss parameters is in progress. At this point, we note that our experimental data for graphNOL obtained under microscale irradiation conditions correlate well with larger scale experiments conducted at the United Technologies Research Center DF laser test facility in East Hartford, CT, using larger spot size irradiations with a 12-15 kW DF laser system.

Figure 5 shows an analysis of the data presented in Figure 4 to determine the effective value of Q* at zero sample thickness. The expected value of this fundamental ablation parameter is 43.9 (± 2.7) kJ/g (using 32.5 kJ/g as the thermochemical enthalpy of ablation, 0.814 as the experimentally determined coupling coefficient, and 1.0 kW/cm^2 as the radiative power loss), approximately 12% lower than our extrapolated value. This small discrepancy is due to the finite sample diameter (1.59 mm), which introduces small radial conduction losses. We expect that further graphNOL experiments using variable sample diameters will yield nearly exact agreement between theory and experiment for this model material.

REFERENCES

1. M. J. Berry, "Carbon Vapor Species," Memorandum dated August 1, 1983 (Rice University, Houston, TX).
2. J. H. Lundell and R. R. Dickey, "The Response of Heat Shield Materials to Intense Laser Radiation," AIAA Paper 78-138, presented at the AIAA 16th Aerospace Sciences Meeting, Huntsville, AL, January 16-18, 1978.
3. C. A. Klein, "Laser Ablation of Graphitic Targets: Scaling Laws," Memorandum Number RAY/RD/M-4146 dated October 31, 1984 (Raytheon Research Division, Lexington, MA) and references cited therein.

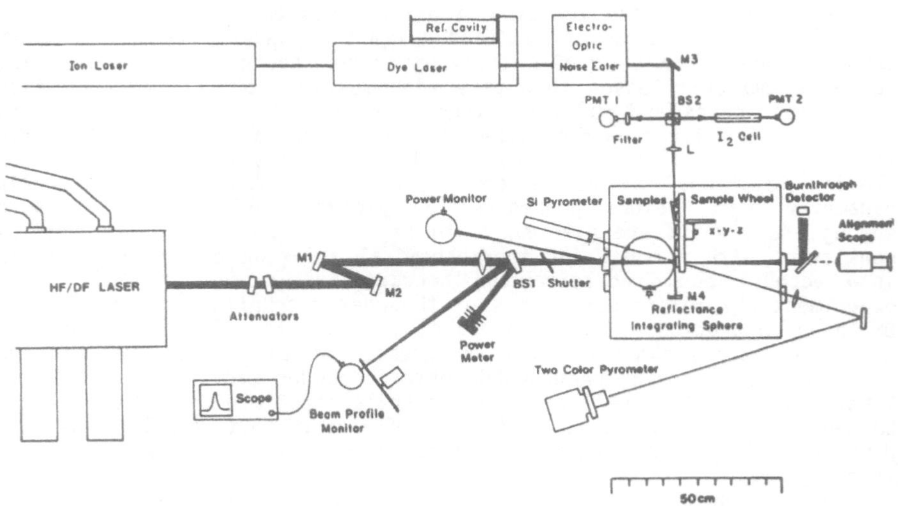

FIGURE 1

FIGURE 1

Microscale laser/materials interaction apparatus. A cw HF/DF chemical laser irradiates samples contained within the vacuum chamber at the far right of the figure. Portions of the laser beam are directed by a beamsplitter BS1 and a wedged chamber window onto diagnostic equipment (a power meter, a fast-response power monitor, and a fast-response beam profile monitor). A fast-acting shutter controls irradiation times on target. An optical delivery system (beam steering mirrors M1 and M2, focusing lens, and attenuators) provides accurately positioned beams on target with controlled and measured intensity distributions. An alignment scope facilitates accurate positioning of the focused laser beam onto the target surface. Realtime sample responses are monitored with diagnostic instrumentation (optical pyrometers for front and back surface temperature measurements, a burnthrough detector, and an integrating sphere plus fast-acting detector for reflectance measurements). Signals from both the laser beam and the sample diagnostics are digitized, recorded, and processed using a minicomputer system.

A laser probe absorption spectrometer is combined with the laser/-materials interaction apparatus. In the top part of the figure, a cw ion laser pumps a single-frequency tunable cw ring dye laser system (Coherent, Inc., Model 699-21) which produces spectral outputs over most of the visible (400-800 nm) spectral region when equipped with the proper dyes and optics. The dye laser system can also be combined with an intracavity second harmonic generator system (Coherent, Inc., Model 7500) to produce tunable ultraviolet spectral outputs. The visible spectral output of the dye laser system is scanned electronically over a 30 GHz region and is passed through an electro-optic modulator (a "noise eater") to obtain stable, low-noise probe signals. A reference cavity within the dye laser system is used to verify single-frequency operation during scans. The low-noise scanned (or fixed-frequency) dye laser probe beam is directed toward the vacuum chamber by mirror M3, passed through beamsplitter BS2, focused to a narrow beam waist in front of the target sample and within the ablated plume by lens L, reflected back through the plume by mirror M4, and detected by a filter (e.g., small monochromator) plus photomultiplier tube (PMT 1) combination. The M3, M4 beam steering mirrors can be translated to position the probe beam accurately for spatial resolution of plume absorptions as a function of distance from the sample surface and of distance from the plume centerline (i.e., the axis of cylindrical symmetry). The dye laser output wavelength is calibrated by monitoring iodine (I_2) cell absorption signals detected by photomultiplier PMT 2.

Other types of probe lasers are used to obtain quantitative measurements on other molecular species and on particles contained in laser-induced plumes.

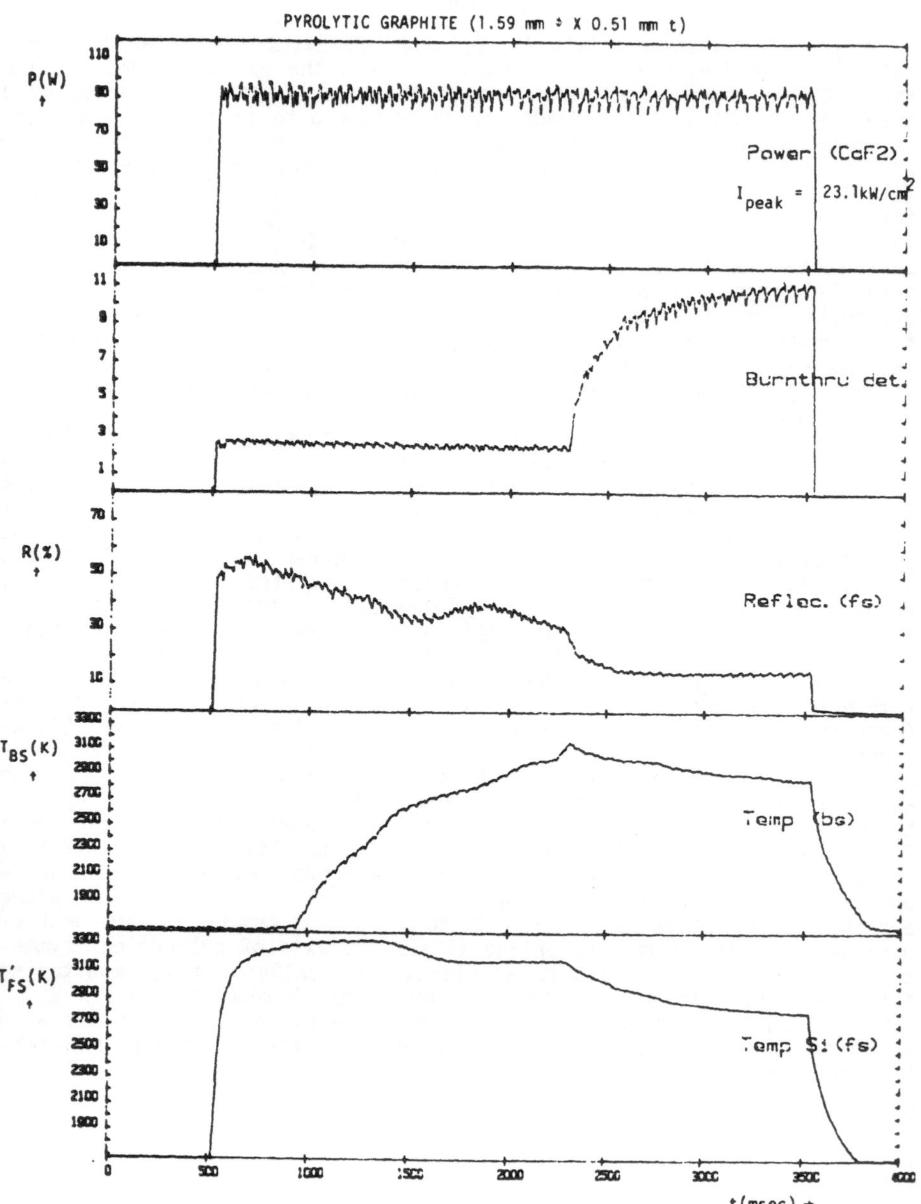
PYROLYTIC GRAPHITE (1.59 mm ⌀ X 0.51 mm t)
P(W)
Power (CaF2)
I peak = 23.1kW/cm2
Burnthru det.
R(%)
Reflec. (fs)
T BS(K)
Temp (bs)
T'FS(K)
Temp Si (fs)
t(msec) →

FIGURE 2

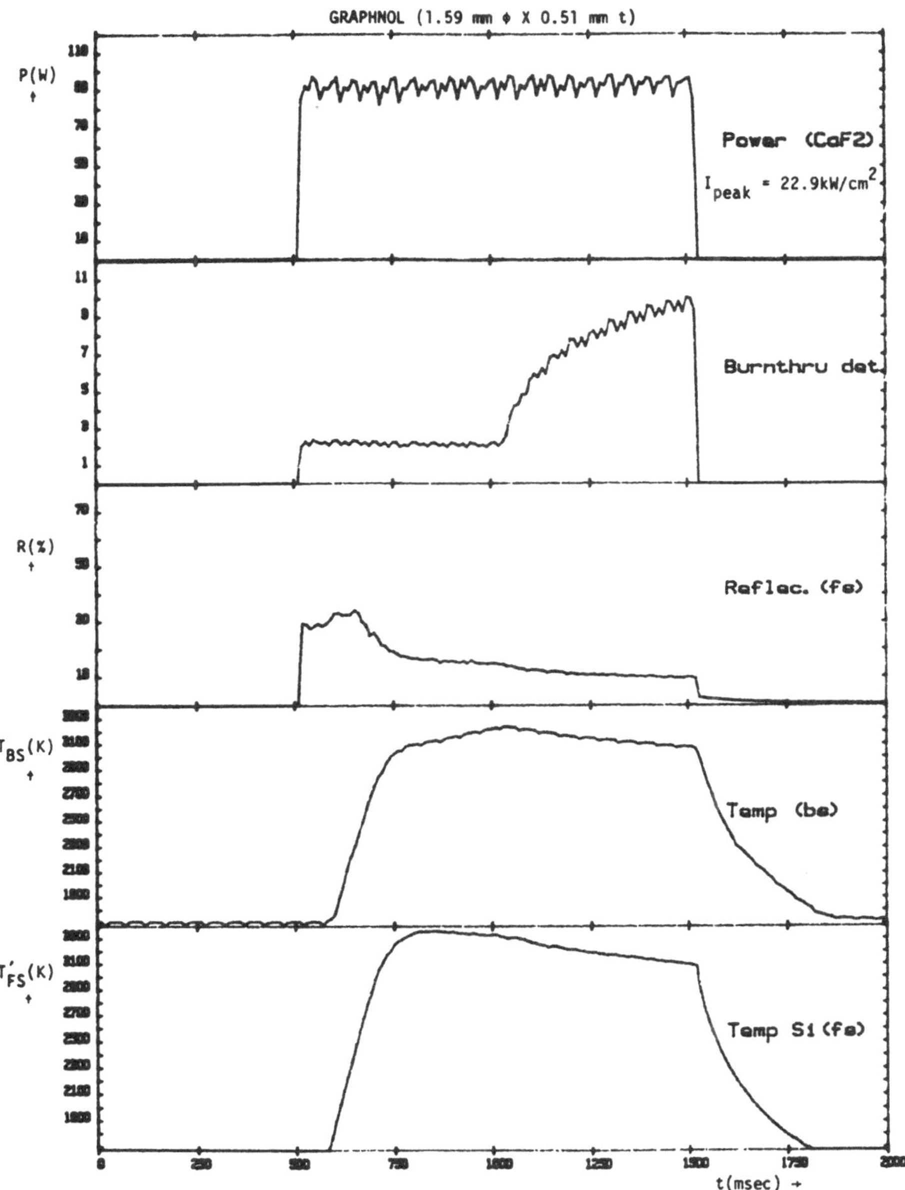
GRAPHNOL (1.59 mm ϕ X 0.51 mm t)
P(W)
Power (CaF2)
I peak = 22.9kW/cm2
Burnthru det.
R(%)
Reflec. (fs)
T BS(K)
Temp (bs)
T'FS(K)
Temp Si (fs)
t(msec) →

FIGURE 3

FIGURE 2

Experimental data traces for a 1.59 mm diameter x 0.51 mm thickness sample of pyrolytic graphite irradiated in a 10 torr Ar atmosphere by 90 W of multiline DF laser power in a near-Gaussian beam profile with a peak intensity of 23.1 kW/cm^2. The sample was oriented so that the incident laser beam was normal to the ab plane.

Top panel: Shutter opening and closing times and laser power during the open shutter period.

Second panel: Burnthrough detector response; burnthrough occurs 1.79 sec after the shutter opens.

Third panel: Front surface reflectance at the incident DF laser wavelengths monitored by a fast PbSe detector mounted in an integrating sphere and calibrated against a gold standard.

Fourth panel: Back surface temperature (averaged within a 0.7 mm diameter spot) monitored by a two-color pyrometer internally calibrated for graphite emissivity.

Bottom panel: Front surface temperature (averaged within a 0.5 mm diameter spot) monitored by a silicon pyrometer uncorrected for the time dependence of the pyrolytic graphite emissivity.

FIGURE 3

Experimental data traces for a 1.59 mm diameter x 0.51 mm thickness sample of graphNOL irradiated in a 10 torr Ar atmosphere by 90 W of multiline DF laser power in a near-Gaussian beam profile with a peak intensity of 22.9 kW/cm^2.

Top panel: Shutter opening and closing times and laser power during the open shutter period.

Second panel: Burnthrough detector response; burnthrough occurs 0.52 sec after the shutter opens.

Third panel: Front surface reflectance at the incident DF laser wavelengths monitored by a fast PbSe detector mounted in an integrating sphere and calibrated against a gold standard.

Fourth panel: Back surface temperature (averaged within a 0.7 mm diameter spot) monitored by a two-color pyrometer internally calibrated for graphite emissivity.

Bottom panel: Front surface temperature (averaged within a 0.5 mm diameter spot) monitored by a silicon pyrometer uncorrected for the time dependence of the graphNOL emissivity.

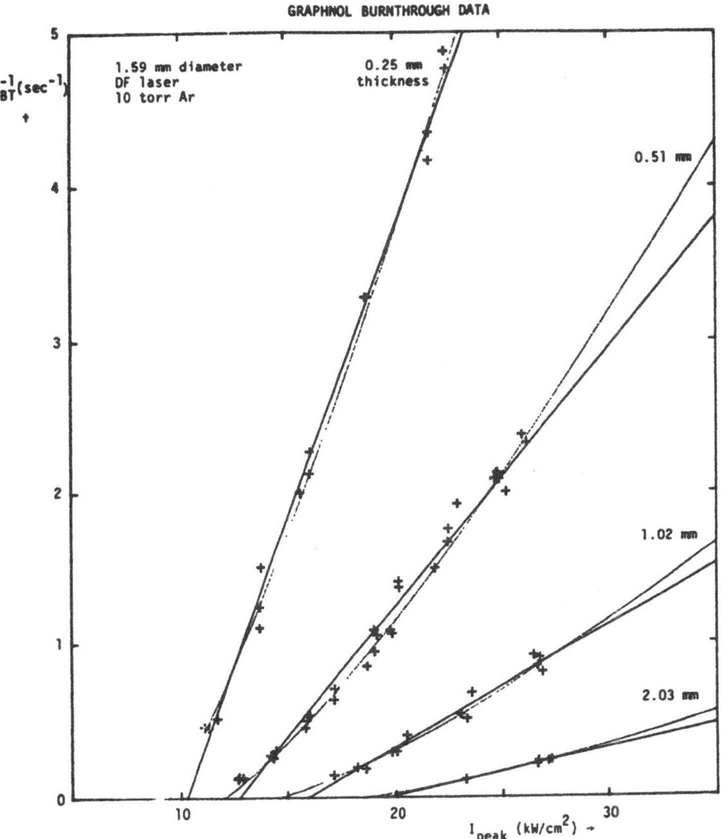

FIGURE 4

Inverse burnthrough times vs. peak intensity for graphNOL samples (1.59 mm diameter, variable thickness) ablated by DF laser radiation under a 10 torr Ar atmosphere. Linear least squares fits (by conventional burnthrough analyses) and nonlinear least squares fits (by Klein analyses) are shown for each data set. For clarity, additional data sets for other sample thicknesses (0.76 mm and 1.52 mm) are not plotted on Figure 4. However, effective figures-of-merit (Q*) obtained from the slopes of all six linear burnthrough fits are plotted in Figure 5 vs. sample thickness.

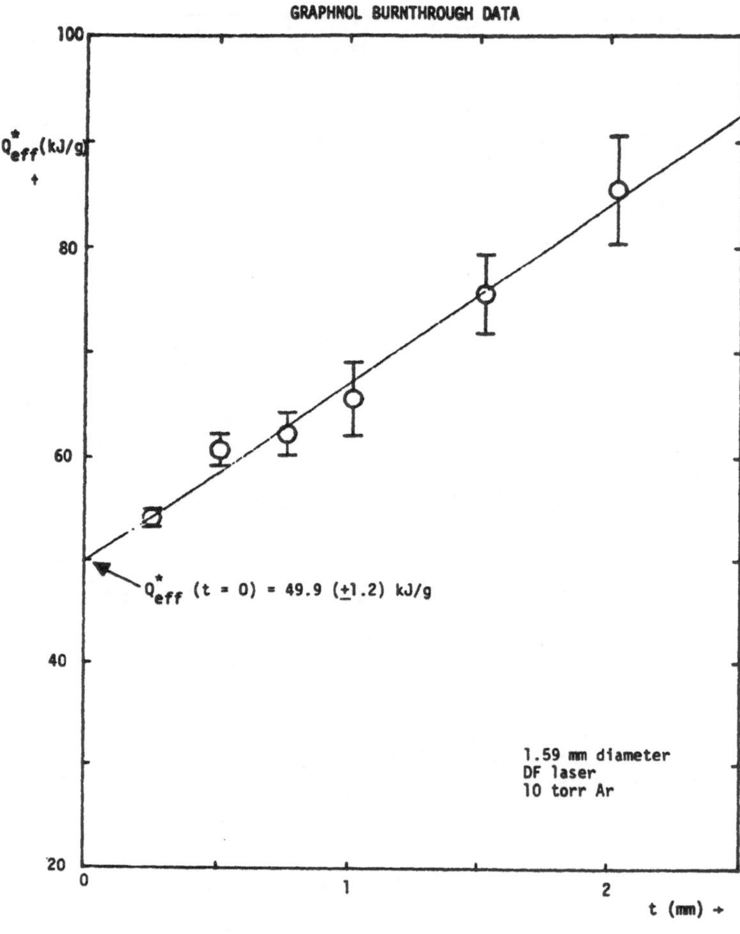

FIGURE 5

Effective figures-of-merit (Q*) vs. sample thickness from slopes of data sets shown in Figure 4 for graphNOL samples (1.59 mm diameter, variable thickness) ablated by DF laser radiation under a 10 torr Ar atmosphere. Statistical uncertainties in each Q* value are shown as error bars for each point. A linear least squares fit to the plotted points is also shown. The intercept (at zero thickness) is equal to 49.9 (± 1.2) kJ/g, approximately 14% larger than the expected value of Q*; see the text for explanation.

SPECTROSCOPIC STUDY OF ATOMIC BEAMS GENERATED BY LASER ABLATION OF MULTI-COMPONENT TARGETS

R. KOPPMANN, S. M. REFAEI* AND A. POSPIESZCZYK
Institut für Plasmaphysik der Kernforschungsanlage Jülich GmbH
Association EURATOM-KFA, 5170 Jülich, FRG

Key Words: lithium, aluminum, ablation

ABSTRACT

An experiment is described where Li and Al beams were generated by ablation of thin, multi-layer targets using a Q-switched ruby laser with a total energy density up to 30 Jcm^{-2}. Measurements using laser-induced fluorescence and mass spectroscopy were combined to analyze the energy and density distribution and the temporal structure of the beams. The maximum translational energy observed was several eV for Li and an order of magnitude greater for Al with a peak particle density in the range of 10^{10} cm^{-3} for both Li and Al.

The targets were analyzed by optical microscopy and secondary ion mass spectroscopy, providing information about the size of the spots and the structure of the metal before and after the ablation experiment.

1. INTRODUCTION

High-power laser irradiation of a metal-film glass interface has been frequently used to generate intense, short bursts of high-intensity energetic atom beams. The injection of such beams into a plasma at pre-selected times allows: (a) study of the effects of impurity ions on hydrogen plasmas, (b) measurement of impurity transport processes independent of impurity ions naturally present in the plasma, and (c) determination of the plasma boundary parameters using the neutral atom beams as a diagnostic tool (1-4).

For the injection of metal impurities the laser blow-off technique has been used successfully to produce 10^{16}-10^{18} particles with energies of 10 eV. A pulsed, high-power, Q-switched solid state laser is normally used to ablate metal-coated glass slides with a coating thickness up to 10 µm from the rear side. Several laboratory experiments have studied the properties of beams produced with this technique (3,5-7).

The following experiment was carried out to determine the characteristics of the various atomic components emitted from irradiated multi-component targets.

2. EXPERIMENTAL

The experimental setup (Fig. 1) consists of (a) a Q-switched ruby laser with a total energy of 0.5 J and a pulse duration of 20 nsec, (b) a HV-chamber and a drift tube with a base pressure of 10^{-6} mbar, (c) a target which can be manipulated from outside without breaking the vacuum, (d) diagnostic systems which will be described in detail later.

---

* Present Address: Department of Physics, Cairo University, Cairo, Egypt.

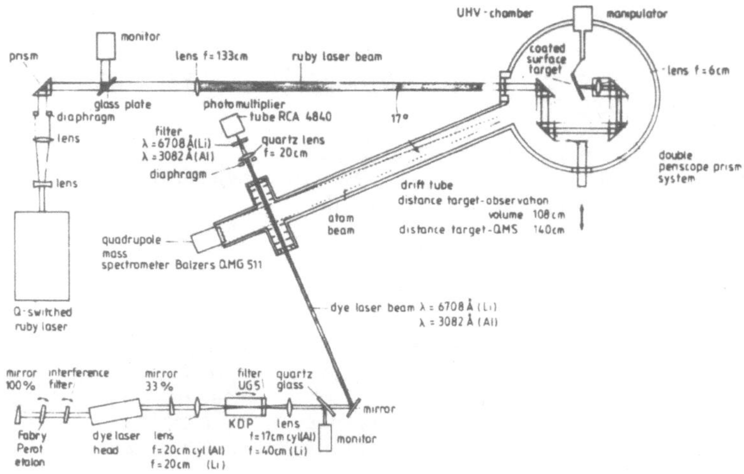

FIGURE 1. Experimental setup.

The ruby laser beam was focused into the vacuum system by two lenses of 133 cm and 6 cm focal length, respectively. During all measurements the laser beam was diverted by a double-periscope prism system and hit the target from the rear side through the glass. The periscope system can be moved to allow shots from the front of the target. In this case the first lens (f = 133 cm) has to be replaced by a lens of f = 63 cm.

The energy density on the target was varied by changing the position of the target along the axis of the ruby laser beam.

The target consists of a 25 x 28 x 1 mm glass slide with vacuum-evaporated metal layers on one side. The thickness of the metal film ranged between 200 nm and 1500 nm.

The target is tilted by an angle of 17° relative to the axis of the ruby laser beam in the direction of the drift tube and can be moved by a manipulator from outside so that a number of spots can be ablated without breaking the vacuum. The size of the spots was nearly circular with a diameter of 1 mm.

The ablated material beam passes through a drift tube to be analyzed by various methods:

- At a distance of 108 cm from the target, the cloud passed an observation volume of 0.18 cm^3, where the atoms in the ground state were excited by a tunable, flash-lamp-pumped dye laser in crossed-beam geometry and were detected by laser-induced fluorescence (LIF) using a photomultiplier tube (RC 4840). For the LIF measurements of the Li atom density, the wavelength of the dye laser beam was adjusted to $\lambda = 670.8$ nm. For the corresponding measurements on Al, a KDP crystal was used for frequency doubling and an optical filter with a cutoff wavelength of ~ 420 nm and optical density of ~ 0.03 was used to block out the visible light. The wavelength was adjusted to $\lambda = 308.2$ nm. Calibration of the absolute densities was done by Rayleigh scattering in argon. This technique is described in detail in Ref. 7.

- At the end of the drift tube, 140 cm away from the target, a quadrupole mass spectrometer (Balzers QMG 511) with electron bombardment ionizer was positioned. The detector was a 14-stage Cu-Be electron multiplier. The signal from the multiplier was fed into a low-capacitance preamplifier and then displayed on an oscilloscope.

3. RESULTS AND DISCUSSION

Lithium has been strongly favored as material for injection, as it has a low mass and therefore a high penetration velocity. Furthermore, the strong resonance transition at λ = 670.8 nm makes Li easily accessible to laser-induced fluorescence techniques.

In this experiment two types of targets were used:

(1) A layer of simultaneously evaporated Li and Al with a total thickness of $<$ 200 nm.

(2) A three-layer sandwich-target (manufactured by LeBow Co., California, USA) with 500 nm Al, 500 nm Li and 500 nm Al, i.e., a total thickness of 1500 nm. The Al layer on top of the Li layer should serve as a protection against oxidation of Li.

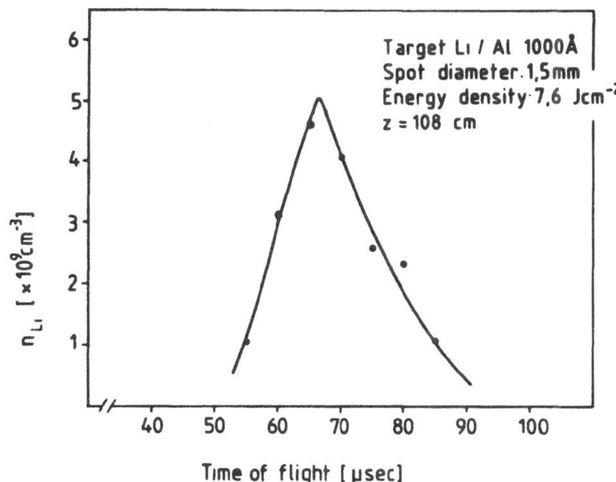

FIGURE 2. Density distribution of Li generated by laser ablation of a Li-Al film obtained by simultaneous evaporation of the metals.

3.1. Experiments with simultaneously evaporated Li/Al

Figure 2 shows the density of Li $n_L(t)$ measured with LIF using a target with simultaneously evaporated Li and Al. The peak density was found to be 5 x 10^9 cm^3, the peak energy 3.24 eV. Comparison of the time of arrival ($\sim$ 70 μsec) with the half width of the pulse ($\sim$ 20 μsec) shows that the distribution is non-thermal. A thermal distribution would be characterized by nearly equal values of time of arrival and half width (see, e.g., Ref. 9). The low density of Li compared with the measurements on Li in Ref. 3 is probably due to the lower amount of Li evaporated during the different preparation processes. The elements on the targets used for the measurements in Ref. 3 have been evaporated successively.

3.2. Experiments with the Li/Al-sandwich targets

3.2.1. Surface analysis. Before installation in the vacuum chamber, a surface analysis of these targets was carried out. The results of this surface analysis using secondary ion mass spectroscopy (SIMS) are shown in Figs. 3 and 4 (10).

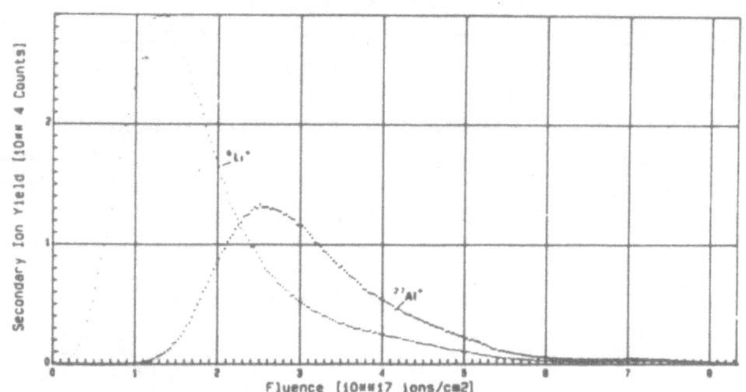

FIGURE 3. Depth profile of Li and Al in the originally three-layer Al/Li/Al target measured by SIMS (linear scale).

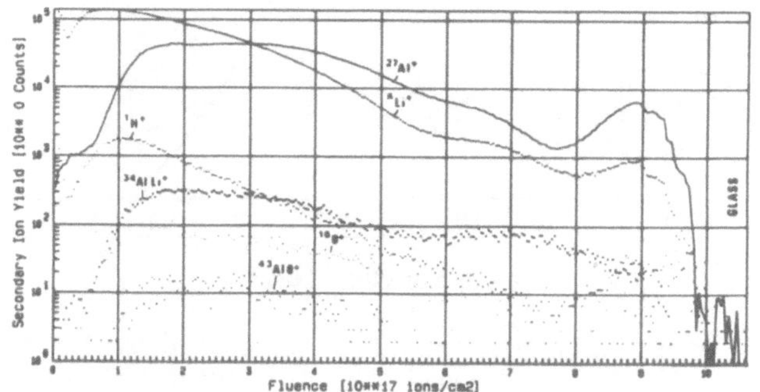

FIGURE 4. Depth profile of Li, Al, LiAl, AlO, H and O in the originally three-layer Al/Li/Al target measured by SIMS (logarithmic scale).

The first depth profile shows that the Li layer has completely diffused to the surface of the metal film. Due to this segregation process the original three-layer target has changed to a two-layer target with 500 nm Li covering 1000 nm Al. The segregation process of binary metal systems is discussed in Refs. 11-13. The surface composition of an alloy of Li and other metals changes with time due to segregation processes depending on the solution enthalpies, the surface energies, the different sizes of the atoms and the temperature. Using the model of Miedema (11), it was calculated that in the case of an Li-Al alloy this effect results in a complete segregation of Li and Al at a temperature of 300°K. The surface concentration of Li reaches a value of 100% (cf. Fig. 5) (14). A similar phenomenon can be observed with these three-layer targets.

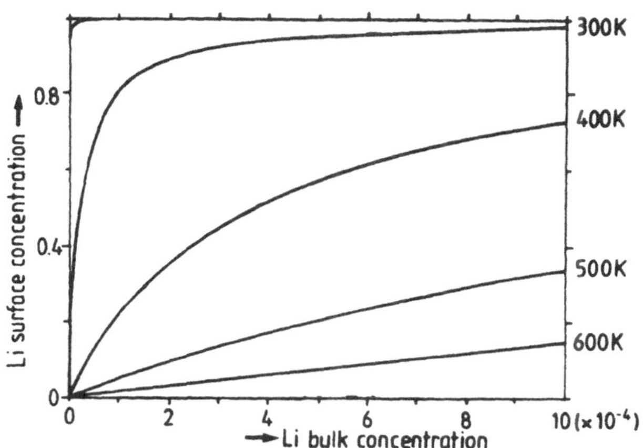

FIGURE 5. Calculation of the Li concentration at the surface of Li-Al alloy as a function of the bulk concentration and the temperature of the probe.

A second depth profile analysis (Fig. 4) shows the presence of six different materials on the same target. The different signal peaks are due to different positions on the target. The SIMS measurements shown in Fig. 3 were made on a lighter part of the light-dark structure, the measurements of Fig. 4 on a darker part on the same target (see below). A part of the Al seems to be oxidized, another part is in the form of LiAl molecules. Hydrogen and oxygen turned out to be the most abundant impurities in the layers. It should be noted that the analysis is only qualitative.

One of the sandwich targets was also analyzed by optical microscopy. The microscopic views (dark-field illumination) showed a light-dark structure on the target, which can also be seen by the naked eye. To stretch the contrast, pictures were made with the light coming from one side only, revealing the light-dark structures as surface features on the target. It can be seen that the thickness of the metal film changes depending on the location of the target. Small "craters" at the target surface are also present (Fig. 6), and in the target material a "bubble"-like structure can be seen (Fig. 7) (see also the picture given in Ref. 15). In air at normal pressure the light-dark structures on the target surface become colored. In the SIMS vacuum chamber with a base pressure in the range of 10^{-10} mbar, part of the metal film scaled off the glass slide.

FIGURE 6. Microscopic view of the surface features of the Al/Li/Al target (illumination from the top). The width of the figure is about 1.5 mm of the sample surface.

FIGURE 7. Microscopic view of the surface of the Al/Li/Al target (dark-field illumination). The width of the figure is about 1.5 mm of the sample surface.

3.2.2. Ablation measurements. The results of the LIF measurements in the case of the sandwich target look quite different from those in the case of the target with simultaneously evaporated Li-Al coating concerning the energy distribution and the density (Fig. 8). The peak densities were found to be 1 x 10^{10} cm^{-3} for Al and

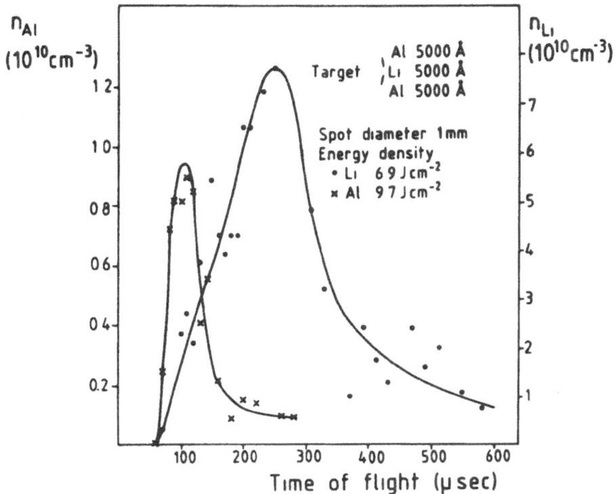

FIGURE 8. Comparison of the density distribution of Al and Li, ablated from a sandwich target.

8 x 10^{10} cm^{-3} for Li. The energies at the density peaks turned out to be about 15 eV for Al and about 1 eV for Li. The half widths were found to be 50 μsec for Al and 200 μsec for Li. The time-of-flight distribution indicates the Li beam has a nearly thermal distribution, while the Al beam is not thermal.

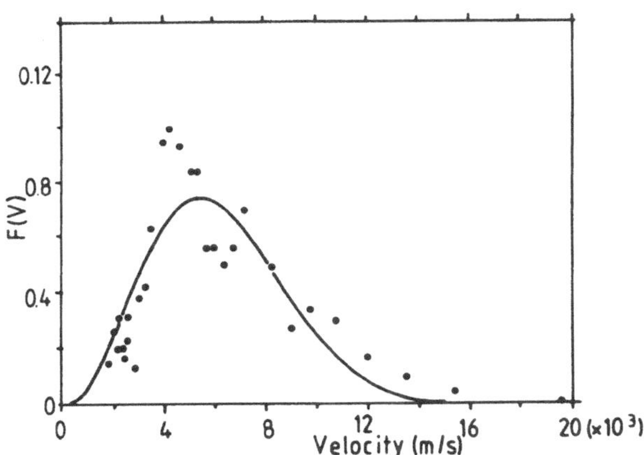

FIGURE 9. Comparison of the energy distribution of Li with a Maxwellian corresponding to a temperature of 1.1 eV.

Figure 9 shows that a Maxwellian of a temperature of 1.1 eV fits the density distribution of Li rather well.

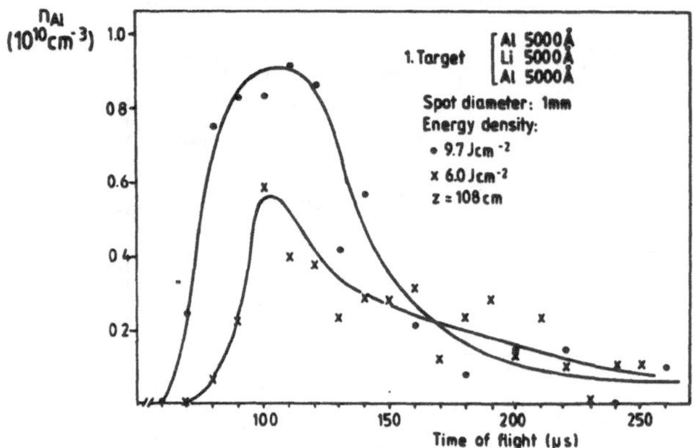

FIGURE 10. Comparison of the distribution of Al ablated with different energy densities of the ruby laser beam at the target.

A comparison of the energy distribution of Al ablated with an energy density of 9.7 Jcm^{-2} and 6.0 Jcm^{-2}, respectively, shows that a slight reduction of the energy density causes only a smaller peak density while the peak energy remains roughly the same (Fig. 10). With an increase of the energy density of 30 Jcm^{-2}, the peak energy of Al changes from 15 eV to 27 eV. This result was also found by Breton et al. (8).

The large scatter in the measurements is because of the variability of the ablation. Due to the limited target area in most cases, one ablated target spot per data point was used.

The increase of the energy density produces a second maximum in the density with a peak energy of 12 eV (Fig. 11). Similar results were reported in Ref. 3 for Li. The results are summarized in Table 1.

In the light of the surface analysis described above, we suggest one possible mechanism which might be an explanation for the ablation characteristics found in our experiment. When the layer is heated by the ruby laser pulse and the temperature of the Al layer reaches values somewhat above the "boiling point" of Li, the Li evaporates from the target, yielding a nearly thermal distribution. The Al layer which is liquid at this temperature is then heated up to still higher temperatures so that the lower part of the layer is in the form of Al vapor between the glass and the liquid surface of the layer. The Al is then ablated at much higher energies than the Li, yielding a sharp non-thermal distribution. The ablation (and evaporation) processes take place in the range of tens of nanoseconds. Since the time of flight from the target to the the observation volume is several hundred microseconds, the Al cloud gets ahead of the Li cloud, reaching the observation volume 150 μs earlier than the latter one. The different distributions (thermal/non-thermal) may arise from the fact that (a) the Li layer is only half the thickness of the Al layer, and (b) the Li layer is the upper layer and can expand

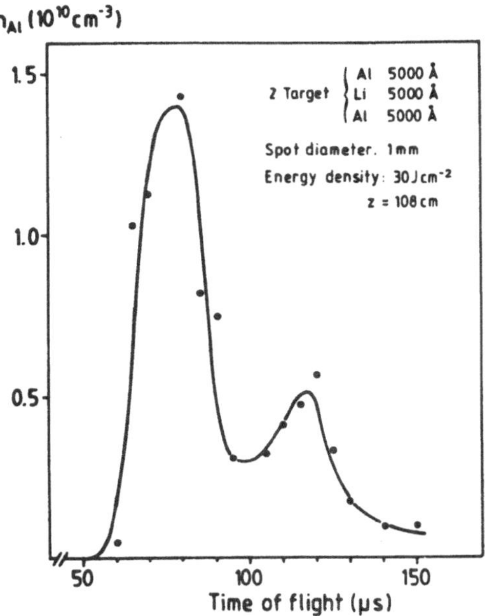

FIGURE 11. Density distribution of Al ablated with an energy density of 30 Jcm^{-2}.

more easily into the vacuum (for details on the ablation mechanisms in the case of laser pulses coming from the front side of the target, see Refs. 16,17.

TABLE 1.

Target	Element Observed	Energy Density Jcm^{-2}	Time of Flight μs	Peak Velocity $x10^5 cms^{-1}$	Peak Energy eV	Peak Density $x10^{10} cm^3$
Li/Al 200 nm	Li	7.6	67	16	3.24	0.5
Al/Li/Al 500 nm ea.	Li	6.9	250	4.8	0.68	8.0
Target 1	Al	9.7	105	10.3	14.8	0.9
		6.0	105	10.3	14.3	0.6
Al/Li/Al 500 nm ea.	Al	29.9	77.5	13.9	26.98	1.4
Target 2	(second max)		(118)	(9.2)	(11.7)	(0.6)

3.3. Comparison of the LIF measurements with quadrupole mass spectroscopy

In addition to the LIF measurements we also used quadrupole mass spectroscopy.

Figure 12 shows a typical QMS signal on mass 27. Earlier investigations showed that both neutral and ionized atoms are generated by laser irradiation, with the ions being typically three times more energetic than the neutrals (6). Due to these measurements Lie et al. (3) supposed that the first peak represents the ionized atoms while the following peaks are due to the neutrals.

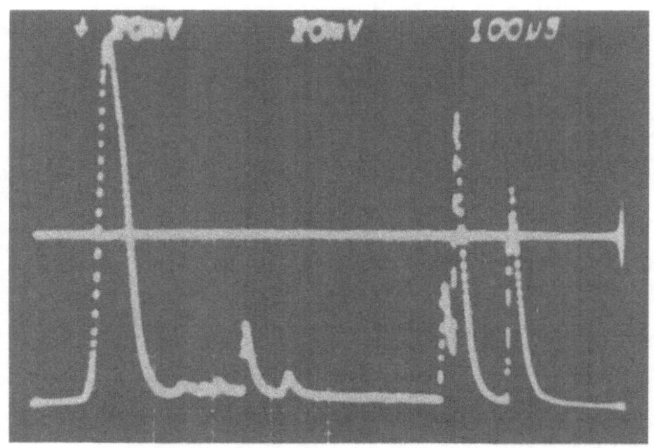

FIGURE 12. QMS signal on mass 27 (aluminum).

According to our measurements the first peak of the QMS signal seems to consist of neutral atoms while the following spikes are due to clusters of atoms as discussed in Ref. 5. The time of flight and the amplitude of these spikes varied by a factor of 2-3 from shot to shot. An explanation for the generation of clusters may be the liquid state of the surface of the Al layer at the time of ablation.

3.4. Optical microscopic analysis

After the ablation experiments the targets were analyzed by optical microscopy. The structure of the spots was compared with the structure of spots of pure Al targets (thickness 3 μm).

The microscopic views show clearly the different ablation processes of a pure Al target (Fig. 13) and a target of Al combined with Li (Fig. 14). In both cases the energy density at the target was 12 J/cm^2.

In the case of the pure Al targets, all material within the area corresponding to the cross section of the ruby laser beam has been ablated, leaving a nearly circular spot of 1 mm in diameter with a sharply defined edge.

In the case of the Li/Al targets ablated under the same conditions, the spots show a roughly circular center where the material is completely ablated, but at the edges exfoliation leaves a structured region of about one spot radius around the ablated center. In the case of the

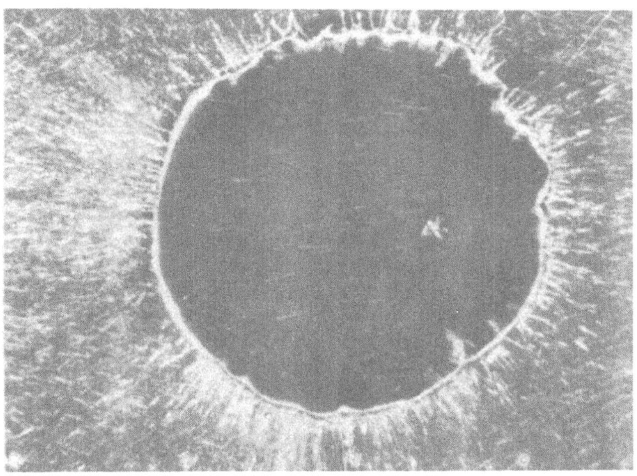

FIGURE 13. Microscopic view of spot ablated from pure Al target (thickness 3 μm). The width of the figure is about 1.5 mm of the sample surface.

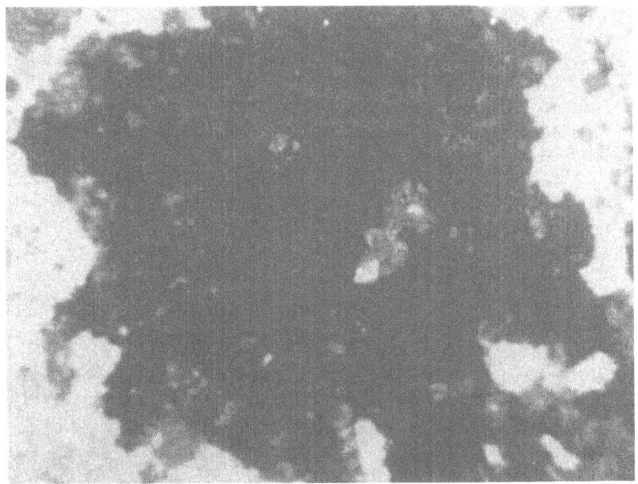

FIGURE 14. Microscopic view of a spot ablated from a Li/Al target (Li 50 nm, Al 80 nm). The width of the figure is about 1.5 mm of the sample surface.

lower energy densities, i.e., larger spot diameter, a part of the material in the center of the spot is left on the glass slide while an annular region is completely ablated. Ablation of the pure Al target under these conditions leaves a larger spot, the area of which is still covered with a thin layer of material.

The microscopic view also shows that a part of the ablated material has been redistributed on the target surface. Probably high field strength produced by the laser beam causes some of the ionized material to fall back onto the target. At a distance of some mm from the spots, radial structures looking like ejected material around lunar craters can be seen.

ACKNOWLEGMENTS

The authors wish to thank Professor E. Hintz for his encouragement and for valuable discussions during this work.

We also thank Mr. S. Musso and Mr. H. Priesent for assisting the experiment and Mr. H. Overkott for preparing some of the targets.

We would like to thank Mr. K. H. Besocke, Mrs. G. Flentje and Dr. K. G. Tschersich of the Institut für Grenzflächenforschung und Vakuumphysik for the surface analysis of the targets.

One of us (S.M.R.) would like to thank Professor L. El-Nadi for the help to get the fellowship and acknowledges gratefully the support of the International Office of the KFA during his stay.

REFERENCES

1. K. Kadota, A. Pospieszczyk, P. Bogen, and E. Hintz, Report No. JÜL 1812, KFA Jülich, Federal Republic of Germany, 1982.
2. K. Kadota, A. Pospieszczyk, P. Bogen, and E. Hintz, IEEE Transactions on Plasma Science (1984), to be published.
3. Y. T. Lie, A. Pospieszczyk, and J. A. Tagle, Fusion Technol. 6, 447 (1984).
4. E. Hintz and P. Bogen, J. Nucl. Mater. 128 & 129, 229 (1984).
5. D. Manos, D. Ruzic, R. Moore, and S. Cohen, J. Vac. Sci. Technol. 20, 1230 (1982).
6. E. S. Marmar, J. L. Cecchi, and S. A. Cohen, Rev. Sci. Instrum. 46, 1149 (1975).
7. P. Bogen and Y. T. Lie, J. Nucl. Mater. 93 & 94, 363 (1980).
8. C. Breton, C. de Michelis, W. Hecq, and M. Mattioli, Rev. Phys. Appl. 15, 1193 (1980).
9. A. Pospieszczyk, P. Bogen, H. Hartwig, and Y. T. Lie, J. Nucl. Mater. 93 & 94, 368 (1980).
10. K. H. Besocke, G. Flentje, and K. G. Tschersich, private communication.
11. A. R. Miedema, Z. Metallkd. 69, 455 (1978).
12. D. M. Gruen, A. R. Krauss, S. Susman, M. Venugopalan, and M. Ron, J. Vac. Sci. Technol. A1, 924 (1983).
13. A. R. Krauss, D. M. Gruen, and A. B. Dewald, J. Nucl. Mater. 121, 398 (1984).
14. R. P. Schorn, private communication.
15. M. E. Drits, E. M. Padeshova, and L. S. Gusej, in Obshchiye Zakonomernosti v Stroenij Diagramm Sostoyaniya Metallicheskich Sistem, (Academy of Sciences of the USSR, Moscow, 1973).
16. J. F. Ready, J. Appl. Phys. 36, 462 (1964).
17. J. E. Rothenberg and R. Kelly, Nucl. Instrum. Methods Phys. Res. 229 (B1), 291 (1984).

CHAPTER 1 - EDITED QUESTIONS

DULEY, KEILMANN, ROCKSTROH, BERRY, KOPPMANN

DULEY

Q. How do you select which experimental data for n and k you will use when calculating R?
A. Data must come from experiments where the surface was clean and in high vacuum.

Q. Do such surfaces have to be flat?
A. Yes, in most cases evaporated films are best.

Q. When you measure the coupling coefficient, does the polarization of the beam have any influence?
A. Yes, but only for non-normal incidence. Normal incidence was used in all my experiments.

Q. What are the typical dimensions of the sample and the duration of the laser pulse?
A. cm and seconds.

Q. Will the pure metals have oxides on them?
A. Measurements were done in a vacuum of about 10^{-2} torr. Oxides will not be important at low temperature but may influence the results at temperatures higher than 900°C.

Q. With the TEA laser, is there a plasma with stainless steel?
A. We tried to avoid plasma formation, but some plasma may have been present at higher sample temperatures.

Q. When grating structures form, can they occur in the solid phase?
A. I think that this may occur very near the melting point when the surface is soft.

Q. Why does roughness affect absorption?
A. Roughness introduces excess defects and any time the crystal structure is distorted, the conductivity goes down. Alloys with a larger defect concentration behave in the same way; that is, they tend to have low electrical conductivity and lower reflectivity.

KEILMANN

Q. Is any of this structure affected by the presence or thickness of the PMMA overlayer?
A. No.

Q. In Figure 3 the period of the surface structures is about 6 μm. Why is it not 10 μm the wavelength of the CO_2 laser light?
A. Because the k vector of the surface wave is not the same as that of the laser light. The period of the structure can be changed by changing the wavelength of the laser.

Q. What acts as the "antenna" to initiate scattering?
A. Any local defect. Even "perfect" crystals will develop such defects sooner or later.

ROCKSTROH

Q. How large are the target samples and what size is the laser beam?
A. The samples are 1-1.5 cm diameter while the laser beam diameter is 2 mm.

Q. Was the normal spectral emittance of the workpiece temperature dependent?
A. Yes, very, but it was taken to be 0.8.

Q. Are your plasmas optically thick?
A. Yes, in the IR but not in the visible.

Q. What was the intensity of the focused laser? How much was absorbed?
A. About 400 kW/cm^2, but we did not measure the absorbed intensity.

BERRY

Q. Why was this experiment performed in 10 torr of argon?
A. This was done so as to match the present experimental conditions to later experiments that involve a 15 kW laser. The same results were obtained in vacuum.

Q. Does the argon pressure have much influence on the number of particles that come off?
A. Not so much coming off, but as you go down the plume, you get soot nucleation in the vapor. Any particles within the plume burn off.

KOPPMANN

Q. How were the films you describe as "targets" prepared?
A. We obtained them from a firm in the US. They were evaporated films.

CHAPTER 2. FUNDAMENTALS OF PHASE FORMATION IN LASER ANNEALING OF METALS

CHAPTER INTRODUCTION - F. SPAEPEN AND P. S. PEERCY

Although the use of lasers for surface treatment of metals predates their use for annealing of silicon, fundamental understanding of the transformation processes in metals and alloys under these unusual conditions is less developed than in the case of silicon. One reason for this, of course, was the perceived technological importance of laser processing of silicon, which led to a broad-based, concentrated study of this problem. Furthermore, many of the physical properties of the phases of silicon, such as their reflectivity and conductivity, are ideally suited for time-resolved measurements of laser-induced transformations; this is much less the case for metallic systems. Finally, the large diversity of metallic alloys and crystal structures, compared to silicon, where only three structures and very dilute alloys must be considered, necessarily delays the emergence of a coherent understanding of the transformations in the metallic state.

The study of laser-induced transformations in metals, however, has benefited greatly from the concentrated effort on silicon. Experimentally, for example, the use of ultra-short pulses (ns or ps) and the transient reflectivity and conductivity techniques which were pioneered in the silicon studies have been recently transferred successfully to the study of metals. Similarly, formulation of the theory of fast transformations under these unusual conditions has also been prompted by the silicon work, which, in this case, benefited from the large body of well-developed transformation theory available in the metallurgical community. In the cost-benefit analysis of the silicon work, discussed briefly by Poate et al. in their introduction to the silicon chapter of this book, these indirect contributions to the study of metals must certainly be taken into account.

The first three papers in this chapter give an overview of the basic mechanisms underlying the laser-induced transformations, most of which start by forming the molten state. A recurring theme here is the distinction between collision-controlled and diffusion-controlled crystal growth. The first one is a very fast process that is thought to occur only for simple crystal structures in partitionless solidification; formation of this type of crystal is unlikely to be suppressed even by the very high quench rates following ps pulsed irradiation. The second process can occur as a result of either long-range diffusion (as in the precipitation of crystals with a composition different from that of the liquid or in eutectic crystallization), or short-range diffusional rearrangements in the partitionless crystallization of relatively complex crystal structures; under these conditions, crystal growth can be suppressed and metallic glasses can be formed. The paper by Peercy illustrates this for the Al-Sb and Al-Ni systems. Peercy also describes effects in two pure metals: defect formation in Al, and formation of metastable phases in undercooled liquid Mn. The paper by Spaepen contains the derivation of the basic crystal growth laws, together with applications to glass formation in ps pulsed laser experiments. The paper by Kaufmann and Wallace outlines, using a number of examples, how control of the crystal growth velocity in cw laser surface melting, combined with heat flow analysis, can be used to obtain numerical values for the parameters in the growth theories. These papers also show that the very high quench rates obtainable by pulsed laser irradiation (up to 10^{13} K/s for ps pulses) can lead to the formation of many novel materials; extended solid solutions, new metastable crystals, and extended glass formation ranges.

The next four papers decribe pulsed laser experiments on pure metallic systems. The paper by MacDonald and Spaepen describes the extension of the transient reflectivity technique, originally developed for the study of silicon, to the melting and regrowth of noble metals, such as Au, Cu, and Au/Cu multilayers, following ps irradiation. Crystallization velocities up to 100 m/s are reported, which indicate that the growth of simple crystals is indeed collision-limited, since the diffusion-limited velocity cannot exceed a few 10's of m/s. The paper by Williamson and Mourou decribes a newly developed, time-resolved electron diffraction technique to study the kinetics of melting of thin foils following pulsed laser irradiation, and reports results on Al. Their finding, however, of a lifetime for the overheated crystal of up to 1 ns following a 20 ps pulse disagrees with the transient reflectivity results, as well as with the transient conductivity measurements on Al reported by Peercy in the silicon chapter, both of which find this lifetime to be much shorter. This clearly needs further investigation.

The paper by Fröhlingsdorf and Stritzker on irradiation of Ga shows clearly how the amorphous phase is formed if the competing crystal growth is diffusion-limited (for the complex α-phase), and is suppressed if the crystal growth is collision-limited (for the simpler β-phase). The paper by Helms et al. reports on the surface defects resulting from irradiation of Mo and Bi; their findings of thermomechanically induced slip are similar to Peercy's results on Al.

The paper by Petit et al. describes a special applicaton of pulsed laser irradiation of a metallic system. An Al/Sb multilayer is heated sufficiently to initiate the reaction of the elements, after which the large exothermic heat of reaction sustains the melting and the formation of semiconducting AlSb. Battaglin et al. describe some attempts at measuring segregation effects during solidificaiton following laser irradiation of Ni-La alloys. Surface segregation was only observed as a result of oxidation; otherwise, all composition profiles could be accounted for by diffusion in the liquid state.

SOLIDIFICATION DYNAMICS AND MICROSTRUCTURE OF METALS IN PULSED LASER IRRADIATION*

P. S. PEERCY
Sandia National Laboratories, Albuquerque, New Mexico 87185

Key Words: pulsed melting, phase formation, ion implantation, electron microscopy

1. INTRODUCTION

As emphasized by many of the contributions to this volume, there is an important and growing technology in laser processing of metals. The more developed aspects of this technology include applications such as cutting, machining, welding, surface hardening, surface alloying, etc. These applications use primarily high-power cw lasers. In contrast, the technology for pulsed laser-metal interactions for laser pulse widths in the nanosecond or shorter time regime is not as well developed; however, studies in this time regime are providing important insight into the processes that control metastable and amorphous phase formation of importance for certain applications. Selected activities in this area will be reviewed in the present paper. When appropriate, systems produced by pulsed surface melting will be compared to related systems produced by ion implantation.

Because the experimental approach used for pulsed laser-metal studies is similar to that for the better known laser annealing of semiconductors, it is instructive to compare the two cases. Important differences between laser irradiation of metals and semiconductors are summarized in Table 1. The most obvious difference is the absorption depth. For most cases of interest semiconductors have absorption depths typically >1 μm, whereas absorption depths for metals are typically one to two orders of magnitude smaller. (There are exceptions for both cases; for example, for semiconductors in the near uv the absorption depth is ≃0.1 μm.) In addition, the thermal conductivity κ is typically an order of magnitude greater for metals than for semiconductors. The consequence of these differences is much faster quench rates leading to faster resolidification velocities in metals than in semiconductors (1). These differences, combined with materials differences such as higher thermal expansion and lower yield stresses for metals than for semiconductors, lead to totally different behavior for epitaxially solidified material under pulsed laser irradiation: For silicon the process commonly referred to as laser annealing can result in defect removal, whereas for metals, in all cases reported to date, laser irradiation of defect-free metals introduces defects. Indeed, defects introduced by the rapid solidification process can improve the strength and toughness of metals (2).

* This work was performed at Sandia National Laboratories supported by the U.S. Department of Energy under contract number DE-AC04-76DP00789.

Draper, C.W. and Mazzoldi, P. (eds.), Laser Surface Treatment of Metals. ISBN 90-247-3405-3.

The well-controlled geometry obtained in surface melting permits detailed theoretical modeling of the melt and solidification process. As a result, studies of surface melting using pulsed lasers are providing fundamental understanding of the dominant mechanisms of importance to rapid solidification. Examples of such studies that will be discussed include the kinetics of metastable phase formation, the formation of amorphous phases in metals and precipitate nucleation and growth on very short time scales.

The microstructures and expected materials properties obtained after pulsed laser irradiation have been classified according to the behavior in the melt by various authors (3). For continuity, we will use the same classification.

(a) Simple single-phase liquid: This system refers to a pure elemental metal which exhibits only a single phase that is stable up to the melting temperature; it is the simplest system which can be considered. A more complex variant of a single phase, elemental metal is one which can undergo one or more crystallographic transformations between room temperature and the melting temperature. Studies of such allotropic systems can provide information on nucleation kinetics (4).

(b) Miscible two-component metals: In increasing order of complexity, the next system is a two-component alloy in which the alloying element is fully soluble in the host liquid. If the system is also fully soluble in the solid phase, the resulting structure is the equilibrium structure that would be obtained by conventional solidification techniques. If the alloy addition is only partially soluble in the solid phase, supersaturated solid solutions and metastable phases can result.

(c) Immiscible mixtures in the liquid: Intermetallic compositions can be prepared, for example, by ion implantation, which are immiscible in the liquid phase. Such compositions can result in either equilibrium or metastable phases after surface melting with a laser pulse. Under certain conditions phase separation without precipitation can occur in the liquid. In that case, the composition after pulsed surface melting will differ from the as-implanted composition.

(d) Amorphous phases: It is well known that amorphous or glassy metals can be produced if appropriate intermetallic compositions are rapidly quenched from the liquid phase. Detailed discussions of the thermodynamic and kinetic conditions necessary for the production of amorphous metals under rapid solidification conditions are presented in the paper by Spaepen (5) elsewhere in this Proceedings.

In the present paper, studies on Al-based alloys will be emphasized. More work has been performed under ultrarapid surface melt and solidification in Al than in any other metal system. In addition, Al is a model system and the results are representative of those for similar metals; it is also of interest as a major constituent for a family of rapidly solidified alloys with high strength-to-weight ratios.

2. DISCUSSION

2.1. Pure metals

Numerous studies of pulsed irradiation of pure metals have been performed by various groups (6-9). In those studies it was observed that, unless the implant damage is very severe, the defect level is always increased by pulsed surface melting; i.e., pulsed irradiation of metals introduces rather than removes defects. This different behavior for metals compared to semiconductors occurs because of the higher thermal expansion and lower yield stress of metals than for semiconductors. The nature and origin of those defects can be illustrated by results for pure Al.

TABLE 1. Order of magnitude comparison of materials parameters important for laser-surface interactions in metals and semiconductors. Laser-dependent parameters refer to 25 · nsec pulsed ruby laser.

Parameter	Semiconductors	Metals
Absorption depth α^{-1} (λ = 0.69 μm)	≃1 μm	≃0.02 μm
Thermal conductivity	≃0.2 W/cm^{2}K	≃2 W/cm^{2}K
Thermal gradient (25 nsec pulse)	≃10^8 K/sec	≃10^{10} K/sec
Solidification velocity	2-3 m/sec	7-15 m/sec
Thermal expansion	≃2 x 10^{-6}/°K	25 x 10^{-6}/°K

If the energy absorbed by the sample from the laser beam is measured calorimetrically (10), the melt threshold energy density E_m can be readily determined. Results of such calorimetric measurements are shown in Fig. 1 for irradiation with a 25 nsec pulse at λ = 0.694 μm. The points are the temperature increase of a thin (≃0.25 mm) sample measured by a small thermocouple attached to the back of the sample. To illustrate the use of this technique to determine the melt threshold energy density, the temperature increase of Al is compared to similar measurements for Si. For Si, the temperature increases linearly with energy density up to ≃0.8 J/cm^2; at higher energy densities, the temperature continues to increase with energy density but with a lower slope. The interpretation of these data is that the slope of the curve at low energy is proportional to the absorption coefficient A_s in the solid phase ($A_s = 1 - R_s$, where R_s is the reflectivity) while the slope at higher energy is proportional to the absorption coefficient A in the liquid phase. For Si, the reflectivity of the molten phase is greater than that of the solid phase. The curvature near E_m is a consequence of the fact that for a 25 nsec pulse the rate of energy loss due to thermal diffusion of heat out of the near-surface region is comparable to the rate of energy input into this region from the laser pulse.

The situation is reversed for Al. The slopes of the temperature versus incident energy density curve are constant in both the solid and liquid phases. Their relative magnitudes, however, are reversed compared to Si because the reflectivity of crystalline Al is greater than that of molten Al. The break in the curve thus identifies E_m as 3.5 J/cm^2. The discontinuity at E_m is a consequence of the high thermal conductivity of Al (10).

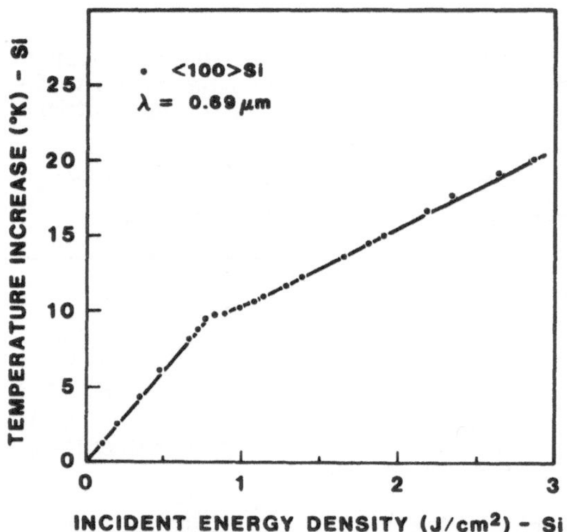

FIGURE 1. (a) Measured temperature increase versus incident laser energy density for Si compared to numerical calculations. The break near 0.8 J/cm^2 is identified as the melt threshold.

As noted above, no effects are observed for pulsed laser irradiation of semiconductors for $E < E_m$. That is not the case for metals, as can be seen from the data (11) for Al shown in Fig. 2. Aligned and random backscattering spectra are shown in Fig. 2a for 2 MeV He incident on <110> Al. Aligned spectra are shown for various energy densities below and above the melt threshold energy density $E_m = 3.5$ J/cm^2. That defects are introduced at incident energy densities below E_m is evident from the increase in dechanneling for energy densities below E_m. The large change in the spectra at energy densities between 3.45 J/cm^2 and 3.5 J/cm^2 is a consequence of melting at the higher energy.

These data can be summarized by plotting the ratio of the channeling yield after laser irradiation to the channeling yield for the virgin sample as a function of incident energy density. The difference in the backscattered yield for depths near the surface for aligned spectra versus incident energy density is shown in Fig. 2b. The channeling yield begins to increase at $E \simeq 0.8$ J/cm^2; this increase continues for E up to E_m, at which point it undergoes a discontinuous jump. These data can be understood as follows: The deposited energy heats the near-surface region of the sample and produces thermal expansion in this region (11). For sufficient thermally-induced strain, the induced stress exceeds the yield stress of Al and the heated region undergoes plastic deformation by slip. Detailed calculations (12) predict that the yield stress would be exceeded at $E_i > 0.7$ J/cm^2, in reasonable agreement with the observations. The plastic strain increases with increasing E; however, for $E < E_m$, much of the strain is removed by stress in the

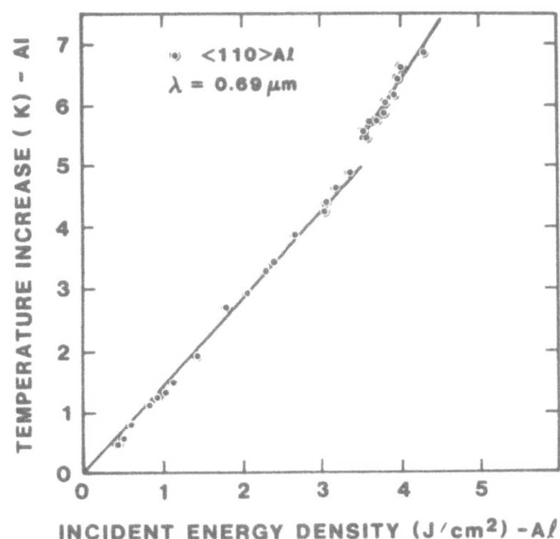

FIGURE 1. (b) Measured temperature increase versus incident laser energy density for electropolished Al compared with numerical calculations assuming the absorption coefficients in the solid and liquid phases of $A_s = 0.104$ and $A_l = 0.13$, respectively. The break near 3.5 J/cm^2 is identified as the melt threshold (Ref. 10).

opposite direction as the sample cools. Apparently motion along the same slip planes relieves much of the stress as long as the surface has not melted, and the discontinuity at E_m occurs because memory of the original slip is lost when the region melts. Thus the total stress must be relieved by new slip, and that process results in the observed discontinuity.

Direct evidence for slip is shown by the SEM micrographs at various magnifications in Fig. 3. For $E < E_m$, the slip lines are relatively faint. Careful examination of the data reveals that the major slip is along the {111} slip planes, as would be expected from the thermal model discussed above. The difference in slip for $E < E_m$ and $E > E_m$ is quite pronounced, as can be seen by comparing the first and second columns in Figure 3. The data in the left column are for $E = 2.9$ J/cm^2, which is less than E_m. The data in the right column are for 3.5 J/cm^2, where channeling indicates maximum disorder. The increase in slip at $E \geq E_m$ is readily evident. The appearance of the surface also demonstrates that melting occurred.

For completeness we note that, in addition to slip, surface melting of Al with a pulsed laser or e-beam quenches in vacancies, which coalesce into loops upon cooling (6,9).

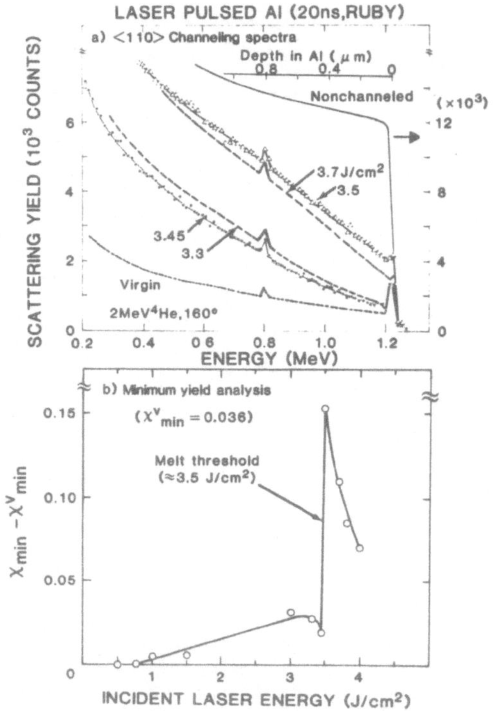

FIGURE 2. Channeling results for laser-irradiated Al for various incident energy densities. (a) 2 MeV ^{4}He backscattering spectra. (b) Increase in minimum yield (at ~1.2 MeV) above that of virgin Al as a function of incident laser energy density (Ref. 11).

2.2. Miscible two-component systems

2.2.1. Miscibility in both the liquid and solid phases. The next level of complexity is represented by two-component systems which are miscible in the liquid phase. Numerous pulsed surface melting studies have been performed in such systems. In general, for this case the solute undergoes simple diffusional motion in the melt. If the solute is also fully soluble in the solid at the concentrations under study, the system solidifies into its equilibrium state. Such systems are typified by Zn in Al (6).

Under the very rapid heating produced by a Q-switched laser, there is evidence that, in addition to normal diffusion, the Soret effect - i.e., the relative atomic motion of two species induced by a temperature gradient - is important (13). Analysis of the atomic motion including this effect provides a qualitatively and quantitatively better fit to the data than do fits including normal diffusion only. For a detailed discussion of diffusion phenomena, including the Soret effect, the reader is referred to the article by Dona dalle Rose elsewhere in this volume (14).

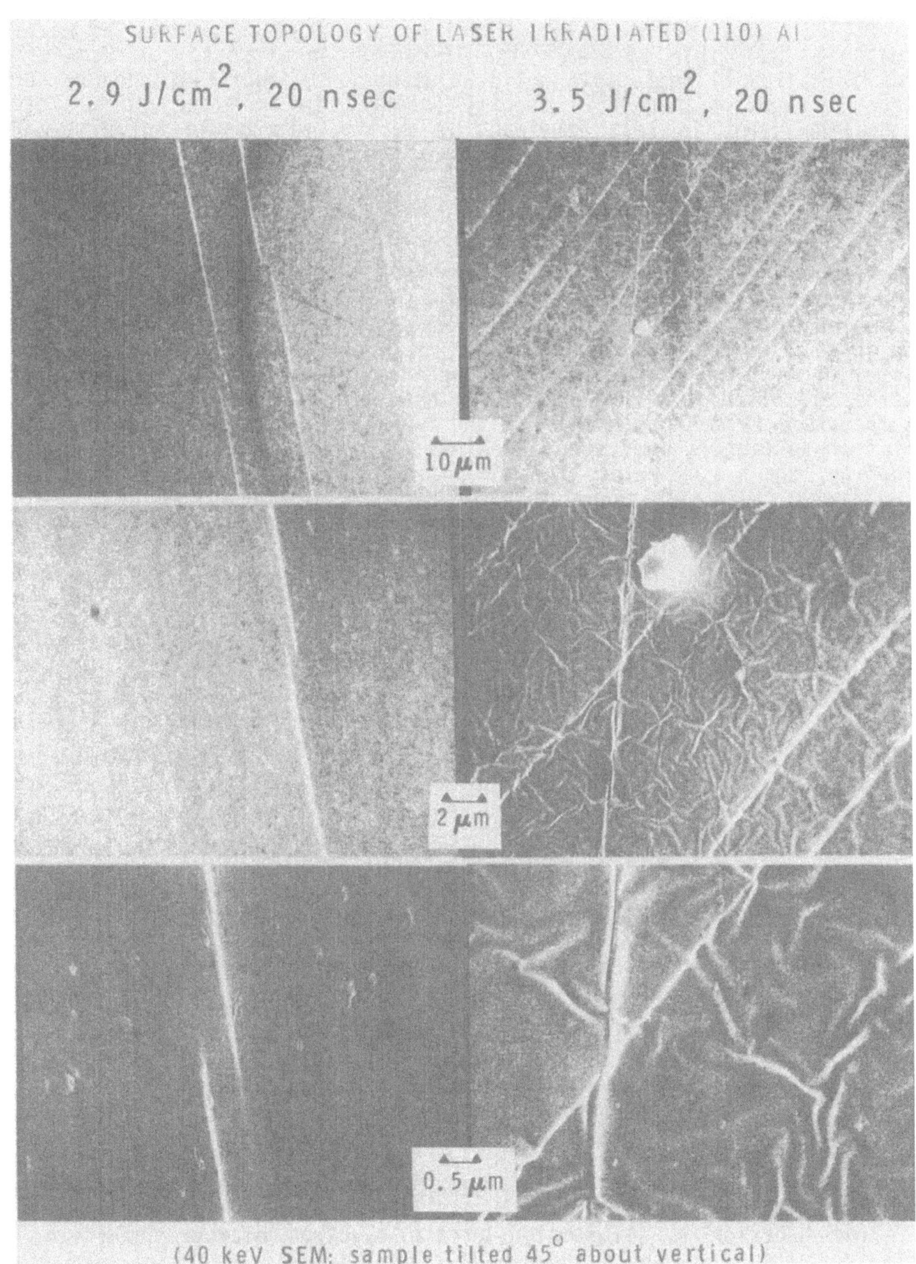

FIGURE 3. SEM Micrographs of laser-irradiated Al for (a) 2.9 J/cm^2 and (b) 3.5 J/cm^2 incident laser energy densities, illustrating slip in the irradiated region below and above the melt threshold energy density (Ref. 11).

2.2.2. Immiscibility in the solid phase. Surface melting of metals that are immiscible in either the liquid or solid phase can result in the formation of metastable solid solutions. In addition, because surface segregation, which is readily observed in Si after pulsed laser annealing (15), is less important in metals, metastable solutions are readily formed. These topics are discussed by Battaglin et al. (16) elsewhere in this volume.

2.3. Immiscible systems

2.3.1. Solid phase precipitation. Phase separation, including precipitate nucleation and growth in the melt, can occur following surface melting of alloys that are immiscible in the melt. One of the cleaner examples of a system that exhibits insolubility in the liquid phase is Sb in Al. The Al-rich region of the phase diagram for the Al(Sb) system is shown in Fig. 4. For an Sb concentration of 2 at.%, melting with either a pulsed laser or e-beam can heat the liquid to ~2000°C. This temperature is well above that of the two-phase regime where the equilibrium phase diagram indicates a mixture of liquid Al and solid AlSb. On cooling, the system enters the two-phase regime at ~750 K; if the system spends sufficient time in this regime for AlSb to nucleate, AlSb precipitates will grow and be frozen into random orientations as the Al solidifies (17).

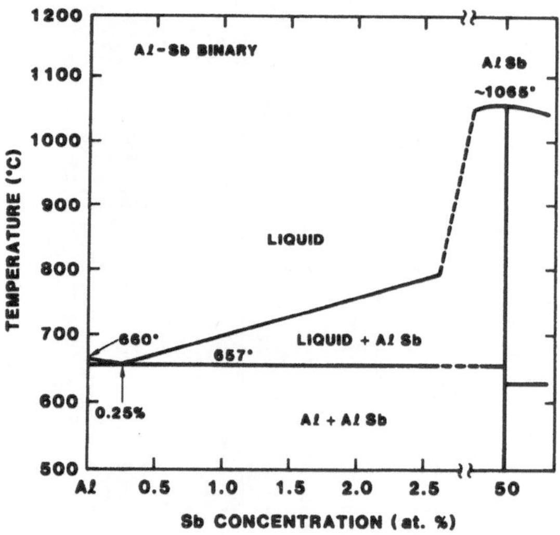

FIGURE 4. Al-rich region of the binary Al-Sb phase diagram.

This behavior is illustrated by the electron micrographs shown in Fig. 5. The four panels show diffraction patterns after ion implantation, after furnace annealing, after melting with a 50 nsec pulse of electrons, and after melting with a 3.7 J/cm^2 pulse from a ruby laser. After implantation, only diffraction spots from the Al matrix are observed. After furnace annealing, extra spots, produced by coherent,

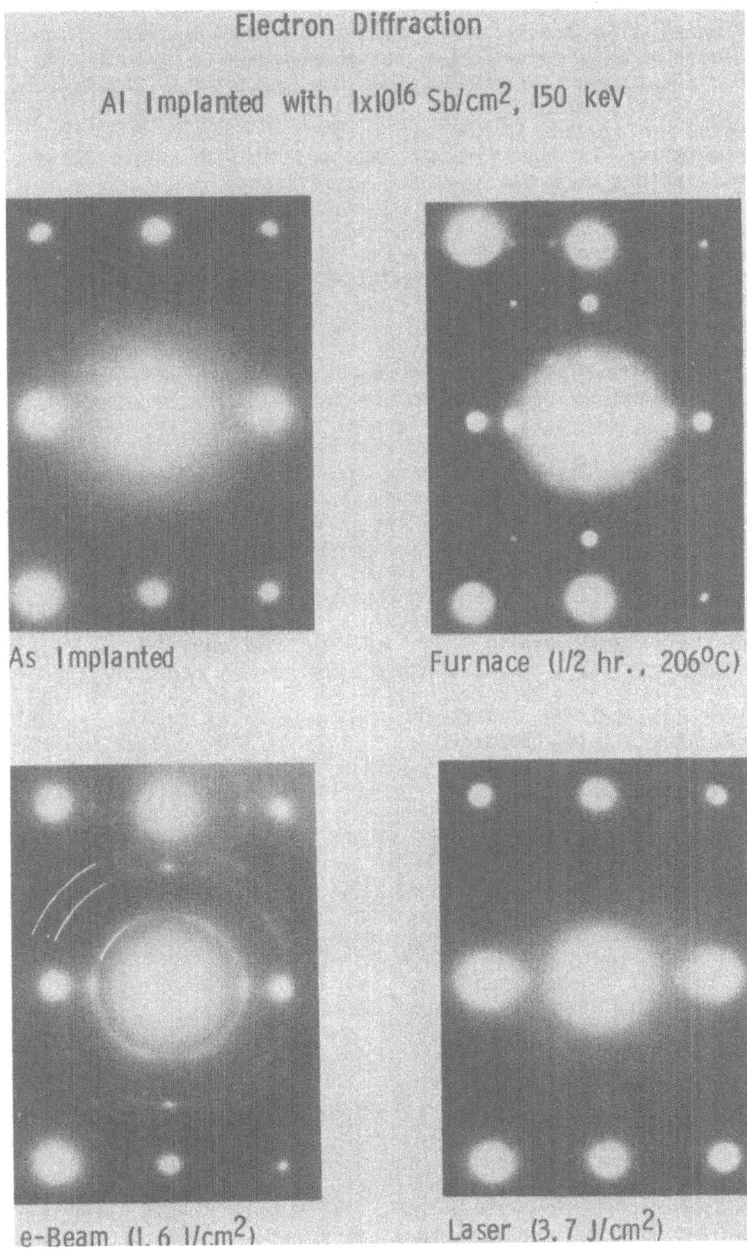

FIGURE 5. <112> TEM diffraction patterns of Sb-implanted Al: (a) as implanted, (b) furnace annealed, (c) melted with an electron beam pulse, and (d) melted with a laser pulse Ref. 17).

oriented AlSb precipitates in the Al lattice, are observed. After the 50 nsec e-beam pulse, ring patterns produced by randomly oriented AlSb precipitates are observed. The ring patterns indicate (17,18) that AlSb precipitates nucleated and grew while the system was in the two-phase region of molten Al and solid AlSb. Because there was no preferred orientation in the liquid, the precipitates were frozen into random orientations when the aluminum solidified.

For surface melting with a 20 nsec laser pulse, however, no precipitates were observed. This result was taken as evidence that the system was not in the two-phase region sufficiently long for the precipitates to nucleate, since the precipitates are expected to grow to easily observable dimensions in <10 nsec after nucleation. Precipitate nucleation times can thus be measured in molten metals in the nsec time regime by increasing the melt duration. Increased melt durations were achieved by laser irradiation at elevated substrate temperatures, which decrease the temperature gradient and therefore the regrowth velocity. TEM and dark field micrographs are shown in Fig. 6 for surface melting at substrate temperatures, T_s, of 100 to 200°C (17).

As in the case of the data of Fig. 5, no randomly oriented precipitates were observed for irradiation at 20°C; however, randomly oriented precipitates are observed for irradiation at $T_s \geq 100$°C. The dark field micrographs indicate precipitates up to 10 nm in size after melting at $T_s = 100$°C and up to 40 nm in size for $T_s = 200$°C.

Nucleation times are estimated for these data by calculating the time-temperature history of the melt. Calculated temperature histories for substrate temperatures T_s of 25, 100 and 200°C indicate that the system was in the two-phase region on cooling for 19 nsec for $T_s = 25$°C, 30 nsec for $T_s = 100$°C and 55 nsec for $T_s = 200$°C. These calculations therefore yield estimates of the nucleation time for AlSb precipitate formation of ~15 + 10 nsec. Such studies thus permit measurements of precipitate nucleation times in the previously inaccessible nsec time regime. Furthermore, the technique can be readily extended to other systems (19).

2.3.2. Liquid phase separation. In some immiscible systems the impurity metal is hardly soluble in the molten phase of the host metal. In this case, pulsed surface melting can lead to separation of the alloy into its nearly pure constituent elements. An example is the Ni(Ag) system in which the melt separates into a Ag-rich region within the Ni-rich host liquid phase, since the miscibility of Ag in Ni is only 6 at.% (at 1437°C). Measurements for <110> Ni implanted with 1×10^{17} Ag/cm^2 to produce a 12 at.% alloy layer are shown in Fig. 7 (20). After irradiation with a Q-switched Nd:YAG laser, the peak concentration decreased to 7 at.%. The effect of the miscibility gap is evident in that, after implantation, the Ag was 80% substitutional, whereas, after subsequent laser irradiation, the substitutionality was reduced to ~50%. TEM measurements revealed Ag dendrites >100 nm in length, which further indicated that phase separation occurred in the liquid (21).

Similar results were observed by Hirvonen et al. (22) in pulsed electron irradiation of Ta in Cu. The Ta was highly substitutional as implanted, but the substitutionality decreased significantly after surface melting by pulsed electron beam irradiation.

2.4. Amorphous metals

For most metals amorphous phase formation requires the addition of alloying components - either metalloids such as B or P, or another metal.

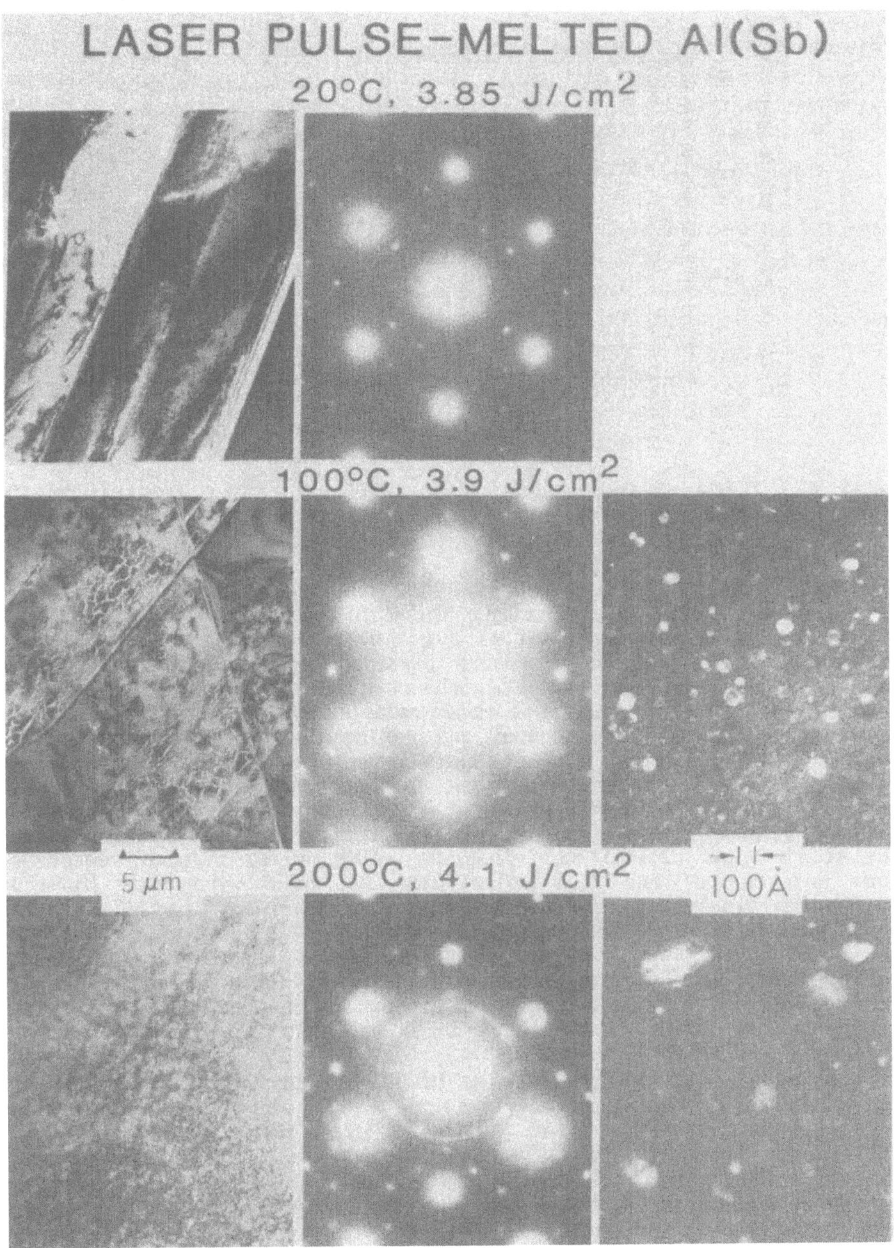

FIGURE 6. Electron diffraction and dark field images of AlSb precipitates in Sb-implanted Al, after melting with a 25 nsec laser pulse, for substrate temperatures of 20, 100 and 200°C (Ref. 17).

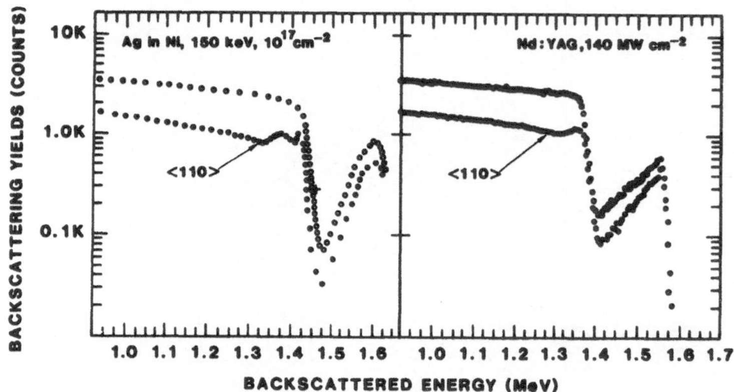

FIGURE 7. <110> channeled and random backscattering spectra for Ni implanted with 1 x 10^{17} Ag/cm^2 at 150 keV before (a) and after (b) melting with a pulsed laser (Ref. 20).

Exceptions are metals which can be found in two or more crystal structures, some of them metastable, at a given temperature; for example, Ga has been produced in the amorphous phase at very low temperatures by both ion bombardment (23) and laser quenching (24).

The Al(Ni) system provides a model metal-metal system for the study of grain refinement and amorphous phase formation, and this system has been studied in detail by both surface melting and ion implantation (25-28). The Ni-rich region of the Al-Ni phase diagram is shown in Fig. 8 (29). Ni has very low (< 0.02 at%) solubility in Al, and the equilibrium phase diagram exhibits a eutectic at 2.7 at% Ni and peritectics at 15.3 and 27 at.% Ni. Thus, as molten Al-Ni with Ni concentrations between 2.7 and 15.3 solidifies, Al and Al_3Ni phases form at equilibrium, whereas for Ni concentrations between 15.3 and 27 at.% the Al_3Ni and Al_3Ni_2 phases are obtained under equilibrium solidification conditions. As will be discussed below, both the Al_3Ni and Al_3Ni_2 phases are suppressed under ultra-rapid solidification conditions. This is attributed to suppression of the nucleation of these rather complex phases in the short time available following pulsed surface melting (28).

In pulsed e-beam melting studies of Ni-implanted Al, Picraux et al. (25) observed epitaxial solidification of fcc Al with supersaturated concentrations of Ni for up to 3 at.% implanted Ni. For higher Ni concentrations, epitaxial solidification breaks down and polycrystalline solidification occurs. Microstructures observed after pulsed surface melting of Al containing 8, 10 and 12 at.% Ni are shown in Fig. 9 (26). Energy densities were chosen to give melt durations of ~12 μsec and solidification velocities of ~7 m/sec. The resulting microstructures are summarized in the bottom panel of the figure and discussed in detail below.

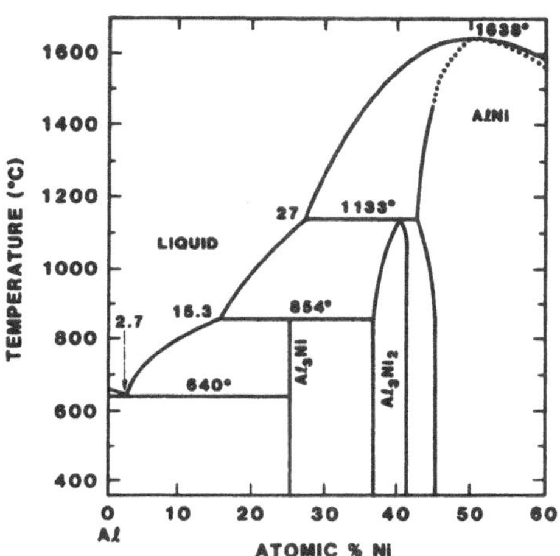

FIGURE 8. Al-rich region of the AlNi phase diagram (Ref. 29).

The polycrystalline nature of the rapidly solidified material is evident from the electron diffraction patterns (upper panels). The microstructures, shown in the dark field images in the center panels, reveal that epitaxial solidificaton is lost for >9 at.% Ni and a high degree of grain refinement occurs. The crystallite dimensions are between 2 and 10 nm for 10 at.% and between 1 and 5 nm for 12 at.% Ni. Such grain refinement has important implications for applications of materials prepared by rapid solidification processing. Most metallurgical modifications to increase hardness are found to decrease ductility and vice versa; however, grain refinement can increase both hardness and ductility (2).

It is natural to ask what occurs for material containing higher Ni concentrations solidified under similar conditions. Studies (30) of samples containing 30 at.% Ni and subjected to similar melt and solidification histories demonstrate that amorphous AlNi forms under these conditions. For this concentration, AlNi precipitates were also observed; however, neither the Al_3Ni nor the Al_3Ni_2 crystalline phase was observed. These phases have rather complex structures with several atoms per unit cell. As noted above, nucleation is expected to be slow under these conditions; indeed, such measurements permitted the nucleation time for these phases to be estimated to be >1000 nsec (28). In addition, for complex crystal structures the growth velocity can be very low if the solidification rate is diffusion limited. Under such conditions, metastable or amorphous phase formation is expected, as discussed by Spaepen elsewhere in this volume (5).

It is instructive to compare the structures obtained by surface melting with those obtained by other techniques which provide rapid quench rates. Ion implantation, which is expected to give "effective quench

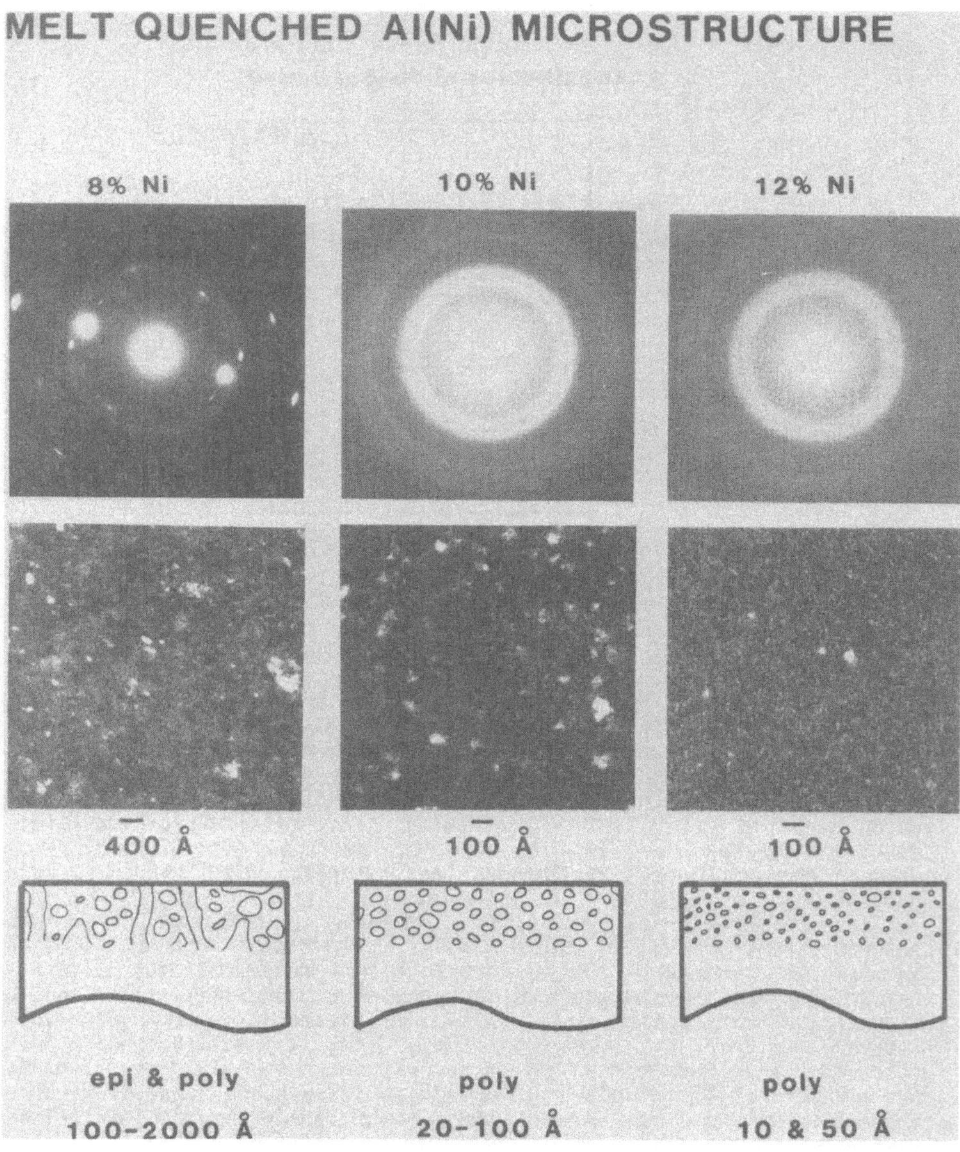

FIGURE 9. TEM results for uniform (left to right) 8, 10 and 12 at.% Ni concentrations in Al after pulsed surface melting under identical conditions. The upper panels show the electron diffraction patterns, the center panels the dark field images of polycrystalline fcc Al grains, and the lower panels schematic cross sections for the melt-quenched layers (Ref. 26).

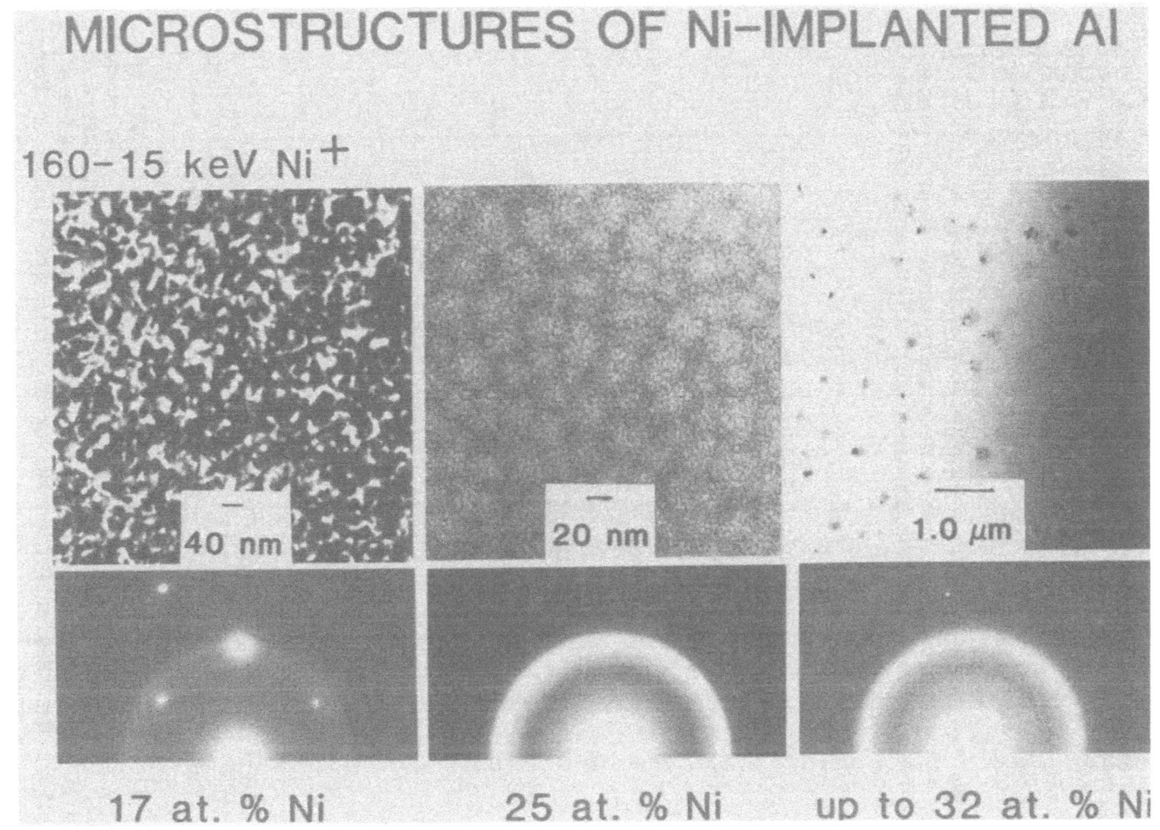

FIGURE 10. TEM micrographs of Al implanted with 17, 25 and 32 at.% Ni. The lower panels show the electron diffraction patterns and the upper panels the dark field images (Ref. 30).

rates" of $>10^{13}$ K/sec, has been studied in the same system. These studies demonstrate that amorphous AlNi can be produced by implanting either Ni into Al (27) or Al into Ni (26). TEM micrographs, taken from the work of Follstaedt and Romig (30), to illustrate the formation of the amorphous phase by ion implantation of Ni into Al, are shown in Fig. 10. The amorphous nature of the implanted material is evident from the broad diffraction rings. A dark field image of the amorphous material, which shows a slight texture, is presented in Fig. 11b. As in the case of rapid solidification, crystalline Al_3Ni and Al_3Ni_2 phases were not observed in the implantation-produced amorphous material. At higher implanted Ni concentrations, however, cubic AlNi precipitates were observed. Measurements of the Ni concentration in the AlNi precipitates produced by ion implantation permitted quantitative values to be obtained for the concentrations in the metastable phase diagram proposed from the earlier surface melting studies (26). This metastable phase diagram is shown in Fig. 11 (30).

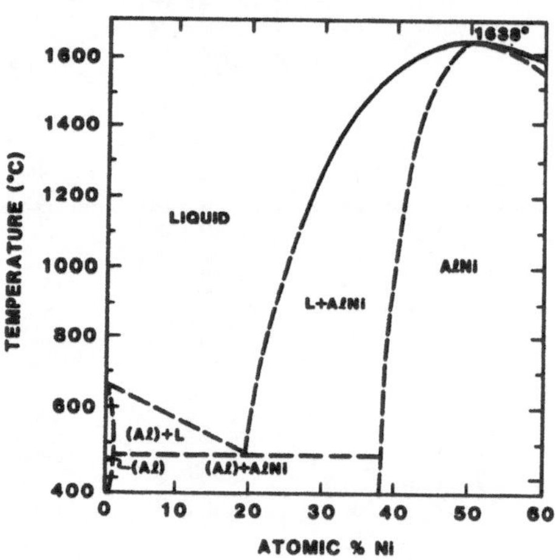

FIGURE 11. Metastable phase diagram for the Al-Ni system, deduced from the ion implantation and pulsed surface-melting studies (Ref. 30).

Since similar suppression of the complex intermetallic Al_3Ni and Al_3Ni_2 phases is observed for all rapid quenching conditions examined to date, this metastable phase diagram appears to be applicable to both surface melting and ion implantation. It is also expected to apply for Al-Ni alloys quenched sufficiently rapidly from the liquid or from the vapor phase by other techniques.

2.5. Melting of allotropic systems: Mn

To date, the vast majority of studies of metastable phase formation using pulsed surface melting have been confined to the formation of supersaturated solutions of the substrate crystal structure or to the formation of thin amorphous layers. In general, supersaturated solutions are observed for host crystals with a simple structure, whereas, with the exception of Ga at very low temperatures, formation of amorphous metallic phases has required alloying of two or more elements. As noted above, the solidification velocity of intermetallic compounds with complex crystal structures can be very slow if the interfacial velocity is diffusion limited. Surface melting in such systems can lead to large undercooling and amorphous phase formation. On the other hand, the simple crystal structures typically encountered in elemental metals at high temperatures are expected to have collision-controlled growth rates. For these metals, the liquid-solid interface is limited by the speed of sound, and the interfacial undercooling is expected to be small for moderate solidificaion velocities. Under these conditions, large interfacial undercoolings cannot be achieved by surface melting.

For a detailed understanding of the effects of interfacial undercooling on the kinetics that control metastable phase formation, pulsed laser melting of Mn was investigated (4). At room temperature, the equilibrium phase of Mn is α; upon heating under equilibrium conditions, Mn undergoes allotropic transformations to the β, γ and δ phases before melting at the equilibrium melting temperature of 1315°C. The calculated free energy differences, relative to the free energy of the melt, along with the equilibrium melting temperatures of the various allotropic phases of Mn, are shown in Fig. 12. Since the curves are plotted

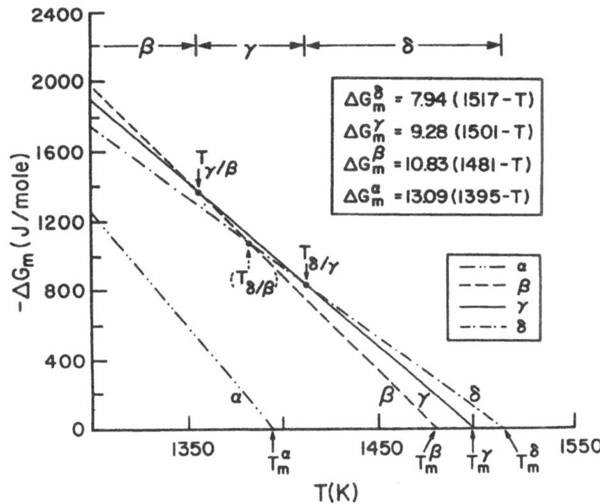

FIGURE 12. Calculated free energy differences, relative to liquid Mn, for the four allotropic phases of Mn. Melting points (T_m^i) and solid phase transformation temperatures ($T_{i/j}$) are indicated; the equilibrium phases are indicated at the top (Ref. 4).

relative to the free energy of the melt, the uppermost curve at any temperature represents the equilibrium phase at that temperature. The solid-state phase transformation temperatures, $T_{i/j}$ from phase i to j and the calculated melting temperatures T_m^j of phase j are given in Table 2.

Under the rapid heating rates available with pulsed laser irradiation, it is possible to kinetically suppress the allotropic transformations to the higher temperature phases (4). Thus laser-induced surface melting of a Mn substrate initially in the α-phase can bypass the β, γ and δ phases to produce a melt at the α-phase melting temperature, which is calculated to be 122°K below the melting temperature of the δ phase. This procedure can therefore yield highly undercooled melts in pure metals. In addition, preparation of substrates in the β-phase by furnace annealing to 900°C and quenching to room temperture at quench rate $dT/dt > 10^4$ K/sec can be used to produce substrates that yield melts at T_m^β to permit this undercooling to be varied.

TABLE 2. Thermodynamic characteristics of Mn allotropes

Allotrope (Structure)	Stability Range (K)	T_m(K)	$T_{i/\alpha}$ (K)	G_m^i(J/mole)	$V_m(m^3/mole) \times 10^6$
α(A12)	0-980	1395*		13.09(1395-T)	7.35+
β(A13)	980-1360	1481*	980	10.83(1481-T)	8.32+
γ(A1)	1360-1410	1501*	1137§	9.28(1501-T)	8.67#
δ(A2)	1410-1517	1517	1209§	7.94(1517-T)	8.79**

* Calculated metastable melting point.

§ Calculated metastable transition temperature.

+ at 300°K; # at 1373°K; ** at 1398°K.

For the case of surface melting of α-Mn, the liquid-solid interface is undercooled by 122 K with respect to the melting point of the phase at the time that the melt front reaches the maximum melt depth. It is also undercooled 106 and 86 K relative to the melting temperature of the γ and β phases, respectively. When the liquid-solid interface starts to return to the surface as the Mn solidifies in the α-phase, this undercooling will increase according to the velocity-undercooling relationship for the α-phase. Because of the complex structure of the α-phase, the solidification velocity might be diffusion controlled; in this case, the additional increase in the undercooling could be significant. These conditions are ideal for the nucleation and growth of other phases in competition with epitaxial solidification of the α-Mn structure. The concept behind the experiments is thus to melt Mn in the α structure and determine if epitaxial solidification of this complex structure occurs, or if the simpler γ and δ phases (fcc and bcc, respectively) form. According to the arguments advanced above in the discussion of the Al-Ni system, nucleation of a cubic structure is expected for sufficient melt durations.

The crystal structures that nucleate after surface melting with a 25 nsec pulse from a ruby laser were determined by electron diffraction. Data for irradiation of α-Mn substrates are shown in Fig. 13 (4). The diffraction pattern on the left shows the α-Mn phase that was retained after irradiation at an energy density of 0.77 J/cm^2, very near the melt threshold energy density (~0.80 J/cm^2). Numerical simulations of the surface temperature during the laser pulse indicated that the temperature in the irradiated region exceeded the transformation temperatures of the β, γ and δ phases. Observation of the α-Mn phase after this irradiation thus suggests that these allotropic transitions can indeed be suppressed kinetically.

At higher incident energy densities, surface melting occurs. The diffraction pattern in the right panel of Fig. 13 was observed after irradiation at 1.16 J/cm^2 to produce a calculated melt duration at the surface of ~45 nsec. Examination of the diffraction patterns reveals that the γ phase nucleates under these conditions. The calculated free energies shown in Fig. 12 indicate that, even though the phase is not the most supercooled phase, it is the phase with the lowest free energy at the melting temperature of the α-phase. While the free energy is important in determining which phases are energetically permitted to form, it is not the sole criterion for determining which phases actually nucleate. It is anticipated that detailed nucleation kinetics, rather than the free energies, are the determining factor in the formation of metastable phases under rapid solidification conditions.

These are preliminary results from the first such studies and illustrate the power of this technique for study of the relative importance of nucleation kinetics and solidificaiton dynamics. Extension of these measurements to the β-Mn system may permit quantitative evaluation of the relative importance of free energies and undercooling in determining nucleation kinetics.

3. SUMMARY

In summary, surface melting of metals by pulsed laser irradiation can lead to the formation of a wide variety of metastable crystalline and amorphous alloys. The phases and microstructures that result are determined by a complex interplay between the thermodynamic driving forces and the nucleation and growth kinetics. Nevertheless, many of the resulting structures can be classified according to the behavior in the melt; for example, supersaturated solutions can be formed if the alloying addition is fully soluble in the liquid but not in the solid. For systems that form compounds in the liquid phase, pulsed melting can be used to measure nucleation times in the nanosecond time regime in molten metals. This technique was illustrated by measurements in the Al-Sb system. On the other hand, if the nucleation of complex intermetallic phases can be suppressed in the melt, metastable and amorphous phases can result. This process was examined in detail in the Al-Ni system. In related studies of solidification kinetics, the undercooling of the melt with respect to stable phases was examined by rapidly heating Mn to bypass the high-temperature allotropes. These measurements were used to determine ease of nucleation for various phases and to estimate nucleation times in highly undercooled melts.

Laser Pulse-Melted α-Mn

0.77 J/cm², 30 nsec
(near melt threshold)
Retains α-Mn

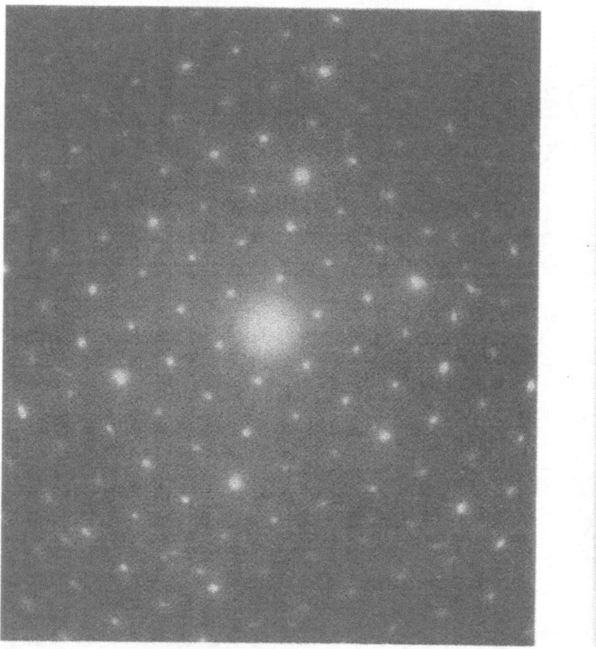

1.16 J/cm², 30 nsec
(above melt threshold)
Quenches γ-Mn

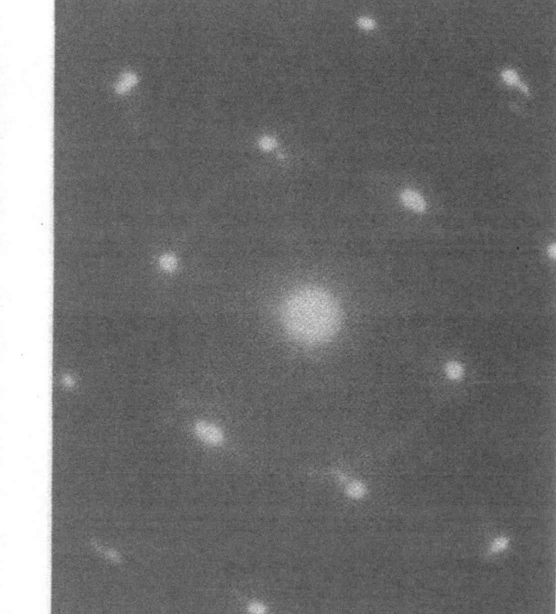

FIGURE 13. TEM electron diffraction patterns from laser-irradiated α-Mn. (a) <111> zone pattern of α-Mn obtained after irradiation with a 0.77 J/cm^2 laser pulse. (b) <110> zone pattern of γ-Mn after irradiation with a 1.16 J/cm^2 laser pulse. A (111) ring at $d = 0.22$ nm is superimposed (Ref. 4).

REFERENCES

1. See, e.g., N. Bloembergen, in Laser-Solid Interactions and Laser Processing, edited by S. D. Ferris, H. J. Leamy, and J. M. Poate, AIP Conference Proceedings No. 50 (AIP, New York, 1979), p. 1.
2. See, e.g., "Amorphous and Metastable Microcrystalline Rapidly Solidified Alloys," National Materials Advisory Board, Publication NMAB-358 (National Academy of Sciences, Washington, DC, 1980), p. 119.
3. See, e.g., D. M. Follstaedt, in Laser and Electron-Beam Interactions with Solids, edited by B. R. Appleton and G. K. Celler (Elsevier North Holland, New York, 1982), p. 377.
4. D. M. Follstaedt, P. S. Peercy, and J. H. Perepezko, Appl. Phys. Lett. (to be published).
5. Frans Spaepen, this volume.
6. L. Buene, J. M. Poate, D. C. Jacobson, C. W. Draper, and J. K. Hirvonen, Appl. Phys. Lett. 37, 385 (1980).
7. W. R. Wampler, D. M. Follstaedt, and P. S. Peercy, in Laser and Electron-Beam Solid Interactions and Materials Processing, edited by J. F. Gibbons, L. D. Hess, and T. W. Sigmon (Elsevier North Holland, New York, 1981), p. 567.
8. L. Buene, E. N. Kaufmann, C. M. Preece, and C. W. Draper, in Ref. 2, p. 591.
9. J. Narayan, in Ref. 3, p. 389.
10. P. S. Peercy and W. R. Wampler, Appl. Phys. Lett. 40, 768 (1982).
11. D. M. Follstaedt, S. T. Picraux, P. S. Peercy, and W. R. Wampler, Appl. Phys. Lett. 39, 27 (1981).
12. P. S. Peercy, unpublished.
13. A. Miotello and L. F. Dona dalle Rose, in Ref. 3, p. 425.
14. L. F. Dona dalle Rose, this volume.
15. See, e.g., C. W. White, B. R. Appleton, and S. R. Wilson, in Laser Annealing of Semiconductors, edited by J. M. Poate and J. W. Mayer (Academic Press, New York, 1982), Chap. 5.
16. G. Battaglin, A. Camera, G. Della Mea, V. Kulkami, P. Mazzoldi, D. K. Sood, and A. P. Pogarny, this volume.
17. P. S. Peercy, D. M. Follstaedt, S. T. Picraux, and W. R. Wampler, in Ref. 3, p. 401.
18. W. R. Wampler, D. M. Follstaedt, and S. T. Picraux, Appl. Phys. Lett. 36, 366 (1980).
19. D. M. Follstaedt, J. A. Knapp, and P. S. Peercy, J. Noncrystalline Solids 61, 62, 451 (1984).
20. C. W. Draper, in Lasers in Metallurgy, edited by K. Mukkorjee and J. Mazumder (TMS-AIME, Warrandale, PA, 1982).
21. L. Buene, D. C. Jacobson, S. Nakahara, J. M. Poate, C. W. Draper, and J. K. Hirvonen, in Ref. 6, p. 583.
22. J. K. Hirvonen, J. M. Poate, A. Greenwald, and R. Little, Appl. Phys. Lett. 36, 564 (1980).
23. M. Holz, P. Ziemann, and W. Buckel, Phys. Rev. Lett. 51, 1584 (1983).
24. J. Fröhlingsdorf and B. Stritzker, this volume.
25. S. T. Picraux, D. M. Follstaedt, J. A. Knapp, and E. Rimini, in Ref. 6, p. 575.
26. S. T. Picraux and D. M. Follstaedt, in Laser-Solid Interactions and Transient Thermal Processing of Materials, edited by J. Narayan, W. L. Brown, and R. A. Lemons (North Holland, New York, 1983), p. 751.

27. D. A. Potter, M. Ahmed, and S. Lamond, in Ion Implantation and Ion Beam Processing of Materials, edited by G. K. Hubler, C. R. Clayton, O. W. Holland, and C. W. White (North Holland, New York, 1984), p. 117.
28. D. M. Follstaedt, S. T. Picraux, P. S. Peercy, J. A. Knapp, and W. R. Wampler, in Mater. Res. Soc. Symp. Proc. 28, 273 (1984).
29. Metals Handbook, Vol. 8, edited by T. Lyman (ASM, Metals Park, Ohio, 1973), p. 262.
30. D. M. Follstaedt and A. D. Romig, Jr., Proc. 20th Annual Meeting of the Microbeam Analysis Society (Louisville, KY, 1985) (to be published).

THERMODYNAMICS AND KINETICS OF METALLIC ALLOY FORMATION BY PICOSECOND PULSED LASER IRRADIATION

FRANS SPAEPEN
Division of Applied Sciences, Harvard University, Cambridge, MA 02138

Key Words: picosecond melting, resolidification dynamics, glass formation

1. INTRODUCTION

Irradiating a metallic surface with a short laser pulse is a method for confining the deposition of thermal energy to a very thin surface layer, which melts and is subsequently quenched at a very high rate. This makes picosecond pulsed laser quenching the fastest melt quenching method available.

In the first part of the paper, the mechanism of heating and quenching in picosecond laser quenching is analyzed in some detail, and simple estimates are made of the basic quantities (cooling rate, melt lifetime, etc.). The possible effects of evaporation are also discussed, and shown to be negligible in this regime.

The second part of the paper deals with the thermodynamic restrictions on the type of transformations that can occur on the very short timescale of the laser quenching process. Which of these allowed transformations actually occurs is determined by the kinetics of the competing solidification processes. Depending on the degree of the structural rearrangement required to form a crystal from the melt, its growth can be collision- or diffusion-controlled. It will be shown that only the simplest crystal structures or dilute solutions exhibit collision-limited growth, which is fast enough not to be suppressed even by picosecond pulsed laser quenching.

In the last part of the paper, a brief review of the work at Harvard on alloy formation is given. The Fe-B system has been investigated most thoroughly, and phase formation (glass vs. crystal) in this system will be analyzed in some detail. Other alloy systems include: Ni-Nb, Mo-Ni, Co-Mo, Co-Nb, Cu-Ag, Cu-Co, and Nb-Si.

2. PICOSECOND LASER QUENCHING MECHANISM

The process of energy deposition, heating and cooling in pulsed laser irradiation of solid surfaces has been analyzed in detail by a number of authors (1,2). Figure 1 illustrates the three stages of the process, using parameters corresponding to the experiments described later.

In the first stage, which lasts for the duration of the pulse, the laser energy is deposited in a layer of thickness α^{-1} (α: absorption coefficient). For optical light metals, α^{-1} is on the order of a few tens of nanometers. Since the transfer of the energy from the electrons, which interact with the laser light, to the lattice occurs on a timescale of less than 1 ps, the process can be described as a thermal one (3). Over the duration of the pulse, t_p, the thermal diffusion length is $\ell_T = (2D_{th}t_p)^{1/2}$. In metals, ℓ_T lies between 25 and 70 nm, depending on the thermal diffusivity ($D_{th} = 10^{-4}$ to 10^{-5} m^2s^{-1}). Deposition of the absorbed laser energy as heat in a layer of thickness ℓ_T results in its melting and overheating to several thousand degress.

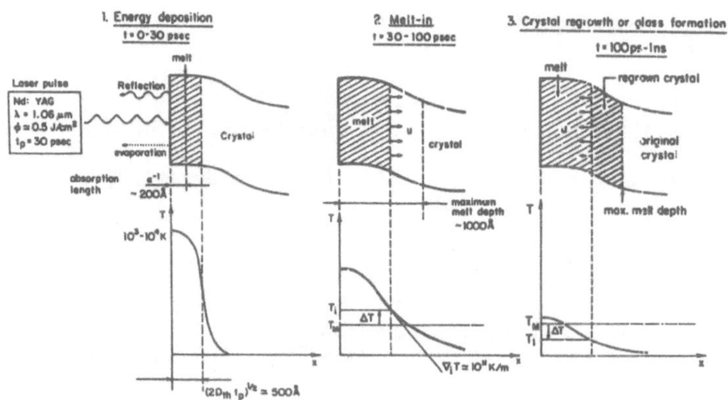

FIGURE 1. Schematic illustration of the mechanism of pulsed laser quenching.

It is worth noting that for pulse durations of less than 1 ps, ℓ_T becomes less than α^{-1}. In this regime, the thickness of the initial molten layer and the thermal gradients become independent of the pulse length. For this reason, femtosecond pulses, which are very useful for time-resolved probing of the irradiation process, do not produce higher quench rates than picosecond pulses. A general discussion of the ℓ_T vs. α^{-1} regimes is given by Bloembergen (1).

In the second stage, which starts at the end of the pulse, more of the underlying crystal is melted, until the overheat of the melt is spent. The crystal-melt interface moves away from the surface until its temperature drops to the equilibrium melting temperature. The maximum melt depth, d, for the conditions of Figure 1 (fluence $\sim$0.5 J cm^{-2}, reflectivity $\sim$0.1) is about 100 nm. Since the thermal gradients in this process are very high (10^{11} K m^{-1}), the melt-in velocity is also large (u $\sim 10^3$ m s^{-1}). The melt-in phase is therefore expected to last only d/u $\sim$100 ps.

In the third stage, the interface temperature falls below the equilibrium melting temperature, and the crystal-melt interface reverses direction. If the crystal regrowth process is fast enough, the entire melt is consumed. Otherwise, i.e., if the melt cools to its configurational freezing point before crystallizing, a glass is formed. The thermal parameters in this regrowth process have been analyzed by sophisticated numerical methods (especially for silicon), but their order of magnitude can easily be estimated from dimensional arguments. The temperature scale is determined by the melting temperature, T_m, which is on the order of 10^3 K. The length scale is set by the melt depth d $\sim 10^{-7}$ m. The average thermal gradient is then $\nabla T = T_m/d \sim 10^{10}$ K m^{-1}, and the corresponding cooling rate is $\dot{T} = D_{th}\, T/d \sim 10^{12}$ K s^{-1}. The lifetime of the melt, τ, is an important experimental parameter, which can be estimated as $\tau = T_m/\dot{T} = 10^{-9}$ s. This estimate is in agreement with transient reflectivity measurements, which show τ to be on the order of a few nanoseconds (4-6). In the analysis of crystal growth rate vs. heat removal, it is useful to know the velocity, u_T, with which isotherms move toward the surface during cooling. A simple linear estimate gives: $u_T = \dot{T}/\nabla T \sim 100\ m\ s^{-1}$.

These parameters are summarized in Table 1. For comparison, the parameters for conventional melt spinning are also listed. The main difference there is the greater thickness of the melt, which brings the cooling rate, $\dot{T} \sim d^{-2}$, down to $10^6\ K\ s^{-1}$.

TABLE 1. Thermal parameters in melt quenching (from ref. 2)

		Laser Quenching	Melt Spinning
Melt temperature	$T_m(K)$	10^3	10^3
Melt thickness	d(m)	10^{-7}	5×10^{-5}
Temperature gradient	$\nabla T(K/m)$	10^{10}	2×10^7
Cooling rate	$\dot{T}(K/s)$	10^{12}	4×10^6
Melt lifetime	$\tau(s)$	10^{-9}	not applicable
Isotherm velocity	$u_T(m/s)$	100	0.2
Heat-flow limited crystal growth velocity	$u_h(m/s)$	230	0.5

The rate of evaporation during laser quenching can be estimated from the kinetic theory of gases. The number of atoms leaving a unit surface per second, which is, in equilibrium, equal to the number arriving from the vapor at a pressure p, is given by $\Gamma = p/(2\pi k_B T\ M)^{1/2}$ (kB: Boltzmann's constant; M: atomic mass). At the boiling point, T_b, p = 1 atm, and $\Gamma = 10^{-23}\ cm^{-2}\ s^{-1}$, or 10^8 monolayers per second. Over the lifetime of the melt this corresponds to a loss of less than a monolayer. During the energy deposition stage, the surface temperature can briefly rise to several thousand degrees above T_b, and the corresponding equilibrium vapor pressure of 10^4 atm. The duration of this extreme overheat is very short, however ($< t_p$ = 30 ps), so that the evaporation loss is at most a few tens of monolayers. The energy loss rate due to evaporation is $\Gamma\Delta h_v/N$ (Δh_v: molar heat of evaporation, $\sim 10^5$ J $mole^{-1}$, N: Avogadro's number), which is at most $10^8\ W\ cm^{-2}$. This is still considerably below the absorbed laser intensity of $10^9\ W\ cm^{-2}$, and hence negligible as an energy loss.

The accuracy of these estimates was checked in a simple experiment (7,8). A thin metallic ribbon was clamped at one end and irradiated with the laser pulse at the other end. The recoil pressure of the evaporation (equal to half the vapor pressure) makes the ribbon oscillate visibly. By measuring the amplitude of the oscillation and the bending stiffness of the ribbon, the recoil pressure could be determined. A value of 10^{10} N m^{-2} was found, which is indeed similar to the peak vapor pressure estimated above.

The holes often found after irradiation of a surface are therefore not the result of evaporation *per se*, but of mechanical displacement of the liquid by the large recoil pressure of the evaporation ("splashing"). Often the morphology of the displaced material around the hole is direct evidence of splashing. Also, in some experiments on thin films supported on a different substrate, substrate atoms are sometimes detected on the top surface of the film in the vicinity of the hole; this, too, can only be explained by splashing.

3. THERMODYNAMICS AND KINETICS

The short timescale of the picosecond melt quenching process puts restrictions on the type of transformations that can occur. For the entire molten layer to be crystallized in the regrowth stage of Figure 3, the crystal-melt interface velocity must be on the order of $u = d/\tau \sim 100$ m s^{-1}. Note that this is also the isotherm velocity, u_T, of Table 1. If the interface lags behind the isotherms, crystal growth may be preempted by glass formation. The time required to crystallize the monolayer of thickness $\lambda = 0.3$ nm at a growth speed u is $t_1 = \lambda/u \sim 3$ ps. The distance an atom can diffuse in this amount of time, $(D_\ell t_1)^{1/2}$, is less than an interatomic distance (D : liquid diffusivity: 10^{-8} to 10^{-9} m^2 s^{-1}). This means that no long-range atomic transport can occur under these conditions, and that the only type of transformation that can occur is partitionless solidification, either by growth of a crystal of the same composition as the melt or by formation of a glass.

The thermodynamic conditions for partitionless crystallization are illustrated on the phase diagram of Figure 2, which contains two primary solid solutions (α,δ) and two intermetallic compounds (β,γ). The free energy diagram at temperature T_1 shows that partitionless crystallization of the liquid (ℓ) to the primary solution δ can only occur for compositions x greater than $x_{o,\delta\ell}$, at the intersection of the free energy curves. The locus of the points $x_{o,\delta\ell}$ for all temperatures forms the $T_{o,\delta\ell}$-line. Partitionless crystallization to the δ-phase can only occur below this T_o-line. For the other phases, similar T_o-lines are shown. At a sufficiently low temperature, T_g, the atomic transport rate (diffusivity) in the liquid state becomes negligibly small, so that no transformations can occur on a reasonable timescale. The liquid is then configurationally frozen and becomes a glass. For a composition in the range x' - x" in Figure 2, no crystallization is possible under picosecond laser quenching conditions, and therefore only glass formation is thermodynamically possible. This thermodynamic criterion for glass formation, however, is only a sufficient one, and not a necessary one as has been claimed by some authors (9,10). To formulate the glass-forming criterion more strictly, it is necessary to consider also the kinetics of partitionless crystallization.

As discussed in a number of previous papers (11,12), the crystal growth velocity, u, can be written as:

$$u = fk\lambda \left\{ 1 - \exp\left\{ -\frac{\Delta G_c}{RT_i} \right\} \right\} \quad (1)$$

where k: atom jump frequency across the crystal-melt interface;
f: fraction of interface sites that can incorporate a new atom;
ΔG_c: difference in molar free energy between crystal and melt (driving free energy, taken positive for undercooling);
T_i: interface temperature.

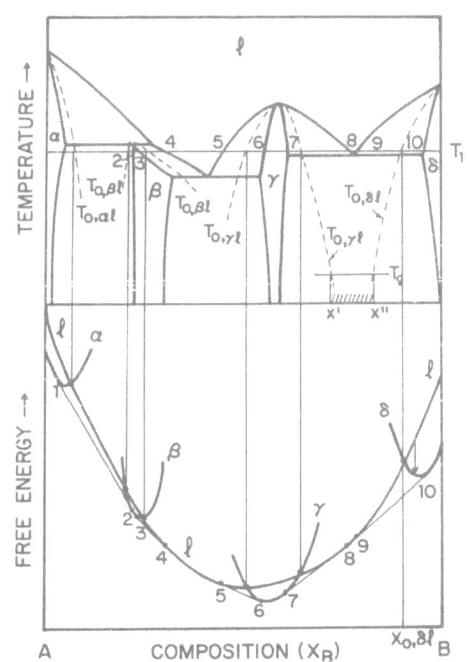

FIGURE 2. Schematic diagram, drawn to a variable scale, of a multilayer film after irradiation with a 30 ps laser pulse with a Gaussian intensity profile. From (25).

If T_i is not too far below T_m, so that the difference in molar entropy between crystal and melt, ΔS_c, can be considered constant with temperature, the driving free energy can be written as:

$$\Delta G_c = \Delta S_c (T_m - T_i) \tag{2}$$

For small ΔG_c, the exponential in equation (1) can be expanded and linearized:

$$u = fk\lambda \frac{\Delta G_c}{RT_i} \tag{3}$$

or, with equation (2):

$$u = fk\lambda \frac{\Delta S_c}{R} \frac{T_m - T_i}{T_i} \tag{4}$$

where, for metals, $f \approx 1$ and $S_c \approx R$.

The crystal growth rate is also determined by the rate at which the latent heat of crystallization, ΔH_c per mole, can be removed. The heat flux corresponding to a velocity u is:

$$\dot{Q} = \frac{u \, \Delta H_c}{\bar{V}} \tag{5}$$

where $\bar{V}$ is the molar volume.

Since this heat must be removed through conduction down the temperature gradient at the interface, $\nabla_i T$, this flux is also:

$$\dot{Q} = \kappa \, \nabla_i T \tag{6}$$

where the κ is the thermal conductivity.

Combining equations (5) and (6) allows definition of a heat flow limited velocity:

$$u_h = \frac{k\bar{V} \, \nabla_i T}{\Delta H_c} \tag{7}$$

Table 1 lists typical values of u_h for Fe, under both laser quenching and melt spinning conditions, using the tabulated value of the temperature gradient for $\nabla_i T$. That u_h and u_T have similar values is a direct result of ΔS_c and the molar specific heat, C, being of the same order of magnitude.

Since the crystal growth velocity in equations (4) and (7) must be the same, they can be combined for metals as:

$$\frac{u_h}{k\lambda} = \frac{T_m - T_i}{T_i} \tag{8}$$

In conventional solidification, the interface kinetics are much faster than the rate of heat removal, so that: $u_{th} \ll k\lambda$, and T_i is close to T_m. The growth is said to be <u>heat flow-limited</u>. In laser quenching, depending on the nature of the interface rearrangements (to be discussed below), the rate of heat removal, due to the very steep gradient, can be much faster than the crystal growth kinetics, so that $u_{th} \gg k\lambda$, and $T_i \ll T_m$. The growth is said to be <u>interface-limited</u>. At such large undercoolings, metastable phases and glasses can be formed.

The value of $k\lambda$ is determined by the nature of the atomic rearrangements necessary to advance the crystal-melt interface. In pure metals, dilute alloys, or crystalline compounds with a simple structure, k can be taken as the thermal vibration frequency. The maximum growth velocity $u_{max,c} = k\lambda$ can then be taken as the speed of sound, u_s, in the liquid. This is the collision-controlled regime, which is treated in more detail in another paper in this chapter (6). Suffice it to point out here that, even in picosecond laser quenching, under the conditions of Table 1, $u_{max} << u_T$, u_h, which makes this type of growth difficult to suppress.

In more concentrated alloys, or compounds with a more complicated crystal structure, which require changes in nearest neighbors upon crystallization, k is a diffusive jump frequency, and can be taken as D/λ^2. The maximum growth velocity in this diffusion-controlled regime is $u_{max,D_\lambda} = D/\lambda$, which is on the order of 10 m/s. Table 1 shows that for picosecond laser quenching, $u_{max,D} << u_T$, u_h, so that this type of growth can easily be suppressed. It follows then from equation (8) that T_i must fall far below T_m, and that glass formation becomes possible. It should also be noted here that the temperature dependence of the liquid diffusivity has a Fulcher-Vogel form $D_\ell = D_0 \exp[B/(T-T_0)]$, which makes D_ℓ, and hence k, become negligibly small in the vicinity of T_0 (i.e., around T_g) (13).

Although the partitionless growth of intermetallic compounds occurs, by definition, without long-range diffusional transport, the growth can still be diffusion-controlled if a drastic rearrangement of the nearest neighbor environment is required to transform the liquid structure into the crystalline one. This is the case if the crystalline unit cell is large, or if long-range chemical order must be established. In the example of Figure 2, if the formation of the compounds β and γ is diffusion-controlled, even below their respective T_0-line, their formation is suppressed in picosecond laser quenching and the intersections of the $T_{0,\alpha\ell}$ and $T_{0,\delta\ell}$ lines with the T_g-line can be used to define a new glass formation range.

This criterion, however, can still be extended, since in many systems glasses can be formed far below the T_0-lines of the primary solid solutions. Several examples will be discussed below. Again, partitionless formation of the primary solid solutions can be diffusion-controlled, and hence suppressed by picosecond pulsed laser quenching, if the change in short-range order between liquid and crystal is considerable.

4. EXPERIMENTAL ASPECTS

The short lifetime of the melt (τ = 1 ns) creates a special problem in obtaining a homogeneous melt, which is necessary for systematic studies of phase formation. The mixing length in the liquid, $(D_\ell\tau)^{1/2}$, is only 3 nm. The alloy components must therefore be mixed on this scale in the starting sample. This can be accomplished in a number of ways, such as ion implantation, co-evaporation, or deposition of multilayers. The latter method is a particularly convenient one that has been used for all the experiments discussed below. A typical sample geometry is drawn in Figure 3. The Al film is evaporated onto the Cu substrate. The multilayer is produced by alternate sputter deposition of the elemental metals, or a metal and an alloy, from two targets [14,16]. The average film composition can be varied conveniently by changing the thickness ratio of the layers. By keeping the repeat length of the multilayers below 3 nm, homogenization is achieved upon

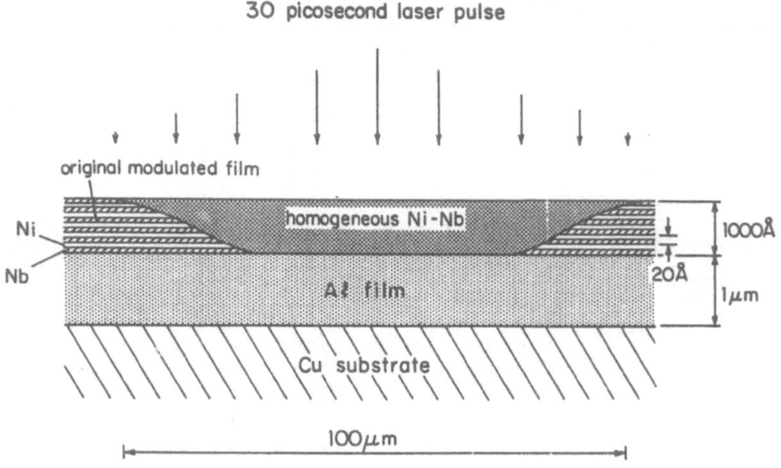

FIGURE 3. Schematic phase diagram (top), and corresponding free energy diagram at temperature T_1 (bottom), illustrating the construction of the T_0-lines for the primary solutions and the intermetallic compounds. In the composition range x'-x" (dashed), only glass formation is possible under conditions of partitionless solidification. The numbers correspond to the same compositions in the top and bottom diagrams.

melting. This was checked experimentally on a Cu-Ag alloy from a Cu/Ag multilayer (7,8). As expected, a metastable fcc solid solution was formed, which had a single lattice parameter, corresponding to the average composition of the film. No evidence of quenched inhomogeneity was found.

After irradiation, the samples can easily be removed from the substrate by dissolving the Al in NaOH. Note that Al is also a good material for a heat sink. Since the films are only 100 nm thick (~ melt depth), they can be investigated by electron microscopy without further thinning.

The reproducibility of the laser system used in the experiments discussed below was insufficient to pre-set the fluence levels predictably. Therefore, on each sample, a series of irradiations were made at different fluence levels. Subsequent investigation was then done on those spots that had a small hole (a few μm) at their center, due to "splashing" induced by the most intense part of the Gaussian beam. These spots were known to have received a fluence large enough to induce melting, and still had a large amount of material available for study.

5. SURVEY OF RESULTS

5.1. Fe-B

This system has been studied in the 12-28 at.% B range (2,17-19). The starting samples consisted of multi-layered α-Fe and amorphous Fe_3B. It was found that alloys containing a minimum of 5 at.% B were amorphous after picosecond laser quenching. Below 5 at.% B, the solidification product was a Fe(B) bcc interstitial solution. The 4 at.% alloy showed a small amount of amorphous material near the top surface of the film (19); it was distributed in a morphology characteristic of an interfacial instability, which could have become possible at the last stage of the solificiation when the crystal growth velocity decreases considerably (20). The redistribution of the B associated with the instability could then have led to glass formation in the B-rich regions.

The T_0-line for the $\ell \rightarrow$ bcc transformation can be calculated fairly accurately from the phase diagram using simple regular solution theory (2,8). The result is shown in Figure 4, and is in agreement with the observation that Fe-B glasses with less than 18 at.% B crystallize into the bcc Fe(B) solution upon heating (21). The crystallization temperature for an 18 at.% B glass is 660 K, which corresponds to 16 at.% B on the T_0-line.

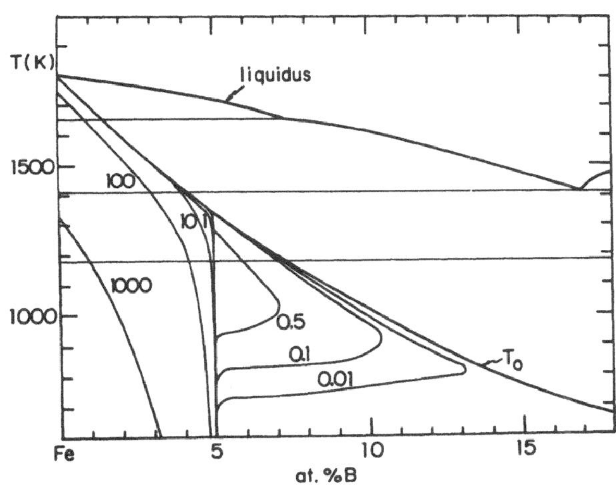

FIGURE 4. The Fe-B phase diagram, showing the T_0 line for the liquid $\rightarrow$ bcc transition. The contours represent the bcc crystal growth speed (in m s^{-1}) as a function of composition and interface temperature, calculated from the model explained in the text. From (2).

The Fe-B glasses clearly form far below the T_0-line (T_0 - T_g is 700 K for a 5 at.% B alloy). As explained above, the growth of the competing bcc phase must therefore be diffusion-controlled in alloys with more than 5 at.% B. Given that the nearest neighbor environment of a B-atom in a Fe-B glass consists of nine Fe atoms in a trigonal prismatic arrangement (22), which is very different from the nearest neighbor environment of an interstitial B in the bcc Fe(B) solution, this diffusional control is to be expected. The glass-forming limit of 5 at.% B suggests that each B atom forms a cluster of about 19 Fe atoms (i.e., one and one-half coordination shells) around it that must be rearranged upon crystallization. The rest of the Fe atoms behave as in pure Fe, and make collisional jumps. The maximum velocity in equation (1) can then be written as (2):

$$fk\lambda = (20x_B)\frac{D_\ell}{\lambda} + (1 - 20x_B)u_s \qquad \text{for } x_B \leq 0.05 \tag{9}$$

$$= D_\ell/\lambda \qquad \text{for } x_B > 0.05$$

where x_B is the atom fraction of B.

Using a temperature dependence for the diffusivity:

$$D_\ell = 1.4 \times 10^{-8} \exp\left\{-\frac{1300}{T - 581}\right\} m^2 s^{-1} \tag{10}$$

obtained by fitting liquid and glass transport data, and a driving free energy:

$$\Delta G_c = (x_{Fe}\Delta S_{c,Fe} + x_B\Delta S_{c,B})(T - T_o) \tag{11}$$

with $\Delta S_{c,Fe}$ = 7.6 J K^{-1} $mole^{-1}$ and $\Delta S_{c,B}$ = 21.8 J K^{-1} $mole^{-1}$, the crystal growth velocity could be calculated as a function of composition and temperature. The results are shown in Figures 4 and 5. Note that crystallization is driven by the undercooling below T_O, not below the liquidus temperature. Figure 5 shows clearly that the isotherm velocity

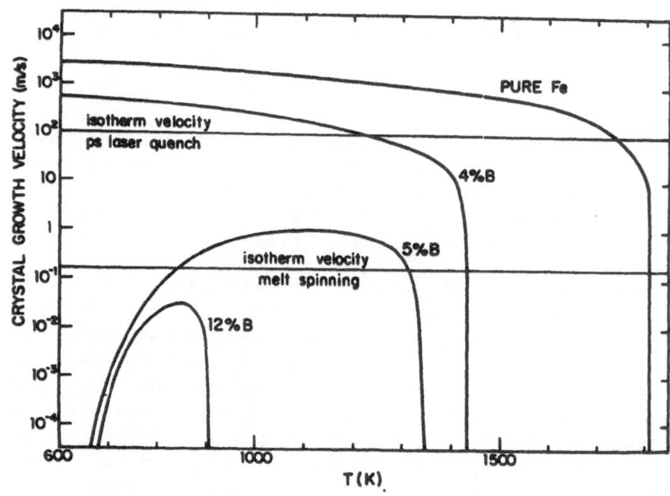

FIGURE 5. Growth velocity of the bcc crystal as a function of interface temperature for four composition in the Fe-B system. From (2).

in picosecond laser quenching is large enough to prevent crystal growth in a 5 at.% B alloy, but not in a 4 at.% alloy. It is interesting that the simple estimates of Table 1 can also account for the minimum of 12 at.% B necessary in melt spinning to obtain a glass (21,23,24).

5.2. Ni-Nb

This system has been studied over the entire composition range (25). The starting materials were multilayers of the elemental metals. As illustrated on Figure 6, a glass was obtained by picosecond laser quenching in the range 23-82 at.% Ni. This range exceeds that for splat quenching (26) ($\sim 10^{10}$ K s^{-1} (27,28)) and for RF sputtering of homogeneous films (29). It is interesting that the cooling rate in the latter process is estimated at about 10^{13} K s^{-1} (30), similar to that for laser quenching. None of the intermetallic compounds, the μ-phase or the Ni_3Nb phase, were formed even if the melt composition was close. This indicates that their growth is diffusion-controlled, which is to be expected for the size of their unit cell and degree of order.

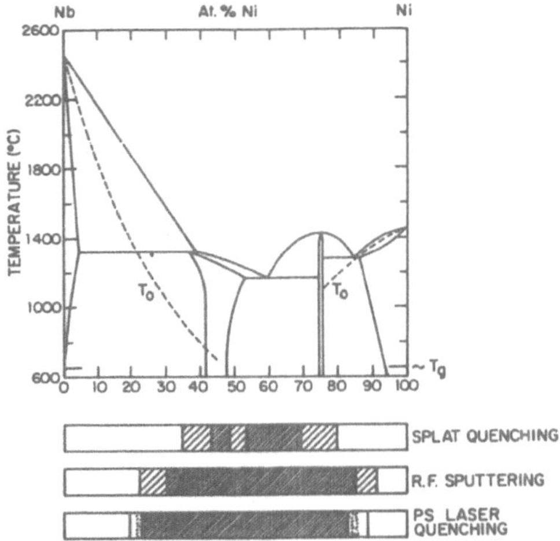

FIGURE 6. Equilibrium phase diagram for the Ni-Nb system, with calculated T_0-lines. T_g indicates the approximate crystallization temperature of nearly equiatomic amorphous alloys (34). The glass-forming ranges for splat quenching (28), RF sputtering (29) and picosecond laser quenching (25) are indicated. Fine hatching: fully amorphous; coarse hatching: mixed amorphous and crystalline; dashed hatching indicates that the glass formation limits for picosecond laser quenching are between the surrounding vertical lines. From (25).

The T_0-lines for the primary solutions on Figure 6 have been calculated from the phase diagram using simple regular solution theory. In this system also, glasses are formed far below the T_0-line ($T_g \sim 940$ K (34)). A mechanism similar to that discussed for Fe-B probably also makes growth of these supersaturated primary solutions diffusion-controlled. That the minimum amount of solute required for glass formation is greater here than for Fe-B may reflect the lesser interaction, and hence smaller cluster size, in metal-metal alloys than in metal-metalloid alloys.

Below 18 at.% Ni supersaturated bcc solutions were formed. Above 89 at.% Ni supersaturated fcc solutions, containing many twins and stacking faults, were formed. The defect density increased with Nb content, probably due to a lowering of the stacking fault energy. Growth twins are also formed in the regrowth of silicon (fcc) from the melt following a laser pulse, at growth velocities intermediate between those of the perfect crystal and the amorphous phase (31).

5.3. Mo-Ni

Glasses were formed, for the first time by melt quenching, in alloys with 30, 50 and 60 at.% Ni (32). The 50 at.% Ni alloy corresponds to an intermetallic compound in equilibrium (δ-phase). Due to its large unit cell (56 atoms Frank-Kasper phase), it is not formed in picosecond laser quenching. The other two glasses again formed far below the T_0-line.

5.4. Mo-Co

A 45 at.% Co alloy was quenched to a glass for the first time by this method (32). The ε-phase, at the same composition, is not formed.

5.5. Nb-Co

A glass was formed at 40 at.% Nb (32). The γ-phase is not formed, even though glass formation probably occurred below the $T_{0,\gamma\ell}$ line.

5.6. Ag-Cu

A disordered fcc phase was formed upon quenching of 35, 50 and 65 at.% Ag alloys (7). This is to be expected, since the crystallization kinetics of a disordered fcc crystal are no different from those of a pure fcc crystal, which are known to be collision-controlled, and hence difficult to suppress. Note that the T_0-line reaches across the phase diagram of Figure 6, so that crystallization of the fcc phase is the dominating process at all compositions.

5.7. Cu-Co

A disordered fcc phase was formed at 50 at.% Co (7). Again, the T_0-line for this phase spans the phase diagram.

5.8. Nb-Si

A fcc phase was formed in the composition range 10-27 at.% Si (33). So far, this phase had only been prepared at 22 at.% Si by shock compression.

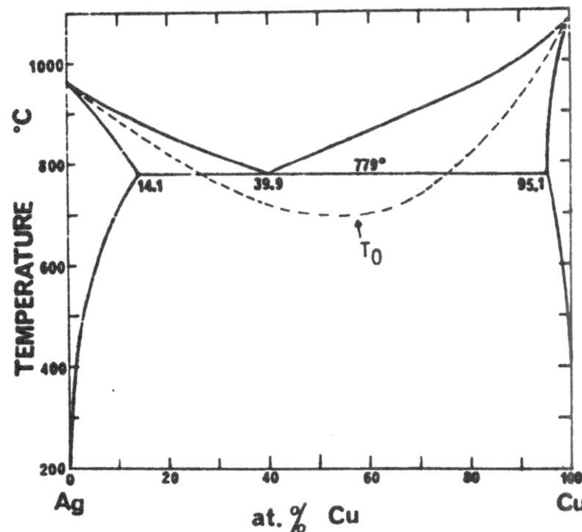

FIGURE 7. Ag-Cu equilibrium phase diagram. The T_0-line has been calculated using the regular solution model. From (8).

ACKNOWLEDGMENTS

The work described in this paper has been performed in collaboration with C. J. Lin and W. K. Wang. It is supported by the Office of Naval Research under Contract No. N00014-83-K-0030.

REFERENCES

1. N. Bloembergen, in Laser-Solid Interactions and Laser Processing, edited by S. D. Ferris, H. J. Leamy, and J. M. Poate (AIP, New York, 1979), p. 1.
2. F. Spaepen and C. J. Lin, in Amorphous Metals and Non-Equilibrium Processing, edited by M. von Allmen (Les Editions de Physique, Les Ulis, France, 1984), p. 65.
3. For a review of these relaxation processes, see W. L. Brown, Mater. Res. Soc. Symp. Proc. 23, 9 (1984).
4. J. M. Liu, R. Yen, H. Kurz, and N. Bloembergen, Appl. Phys. Lett. 39, 755 (1981).
5. P. H. Bucksbaum and J. Bokor, Mater. Res. Soc. Symp. Proc. 13, 51 (1983).
6. C. A. MacDonald and F. Spaepen, this NATO ASI Proceedings.
7. C. J. Lin and F. Spaepen, Mater. Res. Soc. Symp. Proc. 28, 75 (1984).
8. C. J. Lin, Ph.D. Thesis, Harvard University, 1983.
9. T. B. Massalski, Proc. 4th Int. Conf. on Rapidly Quenched Metals, edited by T. Masumoto and K. Suzuki (Jpn. Inst. Metals, Sendai, 1982), p. 203.
10. W. J. Boettinger ibid., p. 99.

11. D.Turnbull, in "Physical Processes in Laser-Materials Interactions," NATO-ASI Proc., edited by M. Bertollotti (Plenum, New York, 1983), p. 117.
12. F. Spaepen and D. Turnbull, in Laser Processing of Semiconductors, edited by J. M. Poate and J. W. Mayer (Academic, New York, 1982), p. 15.
13. For a review of atomic transport in liquids and glasses, see F. Spaepen and A. I. Taub, in Amorphous Metallic Alloys, edited by F. E. Luborsky (Butterworths, London, 1983), p. 231; B. Cantor and R. W. Cahn, ibid., p. 487.
14. M. P. Rosenblum, F. Spaepen, and D. Turnbull, Appl. Phys. Lett. 37, 184 (1982).
15. A. L. Greer, C. J. Lin, and F. Spaepen, Proc. 4th Int. Conf. on Rapidly Quenched Metals, edited by T. Masumoto and K. Suzuki (Jpn. Inst. Metals, Sendai, 1982), p. 567.
16. F. Spaepen, A. L. Greer, K. F. Kelton, and J. L. Bell., Rev. Sci. Instrum. 56, 1340 (1985).
17. C. J. Lin and F. Spaepen, Appl. Phys. Lett. 41, 721 (1982).
18. C. J. Lin and F. Spaepen, in Chemistry of Physics of Rapidly Solidified Materials, edited by B. J. Berkowitz and R. O. Scattergood (TMS-AIME, New York, 1983), p. 273.
19. C. J. Lin and F. Spaepen, Scr. Metall. 17, 1259 (1983).
20. J. W. Cahn, S. R. Coriell, and W. J. Boettinger, in Laser and Electron Beam Processing of Materials, edited by C. W. White and P. S. Peercy (Academic, New York, 1980), p. 89.
21. R. Hasegawa and R. Ray, J. Appl. Phys. 49, 4174 (1978).
22. For a review of the short-range order in metal-metalloid glasses, see J. M. Dubois and G. LeCaer, Acta Metall. 32, 2101 (1984).
23. R. Ray and R. Hasegawa, Solid State Commun. 27, 471 (1978).
24. F. E. Luborsky and H. H. Liebermann, Appl. Phys. Lett. 33, 233 (1978).
25. C. J. Lin and F. Spaepen, "Nickel-Niobium Alloys Obtained by Picosecond Pulsed Laser Quenching," submitted to Acta Metallurgica.
26. R. C. Ruhl, B. C. Giessen, M. Cohen, and N. J. Grant, Acta Metall. 15, 1693 (1967).
27. P. Duwez and R. H. Willens, Trans. Met. Soc. AIME 227, 362 (1963).
28. H. Jones, Proc. 2nd Int. Conf. on Rapidly Quenched Metals, edited by B. C. Giessen and N. J. Grant (MIT Press, Cambridge, MA, 1976), p. 1.
29. T. W. Barbee, W. H. Holmes, D. L. Keith, M. K. Pyzyna, and G. Ilonca, Thin Solid Films 45, 591 (1977).
30. D. Turnbull, Metall. Trans., A 12, 695 (1981).
31. A. G. Cullis, N. G. Chew, H. C. Webber, and D. J. Smith, J. Cryst. Growth 68, 624 (1984).
32. C. J. Lin, F. Spaepen, and D. Turnbull, J. Non-Cryst. Solids 61/62, 767 (1984).
33. W. K. Wang and F. Spaepen, "Face-Centered Cubic Nb-Si Solid Solutions Obtained by Picosecond Pulsed Laser Quenching," to appear in J. Appl. Phys.
34. B. C. Giessen, M. Madhava, D. E. Polk, and J. Vander Sande, Mater. Sci. Eng. 23, 145 (1976).

CRYSTALLIZATION AND NUCLEATION PHENOMENA IN CW SURFACE MELTED ALLOYS

E. N. KAUFMANN AND R. J. WALLACE
University of California, Lawrence Livermore National Laboratory, Livermore, CA 94550, USA

Key Words: T-T-T curves, amorphization, cw laser, e-beam

1. INTRODUCTION

Other contributors to this text have described the thermal history which pulse melting produces in solid surfaces. Also described have been the rudiments of the theory which applies to solidification interface velocities and crystallization phenomena. There are many similarities between the pulsed regime and the continuous wave or cw regime of surface melting. In one respect, however, there is an important difference. With pulsed heating, the isotherm and resolidification velocities depend on the pulse length and thermal properties of the materials. In cw processing, the maximum velocity that the solidification interface or any isotherm can reach is that of the traveling energetic beam. In addition, the dependence of interface velocity on depth from the surface is distinctly different for cw processing as compared to pulse processing. With a greater degree of control over the solidification velocities of interest using the cw alternative and with the aid of finite-element heat flow computer codes, one can hope to identify and understand the various nucleation and growth processes which occur on surface melting. Here, by way of example, we will highlight several phenomena involved in the nucleation and growth of crystalline phases and of glass formation in cw-processed surface alloys.

Once the various phases that might form on surface melting and solidification have been identified from the perspective of thermodynamical accessibility, two kinetic factors must be considered. First, the probability that any given phase will nucleate as a precursor to growth must be taken into account; second, the rate at which a given phase can grow must be evaluated. As an example of the latter, Fig. 1 shows data from Boettinger on the crystallization rate of a Pb-Sn eutectic system as a function of temperature below the melting point (1). One sees from the figure that as the temperature drops below the melting point, i.e., increased interface undercooling, the growth velocity of the eutectic phase increases until reaching a maximum beyond which diffusion of the constituents is hampered by the cooling, thereby slowing the growth rate. The 12 cm/sec maximum growth velocity illustrated in Fig. 1 applies to a relatively complex system where diffusion is necessary at the liquid-solid interface to form the two-phase solid eutectic structure from the single-phase liquid solution. In pure metal systems or in a solid solution, the solidification process involves only collision rather than diffusion-limited processes at the interface and may therefore occur at many meters per second. Once a critical growth velocity is found to be small because of the complexity of the phase formed, other alternatives must be sought. In some instances this will be a crystalline phase which

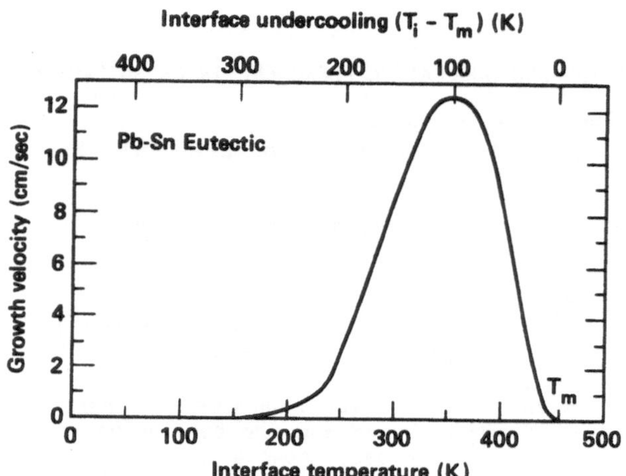

FIGURE 1. The calculated rate of growth of the Pb-Sn eutectic as a function of interface temperature (undercooling) (Ref. 1).

may grow at higher rates. In other instances, with no such phase available, the liquid structure may simply be retained in the form of a glass at low temperature. Figure 2, also taken from Boettinger, provides a schematic illustration of how compositon of an alloy may determine the ultimate product of rapid solidification, depending on the regrowth velocity. It illustrates that at the eutectic composition, one is likely to be forced into forming a glass at high solidification velocities. This would correspond to the Pb-Sn eutectic of Fig. 1. At compositions near terminal solid solutions, one may form, at the highest solidification velocities, metastable extended solid solutions of the primary phases. At intermediate composition ranges, one may find mixtures of crystalline solidification of the terminal solid solution and the eutectic or glass, depending on the velocity.

Nucleation of a phase depends on several factors. Homogeneous nucleation, which depends on fluctuations within the system as a transformation temperature is approached, may be overwhelmed by the effect of heterogeneous nucleation occurring at catalytic sites of varying activities. The sites may be impurities in the melt, inclusions in a solid phase, surfaces, etc. The probability of heterogeneous nucleation depends both on the density per unit volume of the catalytic sites and the potency of each type of catalytic site. Traditionally, the nucleation phenomena are illustrated graphically on TTT or Time-Temperature-Transformation diagrams such as are shown in Fig. 3. Figure 3(a) illustrates a classical situation of quenching from the melt, where a fast quench rate such as $\dot{T}_2$ will miss the nose of the C-shaped curve and allow the metastable retention of a phase such as a glass or a martensite. For a slower quench rate, the system follows a time-temperature path through the C-shaped curve where partial or total transformation toward equilibrium phase may occur. The C shape of the curve on these diagrams arises

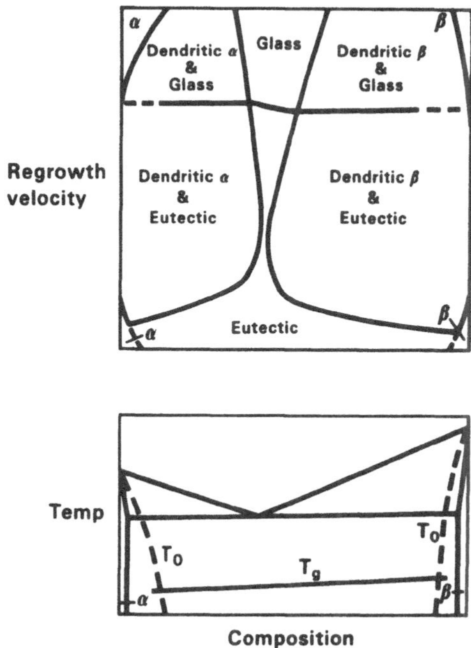

FIGURE 2. Schematic plot of growth velocity versus composition showing microstructure expected for a simple eutectic system (Ref. 1).

from the simple interplay of diffusion and nucleation. At high temperatures, diffusion rates are high, enhancing the growth rate of a phase during transformation, but nucleation rates are low. Conversely, at low temperature, where nucleation rates would tend to be high, diffusion rates are low and prevent rapid growth. Figure 3(b) illustrates time-temperature paths one might follow for heating of a metastable phase, such as glass, in order to allow a transformation.

In practice, there may be several possible phases which can nucleate and which have catalytic sites of varying potency and volume density. Therefore, the TTT diagram of Fig. 4, taken from Perepezko et al., may be more schematically representative of the actual multiplicity of choices (2). In Fig. 4 one sees that higher cooling rates need not make formation of a metastable phase more likely. In Fig. 4 the higher rate $\dot{T}_2$ favors the formation of the phase labeled A which may be the equilibrium phase, whereas the slower rate $\dot{T}_1$ would favor C which may be a metastable phase. Phases A and C differ in their shape and location because curve C represents a metastable phase which has a catalytic site of high potency but relatively lower density, whereas A indicates an equilibrium phase with catalytic sites present in high density but with low potency. With this type of schematic illustration in

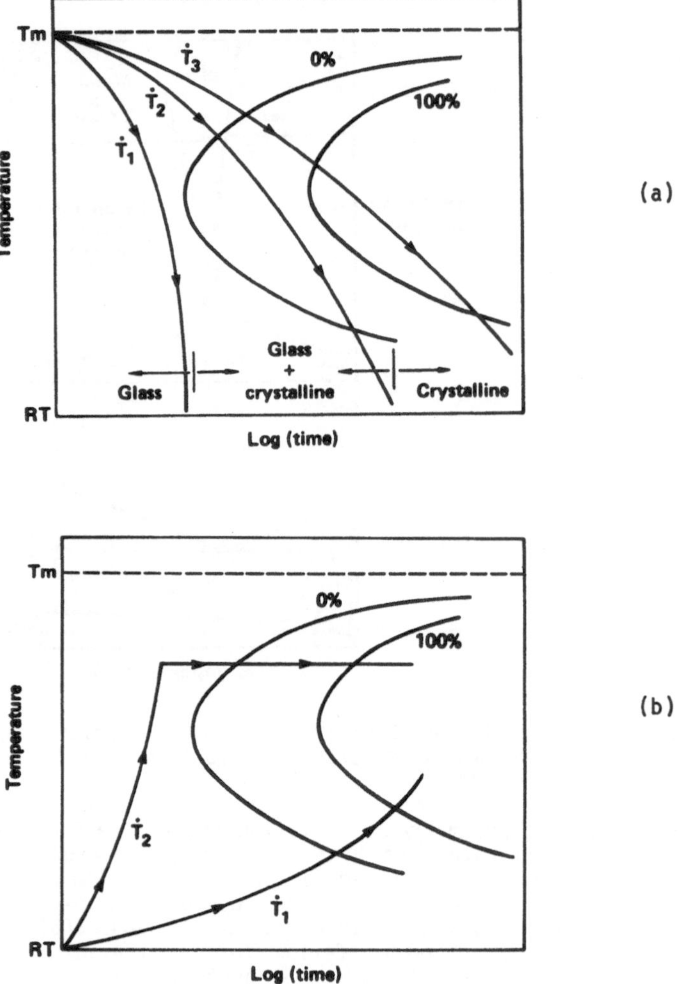

FIGURE 3. Time-temperature-transformation diagram representing (a) quenching from the melt ($\dot{T}_1 > \dot{T}_2 > \dot{T}_3$), (b) heating of a metastable phase in order to allow a transformation.

mind, one can qualitatively understand the great variety of morphologies that one obtains on rapid solidification.

A good example of various kinds of crystallization nucleation that might be seen is given in Fig. 5 taken from Bergmann et al. (3). In Fig. 5(a) one sees a melt pool recrystallizing by nucleation at the melt-solid interface at maximum melt depth and regrowing in an apparent

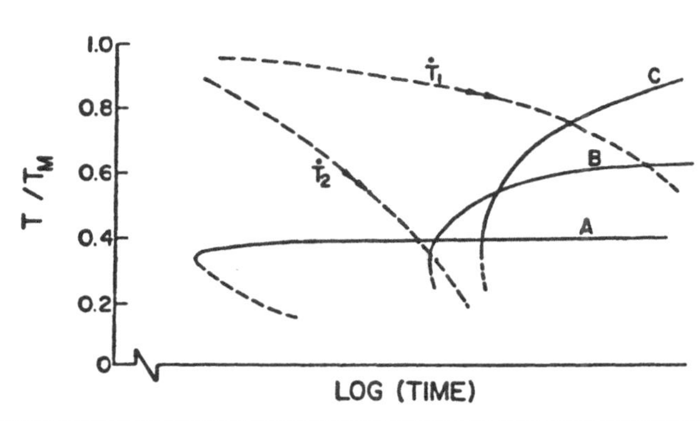

FIGURE 4. Time-temperature-transformation diagram representing different nucleation kinetics that may occur during continuous cooling of an undercooled liquid ($\dot{T}_2 > \dot{T}_1$) (Ref. 2).

epitaxial fashion toward the surface. Thus, nucleation of the crystallizing phase in the melt has occurred at the liquid-solid interface. In Fig. 5(b) one sees dendrites which clearly nucleated within the molten zone, presumably through heterogeneous nucleation on catalytic impurities sites within the liquid itself, and in Fig. 5(c) one sees the result of nucleation of a crystalline phase at the surface of the melt pool with subsequent growth downward into the molten zone.

Another example of the variety of results that one might obtain has been reported by Alden et al. on the Cr-Ta system (4). With samples at the eutectic composition of approximately 10 at% Ta, electron-beam surface melting produced a surface which was a single BCC phase containing approximately 10 at% Ta. Thus a metastable extended solid solution was obtained by melting the eutectic material which was comprised of both the terminal solid solution BCC-chromium phase as well as the Cr_2Ta intermetallic. The micrographs and X-ray diffraction data illustrating these phases are shown in Fig. 6. Also reported in this work, however, was that at higher solidification rates produced by pulsed-laser melting, a new FCC sructure was observed as well as some evidence of glass formation.

Analogous phenomena have been observed in many other systems. For example, in the Pd-Cu-Si system Boettinger (5) showed that, depending on the composition around the eutectic, one forms either glass when the growth rate exceeds the critical velocity or the glass with embedded crystallites of one particularly easily nucleated and fast-growing phase which borders on the eutectic region. The Pd-Cu-Si system shows an extremely low maximum growth velocity of 2.5 mm/sec. Thus it is a very easy glass former in both conventional and surface processing modes. Breinan and Kear (6), among others, demonstrated the easy vitrification of the surface of the Pd-Cu-Si alloy under laser iradiation.

Once a glass layer is formed, one can ask how stable it will be to subsequent thermal excursions, which, for example, will occur in multiple

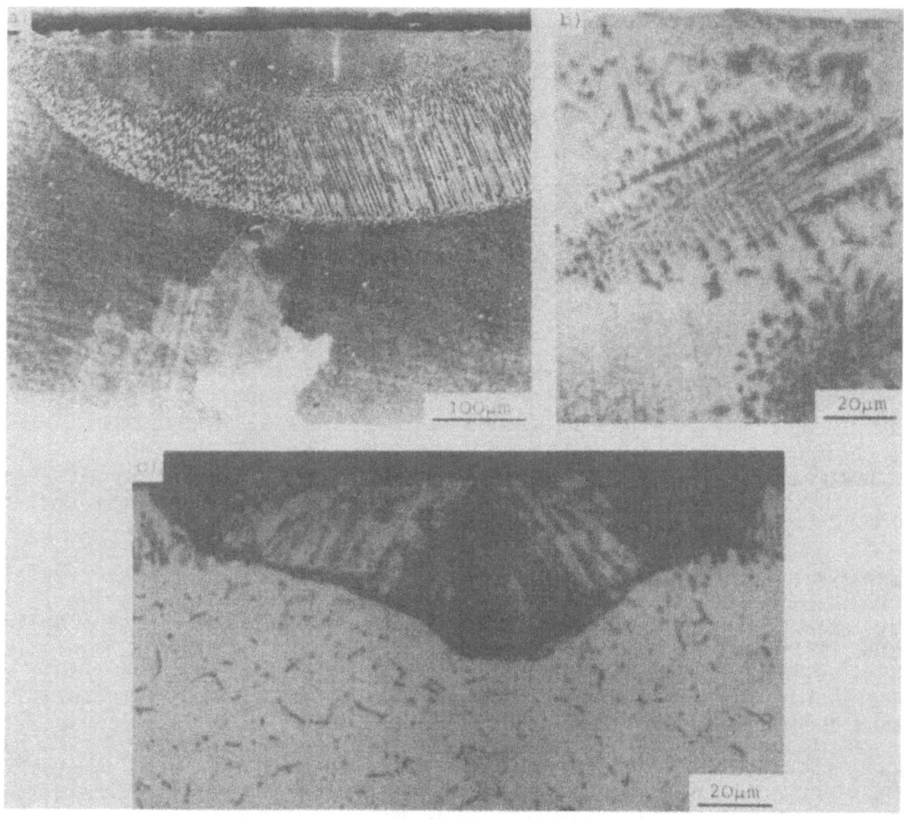

FIGURE 5. Nucleation in laser-melted surfaces: (a) epitaxial crystallization of dendrites (Cu-Be-Co), (b) nucleation within the melt (Ti-Al-V), (c) surface-nucleated eutectic crystals (Fe-B) (Ref. 3).

overlapping passes using a continuous beam. In the case of Pd-Cu-Si, which is a very easy glass former and has a very slow critical growth rate, one might anticipate that this is not a problem. Yoshioka et al. (7) confirmed this by observing no heat-affected zone (HAZ) effects using overlapping passes of CO_2 laser radiation at a traverse rate of 17 cm/sec. Under identical processing conditions the same authors noted that an Fe-Cr-Mo-P-C alloy, on the other hand, which was easily rendered amorphous in single-pass mode, shows crystallization in the HAZ of overlapping melt stripes. The authors were able to explain their results based on the thermal history of the various regions near the overlapping passes in terms of whether the time-temperature path did or did not intersect the C-shaped curve on the TTT diagram. As a general rule, one must heat and cool rapidly enough to avoid touching the nose of the C-shaped curve in order to maintain an amorphous layer. On the other

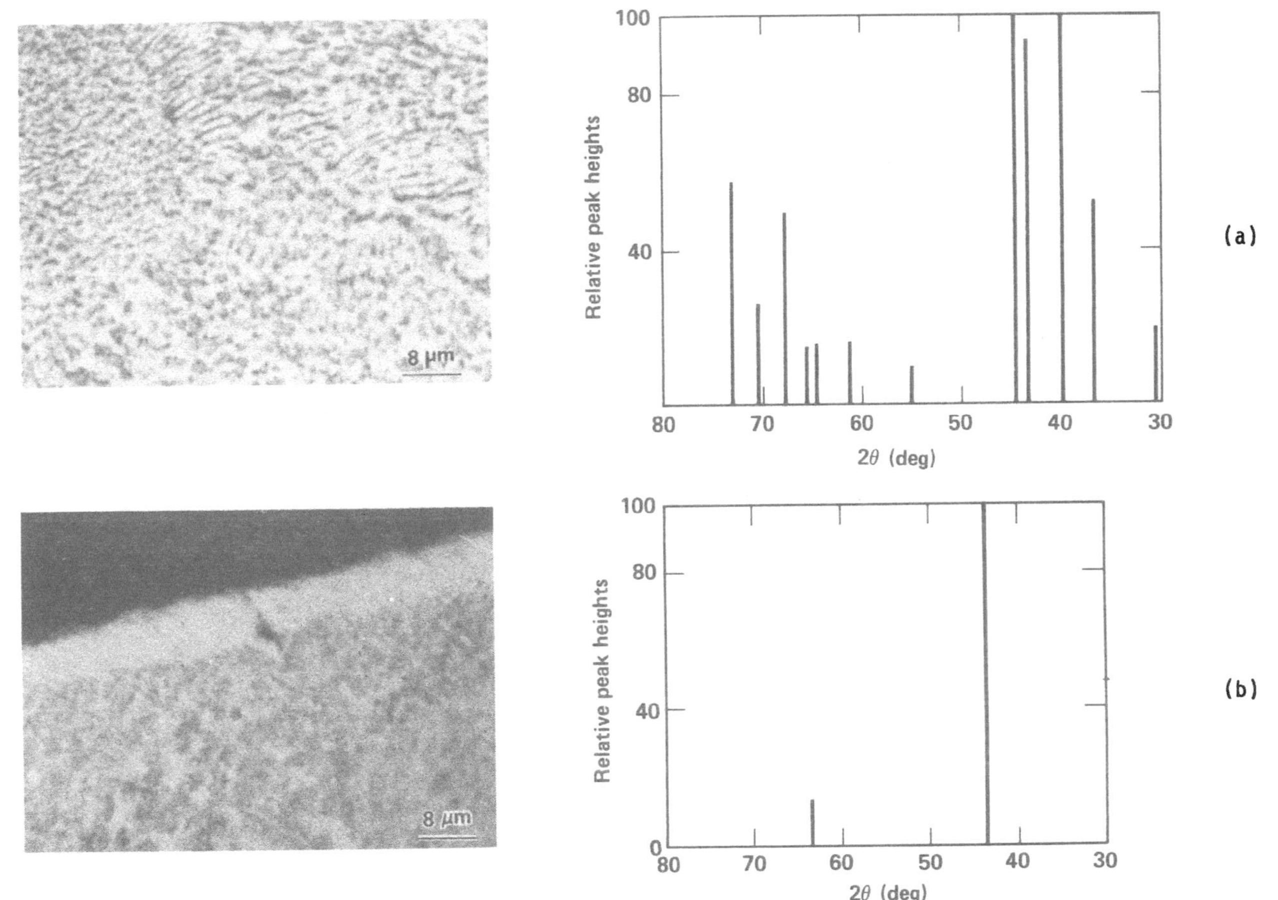

FIGURE 6. Optical metallographic cross section and X-ray diffraction pattern of a Cr–Ta alloy: (a) as case, (b) after cw surface melting.

hand, in many applications where one might be interested in producing an extremely fine crystalline microstructure, the rapid heating and cooling of an amorphous phase in such a way as to just graze the nose of such a curve in a controlled fashion may produce the desired results.

Further examples of some of the behavior discussed above are presented in the following sections.

2. TANTALUM-IRIDIUM SYSTEM

A good illustration of both the composition and velocity dependence of the result of surface melting can be found in work reported on the Ta-Ir system (8). In this system there is a relatively deep eutectic at 55.5 at% Ta and 1950°C. An arc-melted equiatomic alloy, therefore, displays a structure consisting of dendrites of an orthorhombic alpha phase (Ir-rich side of the eutectic) with interdendritic eutectic. A polished sample of this alloy was processed using overlapping passes of a CO_2 laser and subsequently repolished to partially remove the periodic topological features created by melting. Figure 7 shows the result of this procedure where one sees a gradation in the refinement of the crystalline product as well as some featureless and presumably amorphous regions. Based on the original topology and the polishing procedure, one derives that the original surface consisted of the glassy material and that the lateral dimension in Fig. 7 as one moves from left to right, i.e., from the glass to the very fine to the less fine crystallites corresponds to moving in depth from the surface toward the bottom of the melted layer. Figure 8 shows a TEM micrograph obtained from the material shown in Fig. 7 as well as two selected-area-diffraction patterns (SAD). One SAD corresponds to the amorphous surface region and the other corresponds to the neighboring microcrystalline region. An analysis of the microcrystalline diffraction pattern indicates that this region consists of highly strained or twinned grains of the orthorhombic alpha-phase structure. There is no indication of the tetragonal sigma phase that borders the eutectic region on the Ta-rich side.

Judging from the shape of the phase boundary in the binary phase diagram (9) presented in Fig. 9, the rapid cooling of a 50 at% alloy should bring it below the T_0 line rather easily and thus into a region where the partitionless solidification of the alpha phase would be allowed. This is apparently observed. However, at the surface of the material, the maximum crystallization rate for the formation of the alpha phase is apparently exceeded and the glass phase is formed, even though one is presumably below the T_0 line.

The same material was processed using an electron beam and yielded the optical metallographic cross section shown in Fig. 10. The micrograph of Fig. 10 illustrates nicely both the composition dependence of glass-forming ability and the variation of maximum growth rate for a crystalline phase. At the lower left of Fig. 10 one sees the original bulk structure, consisting of dendrites of the alpha phase separated by interdendritic eutectic, and in the band running from the upper left to lower right of the figure, one sees the melted zone. At the surface side of the melted zone, one sees the featureless gray area which is the metallic glass. However, at the base of the melted zone near the maximum melt depth, one sees intermittent pockets of microcrystalline material which favor formation above the alpha dendrites rather than above the eutectic regions. This is clear evidence that the propensity for nucleation of the microcrystalline phase on the alpha phase dendrite is greater than for the nucleation of that phase over the eutectic regions

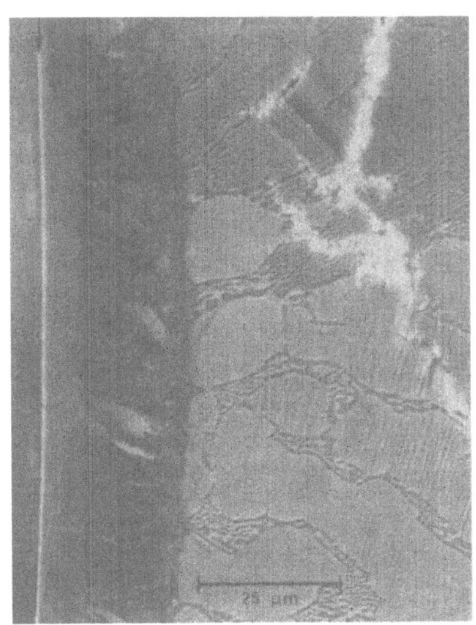

FIGURE 7. Optical metallographic cross section of CO_2-laser processed Ta-Ir specimen showing from right to left, the unmelted bulk (with α_1-dendrites and $\alpha_1 + \sigma$ interdendritic eutectic), a microcrystalline resolidified layer, and a glassy resolidified region. (The arrow indicates the surface of the specimen.)

and that the maximum growth velocity for the microcrystalline phase at the compositon of the alpha dendrite is greater than at the composition of the eutectic. This results in the half-moon shape microcrystalline regions in Fig. 10. Finite-element thermal code simulation for this particular case indicates that the maximum growth velocity is of the order of 1 to 2 m/sec.

It is absolutely necessary to utilize a computer simulation of the heat flow and thermal history of the material as a function of position if one expects to derive quantitative information from such tests.

3. SURFACE-PROCESSED METALLIC GLASS

In order to study both the propensity for glass formation on rapid solidification from the melt and the tendency toward devitrification in the HAZ, a study of a relatively well known, easy-forming alloy was done by Wallace and Kaufmann (10). In that work identically processed ribbons of a Fe-Ni-P-B alloy, both in the amorphous and in the crystallized form, were used.

Electron beam processing was conducted at a variety of powers and traverse rates in order to study the system over a wide range of solidification and thermal transient conditions. The thermal history of the sample was determined by applying a two-dimensional finite element heat flow code in which the parameters were adjusted so as to properly match the experimentally determined maximum melt depth. Typical results of the computer simulation are shown in Fig. 11. Figure 11(a) illustrates

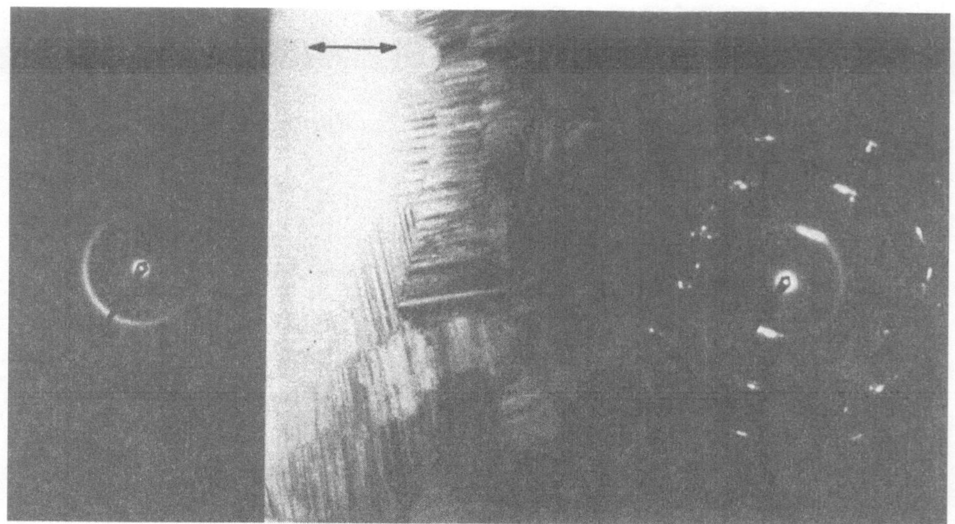

FIGURE 8. Transmission electron micrograph of CO_2-laser processed specimen shown in Fig. 7 with selected area diffraction patterns corresponding to the amorphous and microcrystalline regions. (Marker equals 1000 Å).

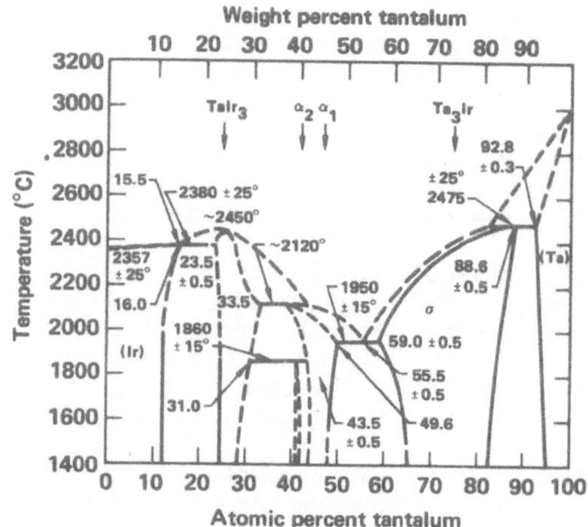

FIGURE 9. Binary alloy phase diagram of the Ta-Ir system (Ref. 9).

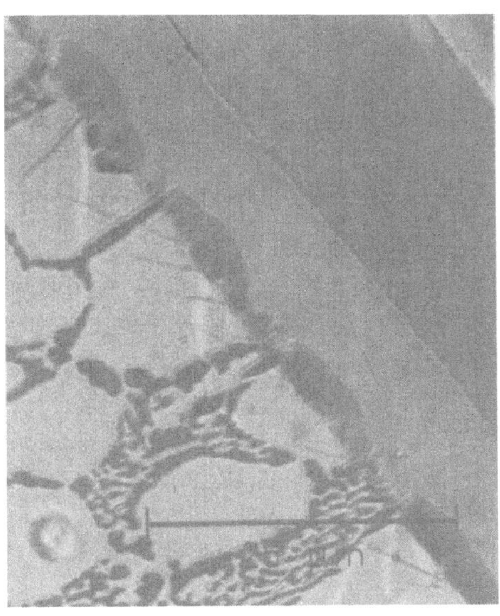

FIGURE 10. Optical metallographic cross section of non-overlapping melt stripe in electron-beam processed Ta-Ir specimen (100 kV, 35 ma, 1420 cm/sec). (The arrow indicates the surface of the specimen.)

the depth as a function of time of the isotherm corresponding to the melting point of the material. Aside from the effects of undercooling, which imply a displacement of the liquid-solid interface from the melting point isotherm, this fairly describes the depth versus time of the liquid-solid interface. Just below the maximum melt depth, the HAZ would experience the largest temperature excursion. Figure 11(b) shows the computed temperature excursion for that point as a function of time. Figure 11(c) shows the heating and cooling rate as a function of time experienced by a point at the maximum melt depth. And, Figure 11(d) shows what would normally be called the quench rate as a function of depth. Note that for cw-beam melting, the quench rate after the initial transient period at the maximum melt depth is essentially constant throughout the resolidified region. Finally, in Fig. 11(e), one sees the computed melting point isotherm velocity as a function of depth for such an experiment. Here one notes that the isotherm velocity, starting from zero at maximum melt depth, accelerates toward the surface and of course can ultimately not exceed the velocity of the electron beam. This velocity behavior is distinct from that observed in pulse melting where, after a rapid transient period, the velocity of the isotherm is essentially constant throughout the melted region.

Optical metallographic cross sections for both the crystallized and amorphous Fe-Ni-P-B ribbons are shown in Figs. 12 and 13. Figure 12 shows the data obtained for crystallized ribbon processed at three

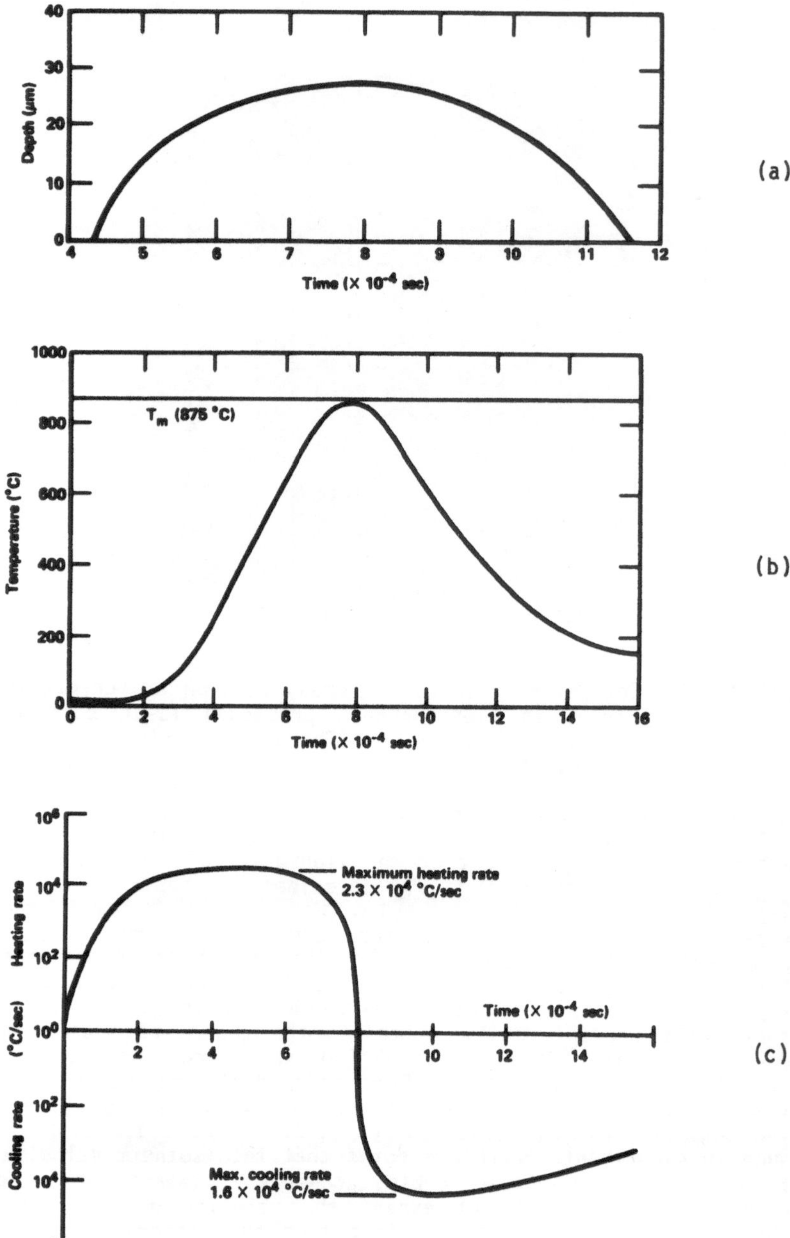

FIGURE 11. Computer simulation of surface processed Fe-Ni-P-B alloy (200 W, 100 cm/sec) showing: (a) depth of melting-point isotherm as a function of time, (b) temperature excursion versus time at maximum melt depth, (c) heating and cooling rate versus time at maximum melt depth.

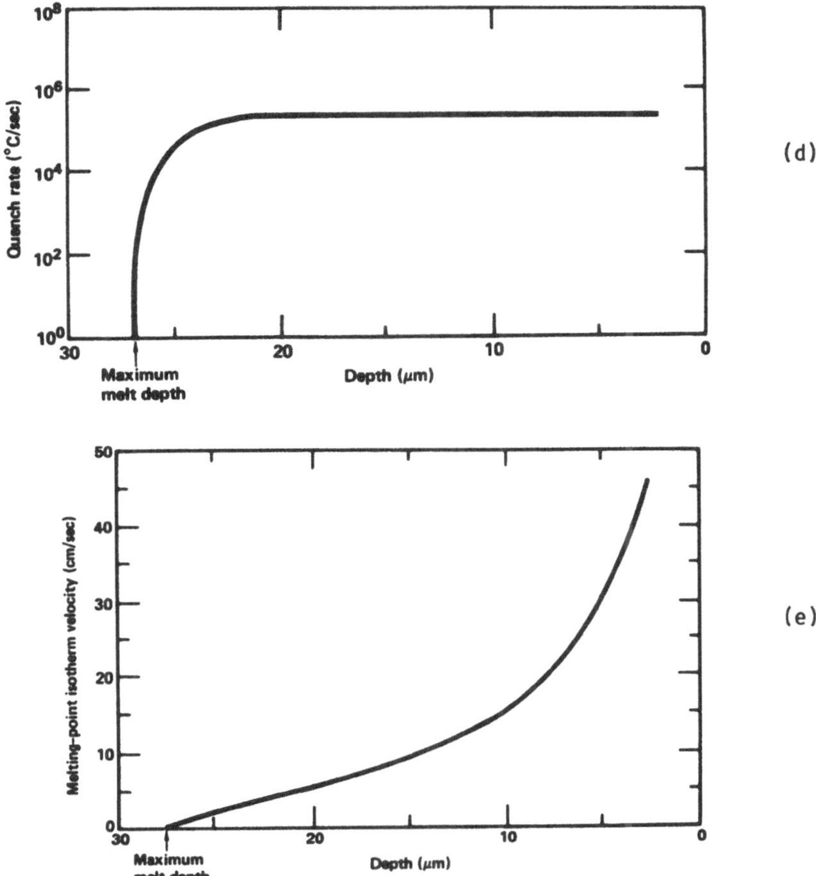

FIGURE 11. Computer simulation of surface processed Fe-Ni-P-B alloy (200 W, 100 cm/sec) showing: (d) quench rate as a function of depth with melted layer, (e) melting-point isotherm velocity as a function of depth within melted layer.

different electron beam traverse speeds. The first and most obvious point to note is that the depth at which glass formation occurs varies with the traverse speed such that at the highest speed the glass formation occurs at the greatest depth. This implies that the solidification rate rises most sharply in that case. Presumably the maximum critical growth velocity for the crystalline phase in this material is a constant. Therefore, one should be able to determine that velocity by comparing these three sets of data. This is done in Fig. 14, where it is seen that the common velocity where glass formation occurs is 5 cm/sec. This form of analysis, coupled with appropriate computer

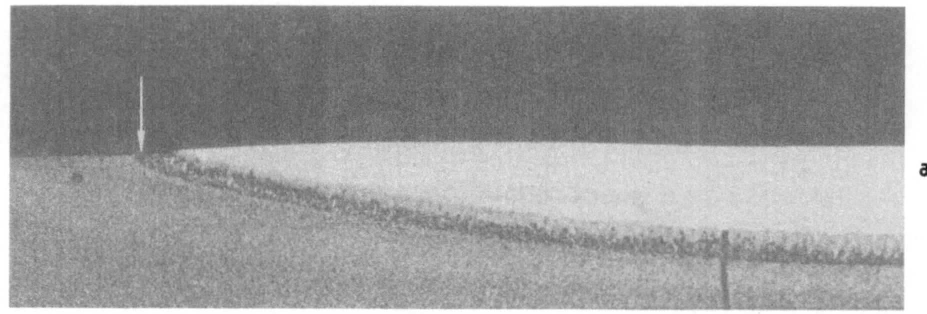

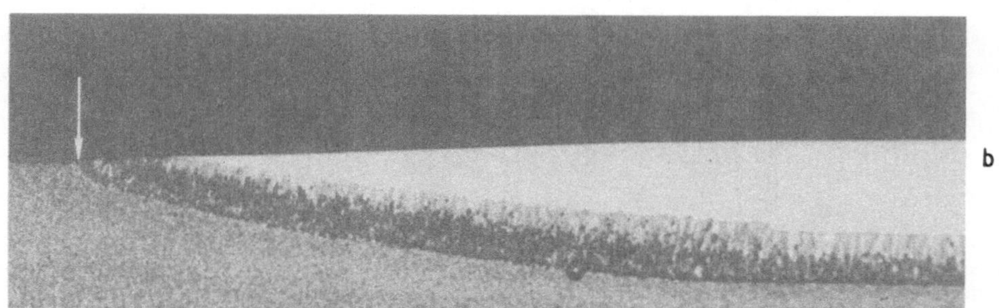

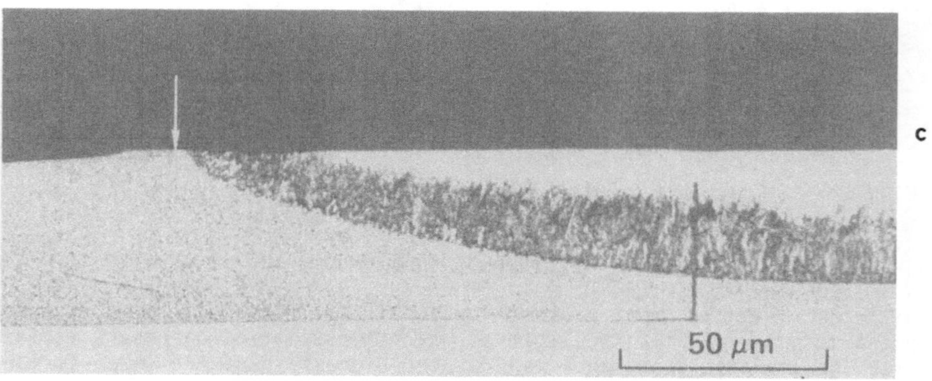

FIGURE 12. Optical metallographic cross section of an electron-beam processed (Fe-Ni-P-B) crystallized specimen at different translation velocities: (a) 100 cm/sec, (b) 50 cm/sec, (c) 20 cm/sec. The arrows define the sample surface and the left side of the melted layer. The uniformly light region at the bottom is the Cu backing.

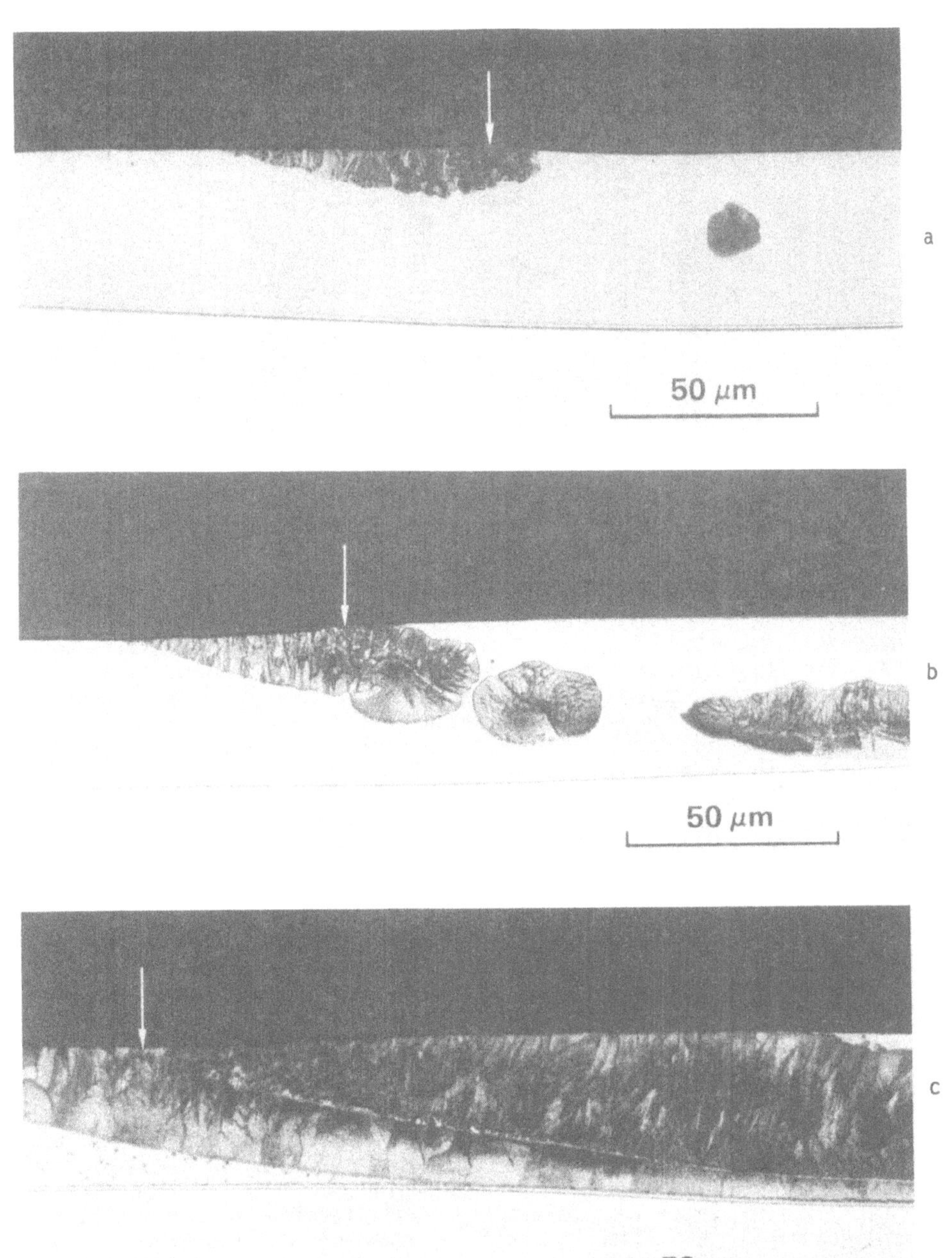

FIGURE 13. Optical metallographic series of cross sections for an amorphous specimen irradiated under the same conditions as in Fig. 12.

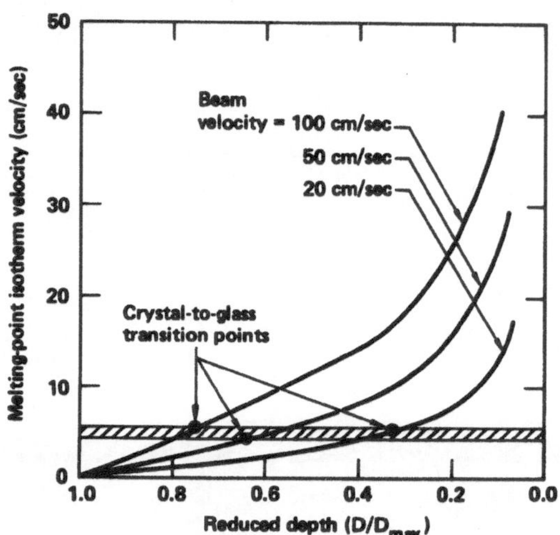

FIGURE 14. The calculated relationship of the retreating melting-point isotherm velocity to the reduced depth (depth within the melted layer in units of the maximum melt-depth) for the irradiation velocities shown in Fig. 12. The measured data for the crystal-to-glass transition has also been plotted on the respective curves.

simulation of the thermal history and isotherm velocities, should be applicable to measurements from this velocity range to quite high velocity ranges in order to develop systematic data on maximum critical growth velocities for a variety of phases. It should also be noted, referring to Fig. 12, that the initial morphology of the resolidifying liquid is that of a microcrystalline material. That is, in all cases the crystalline solid in contact with the liquid acts as a nucleation surface for the growth of crystalline material, and only after that occurs does reversion to glass take place at the appropriate velocity.

Turning to Fig. 13 which displays data taken under identical conditions for the amorphous starting material, one sees quite different results. At the highest velocities, the glass remains glass. That is to say, except for some anomalies near the edge of the melt stripe, there is virtually no evidence that the sample has been processed at all. Presumably the heating process has taken the glass, which is nothing but a viscous liquid, up in temperature to regions of very low viscosity and rapidly down in temperature before any devitrification or crystallization could occur. At the slower velocities, however, the temperature excursion was not sufficiently fast and one sees in the HAZ the characteristics of devitrification from the (viscous) glassy material. The morphology of the crystallites so formed is spherulitic and have clearly formed by nucleation and growth within the glassy phase. At still slower velocities, the devitrifiction of the glass proceeds so quickly that the low viscosity liquid above this region comes in contact with the devitrified glass and thus, replicating the results shown in Fig. 12, will crystallize using the devitrified glass as a nucleating surface.

The observation made for the devitrification of the HAZ can be quantified and summarized on a TTT diagram such as that shown in Fig. 15. This figure illustrates the C-shaped curves which are a result of extrapolation from actual crystallization measurements at lower temperature and longer times for this material. Also shown is the calculated trajectory using the computer simulation of the two fastest passes shown in Fig. 13, that of 50 and 100 cm/sec. One clearly sees that at the 100 cm/sec rate the heating and cooling is sufficiently fast so as to effectively bypass the nose of the transformation curve, whereas at slower speeds one begins to intersect the curve and therefore can explain the partial crystallization observed. Here again, one should point out that with accurate simulations, the validity of the extrapolation of the transformation curves as shown here can be verified, thus augmenting measurements made under more conventional conditions.

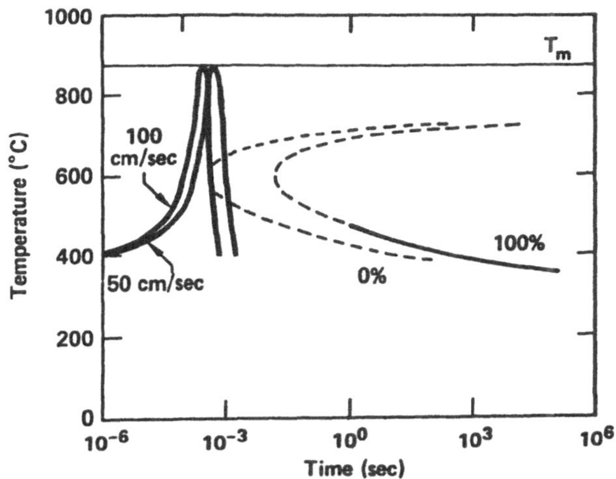

FIGURE 15. Time-Temperature-Transformation data for amorphous Fe-Ni-P-B. The continuous portion of the C-curve represents previously established crystallization kinetics. The dashed portion of the C-curve represents extrapolated start (0%) and finish (100%) times. The continuous lines at the left are the calculated temperature histories below the melted layer for the 50 and 100 cm/sec irradiation shown in Fig. 13.

4. SUMMARY

It has been our intention here to show only by way of example what types of nucleation and growth phenomena one might encounter in rapid surface melting experiments. We have intentionally avoided using the conventional mathematical descriptions of the nucleation and of the growth process. Formalism that has been discussed by other authors in this volume of course applies to everything discussed here. It is, however, noted that these analyses always include a parameterization wherein the value of the parameters is not known a priori. For example, in growth rate considerations, the ratio of the diffusion coefficient to some characteristic diffusion length, be it an atomic distance or a eutectic lamellar spacing, is required to explain observations. Similarly, in analysis of nucleation phenomena, the site densities and potency of catalytic sites are quantities which need to be parameterized. Thus, the suggested approach to the wide variety of problems yet to be resolved in this field is to utilize the form of surface processing illustrated here in a highly controlled way with adequate computer simulations such that the unknown parameters might be determined for a wide variety of cases. Establishing parameter trends in this way should lead to a more fundamental understanding of the parameters involved and eventually to a quantitative microscopic description of the nucleation and growth processes involved.

ACKNOWLEDGMENT

This work was performed under the auspices of the U.S. Department of Energy by Lawrence Livermore National Laboratory under Contract No. W-7405-Eng-48.

REFERENCES

1. W. J.Boettinger, in Rapidly Solidified Amorphous and Crystalline Alloys, edited by B. H. Kear, B. C. Giessen, and M. Cohen, Materials Research Society Symposium Proceedings (Elsevier, New York, 1982), Vol. 8, p. 15.
2. J. H. Perepezko and J. S. Paik, ibid., p. 49.
3. H. W. Bergmann, G. Barton, B. L. Mordike, and H. V. Fritsch, in Rapidly Solidified Metastable Materials, edited by B. H. Kear and B. C. Giessen, Materials Research Society Symposium Proceedings (Elsevier, New York, 1984), Vol. 28, p. 29.
4. D. A. Alden, T. B. Massalski, D. H. Lowndes, and E. N. Kaufmann, Scr. Metall. 19, 67 (1985).
5. W. J. Boettinger, in Proceedings of the Fourth International Conference on Rapidly Quenched Metals, edited by T. Mazumoto and K. Suzuki (Japan Inst. of Metals, Sendai, 1982), p. 99.
6. E. M. Breinan and B. H. Kear, Laser Materials Processing, edited by M. Bass (North-Holland, New York, 1983), p. 235.
7. H. Yoshioka, K. Asami, and K. Hashimoto, Scr. Metall. 18, 1215 (1984).
8. E. N. Kaufmann, R. J. Wallace, K. W. Mahin, C. J. Echer, F. J. Huegel, and C. W. Draper, in Amorphous Metals and Non-Equilibrium Processing, edited by M. Von Allmen (Les Editions de Physique, Les Ulis, France, 1985), p. 59.
9. W. H. Ferguson, B. C. Giessen, and N. J. Grant, Trans. Met. Soc. AIME 227, 1401 (1963).
10. R. J. Wallace and E. N. Kaufmann, "Nucleation and Growth in Surface-Melted Crystalline and Amorphous $Fe_{40}Ni_{40}P_{14}B_6$ Alloys," Journal of Materials Research 1, 27 (1986).

THE KINETICS OF RAPID CRYSTALLIZATION IN PURE METALS

C. A. MACDONALD AND F. SPAEPEN
Division of Applied Sciences, Harvard University, Cambridge, MA 02138

Key Words: transient reflectance, solidification velocity, collision-controlled crystallization

1. INTRODUCTION

Pulsed laser irradiation has been shown (1) to result in the formation and extremely rapid quenching of thin molten layers of both semiconductors and metals. The case of silicon has been extensively investigated. However, the solidification of silicon is also accompanied by a change in the character of the atomic bonding, from metallic in the liquid to covalent in the crystal. This work examines ultrarapid crystallization in metals in order to study the transition from a disordered state to one of long-range order in a system where the bonding is the same in the crystal and liquid. Some evidence exists that this may be a much more rapid process (2-5). One of the first quantitative observations (6) of a phase change in silicon during pulsed laser irradiation employed the transient reflectance technique. The liquid-crystal interface velocity in silicon was later measured directly using the transient change in conductance (7). Both of these experiments were facilitated by the dissimilarity of the crystal and its melt; the reflectance differs by a factor of two and the dc conductivity by several orders of magnitude. In metals the reflectance changes by only about 5% on melting and the dc conductance drops by at most a factor of two. This work employs a standard pump/probe technique to monitor transient changes in the reflectance during pulsed laser irradiation.

2. THEORY

The following kinetic analysis is based on the discussions by Turnbull (8-10). For any material, simple rate theory yields an expression for the crystal growth/melt velocity, u, as a function of the driving free energy of crystallization, ΔG_c:

$$u = f k_i \lambda \{1 - \exp \frac{\Delta G_c}{RT_i}\} \tag{1}$$

where k_i is the attempt frequency, f the fraction of sites in the interface at which incorporation into the crystal/melt is successful, and T_i the temperature of the interface. In the approximation that the (negative) entropy of crystallization, ΔS_c, is constant, one obtains:

$$\Delta G_c \simeq \Delta S_c (T_m - T_i) \tag{2}$$

Thus for small undercooling (or overheating) the velocity is proportional to the deviation from the melting temperature:

$$u = u_0 \frac{\Delta S_c}{R} \frac{(T_m - T_i)}{T_i} \tag{3}$$

where $u_0 = fk_i\lambda$ is the limiting velocity. It is in the nature of this limiting velocity that the solidification of metals can be expected to differ from that of silicon. If the attempt frequency is thermally activated, the growth velocity exhibits a fairly sharp maximum at some finite undercooling, as shown in Figure 1. Usually, the thermally activated process is identified with a diffusive jump similar to that for diffusion in the bulk liquid. In this case the growth velocity is limited by the rate of diffusion in the liquid. In general, in metals the crystal/liquid interface can be considered atomically rough, as its site fraction, f, is nearly unity. This corresponds to the "constant f" plot in Figure 1, which has no discontinuity in the slope of the interfacial velocity versus undercooling curve. For silicon, the site fraction is small, $f \simeq 0.06$, corresponding to a large entropy of crystallization. Thus the interfacial velocity is small for low undercoolings.

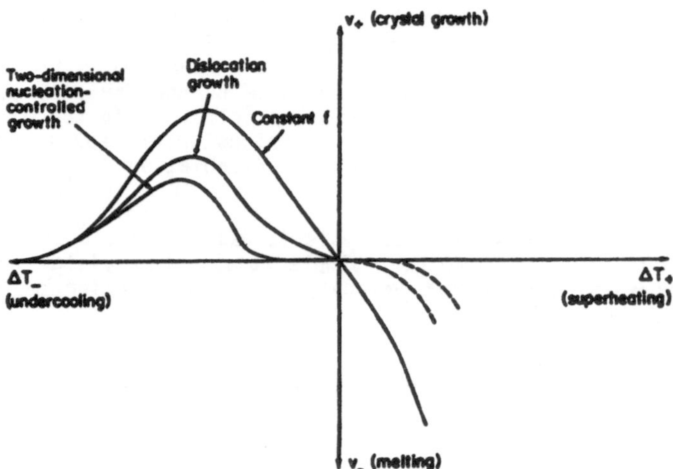

FIGURE 1. Schematic plot of the crystal-melt interface velocity as a function of deviation from the melting temperature for a thermally activated attempt frequency. The upper curve, labeled "constant f," is for an atomically rough interface. The other two curves are for different models on atomically smooth interfaces. From reference (17).

For metallic liquids, crystal growth may not be thermally activated, but rather collision-limited. The attempt frequency, k_i, is then equal to the frequency of thermal vibration and the prefactor, u_0, can be approximated by the speed of sound, u_s, in the liquid. This assumes that u_s is constant for all vibrational wavelengths. In this case the growth velocity continues to increase with decreasing temperature to much larger undercooling and remains non-zero down to very low temperatures.

In this work pulsed laser irradiation is employed to obtain the large thermal gradients needed to drive rapid crystallization. On a timescale of a picosecond or longer, the laser can be regarded as a heat source. The heat is deposited within the optical absorption depth of the surface ($\approx$ 20 nm for visible light in metals) and diffuses into the material under the influence of the resultant large thermal gradient. Using a linear approximation, the gradient can be estimated at the end of a 20 ps laser pulse:

$$\nabla T \approx \frac{T_s - T_r}{\sqrt{2D_{th}}} \approx 2 \times 10^8 \text{ K/cm} \qquad (4)$$

where T_s is the surface temperature ($\approx T_m$), T_r is the ambient temperature, D_{th} ($\approx$1 cm^2/s for gold) is the thermal diffusivity, and τ is the pulse length. The maximum melt depth, L, can be estimated by assuming that all of the energy absorbed from the laser is converted into the latent heat of melting, ΔH_c:

$$E = \frac{F}{(1 - R)} = \Delta H_c L \qquad (5)$$

Using a typical fluence, F, for this experiment of 0.02 J/cm^2, and the reflectivity for gold films at 0.53 µm, R = 50%, yields a value for the maximum melt depth of 100 nm. This provides a length scale to allow the thermal gradient to be estimated at the start of the crystal growth:

$$\nabla T \simeq \frac{(T_m - T_r)}{L} \simeq 10^8 \text{ K/cm} \qquad (6)$$

A simple heat flow analysis can be used to estimate the undercooling that will be produced at the crystal/melt interface by the applied gradient. An interface moving at a velocity u liberates the latent heat of crystallization per unit volume, ΔH_c, at a rate Q given by:

$$\dot{Q} = u\Delta H_c \qquad (7)$$

This heat released by crystallization must be balanced by heat flow due to the thermal gradient:

$$\dot{Q} = -\kappa(\nabla T)_i \tag{8}$$

(where the subscript i denotes values at the interface). Equating yields:

$$u = \frac{-\kappa}{\Delta H_c}(\nabla T)_i \tag{9}$$

Comparing to equation (3), one obtains an expression for the reduced interfacial undercooling, ΔT_r, as a function of the imposed gradient, $(\nabla T)_i$:

$$(\Delta T_r)_i = \frac{T_m - T_i}{T_m} = \frac{1}{u_0}\frac{R}{\Delta S_c}\frac{T_m}{T_i}\frac{\kappa}{\Delta H_c}(\nabla T)_i \tag{10}$$

Using equation (9) with the thermal gradient obtained in equation (6) and the literature values of the thermal conductivity (κ=3 J/cm-K-s), and the heat of crystallization ($\Delta H_c = 1.2 \times 10^3$ J/cm^3) for gold yields a maximum heat flow controlled interfacial velocity of 2.5×10^5 cm/s. Using this value in equation (1) with $u_0 = u_s \simeq 3 \times 10^5$ cm/s, a reduced undercooling of 0.5 is obtained. The crystallization is clearly interface controlled even for a collision-limited process. Note that the gradient calculated in equation (4) for the end of the pulse can be used in the symmetric equations (9) and (10) for the melt-in process to show that solid will be heated well above the melting temperature and that melting is thus also interface controlled.

3. DISCUSSION OF PREVIOUS WORK

A variety of evidence exists to support the hypothesis that crystal growth in pure metals is collision-limited. Nickel dendrites have been observed (2) to grow into the melt at velocities up to 50 m/s. The measured ambient reduced undercooling of 0.1 is an upper limit to the value at the liquid-crystal interface. Since for metals $\Delta S_c \sim R$, equation (2) predicts a velocity of ~300 m/s. Comparison between this estimate and the measured value of 50 m/s sets a lower limit on the velocity prefactor, $u_0 = k_i\lambda f$, of $u_s/6$. Turnbull (10) has noted that crystallization of dilute amorphous metal alloys at temperatures as low as 30 K (3,4), far below the diffusional kinetic freezing temperature, T_g, implies the existence of a faster process for crystallization than diffusion. In addition, there exists indirect evidence for rapid regrowth velocities in metals after pulsed laser melting (5). Large ($\simeq$1 μm) grains were observed in a previously fine grained ($\simeq$50 nm) iron sample after irradiation by a 30 ps pulse. If the regrowth is assumed to have taken place during 1-2 ns, as predicted by a simple heat flow analysis, the regrowth velocity must have been 500-1000 m/s.

In this work the melt duration, and therefore crystal-melt interface velocity, is determined from the time-resolved reflectance measurements of a metal film following pulsed laser irradiation. In a similar experiment on silicon, Liu (6) observed a large (factor of 2) transient increase in the reflectivity corresponding to the metallic melt, followed by a return to the original value as the surface crystallized. The measurements of Thompson et al. (7) of transient conductance in silicon are consistent with these results and also with heat flow calculations. The largest measured crystallization velocity in silicon is ≃15 m/s (11).

Smaller changes in reflectivity are expected in the case of metals because of the similarity of the liquid and solid phases. The Drude theory for an ideal electron gas can be used to preduct the trends of reflectivity with heating and melting. For an ideal gas at zero temperature, the reflectivity is unity for frequencies below the plasma frequency and zero above. Electron-lattice (phonon) interactions soften the transition and decrease the reflectivity below the plasma frequency. Higher temperatures result in more phonon scattering, and thus lower reflectances, similar to the decrease in dc conductivity. Similarly, melting also increases the electron-phonon interaction and decreases the reflectivity. The quantitative value of the change on melting is difficult to compute, and variations occur between samples with different preparation (12-15).

4. EXPERIMENTS

4.1. Optics

Two different lasers are employed to study different time regimes. The first is a 40 ns ruby laser (0.69 μm) used in the setup shown in Figure 2. A continuous wave He:Ne laser is used to monitor the surface reflectivity, transmission, or back surface reflectivity (the latter two for thin films on transparent substrates). The signals from the silicon photo-detectors are observed directly on a fast oscilloscope to achieve a time resolution of 2 ns. A typical reflectance trace is displayed in Figure 3. A slight decrease in the reflectivity is observed, followed by a recovery to the original value in a few hundred nanoseconds.

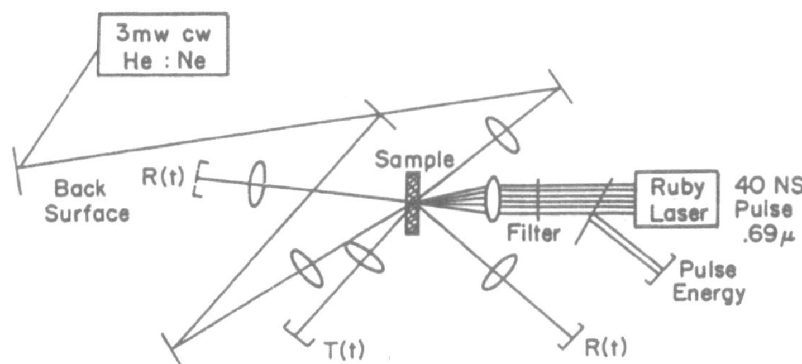

FIGURE 2. Experimental setup for transient reflectance measurements using 40 ns ruby laser pulses to heat the sample.

The second laser, which was used to produce the results to be discussed in Section 5, is a 20 ps Nd:YAG laser with fundamental output at 1.06 μm. The setup for this laser is shown in Figure 4. Part of each

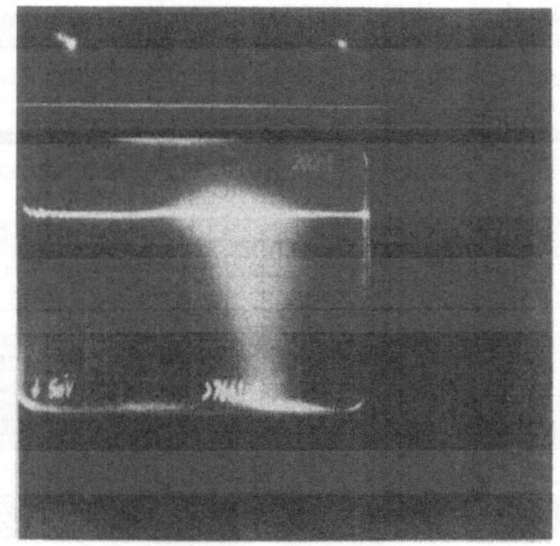

FIGURE 3. Oscilloscope trace of the signal from the He:Ne probe beam reflected off the sample versus time. The ruby laser pulse occurred at the beginning of the trace. A slight initial drop in the reflectivity begins to recover by 500 ns. The time calibration is 200 ns per large division. The zero of the reflectivity is indicated by the start of the vertical bar on the left.

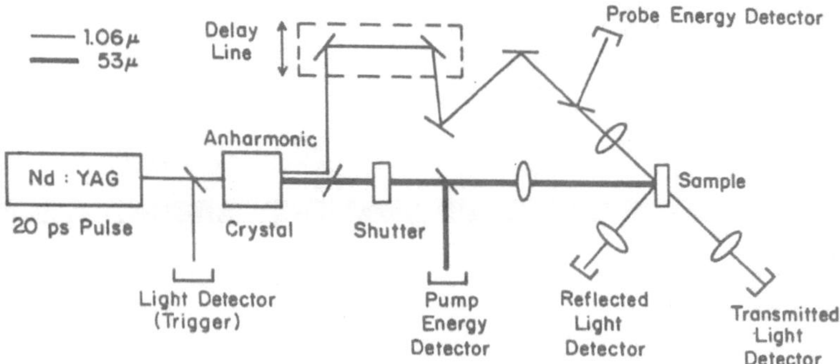

FIGURE 4. Experimental setup for transient reflectance measurements employing 20 ps Nd:YAG laser pulses.

pulse is frequency doubled (to 0.53 µm) and used to melt the sample. The remainder at the fundamental frequency is reduced in intensity, delayed relative to the pump pulse and used to probe the sample. In addition, the sample reflectance is measured before and after each pump shot. A typical plot of reflectivity versus pump fluence for the delay of 2 ns is shown in Figure 5.

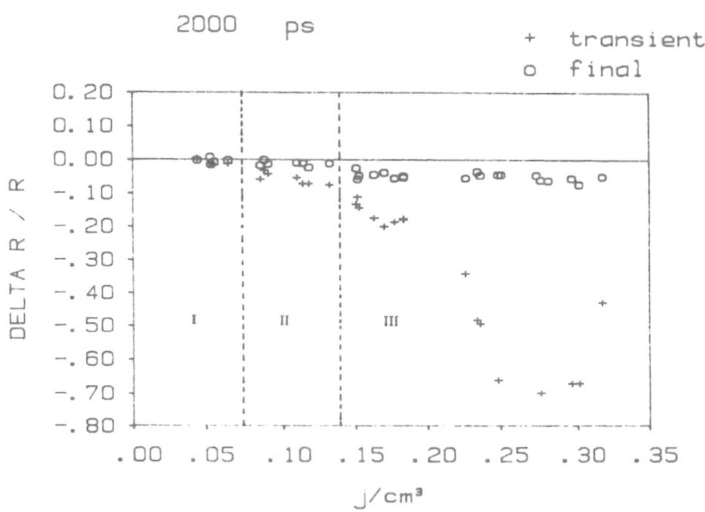

FIGURE 5. Plot of the relative change in sample reflectivity 2 ns (+) and several seconds (o) after irradiation by a 20 ps laser pulse for a variety of laser fluences. Fluence regime I corresponds to solid surface heating, regime II to melting, and regime III to permanent surface damage.

4.2. Sample Preparation

Homogeneous polycrystalline gold films of 20-250 nm thickness were produced by RF sputtering on a variety of highly polished substrates (silicon, sapphire, glass) in a low-vacuum chamber designed for coating SEM samples. Thin copper and aluminum films were produced by vapor deposition. Compositionally modulated thin films were used to determine whether melting had occurred. These thin films (with alternate 2.5-10 nm layers of gold and copper, chosen for complete miscibility) were produced on polished glass or silicon substrates by ion beam sputtering (16). Because the solid state diffusion rates are slow, mixing of the layers can only occur in the liquid state. Mixing of the layers is thus a signature of melting as a result of pulsed laser irradiation. The repeat distance of the as-deposited modulation is verified by observing the angle of the X-ray diffraction satellite. It is usual to observe at least two higher harmonics (indicating sharper than sinusoidal modulation); for one long modulation repeat length (20 nm) film, ten harmonics were observed. Composition versus depth profiles were obtained by Auger spectroscopy on the surface with simultaneous ion beam sputtering to mill away the layers. A typical profile is shown in Figure 6.

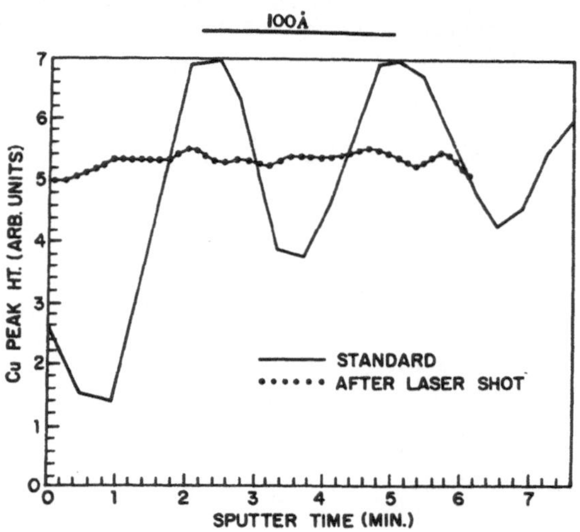

FIGURE 6. Auger spectroscopy profile of copper concentration versus depth in a copper/gold modulated film of 100 Å repeat length. The solid line is for an as-deposited film, the dotted line for the film irradiated at the fluence marked in Figure 5, which was obtained for the same sample. The decay in the composition modulation confirms that melting has occurred at this fluence.

5. RESULTS

Auger analysis and optical microscopy were used to identify the threshold fluence for melting. Unambiguous determination of melting is essential to establish whether transient decays in the reflectivity, as seen in Figure 3, are due to melting or solid surface heating. Microscopic examination of the surface of a 0.25 µm thick gold film after the pulse producing the reflectivity trace of Figure 3 shows some slight damage, indicating that the fluence was above the melt threshold. More convincing evidence is obtained from Auger analysis on modulated films. Figure 5 presents a plot of reflectivity change versus frequency-doubled Nd:YAG laser fluence for a modulated Au/Cu film of 10 nm repeat length. The data can be divided into three fluence regimes. In the first (below 0.04 J/cm^2) no reflectivity change is observed. In the second (between 0.04 and 0.15 J/cm^2) there is a transient reduction in the reflectivity, followed by complete recovery. Above 0.15 J/cm^2 there is no recovery as a result of permanent damage. These features were common to all the materials studied. Auger depth profiles before and after irradiation of the film of Figure 5 are shown in Figure 6. The irradiation fluence is indicated by the mark in Figure 5, and is in the intermediate regime. The mixing of the layers confirms that melting has occurred in this regime.

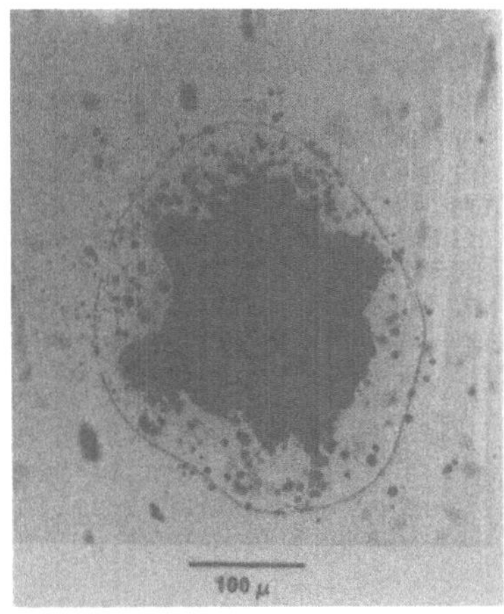

FIGURE 7. Optical micrograph of a damage spot from ps laser irradiation on a compositionally modulated Au/Cu film of repeat length 50 Å and overall thickness of 1000 Å on a glass substrate. The metal has been removed from the dark central area. The rough boundary of the dark region and surrounding speckled area are typical features that also occur in elemental metal films. The sharp circular line is seen only for modulated films.

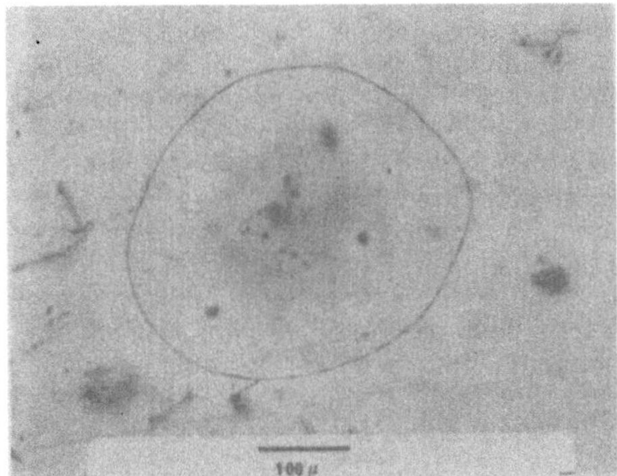

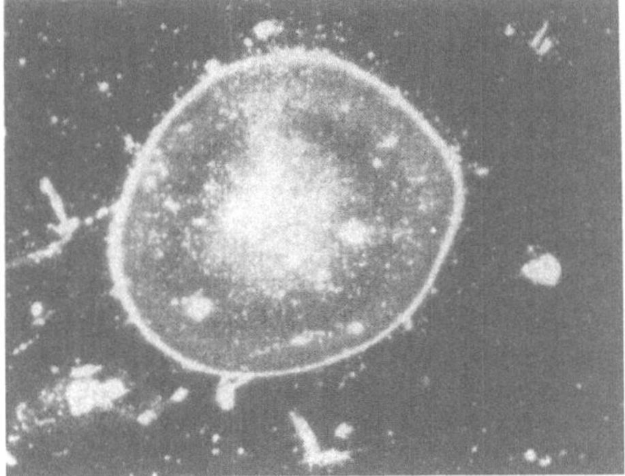

FIGURE 8. Optical micrographs (left) and dark field optical micrograph (right) of a ps laser irradiated damage spot on a Au/Cu film with 50 Å repeat length and 1000 Å overall thickness on a silicon substrate. The sample is the same as in Figure 5. The shot is in the third fluence regime.

Figures 7 and 8 are optical micrographs of typical permanent damage spots (fluence regime III) resulting from ps laser irradiation of a modulated Au/Cu film. Figure 9 is the intermediate regime irradiation spot corresponding to II in Figures 5 and 6. The major feature of Figure 7 is a rough-edged boundary of an inner region in which the metal has been removed from the surface. There is also a surrounding, speckled region. These features are also observed on pure metal films. The sharp circle appearing in Figures 7 and 8 is observed only in compositionally modulated samples. Scanning Auger profiling indicates that the circle may be the edge of a pit from which one or more of the 5 nm layers have been removed. For the sample in Figure 9 the rough-edged boundary was not observed. Note that outside the sharp circle there is a light ring created at lower fluences.

If a surface damage feature can be associated with a particular fluence threshold, then the damage radius, r_d, can be expressed as a function of the applied fluence, f. For a Gaussian beam intensity profile this becomes:

$$f_{th} = f \exp \frac{-r_d^2}{2\sigma^2} \tag{11a}$$

or:

$$r_d^2 = 2\sigma^2 \ln(f) - 2\sigma^2 \ln(f_{th}) \tag{11b}$$

where f_{th} is the threshold fluence. If r_d^2 is plotted versus ln(f) for the sharp circular feature seen in the sample in Figure 8, the result, shown in Figure 10, is reasonably linear, and yields a threshold (0.02 J/cm^2) equal to the start of the third, permanent damage, fluence regime in Figure 5. This implies that circle is the boundary of the damage region, consistent with the Auger profiling results. This damage may be the result of evaporation. Similar results are obtained for the rough boundary of the type seen in Figure 7. The second line in Figure 10 is a plot for the faint circular region seen in Figure 9. In this case, the threshold corresponds to the beginning of the intermediate fluence regime in Figure 5, as does that for the "speckled" region of the type shown in Figure 7. These features, therefore, correspond to melting.

To produce plots of reflectivity, R, the transmitivity, T, versus time the fluence regions such as those shown in Figure 5 were divided into bins. A plot of the relative change in R(t) and T(t) from the initial value at each spot of a 20 nm thick gold film on a sapphire substrate is shown in Figure 11 for two fluences in the intermediate regime. For the lower fluence bin, the reflectivity begins to recover to 400 ps, and recovery is complete in 600 ps. If this recovery is interpreted as due to the movement of the crystal-melt interface, then the regrowth velocity is:

$$u \sim \frac{200 \times 10^{-10}\ \text{m}}{200 \times 10^{-12}\ \text{s}} \simeq 100\ \text{m/s} \tag{12}$$

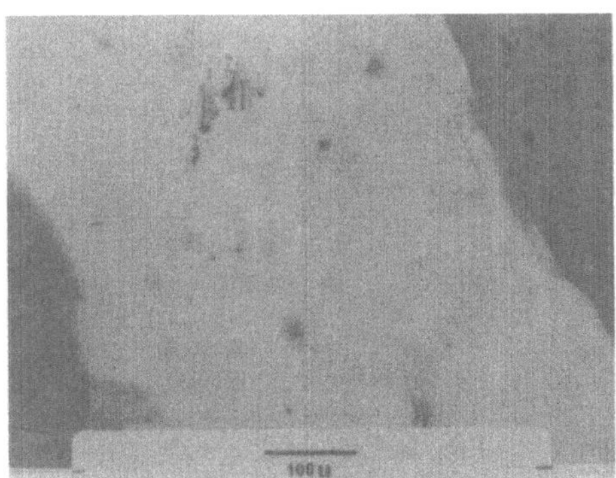

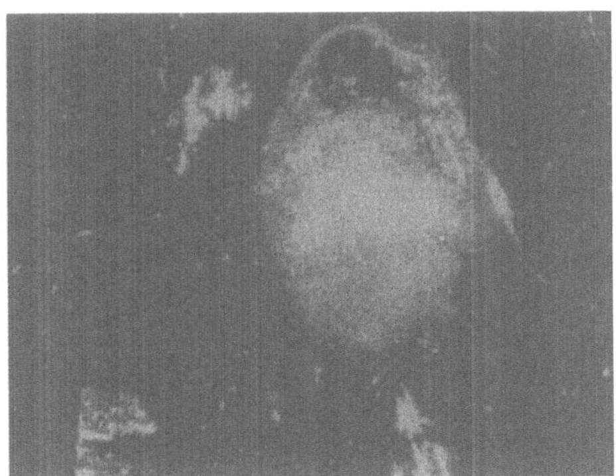

FIGURE 9. Optical (left) and optical dark field (right) micrograph of the laser damage spot profiled in Figure 6. The dark bands in the upper right and lower left are ink marks used to locate the shot. A faint oval outline, roughly one quarter of the picture wide, can be seen just right of center. The interior of the oval is light in the scattered light image.

It should be noted that this result is obtained for a thin film on an insulating substrate. The heat flow, and thus expected interfacial velocity, here is slower than for the bulk case discussed above (Section 2). Figure 12 displays similar results for a bulk copper specimen. Here recovery begins at 600 ps and ends by 1 ns. Assuming that the reflectivity samples a depth equal to the skin depth (~ 25 nm) allows the interfacial velocity for the last stage of crystallization to be estimated at roughly 60 m/s. The peak crystallization velocity for this sample occurred deeper in the specimen than could be sampled. The fluence thresholds for the start of the middle regime in both these cases are similar (0.01-0.02 J/cm^2). The fluence threshold for the bulk is similar to that of the thin film, firstly because the thermal diffusion length during irradiation is only a factor of two or three times larger than the film thickness, and secondly because this may be compensated by a slightly lower reflectivity for bulk copper than for thin film gold. (Actual reflectivities were not measured at the pump frequency but should be on the order of 50%.) In addition, in all the cases in which a transient, recoverable change in reflectivity was observed, the magnitude of the relative change was about 5%. (Absolute probe reflectivities in the infrared varied from 80 to 90%.)

6. CONCLUSIONS

Transient reflectivity measurements can be used to monitor the interfacial regrowth velocities in metals. Optical microscopy and Auger analysis of compositionally modulated films were used to establish that the transient decays in sample reflectivity were accompanied by surface melting. The fastest crystallization velocity measured in this experiment was 100 m/s. This value is the highest known to the authors for

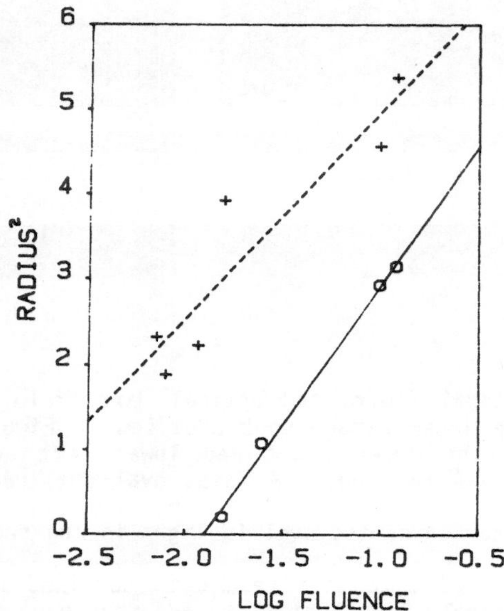

FIGURE 10. Plot of the square of the radius of the sharp circular feature seen in Figure 8 versus the log of the applied fluence (o). The solid line is a least squares fit. The crosses (+) are for the faint outline seen in Figure 9 (which corresponds to the light area outside the circle in Figure 8). The dotted line is also a least squares fit.

any material and is substantially larger than the maximum measured for silicon. This observation supports the theory that crystallization in metals is collision-limited.

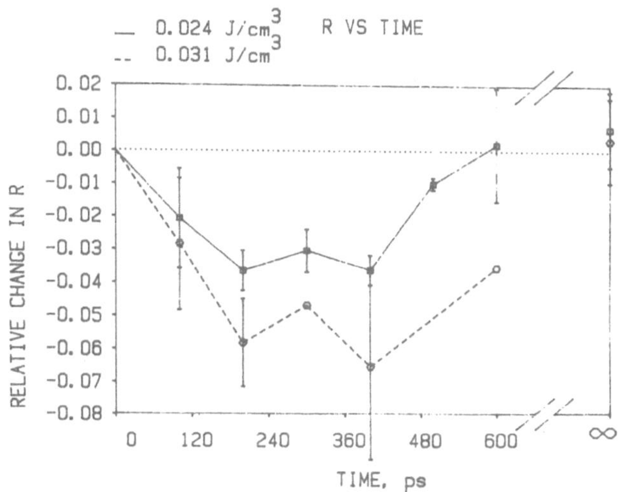

FIGURE 11. Relative change in the sample reflectivity, $(R(t)-R_0)/R_0$, for 20 ps laser irradiation at two different fluences on a 200 Å thick gold film with a sapphire substrate.

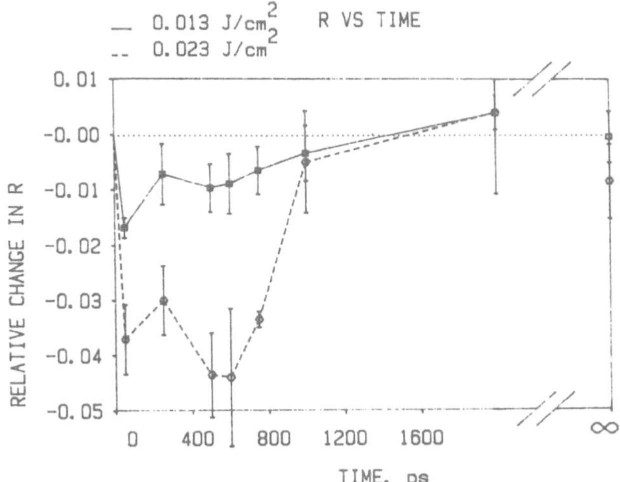

FIGURE 12. Relative change in sample reflectivity versus time for 20 ps laser irradiation on a bulk copper specimen.

ACKNOWLEDGMENTS

The authors acknowledge useful discussions with Prof. D. Turnbull and extensive assistance with the Nd:YAG laser by Dr. A. M. Malvezzi. This work has been supported by the Office of Naval Research under contract number N00014-83-K-0030.

REFERENCES

1. See, for example, Energy Beam-Solid Interactions and Transient Thermal Processing, edited by J. C. Fan and N. M. Johnson (North Holland, New York, 1984).
2. J. L. Walker, in B. Chalmers, Principles of Solidification (Wiley, New York, 1964), pp. 114-115.
3. M. R. Bennett and J. B. Wright, Phys. Status Solidi A 13, 135 (1972).
4. W. Buckel, Z. Physik 138, 136 (1954).
5. C. J. Lin and F. Spaepen, in Chemistry and Physics of Rapidly Solidified Materials, edited by B. J. Berkowitz and R.O. Scattergood (TMS-AIME, 1983).
6. P. L. Liu et al., Appl. Phys. Lett. 34, 864 (1979).
7. M. O. Thompson et al., Phys Rev. Lett. 50, 896 (1983).
8. D. Turnbull, in Physical Processes in Laser-Materials Interactions (NATO-ASI 1980 Pianore, Italy, Plenum Press, 1983).
9. S. R. Coriell and D. Turnbull, Acta Metall. 30, 2135 (1982).
10. D. Turnbull, J. de Physique C4, 1.
11. W. L. Brown in Ref. 1, p. 9.
12. K. Ujihara, J. Appl. Phys. 43, 2376 (1972).
13. S. D. Pudkov, Zh. Tekh. Fiz. 47, 649 (1977).
14. G. S. Arnold, Applied Opt. 23, 1434 (1984).
15. H. G. Dreehsen, J. Appl. Phys. 56, 238 (1984).
16. F. Spaepen et al., Rev. Sci. Instrum. 56, 1340 (1985).
17. F. Spaepen and D. Turnbull, in Laser Annealing of Semiconductors, edited by J. Poate (Academic press, 1982).

GENESIS OF MELTING

S. WILLIAMSON AND G. MOUROU
Laboratory for Laser Energetics, University of Rochester,
250 East River Road, Rochester, New York 14623-1299

Key Words: superheating, nucleation of melt, time-resolved electron-diffraction

1. INTRODUCTION

The fundamental process responsible for initiating the melting of condensed matter has remained a mysterious and, as yet, unsolved problem. The long-standing interest in this most basic of phase transitions has nevertheless resulted in a great number of theoretical interpretations. The key question still to be answered is, what happens on the atomic scale when a crystal melts?

Theories are available that deal with the actual microscopic mechanism of melting (1-4). However, as is often the case, progress on experimental verification has lagged behind. The difficulty that arises is in making a microscopic observation on a time scale appropriate to the ongoing process.

In the past ten years the short-pulse laser has evolved as an ideal tool for studying phase transitions. In addition to supplying energy densities large enough to create a melt in a time much shorter than the transition time, the optical pulse can also be used to probe the melting substance. An important consequence of this feature is that we can now drive a solid to a superheated temperature faster than the system can respond. Figure 1 shows a conventional phase diagram where path 1 is followed under normal equilibrium conditions. If a quantity of energy, E_a, is rapidly deposited into the system, the path taken is that along the equipartition energy line, path 2. Depending on the peak power of the laser pulse and the system in question, the range over which superheating occurs is several thousand degrees. The time τ_{melt}, is then the actual material-dependent melting time. The departure of path 1 from the equipartition line is indicative of defect formation. With the short-pulse laser and a suitable probe, the rate of defect formation even below the melt threshold can be time-resolved.

Several probe techniques have now been developed to time-resolve phase transformations in semiconductors during laser annealing. However, most of these probes (e.g., electrical conductivity (5,6), optical reflection (7,8), optical transmission (9), Raman scattering (10), and time of flight mass spectrometry (11)) supply no direct information about the atomic structure nor the temperature of the material. Probing the structure can reveal when and to what degree a system melts as it is defined by degradation in the long-range order of the lattice. True structural probes based on X-ray (12) and low-energy electron diffraction (13), and EXAFS (14) with nanosecond time resolution, have been developed offering fresh insight into both the bulk and surface dynamics of material structure. Also, a subpicosecond probe based on structural dependent second

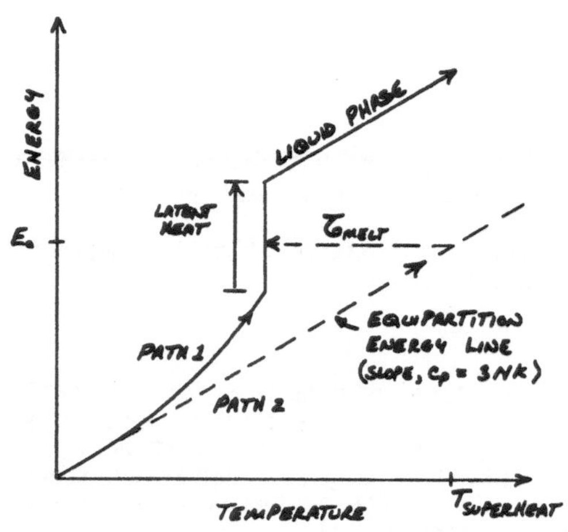

FIGURE 1. Caloric diagram of the solid and liquid phases for a simple metal. Path 1 is followed when the energy is deposited on a time scale slower than the defect formation time. Path 2 is followed when the energy is deposited instantaneously.

harmonic generation (15) has been demonstrated. But at present, only the technique of picosecond electron diffraction (16) can produce an unambiguous picture of the atomic structure on the picosecond time scale.

In this paper we describe an experiment utilizing this instrument to time-resolve the laser-induced phase transition in aluminum. The results are then interpreted in the context of the defect theory of melting.

2. EXPERIMENT AND RESULTS

The technique takes advantage of the strong scattering efficiency of 25 keV electrons in transmission mode to produce and record a diffraction pattern with as few as 10^4 electrons in a pulse of 20 ps duration. The burst of electrons is generated from a modified streak camera that, via the photoelectric effect, converts an optical pulse to an electron pulse of equal duration (17). Also of importance is the fact that the electron pulse can be synchronized with picosecond resolution to the laser pulse (18). The experimental arrangement is illustrated in Fig. 2. A single pulse from an active-passive modelocked Nd^{+3}:YAG laser is spatially filtered and amplified to yield energies up to 10 mJ. The streak tube (deflection plates removed), specimen, and phosphor screen are placed in vacuum at 10^{-6} mm Hg. The electron tube is comprised of the photocathode, extraction grid, focusing cone, and anode. A gold photocathode is used to permit the vacuum chamber to be opened to air. The photocathode is held at the maximum voltage (-25 kV) so that space charge, which can cause significant temporal broadening, is minimized. The portion of the laser irradiating the photocathode is first upconverted to the fourth harmonic of the fundamental wavelength in order to

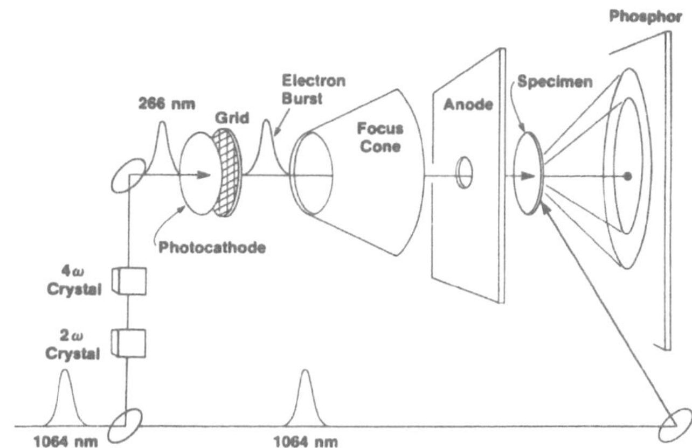

FIGURE 2. Schematic of picosecond electron diffraction apparatus. A streak camera tube (deflection plates removed) is used to produce the electron pulse. The 25 keV electron pulse passes through the Al specimen and produces a diffraction pattern of the structure with a 20 ps exposure.

produce the electrons efficiently. The duration of the UV pulse and thus the electron pulse is ~20 ps. Once the electron pulse is generated, it accelerates through the tube past the anode and then remains at a constant velocity. The specimen is located in this drift region. The electrons pass through the specimen with a beam diameter of 500 μm and come to a 200 μm focus at their diffracted positions on the phosphor screen. A gated microchannel plate image intensifier in contact with the phosphor screen amplifies the electron signal $\sim 10^4$ times.

A metal was chosen over a semiconductor as the specimen because of the ease with which metals can be fabricated in ultra-thin polycrystalline films. The specimens were fabricated by first depositing Al onto formvar substrates and then vapor-dissolving away the formvar. Free-standing films 250 ± 2 nm in thickness were required so that the electrons sustain, on the average, one elastic collision while passing through the specimen. This thickness of Al corresponds to twice the 1/e penetration depth at 1060 nm. It is worth noting that the penetration depth for a metal does not vary significantly from solid to liquid as is the case with a semiconductor where a change in absorption of one to two orders of magnitude is possible. Since the diffusion length $(D\tau)^{1/2}$, where D is the thermal diffusivity coefficient (0.86 cm^2/s) and τ is time, is limited to 25 nm, the temperature in the Al is uniformly established in less than 10 ps. The absorption of the laser by aluminum is 13 ± 1 percent.

The diameter of the laser stimulus is ~4 mm ($1/e^2$) and is centered over the 2 mm specimen. A 1 mm pinhole positioned in place of the specimen facilitates accurate alignment of the laser beam profile to the electron beam. Using a 1 mm pinhole assures accurate measurement of the fluence within the probed region. Synchronization between the electron pulse and the laser stimulus is then accomplished by means of a laser-activated deflection plate assembly (19).

The experimental procedure is then to stimulate the aluminum sample with the laser while monitoring the lattice structure at a given delay. The films are used only once, even though for low fluence levels ($\leq$8 mJ/cm^2) the films could survive repeated shots. Figure 3 shows the laser-induced time-resolved phase transformation of aluminum at a constant fluence of ~13 mJ/cm^2. The abrupt disappearance of rings in

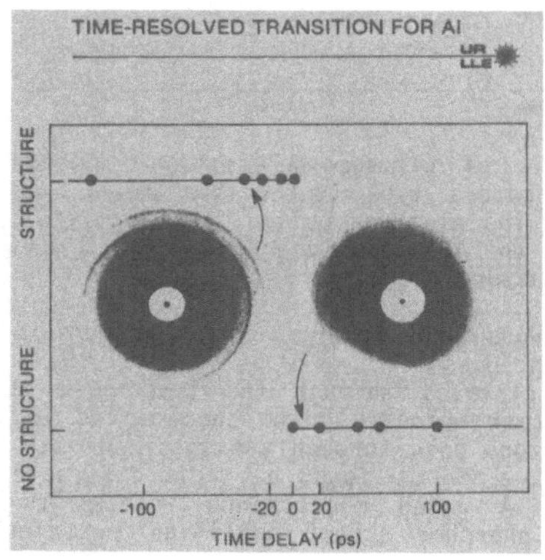

FIGURE 3. Time-resolved laser-induced phase transition in aluminum. The pattern on the left is the diffraction pattern for Al and represents the points along the top line - where the electron pulse arrives before the laser stimulus. The pattern on the right shows the loss of structure in the Al 20 ps (or more) after applying the laser stimulus at a fluence of 13 mJ/cm^2. The fine line background structure occurring in both pictures is an artifact of the circular averaging technique.

the diffraction pattern occurs with a delay of 20 ps. As is evident, the breakdown of lattice order can be induced in a time shorter than the resolution of our probe. However, the fluence required for this rapid transiton exceeds F_{melt}, the calculated fluence required to completely melt the Al specimen under equilibrium conditions (~ 5 mJ/cm^2). At a constant fluence of 11 mJ/cm^2 the phase transition was again observed but only after a probe delay of 60 ps. Figure 4 shows the melt metamorphosis of Al where the points represent the delay time before the complete phase transition is observed for various fluence levels. We see that the elapsed time increases exponentially with decreased fluence

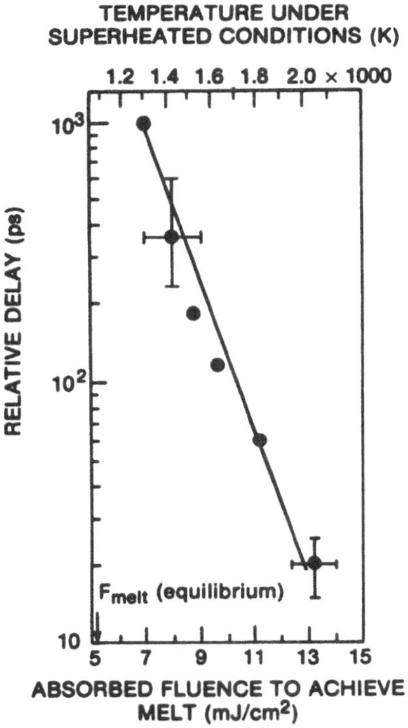

FIGURE 4. Laser-induced melt metamorphosis for aluminum. The points mark the elapsed time for the diffraction rings to completely disappear. The vertical error bar represents the degree of uncertainty in defining the moment of complete melt. The region beneath the curve represents the conditions under which the Al is left in a superheated solid state.

and at 7 mJ/cm^2 the delay is ~1 ns. Because the fluence level that is applied is always in excess of F_{melt}, the observed delay time suggests that the Al is first driven to a superheated solid state before melting. It must be pointed out that as the fluence was decreased, the abruptness with which the rings disappeared became less dramatic. Consequently, determination of the precise delay increases in difficulty with decreasing fluence. The temperature scale represents the temperature of the superheated Al assuming a linear increase in the specific heat with temperature. We see that temperatures in excess of 2000°K are expected with fluence levels near 13 mJ/cm^2. The region beneath the curve represents the conditions under which the Al can be observed in a superheated solid state.

3. CONCLUSIONS

In conclusion, we have demonstrated that the picosecond electron-diffraction technique can be used to provide time resolution of the laser-induced melt evolution in aluminum. We found it possible to melt the aluminum completely in a time shorter than 20 ps if sufficient laser fluence is applied ($\geq 2.6 \times F_{melt}$). The time required to melt the aluminum increases exponentially with decreasing fluence and at $1.4 \times F_{melt}$ the phase transition time increased to ~1 ns. During this time, the two phases coexist as a heterogeneous melt while the superheated solid is being continuously transformed into liquid. We have interpreted the results in the context of the defect theory of melting and found that the activation energy measured agrees with that of Schottky defect formation.

ACKNOWLEDGMENT

This work was supported by the U.S. Department of Energy Office of Inertial Fusion under agreement No. DE-FC08-85DP40200 and by the Laser Fusion Feasibility Project at the Laboratory for Laser Energetics which has the following sponsors: Empire State Electric Energy Research Corporation, General Electric Company, New York State Energy Research and Development Authority, Northeast Utilities Service Company, Ontario Hydro, Southern California Edison Company, The Standard Oil Company, and the University of Rochester. Such support does not imply endorsement of the content by any of the above parties.

We would like to acknowledge the support of Jerry Drumheller, who assisted in the fabrication of the Al films, as well as to thank Hsiu-Cheng Chen for her help during the experiment.

REFERENCES

1. F. C. Frank, Proc. R. Soc. A 170, 182 (1939).
2. J. Frenkel, Kinetic Theory of Liquids (Dover Publications, 1955).
3. J. E. Lennard-Jones and A. F. Devonshire, Proc. R. Soc. A 169, 317; ibid. 170, 464 (1939).
4. D. Kuhlman-Wildorf, Phys. Rev. A 140, 1599 (1965).
5. M. Yamada, H. Kotani, K. Yamazaki, K. Yamamoto, and K. Abe, J. Phys. Soc. Jpn. 49, 1299 (1980).
6. G. J. Galvin, M. O. Thompson, J. W. Mayer, R. B. Hamond, N. Paulter, and P. S. Peercy, Phys. Rev. Lett 48, 33 (1982).
7. D. H. Auston, C. M. Surko, T. N. C. Venkatesan, R. E. Slusher, and J. A. Golovchenko, Appl. Phys. Lett. 33, 437 (1978).
8. C. V. Shank, R. Yen, and C. Hirlimann, Phys. Rev. Lett. 50, 454 (1983).
9. J. M. Liu, H. Kurz, and N. Bloembergen, Appl. Phys. Lett. 41, 643 (1982).
10. H. W. Lo and A.Compaan, Phys. Rev. Lett. 44, 1604 (1980).
11. A. Pospieszczyk, M. A. Harith, and B. Stritzker, J. Appl. Phys. 54, 3176 (1983).
12. B. C. Larson, C. W. White, T. S. Noggle, and D. Mills, Phys. Rev. Lett 48, 337 (1982).
13. R. S. Becker, G. S. Higashi, and J. A. Golovchenko, Phys. Rev. Lett. 52, 307 (1984).
14. H. M. Epstein, R. E. Schwerzel, P. J. Mallozzi, and B. E. Campbell, J. Am. Chem. Soc. 105, 1466 (1983).
15. C. V. Shank, R. Yen, and C. Hirliman, Phy. Rev. Lett. 51, 900 (1983).
16. G. Mourou and S. Williamson, Appl. Phys. Lett. 41, 44 (1982).
17. D. J. Bradley and W. Sibbett, Appl. Phys. Lett. 27, 382 (1975).
18. G. Mourou and W. Knox, Appl. Phys. Lett. 36, 623 (1980).
19. S. Williamson, G. Mourou, and S. Letzring, Proc. 15th Int. Cong. on High Speed Photography, 348 (I), 197 (1983).

AMORPHOUS GALLIUM PRODUCED BY PULSED EXCIMER LASER IRRADIATION

J. FRÖHLINGSDORF AND B. STRITZKER
Institut für Festkörperforschung, Kernforschungsanlage Jülich,
5170 Jülich, Federal Republic of Germany

Key Words: superconducting transition, amorphous gallium

ABSTRACT

Pure crystalline Ga films (α-Ga, β-Ga) have been irradiated at low temperatures (≤ 20 K) with an excimer laser. By measuring the superconducting transition temperature T_c and the residual resistivity ρ_0, the resulting Ga phases (α-Ga, β-Ga, a-Ga) can be identified.

Both crystalline Ga phases can be transformed into the amorphous phase. The threshold energy density for the $\beta \rightarrow a$ transition depends on the film thickness, whereas the $\alpha \rightarrow a$ transition occurs at about 225 mJ/cm^2. This behavior is in agreement with earlier observations that a-Ga can grow on top of the α phase but not on the β phase.

The results of laser quenching are compared with other non-equilibrium techniques for the production of a-Ga, such as vapor quenching and low-temperature ion irradiation.

1. INTRODUCTION

During recent years investigation of metastable metallic systems has attracted great interest because of their remarkable electrical, mechanical or superconducting properties (1). Several different non-equilibrium methods have been used to produce metastable phases. Experiments have shown that vapor quenching and low-temperature ion irradiation result in similar systems because of comparably high quenching rates (10^{14} K/sec) (2), whereas laser quenching with 40 nsec laser pulses is several orders of magnitude slower (3). Therefore, a comparison of laser-quenching experiments to vapor quenching or ion beam irradiation is very interesting.

For such a test Ga appears to be an ideal system for several reasons. First, there is no interfering influence of a second species since it is a monocomponent system. In contrast to typical metals, a high degree of homopolar bonding exists in the lattice of Ga, and therefore it differs rather strongly from a close packed structure. Since vapor quenching results in close packed arrangements, "typical" metals are built up in a crystalline form even at He temperatures, but Ga can be frozen in as an amorphous layer. In addition, it is well known that amorphous Ga films (a-Ga) can be produced by low-temperature ion irradiation (5-7). Another important aspect is that three phases can be clearly distinguished (Fig. 1).

The first one is the amorphous phase formed by vapor condensation onto a substrate at 4.2 K. This phase, with a resistivity ρ_0 of 33 μΩcm and a superconducting transition temperature $T_c = 8.5$ K, is stable until about 16 K. It then transforms into the metastable crystalline β phase (β-Ga) with a resistivity of 3 μΩcm and a T_c value of 6.3 K.

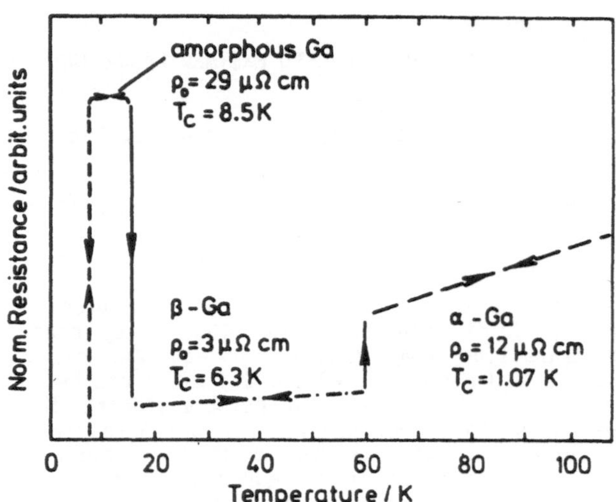

FIGURE 1. Normalized resistance of vapor-quenched gallium (4). The different phases are characterized by the residual resistivity ρ_0 and the superconducting transition temperature T_c.

At about 60 K β-Ga transforms into the stable crystalline α phase (α-Ga) with a resistivity of 12 μΩcm and a T_c of 1.07 K. From these data it is clear that the different phases can be rather well identified by their resistivity and T_c values, but they also show that any laser-quenching experiment intended to produce a-Ga must be performed at low temperatures because of the low crystallization temperature of a-Ga (16 K).

2. EXPERIMENTAL

Ga metal (Koch-light Lab. Ltd., grade 6 N) was evaporated onto quartz substrates at liquid He temperature, resulting in a-Ga. Samples with thicknesses ranging from 15 nm to 70 nm were mounted onto a substrate holder of a cryostat. The resistance was determined by a standard four-point probe technique. The temperature was measured by a calibrated Ge resistor (1 K < T < 50 K) and a Pt resistor (50 K < T). Laser irradiation could be performed *in situ* immediately after quench condensation and suitable annealing to obtain β- and α-Ga (see Fig. 1). The laser used in the experiments was a KrF- excimer laser with 248 nm wavelength, 40 nsec pulse duration and output power of about 0.5 J/cm^2 (without any focusing element).

3. RESULTS

3.1. β-Ga

Ga in the β phase was obtained from a-Ga by heating to 20-40 K. Laser irradiation at low temperatures ($T \leq 4$ K) resulted in transitions β → a-Ga at certain threshold energy densities that depended on the film thickness (Fig. 2a). The results are plotted in Fig. 2b. The energy necessary to amorphize part of the β-Ga film increases with increasing

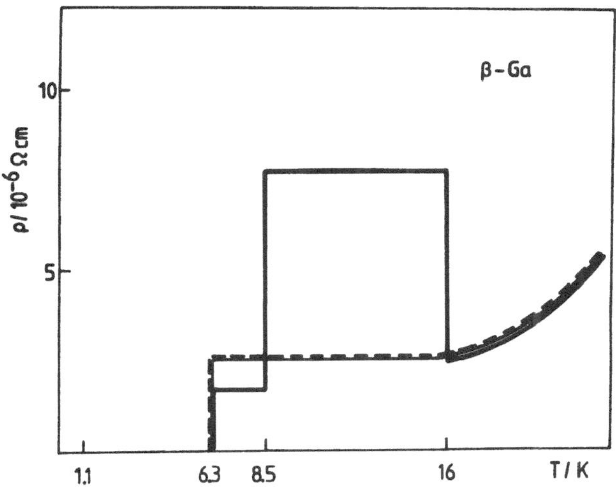

FIGURE 2. (a) Schematic plot of the resistivity of ß-Ga as a function of temperature; crystalline ß-Ga (dashed curve), after 4 K laser irradiation (—) and subsequent heating to 20 K (-).

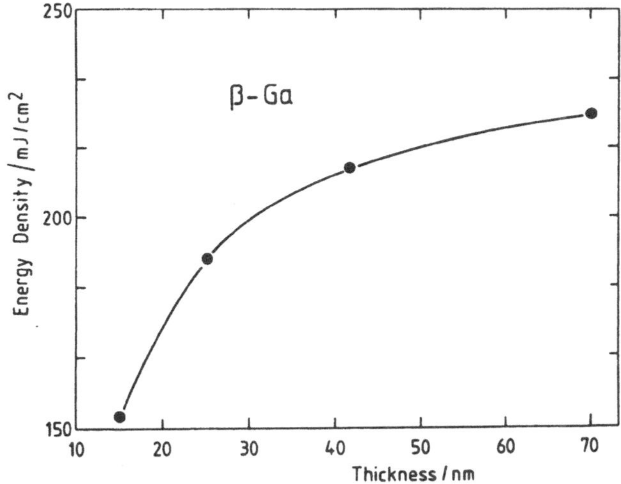

FIGURE 2. (b) Threshold energy densities for amorphization of ß-Ga as a function of film thickness.

thickness of the film. Another surprising result can be seen in Fig. 3. Transformation into the amorphous state as detected by ρ increase can be achieved even at substrate temperatures as high as 20 K. However, in contrast to laser quenching at 4 K, this a-Ga is not stable and has a certain lifetime that decreases with increasing temperature.

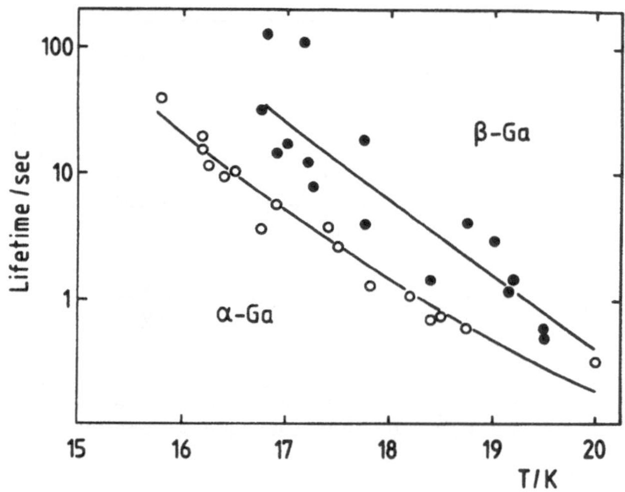

FIGURE 3. Lifetime of a-Ga as obtained by laser quenching of α- and β-Ga at different temperatures.

3.2. α-Ga

α-Ga was produced by warming β-Ga films up to a temperature of about 150 K. Laser irradiation of this stable Ga phase also results in a transition into the amorphous state (Fig. 4a). The results are shown in Fig. 4b, indicating that the α→a transition occurs at about 225 mJ/cm^2, independent of the film thickness. Laser quenching with lower energy densities leads to transitions α→α+β, but no regular behavior has been observed. Laser quenching of films containing both α and β-Ga (i.e., after several pulses without heating to 70 K) changes the onset of amorphization to that of very thin pure β-Ga films (~160 mJ/cm^2). In addition, lifetime measurements of the a phase as obtained from α→a transformations exhibit a temperature dependence comparable to that of β-Ga (see Fig. 3).

4. DISCUSSION

Since these results will be compared to that of low-temperature ion irradiation, the main features of ion beam amorphization of Ga films are briefly reported here (see Refs. 5-7. β-Ga can be transformed into the amorphous phase by Ar^+ irradiation. This is demonstrated in Fig. 5a. T_c and ρ values can be increased up to the corresponding ones of a-Ga by high fluences (2 x 10^{16} ions/cm^2). Ar^+ iradiation of "normal," i.e., α-Ga films, produces the striking result shown in Fig. 5b. At

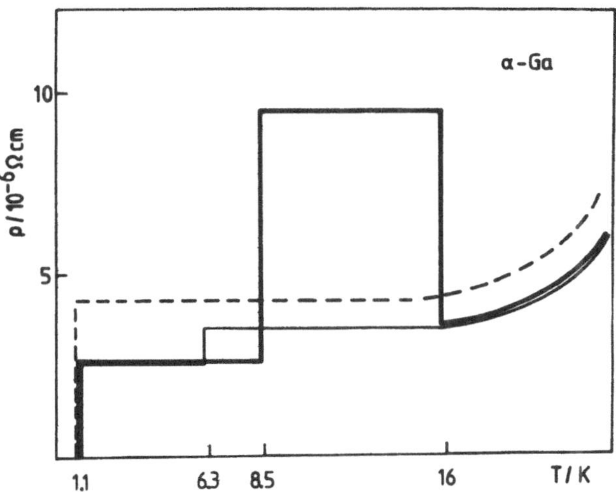

FIGURE 4. (a) Schematic plot of the resistivity of α-Ga as a function of temperature; crystalline α-Ga (dashed curve), after 4 K laser irradiation (—) and subsequent heating to 20 K (-).

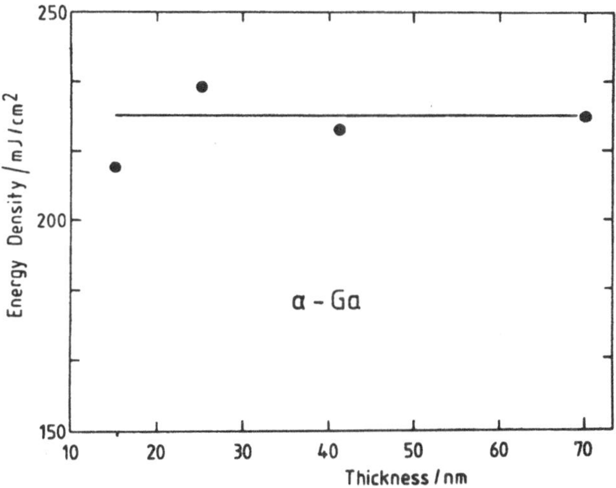

FIGURE 4. (b) Threshold energy densities for amorphization of α-Ga as a function of film thickness.

rather small fluences, $\phi \sim 10^{14}$ ions/cm^2, T_c and ρ increase to nearly the value known for the amorphous state. a-Ga prepared in this way is unstable against further irradiation. It transforms into β-Ga at larger fluences (see Fig. 5b) and the behavior at further increase of fluence is comparable to that displayed in Fig. 5a.

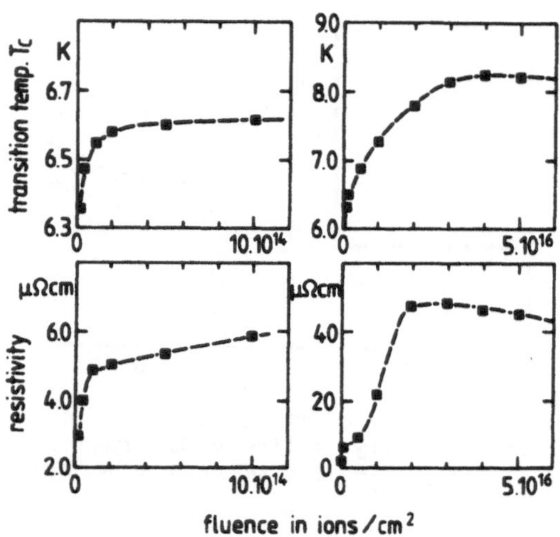

FIGURE 5. (a) Transition temperature T_c and residual resistivity ρ_0 of β-Ga as functions of the fluence of 275 keV Ar ions (7).

Although the results of laser quenching apparently disagree with those of ion irradiation, they can be interpreted in close analogy if the main differences are considered. Low-temperature ion irradiation produces collision cascades (spikes) with energy densities that locally are high enough to exceed the melting energy, so the material is quasi molten and quenched because of rapid energy dissipation. X-ray measurements (8) verify that the short-range order of molten Ga (similar to a-Ga) is closer to that of β-Ga than to that of α-Ga. Thus α-Ga is supposed to act less efficiently as crystallization nuclei than β-Ga. This prediction is confirmed by ion irradiation of Ga at rather small fluences (see Fig. 5a,b). The different behavior of α- and β-Ga concerning irradiation-induced amorphization is in good agreement with vapor quenching experiments (9). The amorphous phase can be obtained by quench condensation onto α-Ga as a substrate, but not onto β-Ga. Again this can be interpreted in terms of the similar short-range order of the "liquid-like" amorphous and the β phase.

Even laser quenching confirms these results. The onset of amorphization of β-Ga depends on the film thickness, i.e., the whole β-film must be molten to avoid recrystallization on β-nuclei. Laser quenching of α-Ga with energy densities ~ 225 mJ/cm^2 results in transitions $\alpha \rightarrow \alpha + \beta$, probably leading to a thin β film on top of an α substrate which would explain the thickness-independent onset of amorphization.

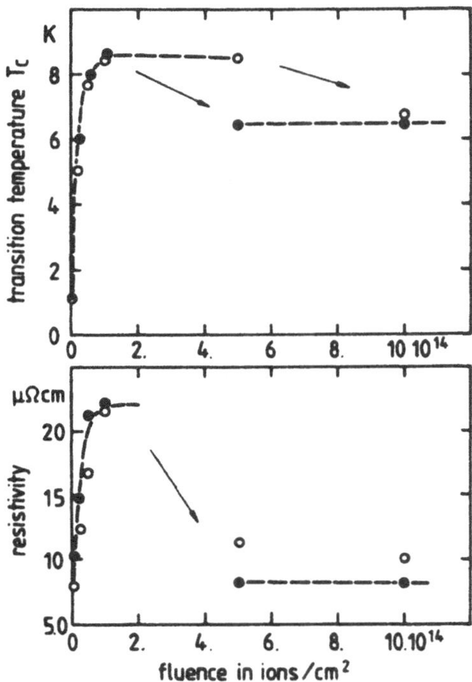

FIGURE 5. (b) Transition temperature T_c and residual resistivity ρ_0 of α-Ga as functions of the fluence of 275 keV Ar ions.

This conclusion is supported by the lifetime measurements. First, α-Ga films containing β-Ga (after pre-irradiation) can be transformed to a-Ga at even lower energies than pure α films, indicating that the whole β-Ga must be molten. Moreover, recrystallization of a-Ga as obtained by laser quenching of α-Ga starts at lower temperatures and proceeds even faster than that of β-Ga (see Fig. 3).

5. CONCLUSION

The experiments give evidence for the first time of the possibility to amorphize a pure metallic element only by laser irradiation, i.e., without a second stabilizing component. Transitions of crystalline (α,β) to amorphous Ga, even at substrate temperatures as high as 20 K, demonstrate that low temperatures are necessary, not only to provide high quenching rates but also to stabilize the amorphous phase. From the results one can conclude that laser quenching is comparable to vapor quenching and low-temperature ion irradiation as indicated in Fig. 6. The internal energy without any temperature dependence is plotted in arbitrary units versus temperature. Equilibrium phases (vapor, liquid, α-Ga) are indicated by solid lines, whereas metastable phases (amorphous and β-Ga) are shown by dashed lines. The similarity of the liquid and

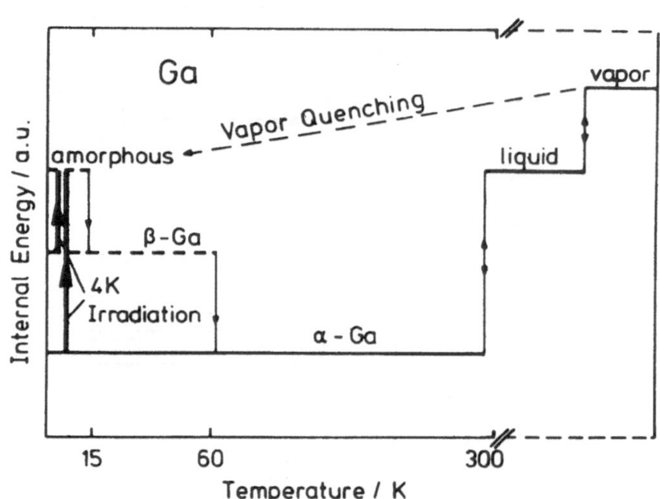

FIGURE 6. Schematic plot of the internal energy of the different gallium phases as a function of temperature (10).

amorphous phases is demonstrated by identical values of internal energy. Included in Fig. 6 are all applicable non-equilibrium techniques. Vapor quenching (dashed arrow) transforms the vapor directly into the amorphous phase; 4 K ion and even laser irradiation (solid arrows) transform both α-Ga and β-Ga into the amorphous phase.

REFERENCES

1. B. R. Appleton, B. Sartwell, P. Peercy, R. Schaefer, and R. Osgood, Mater. Sci. Eng. 70, 23 (1985).
2. B. Stritzker, in Surface Modification and Alloying by Laser, Ion and Electron Beams, edited by J. M. Poate, G. Foti, and D. C. Jacobson (Plenum Publishing Co., New York, 1983), p. 165.
3. Laser-Solid Interactions and Transient Thermal Processing of Materials, edited by J. Narayan, W. L. Brown, and R. A. Lemons, Materials Research Society Symposium Proceedings, Vol. 13 (Elsevier, New York, 1983).
4. W. Buckel and R. Hilsch, Z. Physik 138, 109 (1954).
5. U. Goerlach, P. Ziemann, and W. Buckel, Nucl. Instrum. Methods 209/210, 235 (1983).
6. M. Holz, P. Ziemann, and W. Buckel, Phys Rev. Lett. 51, 1584 (1983).
7. U. Goerlach, M. Hitzfeld, P. Ziemann, and W. Buckel, Z. Physik B 47, 227 (1982).
8. A. Defrain, J. Chim. Phys.-Chim. Biol. 74, 851 (1977).
9. A. Bererhi, L. Bosio, and R. Cortes, J. Non-Cryst Solids 30, 253 (1979).
10. B. Stritzker, in Laser and Electron-Beam Interactions with Solids, edited by B. R. Appleton and G. K. Celler (Elsevier, New York, 1982), p. 363.

DEFECT STRUCTURES ON METAL SURFACES INDUCED BY PULSED LASER IRRADIATION: CHARACTERIZATION BY LEED-SPOT PROFILE ANALYSIS AND He^+ ION CHANNELING

AUBREY L. HELMS, JR., CHIH-CHEN CHO, STEVEN L. BERNASEK
Department of Chemistry, Princeton University, Princeton, NJ 08544

CLIFTON W. DRAPER
AT&T Engineering Research Center, Princeton, USA

DALE C. JACOBSON, JOHN M. POATE
AT&T Bell Laboratories, Murray Hill, NJ 07974

Key Words: molybdenum, bismuth, defects, stress-strain

ABSTRACT

The techniques of LEED-Spot Profile Analysis (LEED-SPA) and He^+ ion channeling have been used to investigate the response of molybdenum and bismuth single crystals to pulsed laser irradiation. Samples of molybdenum with (100) orientations were irradiated with a Q-switched, frequency-doubled Nd:YAG laser under ultra-high vacuum conditions. Good epitaxial regrowth of the melted surfaces was indicated by the appearance of a well-defined LEED pattern. Analysis of the spot profiles as a function of incident electron energy and annealing time at 1000°C indicates the initial formation of random island structures on the surface which coalesce toward a flat surface with prolonged heating. Samples which had been disordered in the near surface region by Ar^+ ion bombardment exhibited a sharp LEED pattern after pulsed laser melting.

The (0001), $(\bar{1}010)$, and $2\bar{1}\bar{1}0)$ surfaces of bismuth were pulsed laser melted using a Q-switched ruby laser. Channeling, Nomarski Interference Contrast microscopy (NIC), and selective chemical etching indicate that the (0001) surface regrows epitaxially with no increase in disorder after pulsed laser melting at low laser fluences. Both the $(\bar{1}010)$ and $(2\bar{1}\bar{1}0)$ surfaces show a marked increase in disorder after irradiation. The responses of these metals and the data are explained using a thermo-mechanical stress model in which the materials plastically deform in response to the high thermal gradients induced during pulsed laser irradiation.

1. INTRODUCTION

The response of solids to high-power laser pulses has been the subject of active research for many years. In contrast to the good epitaxial regrowth observed in semiconductors, metals have been shown to exhibit liquid phase epitaxial regrowth with a marked increase in disorder (1-8). In most of the cases studied to date, a crystallographic orientation dependence was observed, with the most densely packed surfaces generally showing epitaxial regrowth of poorer quality. The extent of the introduced disorder was found to correlate well with laser fluence (3).

The response of metals has taken many forms. Transmission electron microscopy has shown the formation of an extended dislocation network in laser-melted nickel (2). Other modes of damage include slip (5), pitting, dislocation motion and multiplication (7), increased vacancy concentration (8), and cratering (6). The various forms of damage have been found to generally have different laser fluence thresholds.

An interesting class of elements yet to be investigated is Group VB (As, Sb, and Bi). The Group VB semi-metals have rhombohedral crystal structures in which the atoms are arranged in double layers such that each atom has three nearest neighbors and three at a slightly greater distance (9). The bonding within the layers consists of strong, directional covalent bonds, while the bonding between layers is often described as changing from van der Waals to metallic in nature as one increases in atomic number from arsenic to bismuth. This atomic arrangement results in very anisotropic bonding character in different crystallographic directions, which is further evidenced by a large anisotropy in the thermal, physical, electrical, and mechanical properties. Another manifestation of the large bonding anisotropy is the fact that bismuth has only one major slip system, parallel to the (0001) planes.

Paralleling the experimental studies has been an equally intensive theoretical effort (10-14). The laser/solid interaction for large spot-short pulse experiments can be modeled as a semi-infinite slab with one-dimensional heat flow (10). By choosing appropriate boundary conditions, the spatial and temporal profiles of the temperature excursions in the solid may be calculated. Using such a model and concentrating on the near surface region, Musal has calculated the minimum temperature rise at the surface required for the onset of plastic deformation (10). This temperature rise is surprisingly low, being only 20 K for copper (10). In the proposed model, the deformation takes place through thermally activated slip, resulting in steps at the surface.

The development of spot profile analysis applied to LEED over the past decade has made the study of surface defect structures possible (15-21). The angular profile of the diffraction spot in reciprocal space yields information about the atomic morphology of the surface (20). The behavior of the profile as a function of incident electron energy can also be used to make a qualitative assessment of the defect structure. LEED is very surface sensitive, probing only the top 3-4 atomic layers and spot profile analysis allows the distinction between random point defects, ordered terraces, ordered islands, random islands, and facets (17).

An investigation of the pulsed laser melting and epitaxial regrowth of molybdenum and bismuth single crystals is reported here. The crystalline quality of the epitaxial regrowth was monitored using LEED-SPA in the case of molybdenum and RBS and channeling for the bismuth experiments. In both cases, the surface topography was investigated using NIC. The LEED results indicate that the molybdenum surfaces regrow epitaxially with an increase in disorder. The spot profiles and behavior of the FWHM as a function of incident electron energy indicate the formation of random islands on the surface which coalesce back toward a flat surface as a function of heating at 1000°C. Samples which had been disordered by Ar^+ ion bombardment were annealed in a manner similar to the laser annealing of silicon (22). The channeling results indicate that the quality of the epitaxial regrowth for bismuth may be ordered $(0001) > (\bar{1}010) > (2\bar{1}\bar{1}0)$. The (0001) face can be laser surface melted and recrystallized epitaxially with no increase in disorder with the

Q-switched ruby laser much the same as silicon. The increase in disorder observed in the channeling spectra for the $(\bar{1}010)$ and $(2\bar{1}\bar{1}0)$ surfaces is further evidenced in the appearance of prominent slip bands on these surfaces.

2. EXPERIMENTAL

The Mo(100) samples were mechanically polished to a mirror finish using standard metallographic techniques. The samples were spot-welded to thin tantalum foils which were mounted on a specially designed transfer block attached to a sample manipulator. The resistively heated tantalum foil was used to heat the sample to temperatures in excess of 1000°C for cleaning and annealing purposes. The sample temperature was monitored by means of an optical pyrometer focused on the sample through an 8" viewport at the front of the vacuum system. The experiments were conducted in a conventional ion-pumped UHV chamber described previously (23). The samples were transferred out of the main chamber using a magnetically coupled drive system described elsewhere.

The samples were cleaned and characterized in the main chamber and then transferred to the laser chamber. The high-vacuum valves were closed and the laser chamber decoupled from the main system. The chamber was then transported to the laser facilities at the AT&T Engineering Research Center. The samples were irradiated under UHV conditions and returned to Princeton University.

A description of the laser system employed for these experiments has appeared previously (23). To ensure complete coverage, the beam was rastered across the surface by means of optics coupled to computer-controlled linear induction motors. One half of the sample was irradiated five times to ensure uniform modification, leaving the other half to serve as an internal standard.

Samples were irradiated under three different laser conditions. One set of samples was irradiated at 15 MW/cm^2 which is below the threshold for melting. These samples will be designated as "Type A." A second set of samples was irradiated at laser fluences between 25 and 90 MW/cm^2 which were above the melt threshold. The third set were samples that had been Ar^+ bombarded at 3 KeV in 1×10^{-6} torr Ar for one hour at normal incidence. This bombardment produced a disordered surface as evidenced by the absence of a LEED pattern. These samples were irradiated at a laser fluence of 75 MW/cm^2 and will carry the designation "Type C."

The LEED data were collected by photographing the LEED patterns with a 35 mm camera mounted in front of the 8" viewport and focused on the LEED screen. The intensity profiles were evaluated from the negatives by means of a computer-interfaced Vidicon camera system described previously (24). The information collected using this system includes the angular spot profile, spot-to-spot distance, and relative intensity between the spot and the background.

The composition of the surface was monitored using AES. The conditions and instrument parameters were carefully controlled so that all of the spectra were acquired under the same conditions. The surface concentrations of carbon, sulfur, and oxygen were calculated by evaluating the ratio of the peak-to-peak heights of those elements to the peak-to-peak height of the Mo-220 eV transition. The ratios could be compared to literature values to give surface concentrations in units of fractional monolayers (25).

The data accumulation involved characterizing the surface using AES and LEED followed by transfer and laser irradiation. After the sample was returned to the main chamber, the compositional differences between the virgin and irradiated surfaces were determined using AES. The sample was flashed to 1000°C for five minutes to desorb any contamination adsorbed from the background during the transfer process. Photographic LEED data were collected as a function of incident electron energy. The sample was annealed at 1000°C with AES and LEED data collected following 15, 30, 45, 60, 90, 120, and 180 minutes of heating. The AES and LEED data were collected with the sample at room temperature.

The defect nature of the surface was deduced by comparing the spot profiles of the virgin and irradiated surfaces with trends expected from the work of Lagally, Henzler, and others (15-21). By restricting the study to the spot profiles and neglecting the use of integral intensities, they have calculated the expected diffraction profiles for a variety of surface defect structures within the kinematical approximation. Figure 1 summarizes the profiles expected from a variety of defect surfaces. The results described in the following section are derived from qualitative comparisons of their calculated spot profiles and the observed spot profiles under different irradiation conditions.

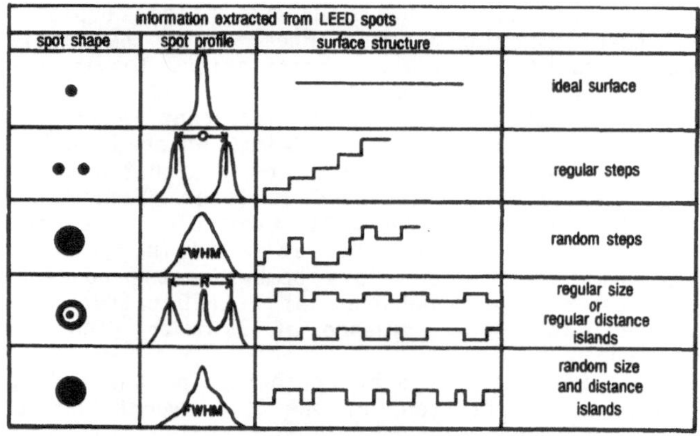

FIGURE 1. Table from Gronwald and Henzler (20) summarizing the information available from LEED-Spot Profile Analysis.

Single crystal slices of bismuth, oriented in the (0001), $(\bar{1}010)$, and $(2\bar{1}\bar{1}0)$ directions, were electromechanically polished to a mirror finish. The electrolyte used for the polishing was a mixture of 10 parts methanol, 2.5 parts HCl, 2.5 parts H_2SO_4, and 1 part glycerin (26). The current density was held at 1 amp/cm^2 and the samples were washed in distilled water followed by an ethanol rinse and dried with air.

The samples were irradiated with a Q-switched ruby laser with a pulse width of 30 nsec. A bent waveguide was used to produce a homogeneous circular output 7 mm in diameter (27). The fluences ranged from

0.5 J/cm^2, which produced a well-defined melt spot, to 0.9 J/cm^2, which resulted in significant evaporation of material.

The crystalline quality of the samples was evaluated by both channeling (28) and selective chemical etching. A solution of 2% I_2 in methanol was used to decorate the intersection of screw dislocations on the Bi(0001) face as triangular pits (29). The pits could then be counted and served as an indication of the extent of deformation or annealing.

3. RESULTS

3.1. Molybdenum

The results for types A and B were similar and will be described simultaneously. For both types, the surface concentrations of carbon and oxygen were observed to increase after returning to the main chamber. This was probably due to the adsorption of background gases during the transportation between Princeton University and AT&T. In each case, the levels of contamination were lower on the irradiated surface, indicating that laser-stimulated desorption occurred during the irradiation phase. This observation correlated well with a slight pressure rise registered on the ion pump controller during the laser processing. The contaminants were easily removed by flashing the sample to 1000°C after transferring to the main chamber.

A clear LEED pattern was observed for both the irradiated and virgin regions of both types of samples. The geometry was consistent with that expected for the (100) surface. The spots for the virgin surface were visually sharper than the spots for the irradiated area. This clearly indicates the introducton of disorder into the surface. The appearance of a LEED pattern for the irradiated region of samples of type B is an indication of liquid phase epitaxial regrowth during the resolidification of the melt.

A comparison of the angular profiles of spots taken from each region indicates that in each case, the half-widths of the spots from the irradiated region were greater than those corresponding to spots from the virgin region (Fig. 2). A plot of the relative half-widths versus incident electron energy for first-order spots from the irradiated region indicated an oscillatory behavior indicative of the formation of stepped structures on the surface (Fig. 3). The amplitude and frequency of these oscillations, as well as the amplitude of the relative half-width, were observed to decrease as a function of accumulated annealing time, suggesting a coalescence of the stepped surface back toward a flat surface. The effects were observed for both types A and B, with magnitudes of the features being larger for type B.

Careful analysis of the shape of the spots indicated that in some instances the spots from the irradiated region contained "shoulders" aligned along the <010> and <001> directions (Fig. 4). These shoulders indicate the orientation of the terrace edges. As with the half-width, the prominence of the shoulders was observed to decrease with accumulated annealing time, indicating the coalescence of the steps.

The LEED patterns in the irradiated regions were slightly expanded relative to the patterns for the virgin areas, as evidenced by an increase in the spot-to-spot distance. The expansion was 3% for type A and 7% for type B. The expansion was isotropic and was determined not to be an experimental artifact due to errors in sample positioning or changes in the incident electron energy. This expansion indicates that the irradiated region is slightly contracted in the plane of the surface in real space.

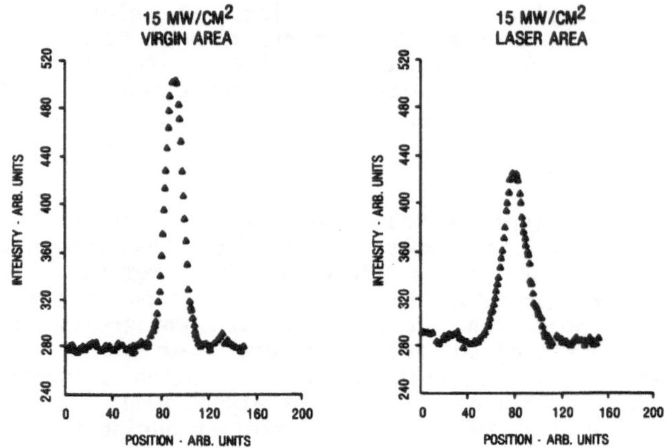

FIGURE 2. A plot of intensity versus position for typical spot profiles for both the virgin and irradiated regions from a sample of type A.

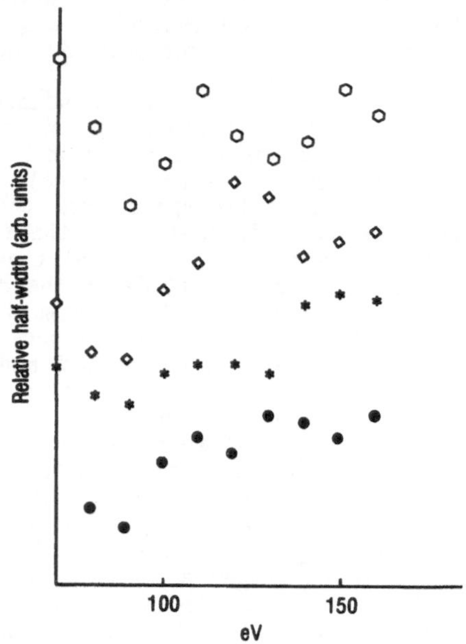

FIGURE 3. A plot of relative half-width (half-width divided by the (0,0)-(0,1) spot-to-spot distance) versus incident electron energy for several heating times: (○) 5 minutes, (◇) 20 minutes, (*) 35 minutes, (•) 80 minutes.

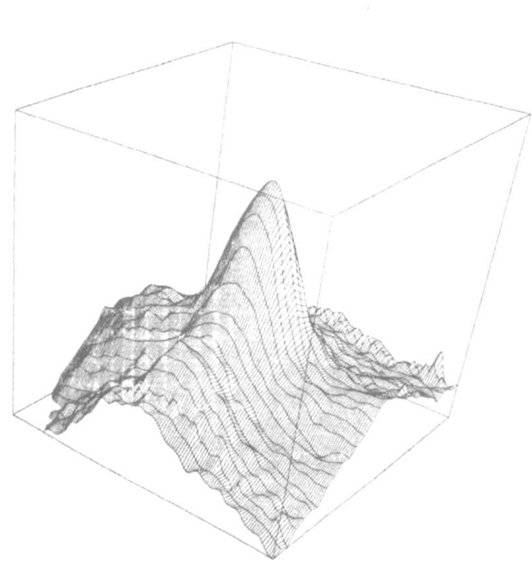

FIGURE 4. A plot of intensity versus position for a spot in the irradiated region of a sample of type B showing the "shoulders."

The AES results for type C followed the same trends as types A and B. A distinct LEED pattern was observed for the irradiated regions of samples of type C. This indicated that the melted region extended beyond the range of damage due to the Ar^+ implantation to the single-crystal substrate below. Liquid phase epitaxial regrowth resulted in a net annealing of the surface. A very poor LEED pattern was observed for the virgin region after a heating time of several minutes, which remained very diffuse relative to the sharp spots observed for the irradiated region throughout the study. For this type, the half-widths of the spots from the irradiated region were smaller than from the virgin region, indicating the extent of the annealing induced by the laser. The irradiated region still showed an increase in disorder relative to the well-annealed surface. As with samples of types A and B, the spot profile analysis indicated some spots with "shoulders." However, unlike the other two types, the shoulders for this type of sample were circularly symmetric. The half-widths of spots from both regions decreased as a function of accumulated heating time, indicating the previously mentioned annealing behavior observed for sample of types A and B.

3.2. Bismuth

The rhombohedral structure may be referenced to a hexagonal basis set. In this notation, the Bi(0001) surface is perpendicular to the C axis, that is, parallel to the planes formed by the covalent double layers. The other two surfaces studied are perpendicular to this face. They were chosen because they form a set of surfaces displaying the anisotropic properties of bismuth (Fig. 5).

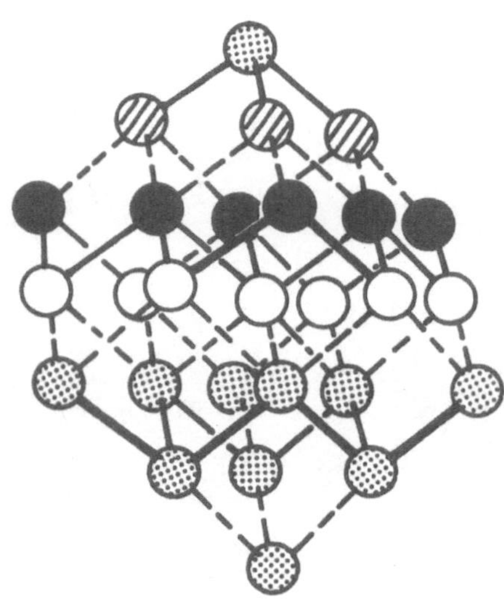

FIGURE 5. The rhombohedral structure of bismuth showing the bonding within and between the double layers.

The regrowth in the (0001) direction is epitaxial and without an increase in the defect density, as evidenced by both channeling and selective etching techniques (Fig. 6). The slight decrease in the χ_{min} for this surface from 9.5% for the virgin surface to 8.7% for the laser-irradiated surface and the scarcity of etch pits observed inside the laser-irradiated areas are attributed to the release of stress, incorporated by polishing, during the liquid phase. The experimental χ_{min} value of 8.7% as compared to a calculated minimum yield of 4.4% (30) indicates that the crystal was of good overall quality. The (0001) half-angle (Fig. 7) was measured to be 0.54 in comparison with the calculated value of 0.46 obtained using Moliere's screening function as outlined in Mayer and Rimini (30).

In the <1010> and <2110> directions the channeling results show epitaxial regrowth but with an increased dechanneling rate which is indicative of increased disorder in the form of dislocations (Figs. 8 and 9). The dechanneling rate does not return to a value equal to that of the virgin crystal, suggesting the crystal is deformed over depths of at least 900 nm. For laser fluences of 0.5 J/cm^2 the ($\bar{1}010$) surface showed a χ_{min} of 16.3% after laser irradiation as compared to 16.1% for virgin surface. The χ_{min} for the ($2\bar{1}\bar{1}0$) surface increased from 7.0% to 11.1% upon irradiation. The observed increase in the χ_{min} for these surfaces is indicative of damage and follows trends as a function of laser fluence observed in fcc, bcc, and hcp metals (3). Figure 8b is a Nomarski Interference Contrast micrograph showing the ($\bar{1}010$) face before and after irradiation above the melt threshold. The (0001) basal slip planes are readily apparent. The number of slip lines did not show any correlation with laser fluence. Trends in the channeling results on crystals irradiated at fluences greater than 0.5 J/cm^2 are consistent with the above results.

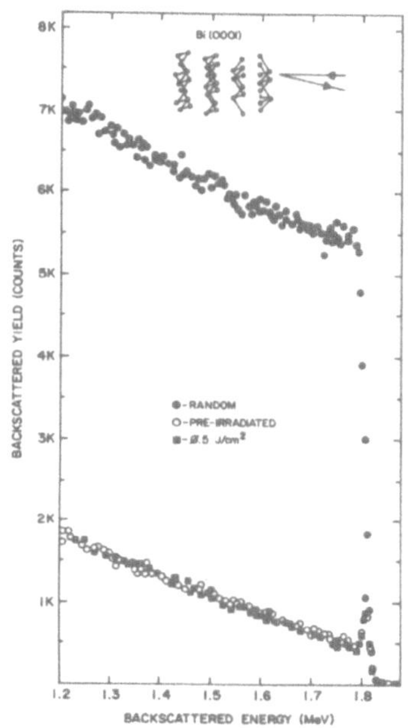

FIGURE 6. (a) RBS/channeling data using a 2.0 MeV He^+ ion beam on Bi(0001) showing preand post-irradiated spectra.

4. DISCUSSION

4.1. Molybdenum

The melt puddles observed in the irradiated region of samples of types B and C using NIC are clear indications that the surface had melted. The appearance of a LEED pattern in these areas indicates that the surface has regrown via liquid phase epitaxy. This is further evidenced by the fact that the geometry of the LEED pattern in these areas is consistent with the original (100) surface. The irradiated surface of samples of type A was visually indistinguishable from the virgin area, indicating that melting had not occurred. The damage in these regions can only be due to thermal effects in the solid phase.

The angular profiles of the spots in reciprocal space yield information about the structure of the surface. The observation of a broader half-width that oscillated as a function of incident electron energy in the irradiated regions indicates the formation of multi-tiered structures on the surface. These trends were observed for both types A and B, implying that the features are not simply due to the macroscopic roughness of the laser-melted region of samples of type B.

The observation of shoulders on the spots indicates the formation of islands with a random size distribution and a random distribution of distances between their centers. The orientation of the shoulders indicates a preferred orientation of the island edges. The circularly

FIGURE 6. (b) Nomarski micrograph for Bi(0001) showing pre- (left) and post-irradiated (right) surfaces showing triangular etch pits at the intersection of screw dislocations with the surface.

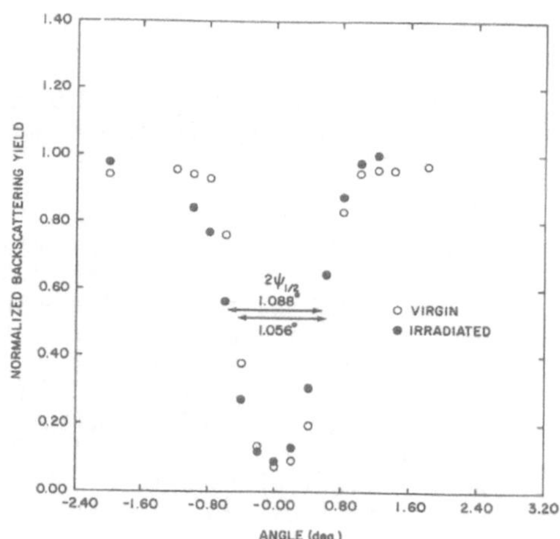

FIGURE 7. Half-angle spectra for pre- and post-irradiated Bi(0001).

symmetric shoulders observed for samples of type C indicate that the preferential orientation of the island edges in these samples is not as strong as in the other two types.

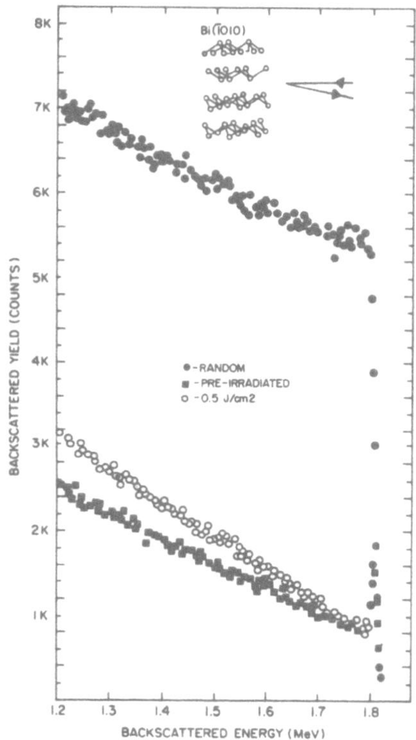

FIGURE 8. (a) RBS/channeling data using a 2.0 MeV He^+ ion beam, on Bi(1̄010) showing pre- and post-irradiated spectra.

It has been shown previously that the damage introduced into metals by pulsed laser irradiation takes the form of dislocation networks (2) and an increase in the number of vacancies (8). This is consistent with the thermomechanical model proposed by Musal (9). The thermal gradients introduced during the pulse cause the heated volume to expand. During the heating phase, this results in compressive stresses accumulated in the heated volume. If the surface melts (types B and C), these stresses are relieved in the liquid phase. After resolidification, the melted volume cools and again stresses are induced by the thermal gradients. If this stress exceeds the critical resolved shear stress (CRSS) for dislocation activation on one of the slip planes of the material, the solid will be plastically deformed through the mechanism of dislocation movement/multiplication. It is well known that the CRSS decreases with increasing temperature, so the hot, resolidified volume is expected to deform before the cooler surroundings. The motion/multiplication of a dislocation can result in the formation of an atomic step at the surface.

The observed LEED results are consistent with the aforementioned model. The major slip planes for the bcc crystal structure are of the

FIGURE 8. (b) Nomarski micrograph for Bi($\bar{1}010$) showing pre- (left) and post-irradiated (right) surfaces.

{211} and {110} families (31). Clear slip patterns are rarely observed in bcc metals because of the cross slip and interaction of these two systems. The edges of the islands may be due to the activation of dislocation sources in one or both of these slip systems. The preferential orientation of the edges seems to indicate that the <110> system is slightly favored over the <211> system. Thus conclusion is derived by noticing that the edges lie along the intersecting lines of the <110> planes with the (100) surface.

4.2. Bismuth

The slip lines and increased dechanneling observed for the ($\bar{1}010$) and ($2\bar{1}\bar{1}0$) surfaces are consistent with the aforementioned model. For these two surfaces, the basal slip system of bismuth is perpendicular to the surface. The slip lines appear where the (0001) basal planes intersect these surfaces. The slip within the melt puddle must be due to compressive stress introduced during the cooling of the hot solid. The appearance of slip lines and the increased dechanneling rate indicate that these stresses were well above the CRSS for dislocation sources lying within the (0001) basal planes. The deep bulk damage, below the melt depth, is due to stress introduced during the heating, melted, and cooling phases of the experiment. The CRSS is a very strong function of temperature for bismuth (32). This may explain why the slip lines on these two surfaces terminate very quickly outside the laser-melted region. The heat flow is poor parallel to the surface, so the temperature profile decreases rapidly as a function of distance beyond the edge of the melt puddle. As the temperature decreases, the CRSS increases dramatically, and the introduced stress may not be sufficient to activate dislocation sources responsible for the slip lines. The behavior perpendicular to these surfaces is similar to that observed of metals,

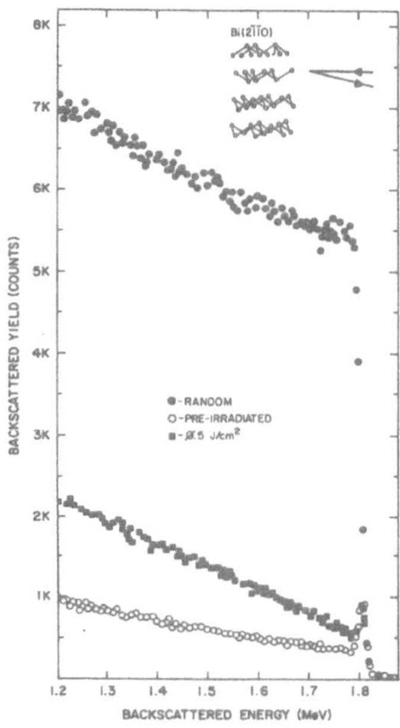

FIGURE 9. (a) RBS/channeling data using a 2.0 MeV He^+ ion beam, on Bi(2$\bar{1}\bar{1}$0) showing pre- and post-irradiated spectra.

and the increased disorder introduced by the pulsed laser melting is consistent with this analogy.

The absence of slip lines on the (0001) surface after pulsed laser melting is due to the fact that the main slip system is parallel to this surface. The stress introduced by the thermal gradients is not sufficient to activate the movement of dislocations perpendicular to the surface. The CRSS for the {01$\bar{1}$1} family of planes, which slip along the <0$\bar{1}$1$\bar{2}$> direction, has been reported to be 50 times higher than the CRSS for slip along the (0001) basal planes (33). This also explains the lack of increased disorder observed in the channeling spectra. The behavior perpendicular to this surface is similar to that observed in the elemental semiconductors, and the high-quality epitaxial regrowth of this surface is also consistent with this analogy.

5. CONCLUSIONS

The response of Mo(100) surfaces to pulsed laser irradiation was studied using the technique of LEED-spot profile analysis. The method has been shown to be very sensitive, indicating damage even at laser fluences below the melt threshold. The behavior of the relative half-width as a function of incident electron energy and the angular profiles of the spots after irradiation suggest the formation of random islands on the surface with edges aligned along the {110} slip planes. The LEED pattern for the irradiated region of the samples which were laser

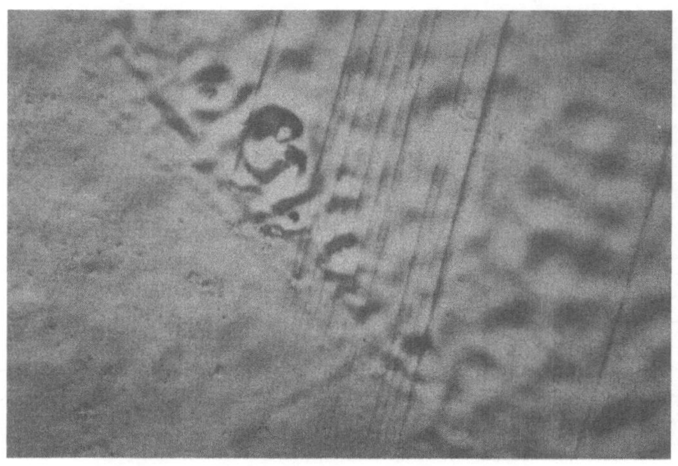

FIGURE 9. (b) Nomarski micrograph for Bi($2\bar{1}\bar{1}0$) showing the edge of the melt puddle.

surface melted indicates liquid phase epitaxial regrowth during resolidification. Furthermore, the appearance of a LEED pattern for the irradiated region of samples that had been disordered by 3 KeV Ar^+ implantation implies that the surface was ordered by epitaxial regrowth from a melt which extended beyond the damaged region to the underlying single crystal. The formation of the islands can be explained using a thermomechanical model in which the metal plastically deforms in response to the introduced thermal stress by the activation of dislocation sources. The movement/multiplication of these dislocations can result in slip and the formation of step edges and multi-tiered structures at the surface.

Epitaxial regrowth was observed for three crystallographic directions for the semimetal, bismuth. A correlation was found between the thermal mechanical character and the quality of the epitaxial regrowth. In the <0001> direction, the epitaxial regrowth is good and without any detectable increase in disorder. The ($\bar{1}010$) and ($2\bar{1}\bar{1}0$) surfaces regrow epitaxially but with some increased disorder visible in the form of slip lines on the irradiated surfaces. The X_{min} and half-angle were measured for the <0001> direction and compare well with calculated values.

ACKNOWLEDGMENTS

The expertise and patience of Ms. Lisa Kennedy '86 of Princeton University and Mr. John Garno of AT&T Bell Labs are gratefully acknowledged in the preparation of high-quality single-crystal surfaces. We also gratefully acknowledge the help of Mr. Randy Crisci of AT&T ERC in the maintenance of the laser system. Special thanks are given to Dr. Everett J. Canning, Jr., of AT&T ERC for helpful discussions on dislocation theory.

REFERENCES

1. A. L. Helms, Jr., C. W. Draper, D. C. Jacobson, J. M. Poate, and S. L. Bernasek, Mat. Res. Soc. Symp. Proc. 35, 439 (1985).
2. L. Buene, D. C. Jacobson, S. Nakahara, J. M. Poate, C. W. Draper, and J. K. Hirvonen, in Laser and Electron-Beam Solid Interactions and Materials Processing, edited by Gibbons, Hess, and Sigmon (Elsevier North Holland, New York, 1981), pp. 583-590.
3. L. Buene, E. N. Kaufmann, C. M. Preece, and C. W. Draper, in Laser and Electron-Beam Solid Interactions and Materials Processing, edited by Gibbons, Hess, and Sigmon (Elsevier North Holland, New York, 1981), pp. 591-597.
4. J. O. Porteus, D. L. Decker, J. L. Jernigan, W. N. Faith, and M. Bass, IEEE J. Quantum Electron. QE-14, 776 (1978).
5. J. O. Porteus, M. J. Soileau, and C. W. Fountain, Appl. Phys. Lett. 29, 156 (1976).
6. M. K. Chun and K. Rose, J. Appl. Phys. 41, 614 (1970).
7. F. Haessner and W. Seitz, J. Mater. Sci. 6, 16 (1971).
8. S. A. Metz and F. A. Smidt, Jr., Appl. Phys. Lett. 19, 207 (1971).
9. J. Donohue, The Structures of the Elements, (Wiley, New York, 1974), pp. 311-316.
10. H. N. Musal, Jr., Symp. on Optical Materials for High Power Lasers, Boulder, CO, 1979, pp. 159.
11. J. H. Bechtel, J. Appl. Phys. 46, 1585 (1975).
12. M. Lax, J. Appl. Phys. 48, 3919 (1977).
13. L. R. Hettche, T. R. Tucker, J. T. Schriempf, R. L. Stegman, and S. A. Metz, J. Appl. Phys. 47, 1415 (1976).
14. E. Rimini, in Surface Modification and Alloying by Laser, Ion and Electron Beams, edited by Poate, Foti, and Jacobson (Plenum, New York, 1981), Chap. 2.
15. M. G. Lagally, Appl. Surf. Sci. 13, 260 (1982).
16. T. M. Lu and M. G. Lagally, Surf. Sci. 120, 47 (1982).
17. M. Henzler, in Electron Spectroscopy for Surface Analysis, edited by Ibach (Springer, Berlin, 1977), Chap. 4.
18. M. Henzler, Surf. Sci. 73, 240 (1978).
19. J. E. Houston and R. L. Park, Surf. Sci. 21, 209 (1970).
20. K. D. Gronwald and M. Henzler, Surf. Sci. 117, 180 (1982).
21. M. Henzler, Appl. Surf. Sci. 11/12, 450 (1982).
22. G. Foti and E. Rimini, in Laser Annealing of Semiconductors, edited by Poate and Mayer (Academic, New York, 1982), Chap. 7.
23. A. L. Helms, Jr., C. C. Cho, S. L. Bernasek, and C. W. Draper, Mat. Res. Soc. Symp. Proc. 48, 3 (1985).
24. T. N. Tommet, G. B. Olszewski, P. A. Chadwick, and S. L. Bernasek, Rev. Sci. Instrum. 50, 147 (1979).
25. M. Salmeron, G. A. Somorjai, and R. R. Chianelli, Surf. Sci. 127, 526 (1983).
26. J. Garno, AT&T Bell Labs, private communication.
27. A. G. Cullis, H. C. Webber, and P. Bailey, J. Phys. E 12, 688 (1979).
28. E. Rimini, in Materials Characterization Using Ion Beams, edited by Thomas and Cachard (Plenum, New York, 1978), pp. 455.
29. L. C. Lowell and J. H. Wernick, J. Appl. Phys. 30, 234 (1959).
30. B. R. Appleton and G. Foti, in Ion Beam Handbook for Materials Analysis, edited by Mayer and Rimini (Academic, New York, 1977), pp. 67-107.

31. D. Hull, J. F. Byron, and F. W. Noble, Can. J. Phys. 45, 1091 (1967).
32. R. E. Reed-Hill, Physical Metallurgy Principles (Van Nostrand, New York, 1964), pp. 121.
33. S. Otake, H. Namazue, and N. Matsuno, Jpn. J. Appl. Phys. 19, 433 (1980).

AlSb FORMATION IN UHV BY LASER ANNEALING OF EVAPORATED Al AND Sb FILMS. CHARACTERIZATION BY AES AND XPS**

E. PETIT*, P. WARNANT, P. A. THIRY, R. CAUDANO
Facultés Universitaires Notre-Dame de la Paix, Namur, Belgium

Key Words: laser-induced reactions, metal-semiconductor transitions

1. INTRODUCTION

Results reported here involve the interaction of a pulsed and doubled Nd:YAG laser beam with multilayer Al and Sb metallic samples (in stoichiometric proportion) which has been studied under ultra-high-vacuum (UHV) conditions. Analyses were performed by Auger electron spectroscopy (AES) and X-ray photoelectron spectroscopy (XPS).

Other people have reported the synthesis of very high purity semiconductor films like AlSb, AlAs and CdTe by laser irradiation of such layered metallic systems. The samples were then protected by a SiO layer, laser treated in the air and characterized by electron diffraction, electrical measurements and optical absorption (1). In contrast with these bulk studies, our paper presents surface analysis observations.

2. EXPERIMENTAL

The UHV chamber system, including a preparation chamber, a transfer chamber and an analysis chamber, has been described elsewhere (1). The sample can be prepared in the preparation chamber, undergo the laser treatment in the transfer chamber and be characterized in the analysis chamber while being maintained under UHV conditions.

The AES analyses were performed using a glancing incidence e-gun and a Varian single-pass Cylindrical Mirror Analyzer (CMA) whose resolution was 0.4% as measured on the elastic peak.

The XPS measurements were obtained with a VSW setup, using Al and MgK_α X-ray lines without a monochromator. The FWHM was approximately 1.5 eV.

Aluminum and antimony metallic films were prepared on glass substrates by electron-beam evaporation at a rate of 0.3 nm/s (Fig. 1). The substrates had been previously rinsed with ethanol and argon sputtered in a glow discharge at 10^{-2} mbar for one hour. AES and XPS spectra (Fig. 2) show that the films are carbon and oxygen free, and although a small amount of Sb was detected in Al films, probably due to a pollution between the melting pots of the evaporator, this pollution does not exceed ten atomic percent at the surface. The layers are, respectively, 15 nm, 64.5 nm and 20 nm thick for the Al-Sb-Al metallic sandwich, as measured by a quartz microbalance. During the evaporations the residual pressure in the chamber stayed below 4×10^{-8} mbar.

---

* Holder of an IRSIA doctoral fellowship.

** Work supported by the Belgian Ministry for Science Policy.

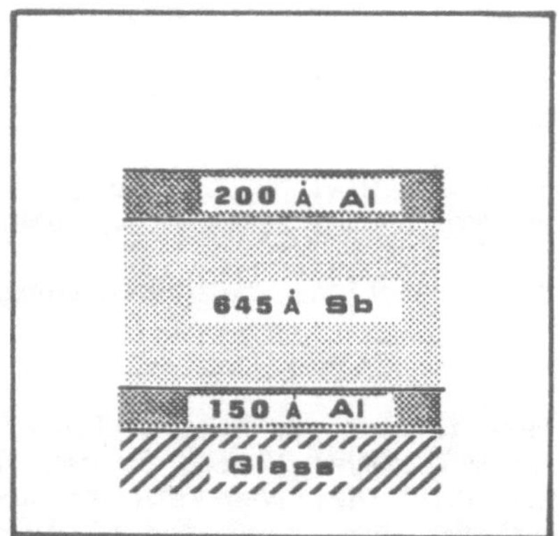

FIGURE 1. The sample was electron-beam evaporated below 4 x 10^{-8} mbar on a glass substrate previously etched in an argon plasma.

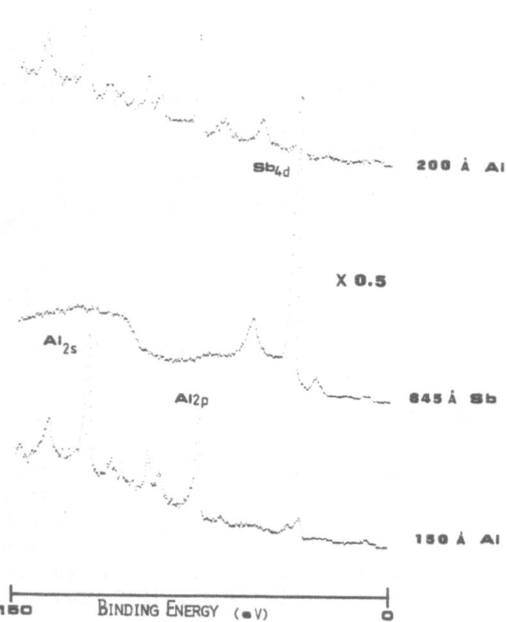

FIGURE 2. Photoelectron spectra performed after evaporations and before laser treatment.

Unfortunately, the uppermost aluminum layer was found to be oxidized because of a pressure rise to 10^{-7} mbar for several hours. Nevertheless, it's well known that a passivation layer of Al_2O_3 quickly grows on metallic aluminum and that it does not exceed 5 nm in this case.

Samples were then pulsed laser treated at 10^{-9} mbar (Fig. 3). At the sample, the laser pulse delivers approximately 2 mJ during 10 ns. The surface area transformed was approximately 0.5 by 5 mm. The fluence is then approximately 80 mJ/cm^2. The laser spot is displaced 0.1 mm and the operation repeated until all the sample is transformed. Transformation is determined by visual inspection since AlSb (a 1.6 eV energy gap semiconductor) is transparent for most of the visible light frequencies.

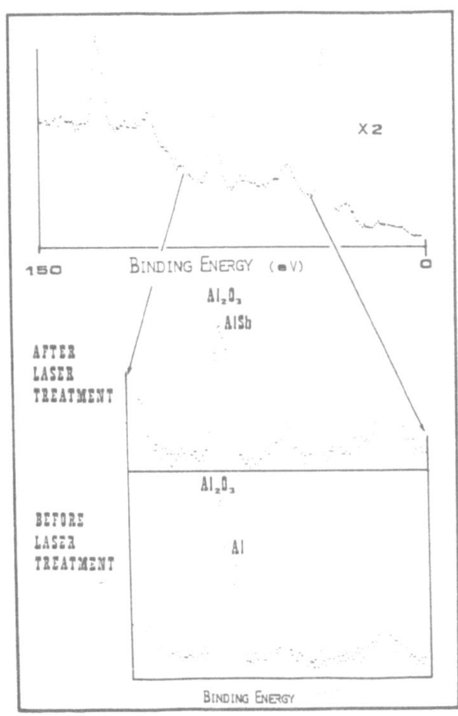

FIGURE 3. XPS spectra after laser treatment in the range extending from 150 to 0 eV (binding energy). The expanded region shows the Al_{2p} line behavior. The sample has been slightly oxidized after evaporations and before laser treatment.

3. RESULTS

By photoemission spectroscopy we observed essentially the Al 2s and 2p lines at 73 and 124 eV, respectively; the Sb 4d line at (32.9-31.9 eV) and the valence band.

The general features reported in the literature (3-5) for the valence band spectra of Al, Sb and AlSb can be observed (Fig. 4). But for the case of AlSb the relative intensity of the three signals at 23, 19 and 14 eV as seen on our energy scale is not the same as those measured on monocrystals. This difference probably occurs because of the polycrystallinity of our sample and the presence of aluminum oxide and antimony at the surface of the sample. These spectra focus our attention on the problems of the Fermi level reference, since for metallic phases it would appear at the same energy as the zero energy.

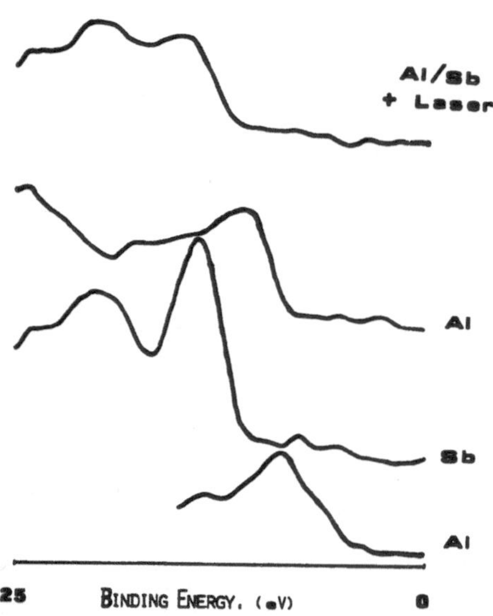

FIGURE 4. Valence bands as seen by XPS.

Evidence of compound formation is seen in the aluminum and antimony signal shift after laser treatment (Fig. 3). Choosing the Al 2p line associated to the oxide at 75.5 eV as a reference (assuming that the oxide is not involved in the laser treatment), we observed the shift of the Al 2p line from 73.0 eV to approximately 74.3 eV.

The Al 2p peak at 75.5 eV seems to not be affected in intensity, although it's difficult to have a precise observation because of the convolution of the Al_2O_3 and AlSb designated peaks in the bulk Plasmon observed on the Sb 4d peak. A change also appears from that of the metallic Sb value of approximately 16 eV to the laser formed compound value of 14.8 eV which is reported in the literature (5) as the AlSb value.

Other evidences of the compound formation are to be observed on AES spectra (Fig. 5b). The general shape of the spectra is obviously changed in the range from 15 to 115 eV, and in the range extending from 1270 to 1450 eV. The Al LMM line which appears at 68 eV for the metallic films is displaced to 58 eV as reported by others (6-8). The higher energy signal seems to be very sensitive to the laser treatment and, as we think, to the AlSb compound formation (since until now, to our knowledge, nothing has been published about these line shapes for AlSb).

The comparison of Al and Sb signal amplitudes in the 15 to 520 eV range show that in the superficial layer there is a 7% excess of Sb compared with the stoichiometric proportions.

The characteristic AES signal of Al oxide may also be observed at its usual place.

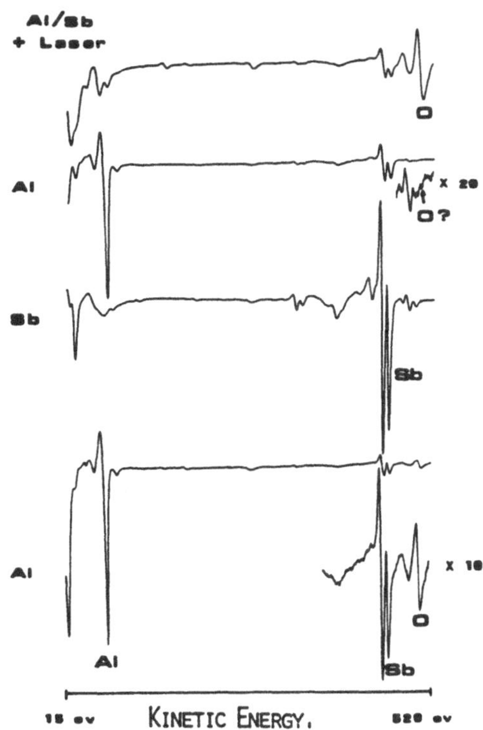

FIGURE 5. Auger spectra after evaporation and after laser treatment.

4. CONCLUSIONS

Many arguments tend to prove that AlSb thin film has really been synthesized by laser mixing of Al and Sb metallic thin film sandwiches. We have observed a segregation of Sb and aluminum oxide at the surface of the sample. Other electrical and optical experiments are still to be done to determine the quality of the film and why the excess of Sb is not included in the AlSb phase.

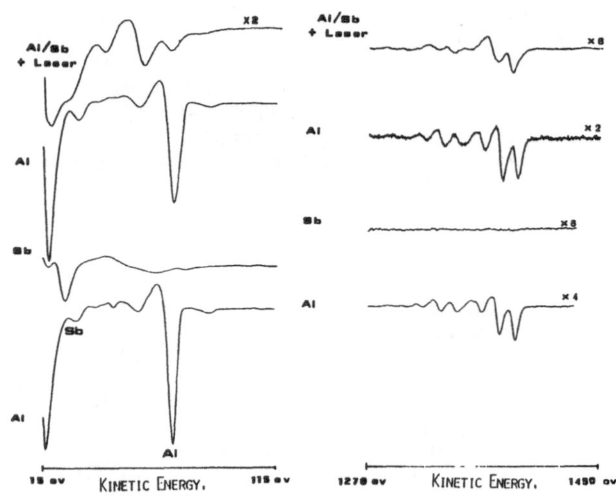

FIGURE 6. Auger spectra after evaporation and after laser treatment (details).

REFERENCES

1. L. Laude, Cohesive Properties of Semiconductors under Laser Irradiation, NATO ASI Series (Martinus Nijhoff, 1983).
2. J. J. Pireaux, J. P. Delrue, P. A. Thiry, and R. Caudano, J. Vac. Sci. Technol., A 2, 1208 (1984).
3. P. Steiner, H. Höchst, and S. Hüfner, in Photoemission in Solids II, edited by L. Ley and M. Cardona, Topics in Applied Physics (Springer Verlag), Vol. 27, p. 369.
4. Photoemission in Semiconductors, p. 106.
5. J. Schenchik, J. Tejeda, and M. Cardona, Phys. Rev. B 9, 2627-2648 (1974).
6. R. Andrew, L. Baufay, Y. Canivez, and A. Pigeolet, J. de Physique 44, 495-499 (1983).
7. J. M. Guglielmacci, F. Charfi, and A. Joullie, Thin Solid Films 76, 69-75 (1981).
8. R. Sporken, J. P. Delrue, and R. Caudano, "Initial Growth Study of Al on Sb(111) Surfaces," International Conference on the Formation of Semiconductor Interface, Marseilles, 1985.

LASER TREATMENT OF La-IMPLANTED Ni SINGLE CRYSTAL

G. BATTAGLIN, A. CARNERA, G. DELLA MEA, V. KULKARNI, P. MAZZOLDI
Dipartimento di Fisica dell'Universita, Via Marzolo 8, 35131 Padova, Italy

D. K. SOOD AND A. P. POGARNY
Microelectronics Technology Center, Royal Melbourne Institute of Technology, Melbourne 300, Australia

Key Words: metastable phases, surface segregation, oxidation

ABSTRACT

The use of pulsed laser irradiation to obtain metastable alloys in metals is now well known. Heat flow model calculations of laser melt transient have led to a good understanding and analysis of solute depth profiles, based on liquid phase diffusion, solute segregation at the liquid solid interface, and thermal gradient-induced diffusion (Soret effect). While segregation effects have been found to give rise to a sharp solute surface peak in many pulsed laser irradiation studies on Si, no such explicit evidence of segregation in metals has yet been shown. A solute surface peak is, however, reported for Hf-, Eu-, and La-implanted Ni after laser irradiation. The origin of the surface peak has been studied by performing laser irradiation in an ambient having reduced oxygen and water content, and on La- and O-implanted Ni samples.

The surface peak formation is attributed to a mechanism involving oxidation and trapping of solute at the surface. The experimental solute profiles are then reproduced with a liquid phase diffusion analysis including such a mechanism.

TEM analysis shows the formation of an amorphous phase in La-implanted Ni, which transforms into a polycrystalline layer after laser treatment.

1. INTRODUCTION

Metastable alloys in metals are obtained by using pulsed laser irradiations (1-4). The characteristics of the heat flow transient (5,6) in the pulsed laser irradiation on metals (high resolidification velocity and large cooling rate) trap solute atoms (7) on the host lattice sites, resulting in solid solubilities extending well beyond the normal equilibrium limits.

Criteria (8) for obtaining a metastable solid solution require miscibility for the components in the liquid phase followed by good liquid phase epitaxy (LPE) under high cooling rates. Defect impurity interaction can influence the final phase formation (9).

Segregation effects in metals under pulsed laser irradiations are not expected. Indeed, a commonly accepted view (10,11) is that the impurity residence time τ_{res} at the regrowing interface is much too long, compared to the regrowth time τ_{reg}, to avoid trapping. $\tau_{res} = \lambda^2/D_i$ is the impurity diffusion coefficient just at the regrowing interface and λ a characteristic layer thickness. In $\tau_{reg} = \lambda/v$, v is the resolidification velocity. In metals, with the rather large values obtained by v, (due to the higher thermal conductivity and lower latent heat of recrystallization which characterize metals with respect to silicon) (12), the condition of the occurrence of segregation $\tau_{res}/\tau_{reg} = \lambda v/D_i << 1$ is seldom satisfied.

A solute surface peak was, however, reported for Hf (13-14), Eu (9) and La (15) implanted in Ni after laser irradiation in air. Such a peak disappeared when the laser irradiation was carried out in vacuum conditions (15).

In this paper we present the results obtained for pulsed laser irradiation of La- and/or O-implanted Ni, in air and in vacuum, for explaining the apparent surface La segregation and the formation of amorphous or polycrystalline surface layers, due to ion implantation and pulsed laser irradiation.

2. EXPERIMENTAL

Electropolished Ni single crystals, <100> orientation, having a damage-free surface and mirror finish have been used in the present experiment for La and/or O implantations and subsequent laser irradiations.

Three types of implanted regions have been produced: (1) implanted with La^{++} at 250 keV energy, (2) implanted first with La^{++} at 250 keV and successively with O^{18} at 35 keV, (3) implanted with only O^{18}. The implantation energy of 35 keV for the O^{18} implants has been chosen in order to produce an O distribution which would approximately overlap the La distribution.

The implanted crystals were irradiated in air or under low-pressure conditions (10^{-2} torr) at various energy densities, E_p, up to 5.2 J/cm^2 by using the ruby laser (pulses of 16 nsec FWHM) of Centro Gas Ionizzati - CNR (Padova).

From the spatially homogenized large laser spot of 16 mm size, a region of 2.5 mm diameter was carefully selected for irradiation which ensured energy uniformity better than $\pm$ 10% over the selected area.

Implanted and irradiated regions have been analyzed by Rutherford backscattering (RBS) and channeling using a 1.8 MeV He^+ beam. The amount of O^{18} was detected by using the $^{18}O(P,\alpha)^{15}N$ nuclear reaction.

The sample surfaces were viewed in a scanning electron microscope (SEM).

Samples for transmission electron microscopy at Melbourne University (TEM) were prepared by jet thinning from the backside, while protecting the irradiated face.

3. RESULTS

3.1. La Profile

In Figure 1 we report the La profiles as obtained by RBS in random and channeling conditions for La-implanted Ni samples, irradiated in air (15). A complete lack of substitutionality is seen in the as-implanted profile (in agreement with previous work (16)) and is found to persist at all energy densities employed in the present experiment.

However, a gradual broadening in the initial La distribution at successively higher energy densities up to 3 J/cm^2 and an almost flat tail (suggestive of convective effects) (17,18) at above 3.5 J/cm^2 are observed.

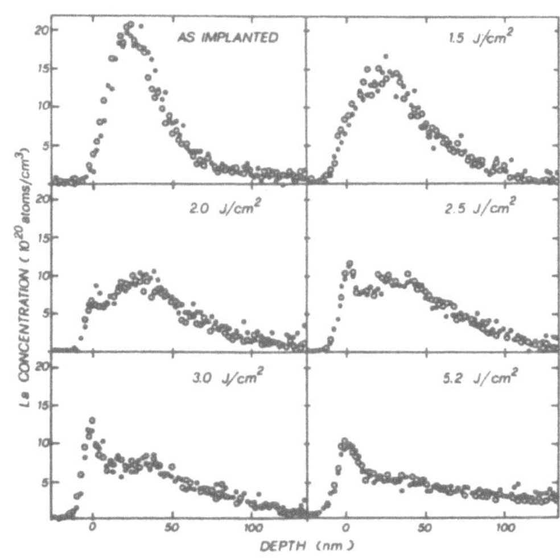

FIGURE 1. Random (•) and <100> aligned (o) depth concentration profiles of La in Ni after irradiation at the indicated pulse energies (15).

In the La depth profile for <1.5 J/cm^2 irradiation, a kink appears at the surface which develops into a clearly defined surface peak at higher energy densities. The La surface peak, which is seen under irradiation in air, is almost absent under low pressure. Figure 2 shows two La profiles as obtained after pulsed laser irradiation in air (open circles) and under low-pressure conditions (full circles), together with the as-implanted distribution (15).

A similar result, reduction in the surface peaking of Hf, was obtained when the irradiation of Hf-implanted Ni was carried out under helium cover gas (14).

By changing the air pressure, we reduced the oxygen and water vapor content in the ambient atmosphere. Since the heat of formation of La_2O_3 is negative and outstandingly large in absolute value, as it is for HfO_2 and other rare earth oxides like Ca, Dy, Gd oxides (presumably Eu oxides, for which no data are available, have the same characteristic), La oxidation is an energetically highly favored process. As a consequence, a strong surface oxidation may be expected for La as soon as it gets at the Ni surface, as well as for Eu and Hf under similar conditions.

In the case of oxygen- and La-implanted Ni samples (Fig. 3), we observed a reduction of La mobility in the liquid Ni matrix, thus supporting our view that oxygen acts as a trapping entity for La.

A fit of the experimental La and Eu (9) profiles has been performed, in cooperation with L. Dona dalle Rose and A. Miotello (15,19) by means of an impurity diffusion equation which takes into account La or Eu capture at the liquid Ni surface, due to oxide formation (i.e., La_2O_3) at the Ni surface with a possible subsequent clustering of oxidized La atoms.

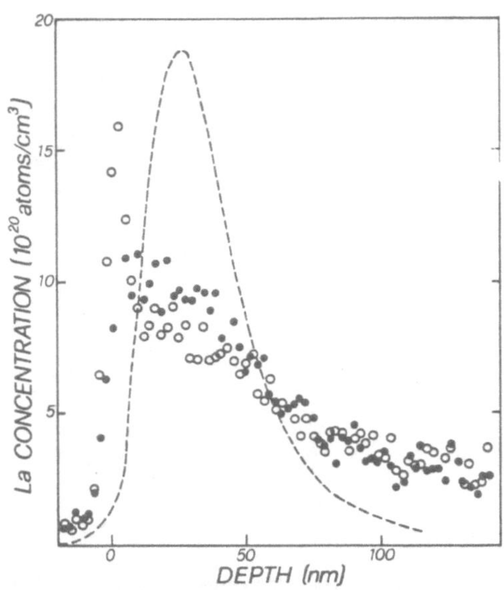

FIGURE 2. Depth concentration profiles of La in Ni obtained after laser irradiation at 4.6 J/cm^2 in air (o) and in vacuum (•). The dashed line shows the as-implanted La distribution (15).

Figure 4a,b shows the calculated convoluted Eu/La profiles together with experimental ones. Through the fit procedure values for the effective capture parameter and the diffusion coefficient are determined. The D values are indicated in the figure and are consistent with the usual liquid phase diffusion coefficients (15,17,20,21).

3.2. Damage

Channeling analysis gives information on the damage introduced in the crystal by implantation and subsequent laser irradiation. Interpretations of such results are sometimes ambiguous. Indeed, either polycrystalline or amorphous surface layers show channeling yields comparable to those obtained in random condition analysis. As a result, TEM investigations can give a clearer picture of the defect distribution and structure of the samples.

In Figure 5 we report the random and <100> aligned channeling spectra for 250 keV La-implanted Ni at a dose of 5×10^{16} ions/cm^2. The Ni aligned to random ratios (χ) for those irradiated (in vacuum) at 2.5 and 3.5 J/cm^2 are reported, as a function of depth, in Figure 6a. The La profiles (aligned and random are coincident) from the same samples are reported in Figure 6b.

The La implantation creates a damage peak with a peak height value comparable to the random value (surface minimum yield $\chi \simeq 100\%$), suggesting the formation of an amorphous layer. At 2.5 J/cm^2 the damage peak becomes very broad while the peak height decreases. At 3.5 J/cm^2 the damage peak height reduces to 70%. Similar results have been obtained for a La implantation dose of 2.5×10^{16} ions/cm^2.

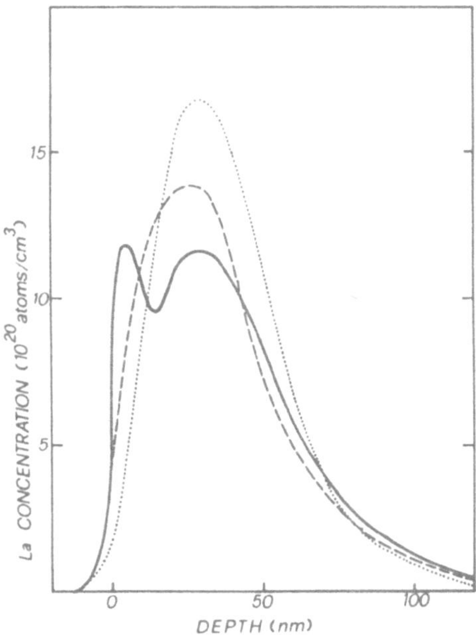

FIGURE 3. Depth concentration of La in Ni, as observed after laser irradiation at 3 J/cm^2, for La-implanted Ni (full curve) and La plus O-implanted Ni (dashed curve). The La profile after oxygen implantation (dotted line) but before laser irradiation is also shown for comparison purposes (15).

For lower implantation doses (15) (10^{16} La/cm^2) the surface peak reaches a maximum value of about 40%, suggesting that the formation of an amorphous layer is obtained only above a critical La concentration. Laser irradiation produces a La redistribution, lowering the impurity concentration. The lack of an amorphous layer, even in the presence of very high cooling rates during pulsed laser treatment (PLT)($\simeq 10^9$ K s^{-1}), is connected to a significant deviation in the melt composition from the glass-forming zone. Similar results have been obtained for METGLAS E4040 (22). Such results are confirmed by TEM analysis.

In Figures 7a,b,c we report the TEM images obtained in the La-implanted Ni at a dose of 5 x 10^{16} ions/cm^2. We observe a buried amorphous layer on top of a polycrystalline layer above the single crystal matrix (see Figs. 7b and 7c). A very thin single-crystal layer with defects and dislocation loops is present at the surface (see Fig. 7a).

No sign of either La or La_2O_3 or any La-Ni intermetallic precipitates is evident in the polycrystalline layer, which is characterized by large grains. Some grains are hcp, indicating the existence of a fcc-hcp transformation.

The La would be present as a Metastable Solid Solution (MSS) either interstitial or substitutional in each grain of polycrystalline Ni. The

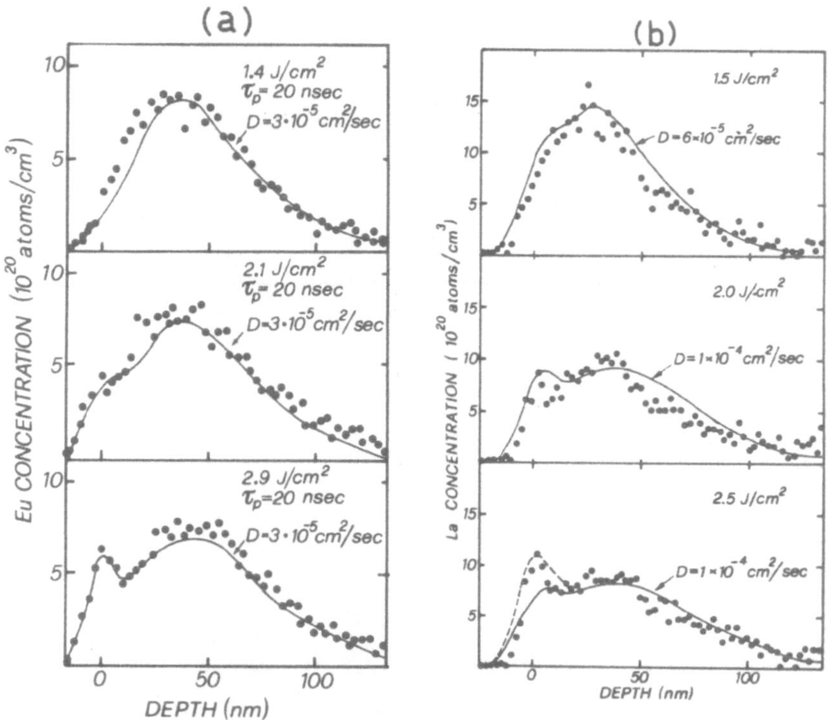

FIGURE 4. Depth profiles of (a) Eu and (b) La at the indicated energy densities. Full curves show the best fit to the depth profiles, obtained from liquid phase diffusion calculations using the indicated diffusion coefficients. In (b) the additional dashed curve for 2.5 J/cm^2 refers to the calculation which also includes a small Ni evaporation (19).

Ni transformation to hcp phase is induced by ion damage. The polyphase is a precursor to amorphization observed in the region of the maximum La concentration, as seen many times in Ni by earlier workers (23).

In Figure 8a,b we show the TEM images obtained for the previous sample after laser irradiation in vacuum at an energy of 2.5 J/cm^2. It would indicate that the critical concentration of La required in liquid phase for its quench to a-phase is not smaller than that for amorphization by ion implantation. The amorphous phase, present in the as-implanted sample, transformed to coarse grain polycrystalline Ni. Each grain probably contains a MSS of La in Ni. Annealing in situ in the microscope showed La precipitates not detected in the initial condition. The ambient concentration of La in the melt seems to be high enough to block Liquid Phase Epitaxy (LPE) at the Liquid Solid Interface (LSI). A thin single-crystal layer is observed at the surface.

At higher laser irradiation energies we detected a very fine grain polylayer. In the case of La- and O-implanted samples the results are similar to those observed for as-implanted La samples. No crystalline oxides are observed.

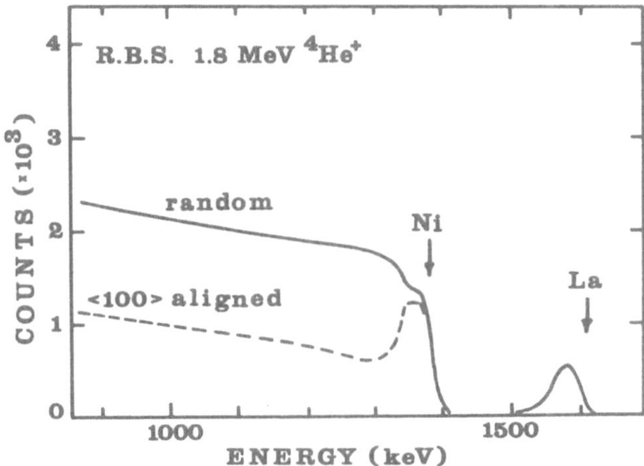

FIGURE 5. Random and <100> axial channeling spectra for 250 keV La-implanted Ni at a dose of 5 x 10^{16} ions/cm^2.

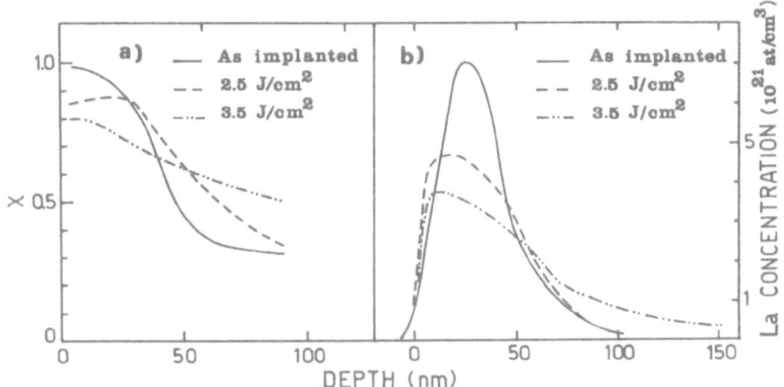

FIGURE 6. (a) Aligned to random ratios (χ) of the Ni spectra for as-implanted, 2.5 and 3.5 J/cm^2 laser-irradiated samples. (b) Depth concentration profiles of La in Ni for the same sample as in (a).

After laser irradiation the amorphous phase transformed to a fine-grain polycrystalline layer containing fcc and hcp Ni crystallites, NiO precipitates, and La_2O_3 precipitates which are more coarse and extend to the surface. Some vacancy loops, or voids, were seen only at 3.5 J/cm^2 laser irradiation. There was weak evidence for competition between La and Ni to react with oxygen in the melt.

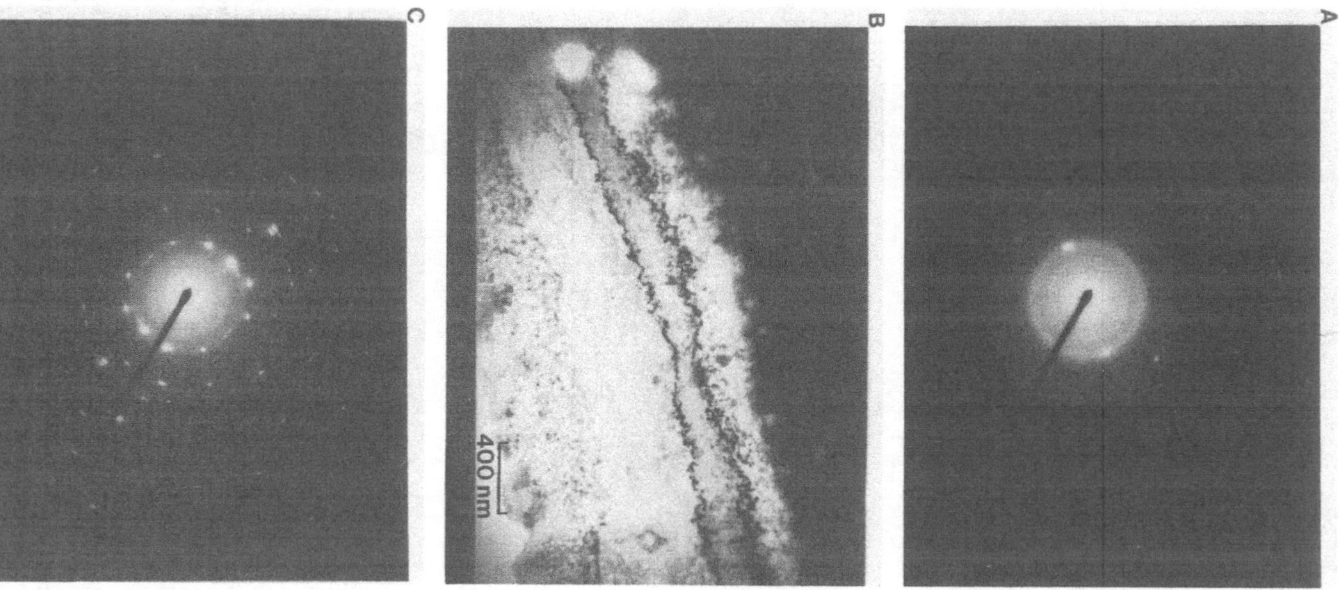

FIGURE 7. TEM images obtained in La-implanted Ni at a dose of 5×10^{16} ions/cm^2: (a) surface region, (b) subsurface region, (c) bulk.

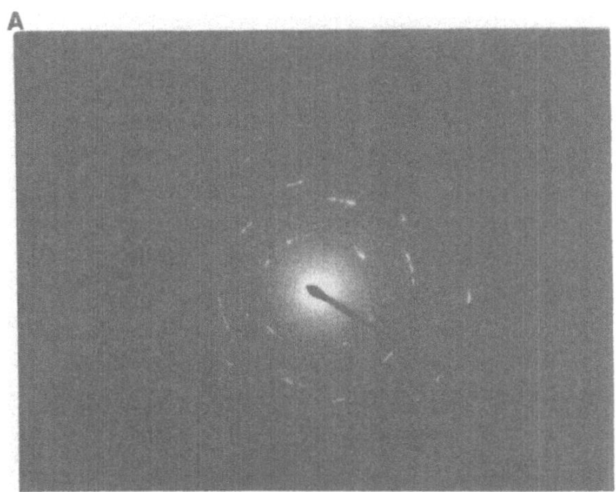

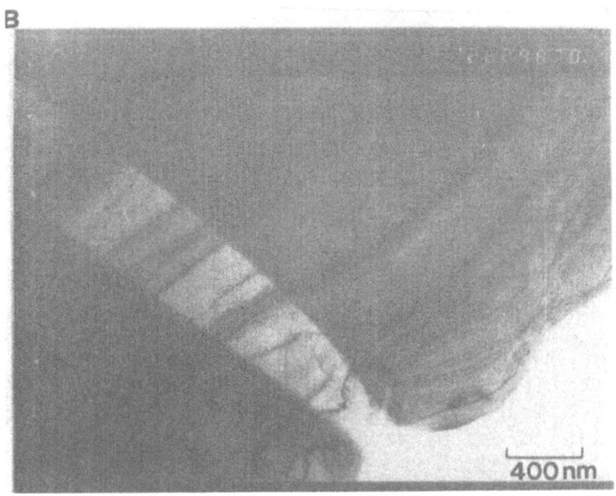

FIGURE 8. TEM images obtained for La-implanted Ni after 2.5 J/cm^2 laser irradiation: (a) EDP, (b) bright field.

Finally, in the case of O-implanted Ni, channeling spectra reported in Figure 9 show a damage lower than that observed for La or La and O implantation, without the surface peak characteristic of an amorphous region. TEM analysis indicates the formation of a buried layer containing polycrystalline Ni, metastable hcp Ni particles and a dense network of dislocations. No NiO phase was detected showing formation of a metastable solid solution of O and Ni poly grains. The top surface had a very thin (<5 nm) single-crystal layer.

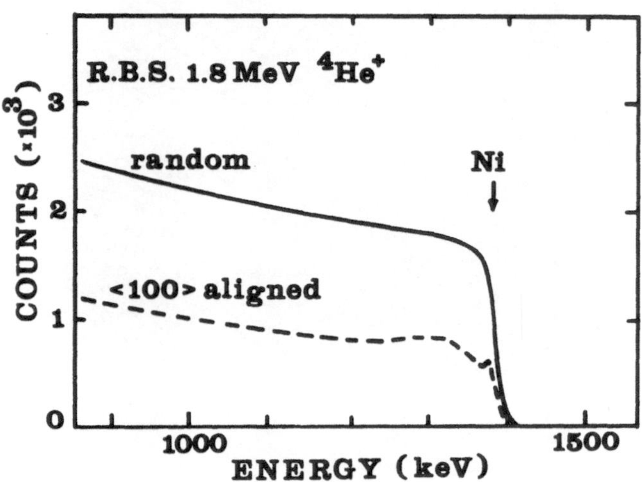

FIGURE 9. Random and <100> axial channeling spectra for 35 keV ^{18}O-implanted Ni at a dose of 5 x 10^{16} ions/cm^2.

Laser irradiation at 2.5 J/cm^2 resulted in the formation of fine-grained, randomly oriented polycrystallites of NiO (10 nm large) (Fig. 10a) and a buried layer of much coarser (about 50 nm) polycrystallites of Ni (Fig. 10b). Increasing the laser irradiation energy, we obtained similar results, with the formation of voids or gas bubbles.

These results are consistent with internal oxidation of Ni in the melt. Laser irradiation produces a molten region well beyond the O implant depth (projected range of 10 nm), with temperatures approaching the boiling point (2730°C) of Ni. Before the solidificaton front arrives, NiO is precipitated out in liquid phase and solidifies at 1984°C well before Ni (at 1455°C (24)). This phase separation could be associated with formation of polycrystalline Ni. We are not able to explain the formation of voids, showing clear black to white contrast change on underfocusing, observed at 3.7 J/cm^2 in the presence of implanted oxygen.

4. CONCLUSIONS

A systematic study of the evolution of La-implanted Ni and O-implanted Ni systems during pulsed laser irradiation has been performed by using RBS and TEM analysis. No segregation effects are evident. An amorphous layer was produced for high implantation doses in La-implanted Ni crystal, which transforms into a poly-layer after laser irradiation. No amorphous phases are evident for O-implanted Ni samples before and after laser irradiation.

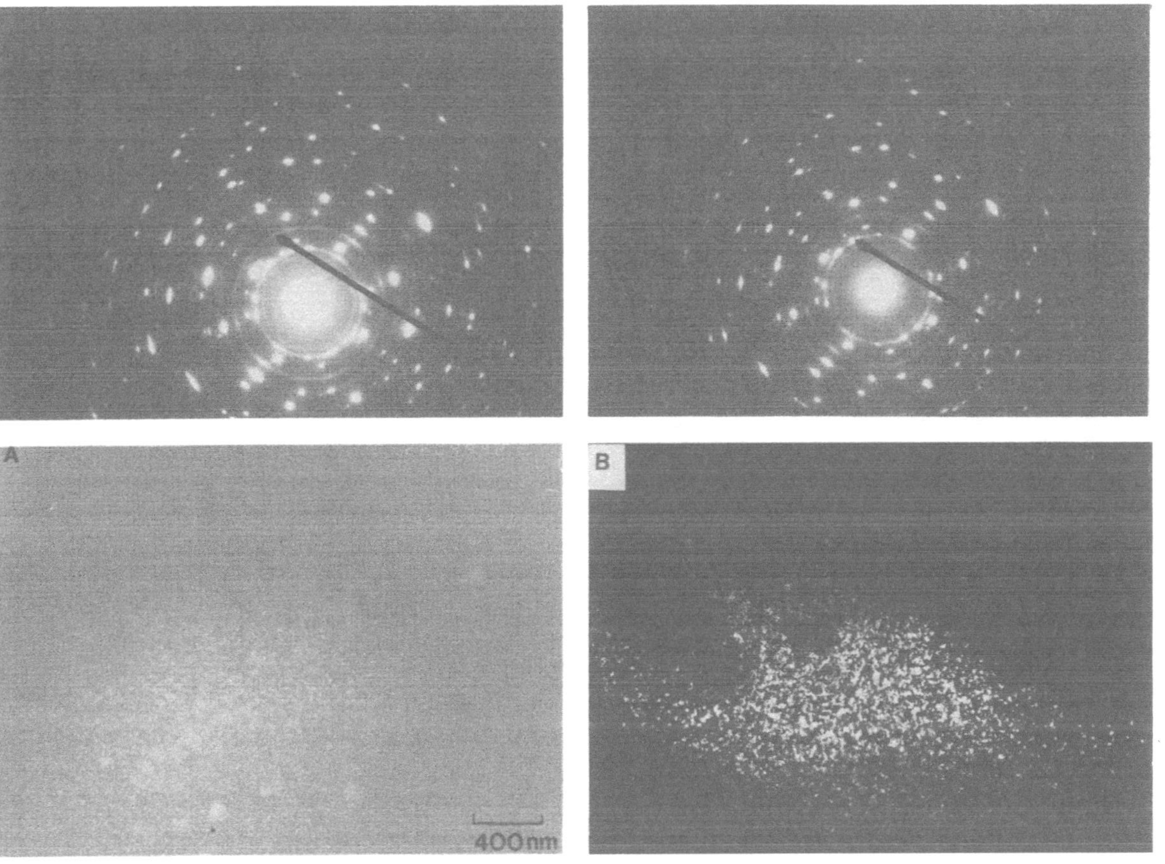

FIGURE 10. Images of (a) randomly oriented polycrystallites of NiO and (b) polycrystallites of Ni in O-implanted Ni after 2.5 J/cm^2 laser irradiation.

REFERENCES

1. Laser-Solid Interactions and Laser Processing, edited by S. D. Ferris, H. J. Leamy, and J. M. Poate, AIP Conference Proceedings No. 50 (AIP, New York, 1979).
2. Laser and Electron Beam Processing of Materials, edited by C. W. White and P. S. Peercy, Materials Research Society Symposia Proceedings, Vol. 1 (Academic, New York, 1980).
3. Laser and Electron Beam Solid Interactions and Material Processing, edited by J. F. Gibbons, L. D. Hess, and T. W. Sigmon (North Holland, New York, 1981).
4. D. K. Sood, Radiat. Eff. 63, 141 (1982).
5. L. F. Dona dalle Rose and A. Miotello, Radiat. Eff. 53, 19 (1980).
6. A. K. Jain, V. N. Kulkarni, and D. K. Sood, Appl. Phys. 25, 127 (1981).
7. K. A. Jackson, G. H. Gilmer, and H. J. Leamy, Ref. 2, p. 104.
8. D. K. Sood, Radiat. Eff. Lett. 67, 13 (1981).
9. G. Battaglin, A. Carnera, G. Della Mea, P. Mazzoldi, A. K. Jain, V. N. Kulkarni, and D. K. Sood, in Metastable Materials Formation by Ion Implantation, edited by S. T. Picraux and W. J. Choyke (North Holland, New York, 1982), p. 333.
10. S. T. Picraux, D. M. Follstaedt, J. A. Knapp, W. R. Wampler, and E. Rimini, Ref. 3, p. 575.
11. P. Mazzoldi, L. F. Dona dalle Rose, and D. K. Sood, Radiat. Eff. 63, 105 (1982).
12. R. F. Wood, J. R. Kirkpatrick, and G. E. Giles, Phys. Rev. B 23, 5555 (1981).
13. L. Buene, E. N. Kaufmann, M. L. McDonald, K. Kothaus, R. Vianded, K. Freitag, and C. W. Draper, in Nuclear and Electron Resonance Spectroscopies Applied to Materials Science, edited by E. N. Kaufmann and G. K. Shenoy (Elsevier North Holland, New York, 1981) p. 391.
14. C. W. Draper, E. N. Kaufmann, and L. Buene, Surface and Interface Analysis 4, 8 (1982).
15. G. Battaglin, A. Carnera, G. Della Mea, L. F. Dona dalle Rose, V. N. Kulkarni, P. Mazzoldi, A. Miotello, G. Jannitti, A. K. Jain, D. K. Sood, and J. Chaumont, J. Appl. Phys. 53, 3773 (1984).
16. D. K. Sood and G. Dearnaley, Radiat. Eff. 39, 157 (1984).
17. G. Battaglin, A. Carnera, G. Della Mea, P. Mazzoldi, E. Jannitti, A. K. Jain, and D. K. Sood, J. Appl. Phys. 53, 3224 (1982).
18. W. K. Chu, J. W. Mayer, and M. A. Nicolet, Backscattering Spectrometry (Academic, New York, 1978), p. 251.
19. G. Battaglin, A. Carnera, J. Chaumont, G. Della Mea, L. F. Dona dalle Rose, A. K. Jain, V. N. Kulkarni, P. Mazzoldi, A. Miotello, and D. K. Sood, J. de Physique C5, 481 (1983).
20. A. Miotello, L. F. Dona dalle Rose and A. DeSalvo, Appl. Phys. Lett. 40, 135 (1982).
21. C. J. Smithells, Metals Reference Book (Butterworths, London, 1975), p. 939.
22. A. K. Jain, D. K. Sood, G. Battaglin, A. Carnera, G. Della Mea, V. Kulkarni, P. Mazzoldi, and R. V. Nandekau, Mater. Res. Soc. Symp. Proc. 13, 703 (1983).
23. Z. Y. A. Al-Tamini, W. A. Grant, and G. Carter, Nucl. Instrum. Methods 209/210, 363 (1983).
24. M. Hansen, Constitution of Binary Alloys (McGraw-Hill, New York, 1958), p. 1024.

EDITED QUESTIONS - CHAPTER 2

PEERCY, SPAEPEN, WILLIAMSON, MAC DONALD, MAZZOLDI, FRÖHLINGSDORF, JACOBSON, HELMS, PETIT, KAUFMANN

PAUL PEERCY

Q. For pure Al what happens in the heat-affected zone below the melt?
A. Damage is introduced in the form of dislocations and slip.

Q. Is there homogeneous nucleation in the melts?
A. We do not know for certain; homogeneous nucleation is rare and one cannot rule out heterogeneous nucleation.

Q. Are there more interstitials in the ion-implanted samples?
A. The samples have been amorphized by the large implant dose; the concept of interstitials is not well defined in amorphous materials.

Q. How do you get by the other phases when you go from α to γ in Mn?
A. By superheating past them with the nsec laser pulse.

Q. How do you know that the Mn α phase did not melt at 0.77 J/cm^2?
A. From transient reflectivity measurements during irradiation and microscopy after irradiation.

Q. What was the composition of the Al-Ni?
A. It ranged from 50:50 Al-Ni to 36 at.% Ni.

Q. Could you force a certain structure by seeding?
A. Most likely, yes.

Q. Do large complicated unit cells have time to form in the short solidification times in this experiment?
A. Icosahedra are believed to form or exist in the liquid phase.

Q. Can you quench it too fast and get amorphous material?
A. Yes.

SPAEPEN

Q. Will photon pressure affect the vapor pressure?
A. No, the photon pressure is negligible.

Q. Is there Al dissolved in the alloys from the underlying layer?
A. No, Al is only found when you blow a hole through the layer and splash the Al.

Q. Isn't most of the energy in the shock wave?
A. One can calculate from the extent of melt depth that most of the energy has gone into melting.

Q. Is there any partitioning of B and Fe?
A. No, not under present quenching conditions; only in the 4 at.% B alloy at the last stages of solidification has possible partitioning been observed.

Q. What is the segregation coefficient for B in Fe?
A. The equilibrium value is very small; most likely, the non-equilibrium value that applies to the present experiments is much higher, which in turn increases the interfacial stability.

Q. How do you check the composition?
A. By knowing the thickness of each layer and the number of layers of each element.

WILLIAMSON

Q. What is the basic parameter?
A. Energy.

Q. What is the Al film thickness?
A. 25 nm.

Q. What was the symptom of fatigue in the Al target?
A. At the lower fluence levels where vaporization is not an issue, the films can be cycled but eventually tear.

Q. When do you turn on the laser?
A. Either before or after the electrons.

Q. What is the synchronization resolution?
A. 20 psec.

Q. When do you stop melting?
A. After 20 psec.

Q. Can you tell if any of the Al transforms to vapor?
A. No, but because the film remains under low fluence levels, we believe only a solid-liquid transition occurs.

Q. Does the film deform?
A. Yes, after the event the films appear to have deformed.

Q. How do you measure lattice parameters when the films are flexible and deformed?
A. On the time scale of interest no deformation has occurred.

Q. Can you use reflection geometry in your electron diffraction to characterize the surface?
A. Yes. In fact, we are developing a system to do that. It will be RHEED.

Q. Does the surface oxide affect the results?
A. We don't know.

Q. Why do you have to signal overage?
A. Because of pulse spreading (electron).

MAC DONALD

Q. Is the orientation of the sample important?
A. No, the probe beam (or the Nd:YAG laser) is within 10° of normal incidence.

Q. Is the measured reflection diffuse or specular?
A. Only the specular component is measured.

Q. Why isn't the damage spot round?
A. The fine scale roughness is due to material non-uniformities. In addition, the actual laser spot is not quite round and varies somewhat on a timescale of several hours.

Q. Have you done heat flow calculations?
A. Heat flow calculations for a variety of substrates are in progress.

Q. Wouldn't you expect the solidification to be faster than it is?
A. In the bulk case the fastest interface velocities would occur for the initial stages of crystallization. We can only measure the regrowth over the last couple of hundred angstroms by which the interface would have slowed considerably. For the thin film case the heat flow and expected interface velocity would be slower than for the bulk.

MAZZOLDI

Q. In the P, B, Fe how thick are the samples?
A. 400 nm.

Q. What is the regrowth velocity?
A. It was calculated to be 20 m/sec.

Q. Were the irradiations performed in a vacuum?
A. Yes.

Q. How deep was the melt?
A. About 400 nm for the higher energies.

FRÖHLINGSDORF

Q. Why are there arrows going in both directions on the phase diagrams?
A. They show the temperatures where the phases are stable and the hysteresis.

Q. Have you used longer laser pulses?
A. No.

Q. Is there any delay in going from α to ß above 16 K?
A. The transition is smeared out over 4-5 K.

Q. What is the difference beteween ion-implanted α and ß phases?
A. In the ß phase there is 4-5% oxygen.

Q. At 4°K are there incorporated gases?
A. Less than 1%.

Q. What is strange about Ga compared to other metals?
A. The bonding in Ga is covalent.

Q. Were you able to measure the time to transform from α to ß?
A. No.

Q. Does any energy go clear through the sample?
A. Yes.

Q. Does the sample get hot?
A. We don't think so.

JACOBSON

Q. Is the As on lattice sites?
A. Channeling does not show that it is.

Q. Does the Stefan-Boltzman equation support ignoring radiative loss?
A. Yes, about 10^3 watt/cm^2 is radiated and the incident power is $>10^8$ watts/cm^2.

Q. Where did you get the thermal constants that you used?
A. From the literature.

Q. What does the resolidified melt area look like?
A. Polycrystalline.

Q. Do you have any end product in mind?
A. No.

Q. Did you see segregation for anything besides As?
A. Yes, segregation was observed for Ge implants as well.

Q. Could large quantities of material be ablating from the surface?
A. The As-implanted data shows that only a few hundred angstroms of material is lost.

HELMS

Q. Did you use overlapping spots in the Mo studies?
A. Yes.

Q. What would you get with one pulse?
A. We did not do that analysis. The laser and the LEED are in different labs ~50 miles apart.

PETIT

Q. From these results, what do we know about the third layer in the Al-Sb-Al samples?
A. After treatment the film is fully transparent. Therefore, there cannot be any metallic Al. This can be confirmed by conductivity measurements.

Q. Is excess aluminum rejected to the grain boundaries?
A. No, it is antimony that is rejected to the grain boundaries.

Q. What is the scenario for mixing?
A. During transformation you need to melt a portion of aluminum with antimony. When melting occurs, the reaction begins immediately and the released energy of formation is sufficient to complete the reaction.

Q. What do the samples look like after treatment?
A. They appear to be polycrystalline AlSb as seen by the SEM.

KAUFMANN

Q. Are the crystals in the near eutectic PdCuSi cross section α phase?
A. Yes, but not nucleating off the substrate. They result from massive solidification below T_0.

Q. Independent of glass transition temperature?
A. If one cuts the C-shaped curve, one gets crystallization (Fig. 3).

Q. What is the concentration of the Ta-Ir alloy? (Fig. 9,10)
A. 75% Ta (near Ta-rich end of the phase diagram).

Q. What is the significance of processing speed? Was there a large difference in traverse velocity?
A. Traverse velocity couldn't be utilized in our CO_2 thermal code model, so we used dwell time which doesn't vary between CO_2 and e-beam cases.

Q. How was the beam diameter measured?
A. From the width of the molten pool.

Q. Does this not vary with interaction time and power?
A. No comment! (Editor's comment - Yes it will, but so will the 1/e optical spot (with power).)

Q. What were the crystallizing conditions for the Metglass ribbon? (Fig. 12).
A. A few hours at elevated temperature is enough to fully crystallize it.

Q. Are you aware of any sort of experiments on magnetic properties of two different viscosity Metglass materials?
A. No.

Q. Can you include convection in your heat transfer codes at LLL?
A. Yes. In addition, the welding group and recently formed stress/strain group have developed a highly sophisticated model together to account also for things such as thermal strains in the sample.

CHAPTER 3. MODELING OF HEAT AND MASS TRANSFER

INTRODUCTION - L. G. DONA DALLE ROSE

This chapter describes the modeling of the heat and mass transfer which occurs during laser irradiation of metals.

The available laser beam specifications supply irradiation times ranging from a few picoseconds to several seconds. On the other hand, the incident energy densities, which can induce observable and reproducible thermal effects, vary in a much narrower range, being on the order of several mJ/cm^2 at the pulsed laser end of the time scale and of some thousands of J/cm^2 at the cw end: This is essentially related to the square root dependence on time of the heat diffusion length, which governs any heating process in the linear regime and the thresholds for different phenomena like, e.g., melting or vaporization. As a consequence, the average power density needed to obtain a given effect is lower at longer laser-material interaction times. When approaching the picosecond end, the heat diffusion length becomes comparable both to the light absorption length, which is on the order of 20 nm in most metals (see Chapter 1), and to the mean free path ℓ of the heat carriers (i.e., the conduction electrons for which $\ell \simeq 20$ nm at room temperature). Under these extreme conditions, the linearity between heat flux and temperature gradient breaks down; higher temperature derivatives in the heat diffusion equation and more careful definitions of the thermophysical parameters are needed (1). At times greater than some picoseconds, heat conduction is correctly described by the heat diffusion equation based on the linear Fourier law for the heat flux.

The energy deposited by the laser beam can be thought of as instantaneously converted into heat (source term). It is also worthwhile noting that the fascinating story of the laser-excited electron gas having a temperature other than the lattice, as proposed and seen for silicon in the subpicosecond regime (1), has no counterpart in the case of metals.

In each time domain, the heat flow exhibits peculiar features, depending on the ratios between the heat diffusion length and the characteristic lengths of the experiment (beam size, sample - or workpiece - thickness); on the incident energy density - or fluence - ; on the phenomenon to be described (heating in solid phase, melting, vaporization, plasma formation, keyholing, radiative and/or convective losses, convective motions in the molten pool, surface alloying, interface mixing, solute redistribution, segregation, undercooling, amorphization,...). For instance, at very short irradiating times (nanosecond regime or shorter) and with a typical beam cross section on the order of a few mm^2, the heat diffusion may be considered as one-dimensional in any practical situation; moreover, any radiative loss from the heating up surface can be neglected as compared to the typical heat fluxes; at longer times, the heat diffusion length is often comparable to the other typical lengths and a three-dimensional heat flow calculation is appropriate; in addition, the typical heat flux in the bulk can become comparable with heat loss rates from the surface (reradiation and convection in the gaseous phase near the surface). As a matter of fact, a one-dimensional approach can also be used at long irradiating times in particular cases: examples are given below in the papers by Mazumder and Gay.

The simplest problem to be tackled is heating of the solid phase: In this case, under a constant incident laser intensity and after a given time, heating is proportional to the combination $(K\rho c)^{-1/2}$ of the material thermophysical properties (thermal conductivity, density and specific heat); such a combination plays the role of an internal, - or bulk -, heating efficiency, describing how much a given metal sample would heat up for a given absorbed energy. A valuable presentation of this property for several metals is given in Figs. 7 and 8 of the Girardeau-Montaut paper. However, in the more general case of heating above melting, as already remarked, the absorbed energy induces several new phenomena, opening up a wide range of modeling possibilities. Broadly speaking, we may distinguish the modeling due to metallurgists, aimed at practical applications (hardening, surface alloying...) and relying upon continuous lasers, from that due to physicists, more involved with basic phenomena. Metallurgists are often interested in (quasi-) steady-state processing conditions, while physicists perhaps prefer (ultra-) rapid transient conditions, under which the onset or the decay of a given phenomenon may exhibit striking behaviors. Much of the heat flow modeling is done through the boundary conditions to which the heat diffusion equation is subjected; this will be illustrated several times in the papers below. Sometimes, as in the case of convective motions in the induced molten pool (see Mazumder paper), the boundary condition couples the heat diffusion equation with the molten fluid momentum equations, which describe the time evolution of the velocity field associated to convective motions.

A conceptually different diffusion mechanism, which may be at work during laser treatment, refers to the mass diffusion of different atomic species in the molten pool. It may be a simple diffusion mechanism in the liquid phase, driven by the concentration and - in some cases - by the thermal gradients, with characteristic diffusion coefficients on the order of 10^{-4} cm^2/s; or it may be a redistribution in the molten pool aided by convective motions and characterized by much higher effective diffusion coefficients. The former process may be rather easily modeled by means of an impurity diffusion equation, whose boundary conditions are detemined by the molten pool specifications as obtained from independent heat flow calculations (see Dona dalle Rose paper). The latter process is far more complex and must be coupled to a calculation of the velocity field in the melt (see Mazumder paper).

In the following, two review papers are proposed: a first one (Mazumder) relating to processes occurring when irradiating with continuous lasers (milli- to one-second regimes) and a second one (Dona dalle Rose) about the effects induced by a single laser pulse in the nanosecond regime. The spirit of these two papers is somewhat different, since the latter is more dedicated to a comparison of the models with experimental results than the former. The Gay paper is an example of a test of the model calculations versus experimental results, in the applicative domain. The Girardeau-Montaut paper explores the issue of heating in solid phase in a rather wide range of times (from 35 ps to seconds), being interested in the heating effect of laser pulse trains, repeatedly shot, mainly with a view to stresses and damage induced in the irradiated solid. This paper is also important in showing how the thermal history depends on the pulse shape details. Finally, the Laufer paper which deals with a CO_2 laser pulse, models, in a very clear and neat way, the tissue-cutting process and the biologically damaged region (i.e., the equivalent, in the metallurgist language, of metal cutting and heat-affected zone).

It must be pointed out that many other lecturers, participants and students of this Study Institute have dealt with heat and mass transfer, from the point of view of both modeling and model testing through experiments. In particular, I would like to mention: on the metallurgists' side, the contribution by Gnanamuthu, which, among other things, discusses the effect of the laser pulse shape on the thermal history (see also Kerrand, who showed a viewgraph with a thermal history exhibiting two peaks), and the contribution by La Rocca, partly devoted to describe a nomogram which summarizes many useful properties of the one-dimensional solution for the heat flow in a semi-infinite slab; on the physicists' side, the Kaufmann paper uses the results from a code, that models the moving source problem in the submillisecond time domain, to interpret experimental results relating to the liquid-to-crystal and liquid-to-amorphous transitions in compound melts. Finally, the Rockstroh paper reports about an effort to model the characteristics of the plasma which develops under a few kW continuous laser irradiating.

Notice. While reading the following papers, pay attention to the notation, since a given symbol often represents different things according to the paper. Moreover, the terminology may be quite different, even when referring to the same concept: for example, the temperature time evolution of physicists is the thermal cycle of metallurgists, the pulse duration is often equivalent to the dwell or interaction or exposure time, etc.

REFERENCES

1. R. E. Harrington, J. Appl. Phys. 38, 3266 (1967).
2. See, e.g., H. Kurz, L. A. Lompré, and M. J. Liu, J. de Physique C5, 23 (1983).

MATHEMATICAL MODELING OF LASER SURFACE TREATMENTS

JOYTI MAZUMDER
Department of Mechanical and Industrial Engineering, University of Illinois at Urbana-Champaign, 1206 West Green Street, Urbana, IL 61801

Keywords: Convection, diffusion, hardening, heat flow calculation: multi-dimensional, keyholing, mass transport

1. NOTATION

c	Constant which defines the interface; dimensionless
d	Diameter of laser beam; mm, [L]
D_{eff}	Effective diffusion coefficient; m^2/sec, [L^2/t]
k	Thermal conductivity; kW/m°K, [ML/^{2}T]
	Length of the rectangular heat source; mm, [L]
p	Pressure; N/m^2, [M/t^2L]
Pe	Peclet number u_o d/ ; dimensionless
q	net heat flux from laser; kW/mm^2, [M/t^2]
Re	Reynolds number u_o d/ ; dimensionless
r_o	Radius of laser beam; mm, [L]
S	Surface tension number; dimensionless
T	Temperature, °K [T]
T_{melt}	Melting temperature, °K, [T]
T^*_{melt}	Dimensionless melting temperature $\frac{T_{melt} - T_{metal}}{qd/K}$; dimensionless
T_{metal}	Temperature of metal when it is not heated; °K, [T]

2. INTRODUCTION

An experimenter is faced with a multi-parameter problem in understanding the laser surface treatment. The interrelationship between the variables is difficult to establish without extensive factorial experimentation. Alternatively, an assumed physical picture of the process can be modeled mathematically, and the model's results can be compared to experimental results to test the model's validity and thus, by inference, the physical model. Therefore, by modeling associated transport phenomena, the required process parameters can be estimated.

Laser surface treatment processes such as surface hardening, surface alloying, cladding, and melt quenching involve energy, momentum (fluid flow) and mass transfer. However, the relative importance of an individual transport phenomenon depends on an individual process. For surface hardening, heat transfer plays the most important role with mass transfer determining the limits of dwell time required for phase transformation. For surface alloying, convection or momentum transfer dominates the process.

In this paper, methods of developing models using transport phenomena are discussed. First, one and two-dimensional analytical solutions with simplifying assumptions, their boundary conditions, methods of solutions, validity and domain of applications will be described. The complexity of the model will gradually be developed by removing some simplifying assumptions and incorporating more appropriate boundary conditions. Numerical techniques will be introduced to develop realistic simulations involving both energy and mass transfer.

3. TRANSPORT PHENOMENA THEORY FOR LASER SURFACE TREATMENT

3.1. Heat conduction

Heat conduction plays an important role for all laser surface treatments, but for surface hardening this is the single most important phenomenon. Several theoretical investigations have been published with the objective of establishing the relationship between process parameters and temperature and hardness distribution. Some of the important models published to date are summarized here to serve as a ready reference for the reader.

3.1.1. Analytical solutions. Different methods for solving the heat conduction equations for various conditions are elegantly and methodically decribed by Carslaw and Jaeger (1). Most of the analytical solutions available are based on one of the many cases solved in their classic text, modified to suit the particular case.

3.1.2. One-dimensional transient model for flat semi-infinite body. Gregson (2) discussed a one-dimensional model using a semi-infinite flat-plate solution for uniform heat source provided by Carslaw and Jaeger (1). He assumed a uniformly intense laser beam profile to be instantly applied and constant in time. Expressions used for the temperature distribution are as follows:

Heating Cycle:

$$T(z,t) = \frac{\varepsilon 2F_0}{K} \sqrt{\alpha t} \cdot \text{ierfc} \left\{ \frac{z}{2\sqrt{\alpha t}} \right\} \qquad (1)$$

$$F_0 \text{ for } t > 0$$

$$F(t) = 0 \text{ for } t < 0$$

Cooling Cycle:

$$T(z,t) = \frac{2F_0\sqrt{\alpha}}{K} \left\{ \sqrt{t} \cdot \text{ierfc} \frac{z}{2\sqrt{\alpha t}} - \sqrt{t - t_L} \cdot \text{ierfc} \left[\frac{z}{2\sqrt{\alpha(t - t_L)}} \right] \right\} (2)$$

$$f(t) = \begin{cases} F_0 \text{ for } 0 < t < t_L \\ 0 \text{ for } t < 0,\ t > t_L \end{cases}$$

where:

T = temperature, °C
z = depth from surface, cm
t = time, s
ε = emissivity $\simeq 1$
F_o = average power density or constant flux/unit time/unit area, W/cm^2
K = thermal conductivity, W/cm °C
α = thermal diffusivity, cm^2/s
t_o = time start for beam power on, s
t_L = time for beam power off, s
ierfc = integral of the complementary error function

These equations are valid if the thickness of the substrates is greater than $(4\alpha t)^{1/2}$. This one-dimensional analysis may be applied to laser heat treatment processes with uniform heat sources which are produced by using optical systems such as a beam integrator, dithered scanning beam, and high-power multi-mode beam with top-hat intensity distribution. One-dimensional solutions provide only approximate thermal distribution. To obtain improved accuracy of thermal distribution, a two- or three-dimensional analysis is required.

3.1.3. One-dimensional transient model for cylindrical bodies. Sandven (3) presented the model which predicts the temperature distribution in the vicinity of a moving ring-shaped laser beam around the periphery of the outer and inner surfaces of cylinders. Sandven (3) developed his model based on the flat-plate solution provided by Carslaw and Jaeger (1) and assumed that the temperature distribution for cylindrical bodies can be approximated by a product solution of the form

$$T = \Theta \cdot I \tag{3}$$

where Θ depends on cylindrical geometry of the workpiece and I is the solution for an equivalent flat plate.

The expression for a cylindrical workpiece is:

$$T \approx (1 \pm 0.43\sqrt{\phi})\,\frac{2Q_o\alpha}{\pi K \cdot V \cdot}\int_{X-B}^{X+B} e^u \cdot K_o(Z^2+u^2)^{1/2}du \tag{4}$$

where

+ = sign is used for heat flow into a cylinder
- = sign is used for heat flow out of a hollow cylinder
Q_o = power density
V = velocity of the source in the x-direction
K_o = modified Bessel function of the second kind, and zero order
u = integration variable
2b = width of the heat source in the direction of motion
B = $Vb/2\alpha$, $Z = Vz/2\alpha$, $X = Vx/2\alpha$
ϕ = $\alpha t/a^2$, a = radius of the cylinder

The integral part of Eq.(4) must be evaluated numerically for $Z > 0$. Graphical solutions for $Z = 0$ for various values of B are provided by Sandven (3) to estimate an approximate hardened depth.

3.1.4. Three-dimensional model for semi-infinite plate. Cline and Anthony (4) determined the three-dimensional temperature distribution for a Gaussian laser beam profile by solving the following equation:

$$\partial T/\partial t - \alpha \nabla^2 T = Q/c_p \tag{5}$$

where Q = power absorbed per unit area and c_p = specific heat. They used a coordinate system fixed at the workpiece and superimposed the known Green function for the thermal distribution of unit point source to represent the Gaussian distribution. The expression developed to determine the temperature distribution is

$$T(x,y,z) = P(c_p \alpha R)^{-1} f(x,y,z,V) \tag{6}$$

where f = distribution function

$$f = \int_0^\infty \frac{\exp(-H)}{(2\pi^3)^{\frac{1}{2}} (1+\mu^2)} d\mu \tag{7}$$

and

$$H = \frac{(X + \frac{\tau\mu^2}{2})^2 + Y^2}{2(1 + \mu^2)} + \frac{Z^2}{2\mu^2} \tag{8}$$

and

R = beam radius
t' = earlier time when laser was at (x',y')
μ^2 = $2\alpha t'/R$, $\tau = VR/\alpha$
X = x/R, Y = y/R, Z = z/R
P = beam power
V = uniform velocity

The cooling rate can be calculated using the following expression

$$\partial T/\partial t = -V[x/\gamma^2 + V/2\alpha \; (1 + x/\gamma)]T \tag{9}$$

where $\gamma = \sqrt{x^2 + y^2 + z^2}$.

3.1.5. Numerical solutions. Numerical methods remove many of the limitations that apply to the analytical methods. For example, the heat source may not have to be assumed to be concentrated in a point, line or plane. Temperature-dependent thermophysical properties and real boundary conditions may be included. In spite of the inherent advantages in numerical methods, only a few numerical solutions for heat flow in laser processing have been developed so far.

The numerical solution to the three-dimensional heat-transfer model for laser materials processing developed by Mazumder and Steen (5) and later modified by Chande and Mazumder (7) allows for temperature-dependent thermophysical properties, spatial distribution of the heat source (Gaussian, uniform or any known distribution), radiative heat losses, convective heat losses, and latent heat of transformation.

The following assumptions were made for this numerical solution (5,6):

1. The laser beam is stationary and is incident at right angles at the center of the substrate width. The substrate moves in the positive x direction (along the length) with a uniform velocity u and is infinite in length but has finite width and thickness.
2. Quasi-steady state is assumed.
3. The power distribution in the beam is Gaussian.
4. The substrate thermal conductivity, specific heat (C_p), thermal diffusivity, and the surface reflectivity are temperature dependent. The substrate density is assumed to be independent of temperature. Specific heat variation accounts for heats of fusion and vaporization (L) by converting them into equivalent step increases in values of specific heat, as, for example,

$$\overline{C}_p \, \Delta \, T_m = \int_{T_o}^{T_m} C_p \, dT + L. \tag{10}$$

5. Surface reflectivity is considered to be zero when the temperature exceeds the boiling point.
6. There is a radiation loss at the upper and lower surface of the workpiece.
7. Convective losses occur at the upper surface due to shielding gas flow.
8. When the temperature at any location exceeds the boiling point, it is considered to have evaporated but remains in the conducting network at a fictitiously high temperature to simulate the effect of high convection and radiation transfer effects from the fast-moving plasma in the keyhole.
9. Radiation penetrating the substrate is absorbed according to the Beer-Lambert law,

$$P_z = P_s \exp(-\,\beta z) \tag{11}$$

where β is the absorption coefficient (m^{-1}) and is considered independent of position within the keyhole and P_z is the absorbed power density at depth z which was of value P_s at the surface.

A control volume approach is utilized as shown in Fig. 1, where the heat is balanced on an axisymmetric control volume. Within the body of the substrate, the heat balance is as follows:

$$\begin{aligned} & - K\,\delta y\,\delta z(\partial T/\partial x)_{PW} - K\,\delta x\,\delta z(\partial T/\partial y)_{PN} - K\,\delta x\,\delta y(\partial T/\partial z)_{PH} \\ & + K\,\delta y\,\partial z(\partial T/\partial x)_{EP} + K\,\partial x\,\partial z(\partial T/\partial y)_{SP} \\ & + K\,\delta x\,\partial y(\partial T/\partial z)_{LP} + \rho\mu C_p\,\partial y\,\partial z[(T_W + T_p)/2] \\ & - \rho\mu C_p\,\delta y\,\delta z[(T_p + T_E)/2] = 0 \end{aligned} \tag{12}$$

where K = thermal conductivity ($Wm^{-1}K^{-1}$), and subscripts W, S, N, H, and L refer to the locations shown in Fig. 1.

Courtney and Steen (8) used this model to predict the depth of the heat-treated zone and thermal cycle time as shown in Figs. 2 and 3. Knowledge of thermal cycle time is essential to calculate the carbon diffusion distance. This model has also been successfully applied for welding (8) and melt quenching experiments. However, the Beer-Lambert coefficient has to be experimentally determined to account for convection which has been neglected.

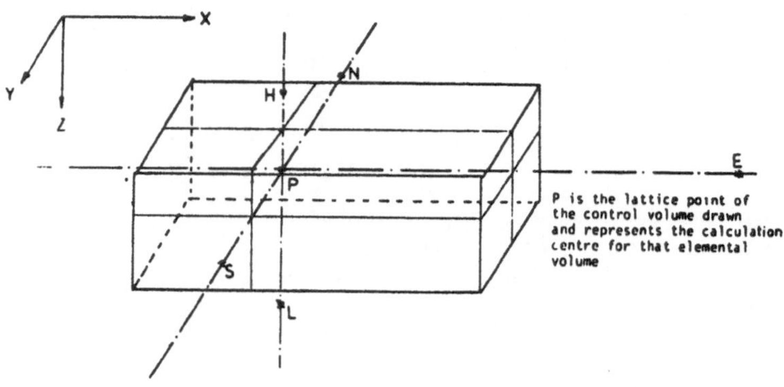

FIGURE 1. Nomenclature used in and around an elemental control volume.

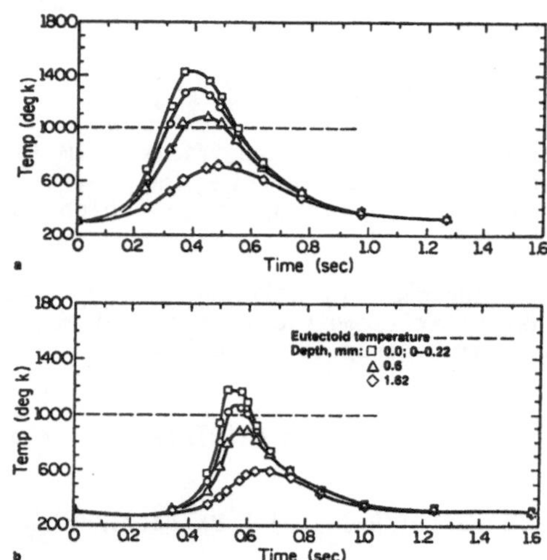

FIGURE 2. Theoretically predicted thermal cycle during laser heating of En8 steel (power = 2 kW, beam radius = 3.0 mm, and reflectivity = 0.4); (a) speed = 22.5 mm/s and (b) speed = 42.5 mm/s (8).

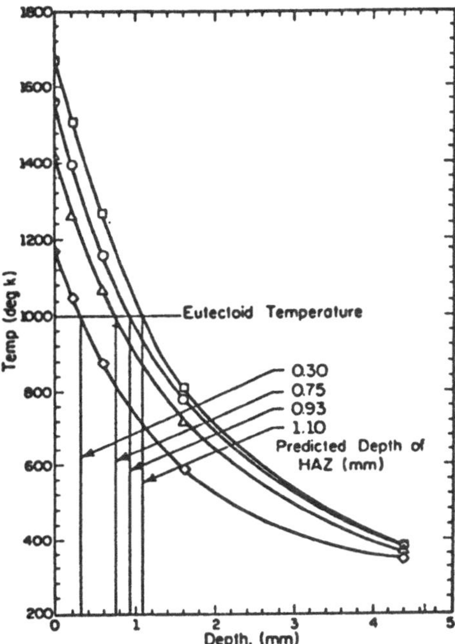

FIGURE 3. Theoretically predicted thermal profiles (power = 2 kW, beam radius = 3.0 mm, reflectivity = 0.4) (8). Speed, mm/s: □ 8.0; ○ 15.0; △ 22.5; ◇ 42.5

3.2. Convection

Convection is the single most important factor influencing the geometry of the pool, including its shape, undercut, and ripples, and can result in defects such as variable penetration, porosity, and lack of fusion. Convection is also primarily responsible for mixing and, therefore, affects the composition of the melt pool. The heat transfer and thus the cooling rate is greatly enhanced in the presence of convection (9). This in turn will affect the microstructure. The homogeneity of solute redistribution during laser surface alloying as reported by Chande and Mazumder (7) can only be explained by the presence of convection current.

Surface tension-driven flow has been identified to be responsible for convection within the molten pool. While most of the work to date has been convection, a quantitative understanding of the effect of convection on pool shape and mixing is of importance. Anthony and Cline (10) did an analysis on the surface tension-driven flow within the molten pool. It is essentially a one-dimensional problem, and the flow field thus obtained is not coupled to the energy equation. Therefore, no additional information is obtained as far as the heat transfer process is concerned. Oreper et al. (11) developed a two-dimensional convection model. Buoyancy, electromagnetic and surface tension forces are considered. Numerical solutions were obtained based on a specified pool profile. It was found that the surface tension gradient is the dominant factor in many cases. However, the solid-liquid interface, i.e., the pool shape, is not known a priori. It is part of the problem to be solved. A two-dimensional transient model for laser surface-melted pool was developed by Chan, Mazumder, and Chen (12,13). It is shown that surface tension is responsible for the fluid flow and convection. The cooling rate at the edge of the pool is found to be higher than that at the bottom of the pool along the centerline. This agrees with the experimental findings that the microstructure is finer at the edge of the pool than at the bottom of the pool. It is also predicted that the recirculating velocity is one or two orders of magnitude higher than that of the scanning velocity.

3.2.1. The two-dimensional transient model. A two-dimensional analysis is presented, modeling a laser beam having a defined power distribution striking the surface of an opaque material of infinite width, thickness, and length (Fig. 4). Some of the incident radiation is reflected while the rest is absorbed. The heat absorbed developed a molten pool. Owing to the high temperature gradient on the surface in the transverse

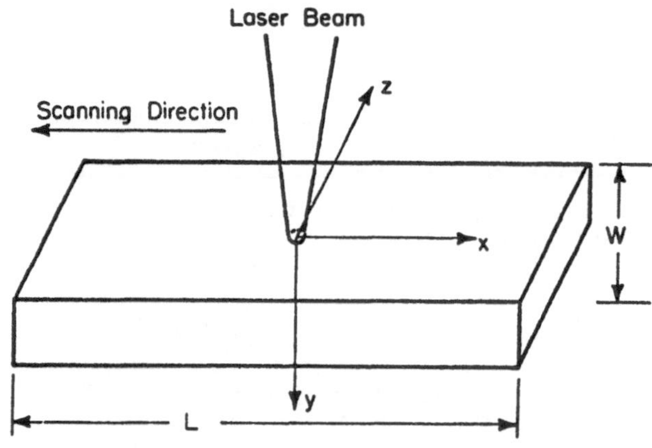

FIGURE 4. Schematic diagram of the process.

direction, a surface tension gradient is developed. It is this mechanism that drives the flow. As the flow develops, energy transfer mechanism becomes a convective problem with the flow driven by the surface tension gradient. The basic assumptions are:

1. The liquid metal is considered to be Newtonian so that the Navier-Stokes equation is applicable.
2. All the properties of the liquid metal and solid metal are constant, independent of temperature (except the surface tension). This allows simplifications of the model; however, variable properties can be treated with slight modifications. The dependence of surface tension on temperature, the driving force of the flow, is assumed to be linear.

3. The latent heat of fusion is neglected since the energy liberated is small compared to total enthalpy change associated with temperature differences.
4. Thermal conductivity is assumed to be the same for both liquid and solid phases for the sake of simplicity of the model.
5. The surface of the melt pool is assumed to be flat to simplify the surface boundary condition and, hence, surface rippling is neglected.

4. MATHEMATICAL FORMULATION

The appropriate governing equations are:

Energy equation

$$\partial T/\partial t + (\underline{u} \cdot \underline{\nabla})\, T = \kappa\, \nabla^2\, T \tag{13}$$

Continuity

$$\underline{\nabla} \cdot \underline{u} = 0 \tag{14}$$

Momentum equations

$$\partial u/\partial t + (\underline{u} \cdot \underline{\nabla})\, u = -(1/\rho)(\partial P/\partial x) + \nu\, \nabla^2\, u \tag{15}$$

$$\partial v/\partial t + (\underline{u} \cdot \underline{\nabla})\, v = -(1/\rho)(\partial P/\partial y) + \nu\, \nabla^2\, v \tag{16}$$

Boundary conditions at the surface are

$$y = 0,\ v = 0,\ \mu(\partial u/\partial y) = -\sigma'(\partial T/\partial x)$$

$$k(\partial T/\partial y) = \begin{cases} -q, & |x| \le d/2 \\ 0, & \text{otherwise} \end{cases} \tag{17}$$

At the liquid-solid interface

$$q = \frac{\text{total absorbed power}}{\text{length } (\ell) \text{ x width } (d) \text{ of laser beam}} \tag{18}$$

$$f(x,y,t) = C; \quad u = v = 0, \quad \text{when} \quad T = T_m$$

and

$$|x|,\ y \to \infty,\ T \to T_{metal} \tag{19}$$

Introducing the dimensionless variables as follows:

$$(x^*,y^*) = (x,y)/d,\ t^* = t/(d/u_o),$$

$$(u^*,v^*) = (u,v)/u_o$$

$$P^* = P/\rho\, u_o^2, \text{ and } T^* = (T - T_{metal})/(q\ d/k) \tag{20}$$

The governing equations then become:

$$\frac{\partial T^*}{\partial t^*} + u^* \frac{\partial T^*}{\partial x^*} + v^* \frac{\partial T^*}{\partial y^*} = \frac{1}{Pe}\, \nabla^2\, T^* \tag{21}$$

$$\frac{\partial u^*}{\partial x^*} + \frac{\partial v^*}{\partial y^*} = 0 \tag{22}$$

$$\frac{\partial u^*}{\partial t^*} + u^* \frac{\partial u^*}{\partial x^*} + v^* \frac{\partial u^*}{\partial u^*} = - \frac{\partial p^*}{\partial x^*} + \frac{Pr}{Pe} \nabla^2 u^* \tag{23}$$

$$\frac{\partial v^*}{\partial t^*} + u^* \frac{\partial v^*}{\partial x^*} + v^* \frac{\partial v^*}{\partial y^*} = - \frac{\partial P^*}{\partial y^*} + \frac{Pr}{Pe} \nabla^2 v^* \tag{24}$$

subject to the boundary conditions,

$$y^* = 0,\ v^* = 0,\ S \frac{\partial T^*}{\partial x^*} = - \frac{\partial u^*}{\partial y^*}$$

$$\frac{\partial T^*}{\partial y^*} = \begin{cases} -1 & |x^*| \le 1/2 \\ 0 & \text{otherwise} \end{cases} \tag{25}$$

and at the liquid-solid interface,

$$f^* (x^*,y^*,t^*) = C.$$

$$u^* = v^* = 0, \text{ when } T^* = T^*_m \tag{26}$$

and

$$T^* \to 0 \text{ as } |x^*|,\ y \to \infty \tag{27}$$

where

$$Pe = u_o\, d/\kappa,\ Pr = \nu/\kappa$$

$$S = \frac{\sigma'\, qd}{\mu\, u_o\, k},\quad T^*_{melt} = \frac{T_{melt} - T_{metal}}{q\, d/k} \tag{28}$$

It is important to point out that the four dimensionless parameters, namely, Pe, Pr, S, and T^*_{melt} are independent. They arise naturally from the general three-dimensional equations. Reynolds number and surface tension number can be grouped together, their product as one parameter. We consider these four dimensionless parameters to understand the convection in the pool. This particular way of nondimensionalizing the equations also permits a simple transformation to obtain the scanning process. A computer program SOLA (14) is employed. The basic method of the algorithm is presented in Hirt's report (14).

5. DISCUSSION OF THE MODEL

The governing parameters arising from the dimensionless equations are Peclet number (Pe), Prandtl number (Pr), Surface tension number (S), and Dimensionless melting temperature (T^*_m). Each of these affects the characteristics of the solution and each has its own physical interpretation.

The Peclet number Pe signifies the ratio of the rate of convection associated with the scanning speed and the rate of conduction. Thus, if thermocapillary motion were not present, higher Pe would imply smaller conduction-induced melt zones. In the presence of thermocapillary convection in the melt, the melt zone is also influenced by surface tension parameter S, which is a measure of the ratio of thermocapillary velocity and the scanning velocity. For a fixed scanning velocity, an increase in S signifies an increase of thermocapillary flow, although a direct proportionality relationship should not be assumed due to the complexity of the processes involved. Since the thermocapillary effect is caused by the temperature gradient, an increase in heating power, a decrease in beam diameter, or an increase in the negative temperature coefficient of the surface tension leads to an increase in S. The Prandtl number Pr, a fluid property, is the ratio of kinematic viscosity and heat diffusivity, and hence, signifies the relative speed of momentum and heat diffusion. The physical properties used and values of Pr for steel, aluminum, and sodium nitrate, a material used frequently in melt pool modeling, are shown in Table 1. The orders of magnitude of the governing parameters are tabulated in Table 2. The estimation is based on process parameters in the work by Chande and Mazumder (15).

TABLE 1. Physical property of steel, Al, and $NaNO_3$

	Steel	Al	$NaNO_3$
ρ	7.0×10^3 kg/m^3	2.385×10^3 kg/m^3	1.904×10^3 kg/m^3
μ	5.6×10^{-3} N s m^{-2}	2.8×10^{-3} N s m^{-2}	2.78×10^{-3} N s m^{-2}
ν	7.84×10^{-7} m^2/sec	1.17×10^{-6} m^2/sec	1.46×10^{-6} m^2/sec
k	31 W/mK	100 W/mK	1.0×10^{-5} W/mK
K	1.0×10^{-5} m^2/sec	6.0×10^{-5} m^2/sec	5.6×10^{-7} m^2/sec
Pr	0.078	0.02	2.6
T_m	1500°C	600°C	306.8°C
σ'	-0.112×10^{-3} N/m/K	-0.35×10^{-3} N/m/K	-0.7×10^{-4} N/m/K
λ	205×10^{-3} J/kg	393×10^{-3} J/kg	----

The Reynolds number Re = Pe/Pr is not an independent parameter here and does not have a clear physical meaning. However, it is interesting to note in Table 1 that the kinematic viscosities of the three materials listed are all approximately equal to 10^{-6}. Accordingly, holding the Reynolds number constant is equivalent to holding the beam diameter and scanning velocity constant. This provides a convenient basis for comparing the effects of different parameters. For example, with Re held constant, the effects of different materials are reflected as Prandtl

TABLE 2. Order of magnitude of parameters.

	Steel	Al	$NaNO_3$
Re	2.55 to 8.29	17 to 55	14 to 45
Pe	2 to 6.5	0.3 to 1.0	36 to 120
S	5×10^4 to 2.5×10^5	10^5 to 5×10^5	2.0×10^8 to 10^9
T_m^*	0.05 to 0.1	0.006 to 0.016	3×10^{-10} to 7×10^{-10}

number effects, and the effects of increasing heating power are reflected as effects of increasing S. S is also influenced by the temperature coefficient of the surface tension. T_m^*, the dimensionless melting point temperature, is a measure of the melting point temperature as compared to the peak temperature in the melt pool. Consequently, a small value would imply a large melt pool.

This two-dimensional convective heat transfer and fluid flow analysis has revealed many important aspects of the surface tension-driven fluid flow in the surface-melted pool and its effect on pool shape, cooling rate, velocity field and solute redistribution. The important findings are as follows:

1. Recirculating velocity is predicted with the flow near the surface one or two orders of magnitude higher than that of the moving heat source. There are two counter rotating vortices except in the high Prandtl number case.
2. Surface temperature gradient, which is the driving force for the fluid flow, is maximum at the edge of the beam leading to the most vigorous outward velocity.
3. As Prandtl number increases, the aspect ratio (width divided by depth) increases.
4. As surface tension number increases from 30,000 to 55,000, the aspect ratio increases. However, when it increases from 55,000 to 100,000, the aspect ratio decreases leading to "deep penetration" due to the counter rotating vortex.
5. The cooling rate at the edge of the pool is found to be higher than that at the bottom of the pool along the centerline. This implies that the solidification will proceed from the edge of the pool.
6. As the Prandtl number increases from 0.02 to 0.1, the cooling rate at the edge of the pool decreases. But it increases when the Prandtl number increases from 0.2 to 2.6.
7. The cooling rate at the edge of the pool increases with the surface tension number.
8. Because of the high recirculating flow, uniform solute redistribution is expected. The existence of the counter rotating vortices in the pool implies that segregation, if any, might be expected at the location where the vortices meet.

6. MASS TRANSPORT

For processes such as laser surface alloying and cladding, mass transport is a very important phenomenon. A mathematical model for mass transport during laser surface alloying would help clarify several aspects of the problem. The mass flux necessary to obtain a desired average composition in the liquid state could be computed. Powder loss during alloying would then be estimated, knowing the actual mass flux during laser processing. The model could be used to simulate the effect of varying the method of supplying alloying elements. Having predicted an average liquid pool composition and measured the actual solid state composition, the effective solute partitioning coefficient C_s^* at the solid-liquid interface could be calculated. This effective C_s^* could then be compared to the value determined from the equilibrium phase diagram to check if conditions of local equilibrium existed ahead of the solid-liquid interface. This would be a useful check, as local equilibrium is assumed in predicting possible compositions during rapid solidification from equilibrium phase diagrams.

Chande and Mazumder (16) used the momentum transfer model described in the last section and coupled that with the diffusion equation to estimate the mass transfer during laser surface alloying since convection dominates the process.

For mass transfer calculations, the following assumptions are made:

1. The effect of alloying on solute mass diffusivity was neglected because accurate high-temperature data were unavailable; mass transport by diffusion was negligible compared to that by convection ($u_0\ d/D > 100$) and it simplified the formulation.
2. Mass flux was constant and uniform across the width of the pool at the surface. This rate and distribution could be altered to allow for any other experimental condition (e.g., wire feed or nonuniform powder addition into the melt pool).
3. There was no transfer of alloying elements across the solid-liquid interface. This was a very good assumption that was verified experimentally using Electron Probe Micro Analysis technique.

Melting of powder particles introduced into the melt was found to be practically instantaneous (16). Thus mass flux could be considered as being added in the liquid state.

The governing equation for two-dimensional convective diffusion of mass for constant substrate properties could be written as

$$D\left(\frac{\partial^2 C}{\partial x^2} + \frac{\partial^2 C}{\partial y^2}\right) - \left(u\frac{\partial C}{\partial x} + v\frac{\partial C}{\partial y}\right) = \frac{\partial C}{\partial t} \tag{29}$$

where D is the diffusivity of the alloying material in molten substrate (m^2/s), C is the concentration of solute (kg/m^3), and u and v are the local components of the fluid velocity field along the x and y directions, respectively (m/s). The initial and boundary conditions are:

$$t = 0,\ C = 0,\ \text{all } x \text{ and } y, \tag{30}$$

$$t > 0,\ C = 0,\ \text{for all } x \text{ and } y \text{ beyond interface}, \tag{31}$$

$$\partial C/\partial x = 0,\ x = 0 \text{ along centerline}, \tag{32}$$

$$D(\partial C/\partial y) = -\ j, x < x_{SL},\ y = 0 \tag{33}$$

surface flux across melt pool,

$$\partial C/\partial x = \partial C/\partial y = 0 \text{ at solid-liquid interface.} \tag{34}$$

These equations were numerically solved using alternate direction implicit methods. The result of the mass transfer calculations indicates the importance of fluid flow in determining solute distribution during laser surface alloying. The small effect of changing solute diffusivity on its distribution, the uniform mixing even when mass flux was present over only a part of the pool surface, and the nature of the three-dimensional plots all show that the pattern of fluid flow controls the resultant solute distribution.

7. CONCLUDING REMARKS

Although laser surface treatments are complicated processes, proper understanding of mechanisms can be obtained by methodical modeling. The problem can be first approached in simplified form with proper assumptions. Each step will be useful for a range in spite of their limitation. With gradual removal of simplifying assumption, even a complicated process such as this can be studied.

REFERENCES

1. H. S. Carslaw and J. C. Jaeger, Conduction of Heat in Solids, 2nd ed. (Oxford Univ. Press, 1959).
2. V. Gregson, "Laser Heat Treatment," in Laser Materials Processing, edited by M. Bass (North Holland, 1983).
3. O. A. Sandven, Proc. SPIE 198, 198 (1979).
4. H. E. Cline and T. R. Anthony, J. Appl. Phys. 48, 3895 (1977).
5. J. Mazumder and W. M. Steen, J. Appl. Phys. 51, 941 (1980).
6. J. Mazumder, Ph.D. Thesis, London University, 1978.
7. T. Chande and J. Mazumder, Lasers in Metallurgy, edited by K. Mukherji and J. Mazumder (The Metallurgical Society of AIME, Warrendale, PA, 1981), p. 165.
8. C. G. H. Courtney and W. M. Steen, Met. Technol. 6, 456 (1979).
9. T. Chande and J. Mazumder, Appl. Phys. Lett. 41, 42 (1982).
10. T. R. Anthony and H. F. Cline, J. Appl. Phys. 48, 3888-3894 (1977).
11. G. M. Oreper, T. W. Eagar, and J. Szekely, Welding Journal 63, 307 (1983).
12. D. Chan, J. Mazumder, and M. M. Chen, Applications of Lasers in Materials Processing, edited by E. A. Metzbower (ASM, 1983), p. 150.
13. C. Chan, J. Mazumder and M. M. Chen, Metall. Trans., A 15, 2175 (1984).
14. C. W. Hirt, B. D. Nichols, and N. C. Romero, "A Numerical Algorithm for Transient Fluid Flows," UC-34 and UC-79d, April 1975.
15. T. Chande and J. Mazumder, Metall. Trans., B 14, 181-190 (1983).
16. T. Chande and J. Mazumder, J. Appl. Phys. 57, 2226 (1985).
17. L. Peterson, M.S. Thesis, University of Illinois at Urbana-Champaign, 1984.

REFERENCES

1. [illegible]
2. [illegible]
3. [illegible]
4. [illegible]
5. [illegible]
6. [illegible]
7. [illegible]
8. [illegible]
9. [illegible]
10. [illegible]
11. [illegible]
12. [illegible]
13. [illegible]
14. [illegible]
15. [illegible]
16. [illegible]

APPLICATION OF MATHEMATICAL HEAT TRANSFER ANALYSIS TO HIGH-POWER CO_2 LASER MATERIAL PROCESSING: TREATMENT PARAMETER PREDICTION, ABSORPTION COEFFICIENT MEASUREMENTS

PAOLO GAY
Centro Ricerche Fiat, Orbossano, Italia

Key Words: Absorption coefficient, coating, hardening, heat flow calculation: multi-dimensional, melting, steel, surface alloying

1. INTRODUCTION

During the heat-treating and alloying processes, the laser spot has dimensions of the order of 1 cm, power densities of 10^3-10^4 W/cm^2 and interaction times of about 1 sec. Since the radiation is absorbed in a very thin layer, the subsequent processes can be conveniently described on the basis of heat conduction physics, by equating the laser beam to a heat flux entering the surface.

The main purpose of the mathematical models, here presented, is the prediction of phase transformation depths, and of melting depths in order to forecast laser processing parameters such as laser power, beam shape and relative velocity between workpiece and laser beam.

As the absorption coefficient is the most critical model parameter, experimental techniques to measure it were developed. A description of absorption coefficient measurements of samples at different surface temperatures is presented.

The discussion of some comparisons between experimental depths and calculated results is also presented in order to evaluate the effectiveness of different models.

2. MATHEMATICAL MODELS

2.1. Simple one-dimensional

A first useful approach for the study of material-radiation interaction is offered by the one-dimensional model (1). The treated material is assumed to occupy a semi-infinite space with a constant incident energy flux at the surface for a certain interaction time τ, sec. The model uses a Fourier heat transfer equation with the following boundary conditions:

$$Q_s = K \frac{\partial T}{\partial x}\bigg|_{x=0}$$

where Q_s is the entering heat flux, T is the temperature and x the coordinate orthogonal to the surface. In this equation the main physical property of the material, the thermal conductivity K, appears. The second most important property is the thermal volumetric capacity ρC_p (ρ, density, C_p, specific heat). With the ratio between these parameters one can define the thermal diffusivity connected to temperature propagation in the material. These parameters are considered constant to the first approximation.

The main results of the model are:

- Prediction of the maximum surface temperature to be compared with the temperature of phase transformation, of melting or vaporization,
- Prediction of hardened depth, based on the thickness of material heated above the austenitic phase transformation temperature,
- Prediction of melting depth, based on the thickness of material heated above the melting point,
- Prediction of heat penetration depth $D_i = 2(\alpha \tau_s)^{1/2}$ during interaction time; this is equal to the depth at which the temperature reaches 10% of the surface temperature.

2.2. Three-dimensional model

When the thickness of the workpiece or the linear dimensions of the laser spot are of the same order of magnitude as the depth of heat penetration, then the one-dimensional hypothesis is no longer adequate.

To show the effect of these factors, a three-dimensional model has been developed. This model considers a plate of finite thickness moving at constant velocity under a rectangular-shaped incident laser beam of uniform power density. The initial temperature of the plate is constant and the temperature field is calculated from the steady-state case. The physical parameters are considered constant as temperature vaires. The model is based on the image method and considers a reference system in translation.

The calculations provide the temperature behavior in time for each point and of heating and cooling speeds in the austenitic field, thereby estimating the depth and shape of the hardened zone.

2.3. Bidimensional axial symmetric

The model calculates the axial and radial temperatures with the finite difference method with the following boundary conditions: constant input heat flux on a circular area on the upper side, convection heat exchange on the whole upper surface, adiabatic conditions on lateral and lower surfaces.

The mathematical model allows both a time variation of the input flux density and an independent variation of heat capacity and conductivity. To take into account the latent heat of fusion, the near melting temperature specific heat capacity was properly modified.

The program was implemented for a PDP 11/70 computer and typical computation time was a few minutes.

2.4. One-dimensional with physical parameters variation

Especially with a laser surface melting process, in order to correlate experimental and calculation results, it is necessary to consider the variation of thermophysical material properties with temperature.

The model considers a plate of finite thickness and takes into account the variations with temperature of thermal conductivity, specific heat and absorption coefficient. The latent heat of fusion is also taken into account.

Finite difference numerical technique is used.

3. EXPERIMENTAL FACILITIES

3.1. High-power laser application laboratory

The laser application laboratory is equipped with two CO_2 lasers. One supplied by Volfivre, Florence, generates either a 500 W continuous or a 2 kW pulsed beam. It has an automatically controlled 6" x-y axis table with a maximum speed of 4.8 m/min. The second system was partially supplied by AVCO Everett (USA). It provides a continuous beam from 1 to 15 kW. The 15 kW system consists of the HPL6 source and two work stations. The first station is used for welding and cutting, and has an x-y table and two rotating heads. The second is used for heat treatments and surface alloying, and has an x-axis table and two rotating heads.

The heat treatment optical system has eight mirrors, two of which can be vibrated. Electrical adjustment of the degree of vibration is used to form rectangular beams measuring from 5 to 20 mm per side. It is possible to use a mask to have a circular beam on the work table.

The workpieces are automatically moved by a C.N.C. which also varies the laser power.

3.2. Calorimeter

To measure absorption coefficients at low surface temperature, a calorimeter was developed (2). The calorimeter is based on the measurement in steady-state conditions of the thermal jump induced in the cooling fluid in thermal equilibrium with the irradiated surface. This temperature difference, which is proportional to the power absorbed by the surface under test, can be measured directly or compared with a reference thermal jump electrically induced (e.g., by an electrical dissipator). The cooling fluid (nearly always distilled water) from the thermostat is sent via a pump and a flowmeter to the laser radiation absorber. This can be a cooled mirror or a support for a sample, built in such a way as to guarantee a good thermal exchange between the water and the irradiated surface. The dissipator was made of a Chromel spiral dipped in the cooling water. The thermocouples measure the thermal jump induced by the absorber and by the dissipator. Chromel-Alumel functions having a sensitivity of 40 μV/°C were used. The absorption measurements of steel SAE 1045 samples were carried out using the 500 W laser source with a typical water cooling rate of 1 liter/min.

3.3. Absorption measuring technique

To have meaningful absorption data for surface temperatures just lower and higher than the melting point, an experimental technique utilizing power densities and interaction times typical of laser heat treatment and alloying processes was developed (3). The basic idea was the measurement of the incident power and the resultant temperature distributions at the same time to evaluate the input heat flux during a laser process itself.

To avoid some mathematical difficulites, a simple cylindrical geometry and stationary source were chosen.

The experimental work was carried out on the heat-treating station of a 15 kW laser system. Figure 1 shows the experimental setup. A circular laser beam was directed into a cylindrical metal surface. The incident laser power was measured calorimetrically, and sample heating was evaluated using two thermocouples located at different depths. Surface temperatures were measured with an IRCON pyrometer Model 6000, taking into account emissivity coefficients measured in an oven. To increase

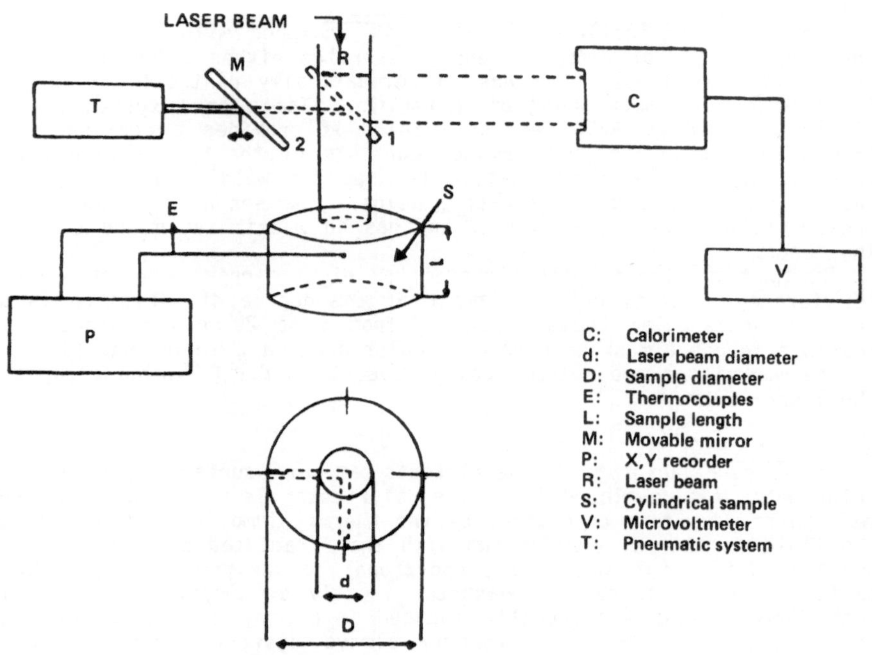

FIGURE 1. Schematic of the experimental system used for absorption coefficient measurements.

measurement precision and reduce data processing time, an automatic data acquisition system, implemented with an HP85 personal computer, was used.

For all tests two base materials were used, and to increase measurement accuracy, the same experimental condition was repeated on five samples. Base materials were nodular cast iron and SAE 1045 carbon steel.

For experiments with temperature lower than melting point, the following conditions were kept constant: sample geometrical dimensions (diameter 50 mm and height 20 mm), axial thermocouple distance from surface (1 and 4 mm), beam dimensions (diameter 16 mm), incident power ($\sim$ 900 W) and interaction time (4 seconds). The following surface conditions were tested: sandblast, graphite, phosphate and titanium oxide.

In order to increase power density (5×10^4 W/cm^2) for experiments with temperature higher than melting point, the beam diameter was decreased to 14 mm and input power increased up to 3 to 5 kW. These sample conditions were: base material surface melting and alloying with stellite F or Eatonite 3.

4. RESULTS AND DISCUSSION

4.1. Phase transformation depth prediction

A typical comparison between experimental data of phase transformation depth and calculation with a one-dimensional simple model is shown on Figure 2. For interaction times up to 1.3 sec and beam dimensions of 12 x 12 mm, the fitting is adequate by using proper absorption coefficient and austenitic transformation temperature (4).

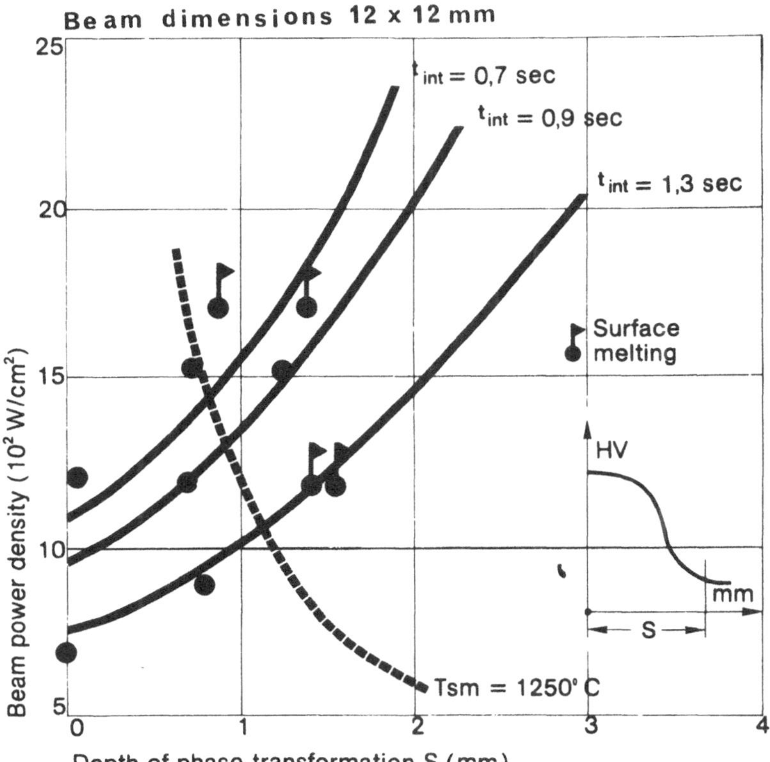

FIGURE 2. Use of a simple one-dimensional model to predict phase transformation depths.

With higher interaction times and limited workpiece thickness, a better prediction of the phase transformation depth is achieved with the three-dimensional model.

Some examples are given here to show a comparjson between results obtained by calculation and by experiment for the case of flat medium steel samples of normalized SAE 1045 in the absence of surface melting. Figure 3 shows the calculated temperature distributions in the transverse sections corresponding to the maximum temperature. The 800°C

Hardened sample sections

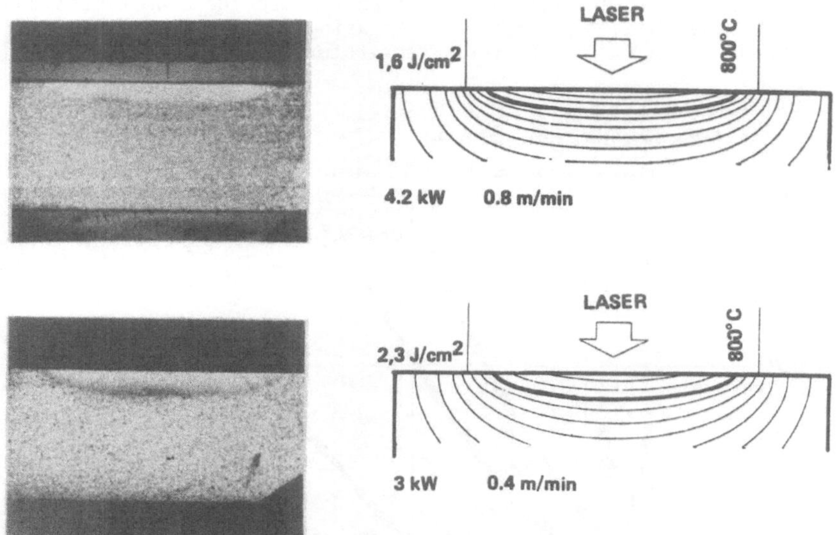

FIGURE 3. Sections of treated samples and calculated isotherms.

Experimental tests

Material	SAE 1045
Coating	phosphate
Plate thickness (mm)	15
Beam dimension (mm)	16 x 16
Power (kW)	6-10
Velocity (m/min)	0.4-1.5
Melted depth (mm)	0
Hardened depth (mm)	0-1.7

isotherm corresponding to the austenitic phase transformation temperature, is shown in the diagrams. The shapes delineated by these isotherms are seen to correspond to the hardened zones found in cross-sectioned samples. Depths and widths are within 5 to 10% of the measured values for different values of laser power (2 to 6 kW). The simple one-dimensional model, on the contrary, gives depth values 30 to 50% greater than those obtained experimentally.

4.2. Absorption coefficient measurements

4.2.1. Coating at ambient temperature. The results of calorimetric measurements of absorption coefficients of some SAE 1045 samples with different surface conditions are reported in Table 1.

TABLE 1. Absorption coeficients of some SAE 1045 steel samples with different surface conditions and finishing.*

Surface Condition	Incident Power (W)	Absorbed Power (W)	Absorption Coefficient
Polished	257	29	0.11
Blasted	257	88	0.34
As received	257	95	0.37
Blackened	257	132	0.51
Phosphate	257	239	0.93

* Chemical composition % in weight 0.45C, 0.8 Mn, 0.3 Si, 0.1 Cr, 0.02 P, 0.02 S.

As the absorption of pure iron is about 4.5%, the polished steel sample exposed to atmosphere absorbs almost twice as much as a film of pure iron evaporated on a substrate at a pressure of about 10^{-6} mm. This confirms the importance of the oxide films forming on the surface of metallic specimens exposed to air. A maximum absorption value of 0.93 was measured with phosphate coating.

4.2.2. Surface temperature lower than melting point. Thermophysical material properties and their variations with temperatures were the most important parameters of the computer program. Then a secondary result of absorption coefficient measurements was the determination of thermal conductivity of the materials under investigation, up to the melting temperature (Figure 4). The fact that the thermal conductivity of carbon steel is nearly double that of nodular cast iron explains the different absorption coefficients resulting from the same type of coating. In fact, with the same input laser power, different surface temperatures and different modifications of the surface physical properties were reached in the two materials.

In Table 2 the absorption coefficient values determined for different coatings and base materials are given. The values vary from a minimum of 0.33 to a maximum of 0.89 changing from sandblast to phosphating. For the same coating, absorption coefficients on carbon steel are 25% higher than that of nodular cast iron.

A typical comparison between calculated and measured temperatures versus time is shown in Figure 5 for phosphate coating on nodular cast iron with 350 W of laser incident power. The agreement is fairly good.

4.2.3. Surface temperature higher than melting point. For experiments with surface temperature higher than melting point, a typical comparison between calculated and measured temperature is shown in Figure 6. The sample of carbon steel, initially phosphate coated and without added surface layer, was melted with 3.3 kW of laser incident power. The agreement is still good if the finite response time of thermocouples is considered to explain the discrepancy on the cooling phase.

TABLE 2. Summary of test data and results for surface temperature lower than the melting point.

Material	Surface Treatment	Average Incident Power Pinc. ± 5% (W)	Average Absorption Coefficient $A = \frac{Pab.}{Pinc.} + \bar{A} \pm A\%$	Max. Temp. 1 mm below Heated Surface(°C)
Nodular	Phosphate	964	0.59 ± 14%	486
Cast iron				
" "	Graphite	916	0.64 ± 4%	479
" "	Sandblast	952	0.33 ∓ 18%	265
" "	Titanium oxide	911	0.71 ∓ 4%	564
AISI 1045	Phosphate	870	0.89 ± 9%	436
" "	Graphite	879	0.81 ∓ 23%	396
" "	Sandblast	932	0.46 ∓ 18%	218

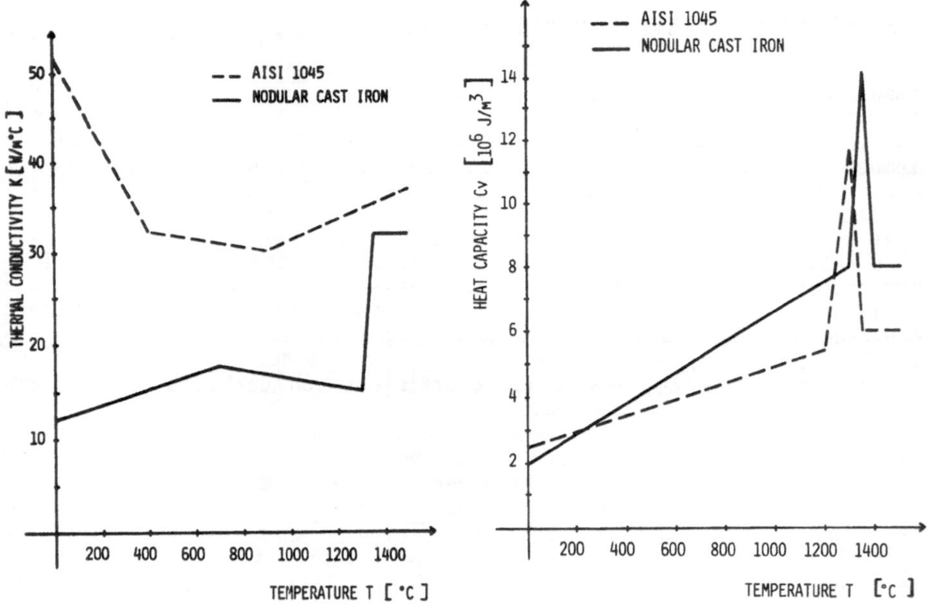

FIGURE 4. Thermal conductivity and heat capacity versus temperature for nodular cast iron and carbon steel (SAE 1045) as determined by the fitting of experimental and calculated results.

TABLE 3. Summary of test data and results for surface temperatures higher than the melting point.

Material	Average Incident Power Pinc. ± 5%(kW)	Average Absorption Coefficient $A = \frac{Pab.}{Pinc.} + \bar{A} \pm A/\%$	Notes
Nodular cast iron	3.01	0.287 ± 7%	Base material surface melting
Nodular cast iron	5.02	0.160 ± 9.5%	Alloying with Stellite F
Nodular cast iron	4.13	0.188 ± 11%	Alloying with Eatonite 3
Carbon steel AISI 1045	3.17	0.369 ± 7%	Base material surface melting
Carbon steel AISI 1045	4.77	0.180 ± 8.5%	Alloying with Stellite F
Carbon steel AISI 1045	4.3	0.24 ± 11%	Alloying with Eatonite 3

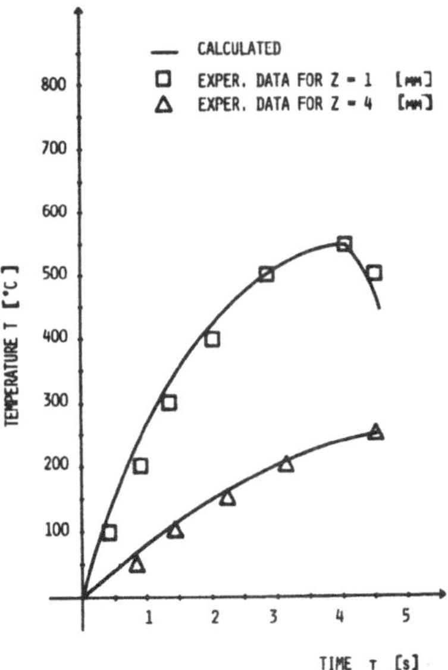

FIGURE 5. Temperatures versus time trends at different depths for measured and calculated conditions for a phosphated nodular cast iron sample with 950 W of incident power.

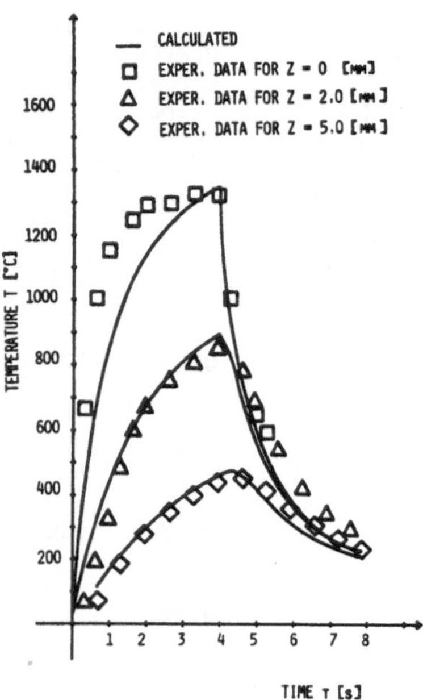

FIGURE 6. Temperatures versus time trends at different depths for measured and calculated conditions for a phosphated nodular cast iron sample with 3.3 kW of incident power.

As shown in Table 3, absorption coefficient values vary from 0.37 to 0.16 for different melting processes. For base material melting, variations are from 0.3 to 0.37, with a 70% decrease of values measured for surface temperatures below the melting point. For alloying with Stellite F and Eatonite 3 powders, still lower values were measured (0.16 to 0.24). As for surface tempertures below the melting point, absorption coefficients for carbon steel are 25% higher than for nodular cast iron.

4.3. Melting depth prediction

To predict laser melting depths, it is necessary to use one-dimensional models with physical parameters and absorption coefficient variations with temperature.

Figure 7 shows a comparison of melting depth predictions with different one-dimensional models and experimental results. The experimental conditions were: base material lamellar cast iron, constant power density (3 kW/cm^2), beam spot size 10 x 10 mm, interaction time variations from 0.75 to 3 seconds.

For an interaction time of 2 seconds, the prediction of the melting depth with a simple one-dimensional model is nearly five times the experimental value of 0.5 mm. Taking into account thermal conductivity

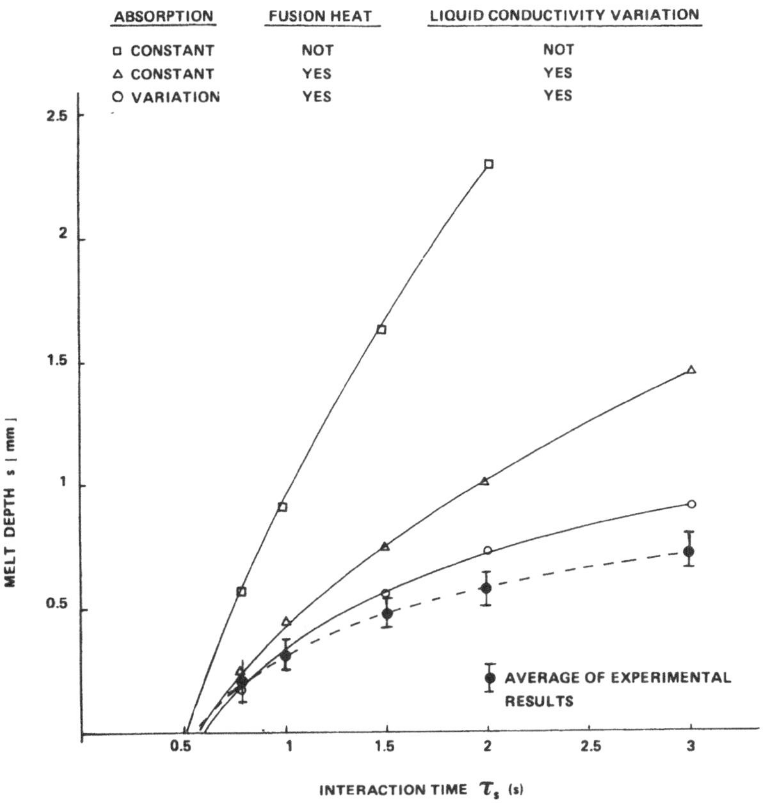

FIGURE 7. Use of monodimensional models for melting depth prediction.

variations from 60 to 25 W/m °C, fusion latent heat, and absorption coefficient variation from 0.60 to 0.28, melting depth predictions are only 1.4 times the experimental value. The one-dimensional model, taking into account only conductivity variation and fusion heat, does not explain the low slope of the melted depth for interaction times more than 1.5 seconds.

5. CONCLUSIONS

Absorption coefficients for heat treating and alloying processes were measured with an experimental and mathematical approach based on heat transfer analysis.

The experimental data presented support the present description of the heating process of metal samples exposed to laser radiation. At low surface temperature the process is determined only by the coating specifications. At higher temperature, below the melting point, the process is determined by the interaction between coating, base material and ambient gas with a physical and chemical variation of surface properties. At melting temperature the heating process is determined mostly by the liquid phase which presents absorption conditions close to those of a pure metal.

Therefore, while the prediction of phase transformation depth can be achieved also with a simple one-dimensional model, the prediction of melting depth can be achieved only with more complete dimensional models. These models take into account the variations with temperature of either physical properties or absorption coefficient.

ACKNOWLEDGMENTS

The author wishes to thank Mr. Appiano of CRF for his help in this work.

REFERENCES

1. G. Alessandretti, P. Gay, G. Manassero, Proceeding IV Gas Chemical Laser, Sept. 82, Stresa, Italy.
2. F. Crescenzi, A. Cutolo, P. Gay, S. Solimeno, Optical Engineering 21 (3), 511-516 (1982).
3. P. Gay, G. Manassero, Proceedings ICALEO, Nov. 1983, Los Angeles, USA.
4. P. Antone, A. Blarasin, M. Castagna, and P. Gay, La Metallurgie Italiana, No. 1, 10 (1980).

HEAT AND MASS TRANSFER IN PULSED LASER HEATING

L. F. DONA DALLE ROSE
Dipartimento di Fisica "G. Galilei" and C.I.S.M., Padova University, I-35131 Padova, Italy

Key Words: boiling, convection, diffusion, evaporation, heat flow calculation: one-dimensional, mass transport, melting, resolidification

ABSTRACT

Under a laser-induced ultrarapid heat flow transient, a number of different regimes and phenomena may occur, according to the values of the incident energy density and the pulse time duration.

Computer codes allow rather careful modeling of such a transient in a given sample on the basis of the heat flow equation and of the appropriate boundary conditions. The heat flow transient may then be characterized by means of quantities such as the molten phase duration, the heating and cooling rates, the maximum molten depth, and the evaporated thickness.

Many observed after-transient properties of an irradiated sample can be interpreted in terms of the heat flow transient structure and quantitatively related to its details. As an example of this, normal and Soret diffusion, precipitation, surface oxidation and non-equilibrium segregation will be discussed. Other experiments, involving higher absorbed energies, exhibit material losses or unusual diffusion properties. These findings will be discussed on the basis of transient evaporation, boiling and convection, in order to assess the occurrence of such phenomena in metals and their relevance under ultrarapid laser irradiating.

After eight years of both theoretical and experimental work (1-3) on ultrarapid (laser or e-beam induced) thermal transients in metals, we can say that many questions have been settled out; there are, however, rather as many problems which are still open and deserve a clarifying effort.

1. INTRODUCTION: THE HEAT FLOW EQUATION

The main tool for interpreting the different kinds of experimental data is the one-dimensional heat diffusion equation (4)

$$c\varrho\frac{\partial T}{\partial t} = \frac{\partial\left[K(T)\frac{\partial T}{\partial x}\right]}{\partial x} + Q(x,t) \tag{1}$$

where c, ρ and K are the sample specific heat, density and thermal conductivity (depending on the temperature $T = T(x,t)$, on the state, whether solid or liquid, and possibly on the amount of embedded impurities, damage and composition). $Q(x,t)$ represents the source term (a laser pulse in the present context; another frequently used facility is afforded by an e-beam pulse). Equation (1), together with several appropriate boundary conditions, has been solved numerically by means of computer codes (5-8). The simplest and most obvious boundary conditions refer to the initial sample temperature, the limiting temperature down in the bulk depth and the radiative loss at the surface, i.e., respectively

$$T(x,0) = T_0 \; ; \qquad T(\infty,t) = T_0 \; ; \qquad \left.\frac{\partial T}{\partial x}\right|_{x=0} = 0 \tag{2a,b,c}$$

where T_0 is the thermal bath temperature.

During the time evolution of the thermal transient several additional constraints must be satisfied at the interfaces where phase transitions occur. Each one of these new boundary conditions is best expressed in terms of two equations, a first one keeping into account heat conservation during the heat flow and a second one of thermodynamical nature relating to other physical constraints at work in the process.

In the case of melting or resolidification, the two equations are (x-axis directed toward the sample interior):

$$\varrho H_{fus}\dot{X} = K_{sol}\left.\frac{\partial T}{\partial x}\right|_{X+} - K_{liq}\left.\frac{\partial T}{\partial x}\right|_{X-} , \tag{3a}$$

i.e., a Stefan moving boundary condition, where $X = X(t)$ is the instantaneous melting/resolidification front position along the x-axis, and H_{fus} is a positive constant equal to the latent heat of fusion/ resolidification; moreover

$$\dot{X} = F(T_i - T_m), \tag{3b}$$

where F is a function of the difference between the solid-liquid interface temperature T_i and the equilibrium melting temperature T_m (i.e., of the solid superheating during melting and of the liquid undercooling during resolidification). The actual form of F is determined by the crystal melting or growth thermodynamics.

Usually, in the case of metals and in the nanosecond regime, Eq.(3b) has been neglected, this corresponding to a simple heat flow-controlled process on the basis of Eq.(3a). The argument runs as follows. In the case of melting, it is a generally accepted view (9,10), that superheating of solids above T_m does not occur to any appreciable extent, since the formation of a liquid skin at the surface, once this is heated up to T_m, always minimizes the free energy of the solid. Recently, a very interesting experiment (11), on some very thin self-sustaining Al films, has shown the occurrence of considerable superheating and of some delay effects in the film melting under irradiating in the picosecond regime. The delay time is about 1 ns after the laser shot, at a superheating of about 350°C above T_m, and it falls down to ~ 20 ps at 1200°C. Nevertheless, when irradiating a bulk sample in the nanosecond regime, the above observed effects ought in general play no role since the transient time scale is much longer. Moreover, in most cases, the heating rate is so high that a very short time (~ 1 ns) is spent in the range of the observed superheatings.

In the case of resolidification, from regrowth thermodynamics, one gets (12)

$$v_{res} = -\dot{X} = f\lambda k_u \frac{H_{fus}M}{k_B T_m} \frac{T_m - T_i}{T_i},$$

where f, i.e., the fraction of interfacial growth sites, is ≤ 1; λ equals a monolayer thickness, f is the configurational rearrangement frequency, and M the atomic mass. The quantity $H_{fus}M/k_B T_m$ is nearly unity for most metals (except a very few cases); k_u can hardly exceed the sound velocity limit (13), so that

$$v_{res} \lesssim v_{sound} \frac{\Delta T_i}{T_i}, \qquad \Delta T_i \equiv T_m - T_i \ . \tag{4}$$

In Al, e.g., $v_{sound} = 5 \times 10^3$ m/s (14), so that $T_i = 3.7°K$ if $v_{res} = 20$ m/s. For small undercooling in metals, then

$$v_{res} = \frac{1}{\beta}(T_m - T_i) \ , \qquad \beta \simeq T_m / v_{sound} \ . \tag{5}$$

Therefore, the constant β is on the order of 10^{-3} °K $(cm/s)^{-1}$ (in Si $\beta \sim 10^{-1}$°K $(cm/s)^{-1}$, cfr. (5)). For Al β equals 1.87×10^{-3}°K $(cm/s)^{-1}$; the largest values of β occur for metals like Au, Pt, W (6.6, 7.3 and 8.0 x 10^{-3}°K $(cm/s)^{-1}$, respectively).

As a consequence, the interface temperature in metals can be to most purposes consistently assumed equal to T_m and v_{res} becomes a heat transport limited rate, through the Stefan problem (3a); see, however, (13). In Figure 1 we report the time evolution of the heat fluxes Φ^- and Φ^+, which respectively go inward and outward from the liquid-solid interface, as calculated (15) assuming (3a), in the case of an Al sample under ruby laser irradiating (the absorbed energy is 0.315 J/cm^2 and $\tau_p = 15$ ns). The time at which the two curves cross each other corresponds to a position of the interface equal to the maximum molten depth. Earlier the balance of the two fluxes yields a nonvanishing melt front velocity; later it yields the resolidification velocity. Clearly, at a certain time, towards the end of the transient in the liquid phase, Φ^- goes to zero; afterwards, we can put, from Eq.(3a)

$$v_{res} \equiv -\dot{X} = -\Phi^+/\varrho H_{fus} = -K_{sol} \frac{\partial T}{\partial x}\Big|_{X^+} \Big/ \varrho H_{fus} \equiv v_{res}^{Stefan} \ , \tag{6}$$

where the superscript Stefan reminds that $T_i = 0$.

We can say that Eq.(6) holds when the absorbed energy is such that the molten phase duration largely exceeds the pulse duration. In this case, it is easily seen that

$$v_{res} = C/E_{abs} \ , \qquad C = cK_{sol}(T_m - T_0)^2/H_{fus} \ , \tag{7}$$

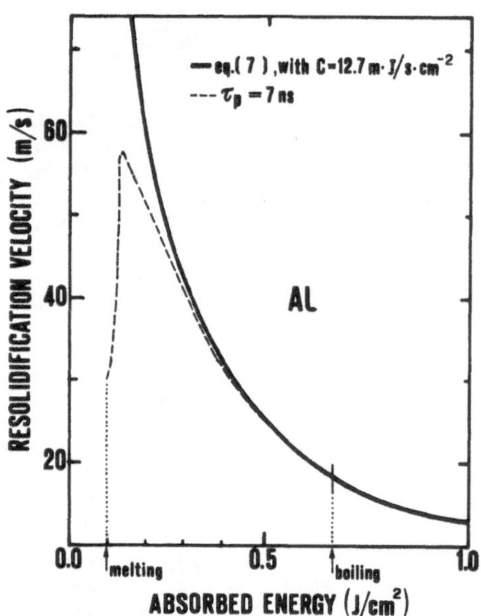

FIGURE 1. Calculated heat fluxes at the liquid-solid interface. Φ^- and Φ^+ are the fluxes from the liquid and to the solid phase, respectively. Calculations were carried out numerically on a moving grid (15).

i.e., the resolidification velocity is inversely proportional to the absorbed energy and independent of the pulse duration , being controlled by the parameters which appear in the definition of the constant C. At the lowest absorbed energies which produce melting, however, Φ^- effectively contrasts Φ^+ and v_{res} decreases with decreasing E_{abs}, thus showing a maximum.

In Figure 2 the general trend (dashed line) of v_{res} as a function of E_{abs} is given for Al. A solid line is superimposed to the dashed line; it shows schematically the velocities which can be actually swept with a laser pulse of given duration, and therefore of given melting and boiling thresholds (see below). In fact, such thresholds are approximately given by simple heat conserving balances (see, e.g., (16)) as

$$E_{abs}^{melt} \sim \varrho c(T_m - T_0)\sqrt{2D_S\tau_p}\ , \qquad E_{abs}^{boil} \sim \varrho c(T_b - T_0)\sqrt{(1+b)D_S\tau_p}\ , \qquad (8)$$

where D_s is the solid phase heat diffusivity (i.e., $K_{sol}/\rho c$), $b = K_{liq}/K_{sol}$ and T_b the boiling temperature at one atmosphere.
For example, the melting threshold at τ_p = 15 ns can be as low as a

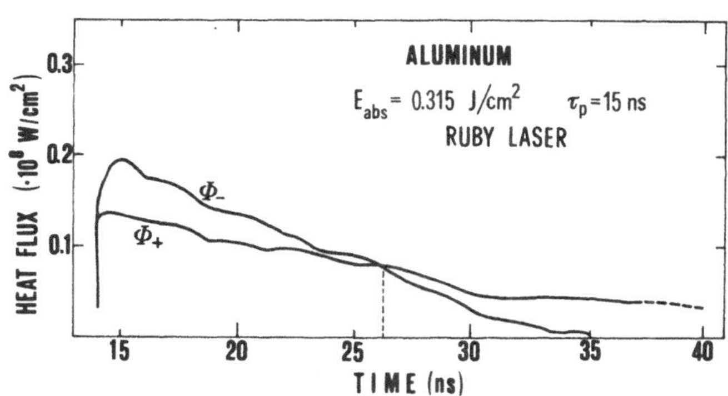

FIGURE 2. General behavior of the resolidification velocity as a function of the absorbed energy (solid line). The dashed lines refer to the actual behavior within the melting and boiling thresholds for the given pulse duration.

few tens of mJ/cm^2 in the case of Pb and Sb or as high as about $0.5\ J/cm^2$ for Cu. The range in E_{abs} from E_{abs}^{melt} to E_{abs}^{boil} again varies from about $60\ mJ/cm^2$ for Sb to about $0.6\ J/cm^2$ for Al, Cu, Au, Pt. Of course the actual range of pulse fluences is much larger, being equal to the absorbed energy range divided by $(1 - R)$, where R is the (average) reflectivity coefficient for the laser pulse wavelength during the transient. (Recall that for many metals R can be quite near to unity).

Another phase transition which may occur under pulsed laser irradiating is surface evaporation and/or boiling. The two equations for the evaporation front, similar in nature to Eq.(3a,b) for the case of the solid-liquid interface, are as follows(17): If the front instantaneous position, with respect to a reference frame fixed in the bulk of the sample, is denoted by $S = S(t)$, then

$$\varrho H_{vap}\dot{S} = K_{liq}\frac{\partial T}{\partial x}\bigg|_{x=S^+} , \tag{9}$$

where H_{vap} is the (constant) heat of vaporization; moreover, a thermodynamical condition relates S to the surface temperature $T_S = T_S(t)$, being either (thermodynamical surface vaporization)

$$\dot{S} = U\exp(-MH_{vap}/k_BT_S) , \tag{10a}$$

or (ordinary boiling process, cfr. (7))

$$\dot{S} = \begin{cases} U\exp(-MH_{vap}/k_BT_S) & \text{when } T_S < T_b, \\ \text{as given by eq.(1) plus the b.c. for the heat flux at the surface, i.e. } \Phi = \rho H_{vap}\dot{S} \text{ [compare with eq.(9)]} & \text{when } T_S = T_b. \end{cases} \quad (10b)$$

Here $U = P_o \exp(MH_{vap}/k_BT_b)/\rho_{liq}\sqrt{2\pi k_BT_S/M}$, with P_o = boiling pressure, is a velocity on the same order as sound velocity (17). Eq.(10a) describes the vaporization rate from the sample surface that always occurs while heating up; the only practical limit for the maximum attained temperature is T_{cr}, i.e., the critical temperature; $\rho_{liq}\dot{S}$ correspondingly represents the maximum vaporizing flux for a given molten sample, whose surface temperature is T_S. On the other hand, Eq.(10b) simulates a condition under which at $T = T_b$ "bulk evaporation" occurs, because of some mechanisms which enhance the actual evaporating surface (e.g., vapor bubble nucleation in the bulk, preexisting bulk cavities filled with saturated vapor and moving to the evaporation front; convective motions;...). Some authors (18) claim that the latter process has no special meaning for heatings which are either of short duration or take place in vacuum (see however below).

Process (10a) may give origin to a wealth of different transients depending on the value of the pulse duration τ_p and of the fluence E_p (or, for a given τ_p, of the average irradiating intensity $I = 1/2\ E_p/\tau_p$). If the laser pulse intensity I is above a threshold value given by

$$I_{thr} = (\varrho H_{vap}/(1-R)\sqrt{\tfrac{1}{2}(K_{sol}+K_{liq})/\varrho c\tau_p},$$

(here R is again the reflectivity of the sample under irradiating), then an intense evaporation regime set in (19), i.e., a regime which is characterized by a stationary temperature T_S^* of the vaporization surface front

$$k_BT_S^* = MH_{vap}\Big/\ln\left[\varrho H_{vap}U/I(1-R)\right]$$
$$= MH_{vap}\Big/\ln\left[\varrho H_{vap}2U\tau_p/E_{abs}\right] \quad (11a)$$

and by a stationary front velocity

$$\dot{S}^* = (1-R)I/\varrho H_{vap} = E_{abs}/2\tau_p\varrho H_{vap} \quad (11b)$$

In the l.h.s. of Fig. 3, T_S (abscissa axis) is plotted as a function of I (vertical axis), for Sb, Al and Ni, up to their critical temperature (8600°K for Al (20) and estimated to be 4-7 times T_b in other cases (21)). In the r.h.s. of the same Fig. 3, I_{thr} is plotted as a function of the pulse duration τ_p: The dashed region here represents the (I,τ_p) conditions which characterize nanosecond pulsed laser irradiating. For a given (I,τ_p) pair, one may enter Fig. 3 from the intensity axis, check whether τ_p is long enough to attain the intense evaporation regime (i.e., whether the point (I,τ_p) lies above the threshold line for the chosen metal) and finally check whether the surface front temperature is below T_{cr} or not. The different possibilities ought to exhibit quite a range of evaporation behavior.

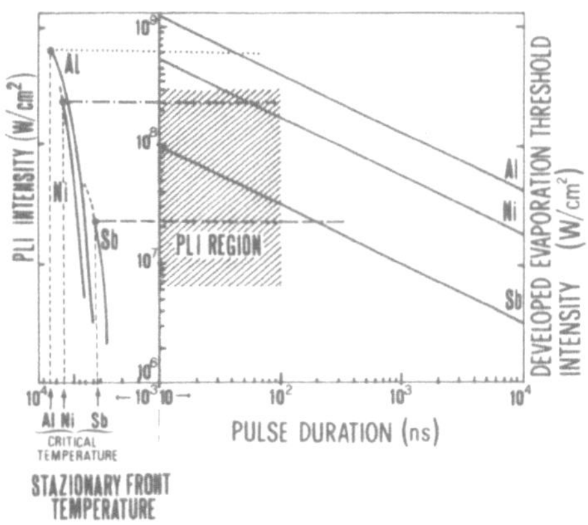

Element	T_b (°K)	T_{cr} (°K)
Si	1861	3250-5900
Ni	3188	6200-11250
Al	2740	8650

FIGURE 3. (r.h.s.) Developed evaporation regime intensity thresholds as a function of the pulse duration for Al, Ni and Sb, together with the pulsed laser irradiating region; (l.h.s.) stationary evaporation front temperature (abscissa) as a function of the incident laser intensity (ordinate); arrows refer to critical temperatures (see table).

In Table I we report (22) the ratio R between the energy used for surface vaporization and the total absorbed energy for pulsed laser irradiating of Sb samples (R = 0.63, τ_p = 7 ns) at two fluences which show clearly the difference between normal and intense evaporation regimes; the maximum attained temperature T_{max} and the evaporated thickness S_{ev} are also reported.

Table I

E_p (J/cm^2)	E_{abs} (J/cm^2)	$\mathcal{R}$	$\hat{T}_{max}$ (°C)	S_{ev} (Å)
0.41	0.152	2%	2360	negligible
2.10	0.777	81%	5675	3376

In Table II we report the evaluation of similar quantities for an Al sample (R = 0.79, τ_p = 15 ns), comparing the surface vaporization with a a boiling process at E_p = 5. J//cm^2, i.e., E_{abs} = 1.05 J/cm^2 (recall from Eq.(8) that E_{thr}^{boil} = 0.7 J/cm^2 for Al). Notice that the maximum maximum molten depth L_{max} is consistently lower in the boiling off case, since then it saturates to a practically constant value, as a function of E_{abs} (see Ref. 7).

Table II

process	$\mathcal{R}$	$\hat{T}_{max}$(°C)	S_{ev} (Å)	L_{max} (Å)
surface vaporization	6%	3963	100	18900
boiling	51%	2467 *(i.e. T_b)*	900	13300

As a conclusion we expect that surface vaporization is a poor thermal sputtering mechanism for most metals. A convection-aided boiling process might, however, be important if present. As an alternative, in the absence of a clamping of the surface temperature to a fixed boiling temperature (whatever physical phenomenon this represents), the surface temperature may achieve quite high values, up to the critical temperature; several new physical proceses may then be imagined (19,23,24,...), including plasma formation (25). In this respect the reflectivity, a crucial parameter in the present discussion, may vary considerably during the transient and greatly affect the actual energy absorption and hence the overall transient quality.

Before leaving this introductory section, it is important to realize and to keep in mind for the following discussions that the transient has a definite structure both in time and in space. In Fig. 4 we schematically report the time intervals which are relevant for the discusson below. Notice, in particular, that the evaporating transient lasts for a time much shorter than the molten phase duration, and it is always located in the early stage of the liquid phase transient.

As to the space variations, notice that the solid phase thermal length $\sqrt{2\ K_{sol}\tau_p/\rho c}$ is on the order of 1000 nm at τ_p = 15 ns for many metals. The steepest temperature gradients occur in liquid phase, at the beginning of the molten phase transient ($\sim 10^7$-10^8 °K/cm), while those in solid phase, which are responsible of the high resolidification velocity, are 10^5-10^6 °K/cm. All these quantities are a function of the laser pulse specifications E_p, τ_p and there are simplified formulae which reproduce the main dependencies (16): see Table III, where E_p enters through E_{abs}; with some caution some of these formulae (e.g.,

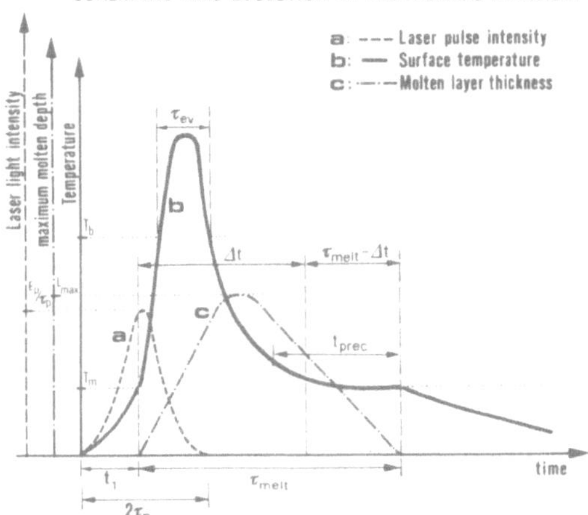

FIGURE 4. Schematic time evolution of the thermal transient: (a) laser pulse intensity, (b) surface temperature, (c) molten layer thickness.

L_{max}, v_{res}), may be used also when the source term is an e-beam pulse (16A).

As a final remark, heat transients in metal can be calculated by using appropriate average values for c, ρ and K_{sol}, K_{liq}, which are slowly varying functions of T in a given phase (solid or molten). Taking into account their actual temperature variation would only change the results by several percent, while significantly increasing the computer time.

2. REVEALING THE THERMAL TRANSIENT STRUCTURE IN METALS (at lower absorbed energies)

Experiments which involve lower absorbed energies, at which no mass loss phenomena occur, allow the simpler test of the computed heat flow transient structure. The latter quite depends on the used energy source (whether laser or e-beam pulse). Roughly speaking, the molten phase duration may be divided into two subsequent stages (see Fig. 4), an earlier one, which is quite warmer (its average temperature being at an intermediate value between T_m and T_b) and a second one characterized by an almost constant temperature, i.e., T_m, all over the molten layer. In the case of a laser source term, the former stage, as already remarked, exhibits very high thermal gradients in liquid phase. The existence of these two stages may be experimentally evidenced by looking at the behavior of probe impurities embedded in the host metal sample through either implantation or sandwiching of a very thin impurity layer. More precisely, the measured impurity profile before irradiating is compared with the after transient one, on the assumption that one can go from the former to the latter in terms of diffusion mechanisms or other processes going on during the transient. While

TABLE III. Analytical simplified formulae for some of the quantities that characterise a heat flow transient,in terms of the laser pulse parameters $E_{abs} = (1-R)E_p$ and τ_p. The quantities $\alpha_1, \alpha_2, \eta_2, \gamma_M, \beta_d$ are constants on the order of unity for a given metal [a]; β_u is a slowly varying function of E_p and τ_p,again on the order of unity [16].

Quantity	*Description*	*Simplified formulae*
τ_{melt}	molten phase duration [b],[e]	$\tau_{melt} = \alpha_2 E_{abs}^2 \Big/ 2D_S \left[\varrho c(T_m - T_0)\right]^2$
t_1	time necessary for the onset of melting	$t_1 = \alpha_1 \tau_p^{4/3} \Big/ (\tau_{melt})^{1/3}$
τ_{ev}	effective duration of the thermodynamical vaporisation transient[c]	$\tau_{ev} \simeq (4k_B \hat{T}_{max}/MH_{vap})\tau_p$
τ_{boil}	boiling off duration [d],[b],[e]	$\tau_{boil} \simeq E_{abs}^2 \Big/ 2D_L \left[\varrho c(T_m - T_0)\right]^2$
$T_{max} - T_m$	maximum temperature [e] attained (neglecting evaporation / boiling)	$T_{max} - T_m = \eta_1 E_{abs}^2 \Big/ \left[\tau_p K_L \varrho c(T_m - T_0)(1 + \frac{H_{fus}}{c(T_m - T_0)})\right]$ $\eta_1 = 0.293(\gamma_M/\beta_u)(\sqrt{2} - t_1/\tau_p)$
L_{max}	maximum molten depth	$L_{max} = \begin{cases} \eta_2 \dfrac{E_{abs}^3/4D_S\tau_p\left[\varrho c(T_m - T_0)\right]^3}{1+\frac{H_{fus}}{c(T_m - T_0)}\left(1+(\beta_d\eta_2/\alpha_2)\frac{\tau_{melt}}{\tau_p}\right)}, & \text{general case;} \\ E_{abs}\Big/2\beta_d \varrho H_{fus}, & \text{if } \tau_{melt}/\tau_p \gg 1. \end{cases}$
v_{res}	resolidification velocity (when $\tau_{melt}/\tau_p > 1$)	$v_{res} \simeq K_S \dfrac{c(T_m - T_0)}{H_{fus}} / E_{abs}$

[a] the values for Al are given in table II of ref.[16].
[b] $D_S = K_S/\varrho c, D_L = K_L/\varrho c$.
[c] see ref [18]; here $\hat{T}_{max}$ is the maximum achieved temperature, in a heat flow transient which includes vaporisation,and it is slightly smaller than T_{max} given below.
[d] formula obtained from an argument similar to that yielding τ_{melt} (cfr. [16]).
[e] notice that this quantity is directly proportional to the square of the so called heating efficiency $2(1-R)/(K\varrho c)^{1/2}$ (see [18]).

normal diffusion may occur during both stages, there are other phenomena which are characteristic of one stage or the other. The first stage offers the unique combination of high concentration gradients (as due to ion implantation or mixing of a layered structure) and extreme liquid phase temperature gradients. In a dilute solution the impurity flux may be expressed (26) in terms of the impurity concentration $n(x,t)$ and of the sample temperature $T(x,t)$ as

$$J_{imp} = -D\frac{\partial n}{\partial x} - DS_T n\frac{\partial T}{\partial x}, \tag{12}$$

where D is the ordinary diffusion coefficient, S_T the Soret coefficient of the process (both are supposed to have constant effective values in a given transient); when $S_T = 0$, one recovers the ordinary diffusion flux. The impurity diffusion equation is

$$\frac{\partial n}{\partial t} = -div(J_{imp}) = D\frac{\partial^2 n}{\partial x^2} + DS_T\frac{\partial n}{\partial x}\frac{\partial T}{\partial x} + DS_T n\frac{\partial^2 T}{\partial x^2}\,. \tag{13}$$

In the r.h.s. the first term is an ordinary diffusion term, the third term may be shown to play no role; the second term is the Soret diffusion term governed by both the concentration and temperature gradients. Equation (13) has to be solved (numerically) by using a molten phase (time dependent) depth and a total duration (either Δt or τ_{melt} (when $S_T = 0$), see Fig. 4), that must be computed previously by means of an appropriate heat flow calculation. As compared to ordinary diffusion, Soret diffusion with the positive S_T coefficient yields a concentration depletion in the near surface region and a small thermal shift of the profile towards colder regions. Evidence for positive S_T Soret diffusion has been found for Cu and Zn in Al, and Au in Ni (27). The lack of negative S_T observed cases may be simply due to the fact that on a microscopic ground the S_T sign is largely dominated by the mass difference between impurity and matrix atoms (28); a negative sign implies heavier matrix atoms, this being unobservable when Rutherford backscattering (RBS) is used. But the most frequent case is $S_T = 0$. Many after transient impurity profiles have been fitted by means of an ordinary diffusion process, along τ_{melt}, always yielding a D coefficient in the 10^{-5}-10^{-4} cm^2/s range (see, e.g., (1), (2) and several papers in (3)).

In principle, the second stage of the molten phase transient lends itself to the occurrence of many different phenomena. We recall here impurity segregation at the resolidification interface, impurity precipitation, liquid phase epitaxy, damage trapping, damage-impurity interaction, amorphization of heavily implanted regions,...

The impurity precipitation has been observed in Sb implanted Al, at an Sb concentration of a few atomic percent (29). The Sb precipitation may be understood by looking at the Al-rich portion of the equilibrium phase diagram for the Al-Sb binary and by noticing that the time - spent (cfr. T_{prec} in Fig. 4) by the cooling Al molten phase within the temperature interval associated with a two-phase state (i.e., liquid plus Al-Sb precipitate) at the given Sb concentration - may be long enough to cause precipitation in certain transients and thus allow observing of submicrosecond nucleation times.

As to non-equilibrium impurity segregation occurring at the resolidifying liquid-solid interface, in metals it exhibits features that are much simpler than those observed, e.g., in silicon. While in the latter case (cfr. Ref. (1), Chap. 4), the equilibrium segregation coefficient changes, in laser-induced transients, to a value which is always different from unity and such that the moving resolidification front generates measurable effects (e.g., a pronounced surface peak) in the impurity profile (whose shape would be otherwise determined by ordinary diffusion). In the case of metals the segregation coefficient turns out to be essentially equal to unity, because of the higher resolidification velocities involved in the nanosecond regime (see (8) and references therein). As a consequence, the diffusion (both ordinary and Soret-like) profiles are simply frozen in the solid phase and no instability in the planar resolidification front leading to the formation of a cell structure (see, e.g., (30)) has yet been detected.

We shall not discuss in this review the other phenomena occurring in the second stage of the molten phase and mentioned above. Details and other references may be found in Ref. 1, mainly Chapter 11.

Let's only discuss another phenomenon which may occur along both stages, i.e., impurity surface oxidation. This is, of course, limited to irradiating conditions in air or O_2 atmosphere. This phenomenon is interesting since it may give origin in metals to a surface peak of those kinds of impurities which have a large negative heat of formation for the corresponding oxide. Examples are some rare earth impurities (e.g., La, Eu, and also Hf) in Ni (31,32). In the case of La implanted Ni, the RBS La spectra have been successfully reproduced by assuming: (1) La diffusion during a molten phase transient, whose parameters (maximum molten depth, resolidification velocity, and duration) were independently calculated on the basis of a heat flow calculation; the La diffusion coefficient is considered to be a free parameter for a given profile; (2) La capture at the Ni surface in small oxide clusters at a rate which was used as a second free parameter, assumed to be equal for all the fitted profiles.

As a conclusion to this section, we can say that many qualitatively different phenomena and explanations confirm a well-defined structure in the heat flow transient in a given metal sample. This is important, since it affords an established starting point for more complex situations like: (a) transients at higher absorbed energies, (b) transients in layered structures, (c) laser irradiating with a pulse train.

3. OPEN PROBLEMS

Many questions are still open and deserve a clarifying effort. I think that some points are:

- Thermal sputtering during a single laser shot,
- Role of the convective motions and conditions for their onset,
- Work on samples acting as a substrate and covered by thin films, in order to clarity such questions as thermal contact resistance, film melting threshold and dynamics, mixing (at eutectic points, in liquid phase,...).

Some of these points, together with the study of stresses induced in solid phase during heating, are also important in connection with the understanding of multiple shot laser iradiating (see, e.g., (18)).

3.1. Thermal sputtering

In Ref. 33 this name is given to any material removal which occurs when a beam of energetic particles, photons included, strikes a solid or liquid target. In the case of laser-induced sputtering many different removal mechanisms exist, such as vaporization, ablation, exfoliation, boiling off, desorption, decomposition, etching, photolysis, hydrodynamical sputtering,... Even though some authors (ibidem) think that the different mechanisms are not easily distinguishable - e.g., by estimating their rates analytically - we think that several experiments made at varying laser fluences give quite a lot of workable information. Since we are dealing with metals, some removal mechanisms may be excluded; in the spirit of the above introduction we shall here limit ourselves to discuss mainly vaporization and boiling off. Evidence for thermal losses in single-shot experiments is widespread (2). Among the more recent data, I would like to mention some data concerning pure Si molten samples and, in the case of metals, data referring to Al and Ni covered by thin metal films. Already Stritzker et al. (34) by using a time of flight technique, showed that the emitted silicon ions under ruby laser irradiating in vacuum (τ_p = 20 ns, fluences from 0.8 up to 2.5 J/cm^2) exhibit a velocity and an emission rate which is consistent with a simple heat flow thermal model in Si, and with a vaporization rate exponentially increasing with the Si molten surface temperature. The maximum attained temperature is about 3000°K in this experiment. Later experiments (35) made with a UV laser in the picosecond region (30 ps) under good vacuum conditions, measured both the total Si ion emission per cm^2 and the ion velocity as a function of the laser fluence. Two emission regimes were actually found. In a first one, at fluences between 25 mJ/cm^2 (threshold for melting) and $\sim$150 mJ/cm^2, again a thermal model, including thermodynamical vaporization, can consistently explain the Si ion loss; if the model is true, it implies the achievement of Si sample temperatures as high as the critical one ($\sim$5000°K). In the second regime (above 150 mJ/cm^2), a completely new, highly non-linear mechanism for ion generation and acceleration sets in, which is presumably related to the formation of an optically dense plasma in front of the surface. In this regime the emitted charge density may correspond to an "evaporated/ablated" thickness as large as $\sim$120 nm.

To our knowledge, no experiments similar to the ones just decribed have been performed on metals. Several irradiating experiments have, however, been performed in air on samples either covered by metal films or implanted with a metal impurity (see, e.g., Ref. 2). Generally speaking, the main aim of the related work was to find the mixing properties of the film into the substrate or the diffusion behavior of the impurity in the matrix.

Nevertheless, meaningful loss data have been measured by means of RBS spectra. Early work dealt with Sb and Pb films over an Al substrate (36,37). A distinct feature of the film loss vs. fluence plot was that above a certain fluence value the loss saturated to a constant value. At lower fluences the loss was higher. The topography of the surface showed globule formation in the Sb case, pratically at all used fluences; globules were not observed with Pb films at the investigated fluences and the surface aspect was greatly varying with the fluence.

The Pb (75 nm) over Al system was later investigated (38) with a 25 keV electron beam pulse having a 50 ns (fwhm) duration and corresponding to absorbed energies varying from 0.15 up to $\sim$2.3 J/cm^3 (cf. Fig. 5a). As it is known, because of the much larger energy deposition

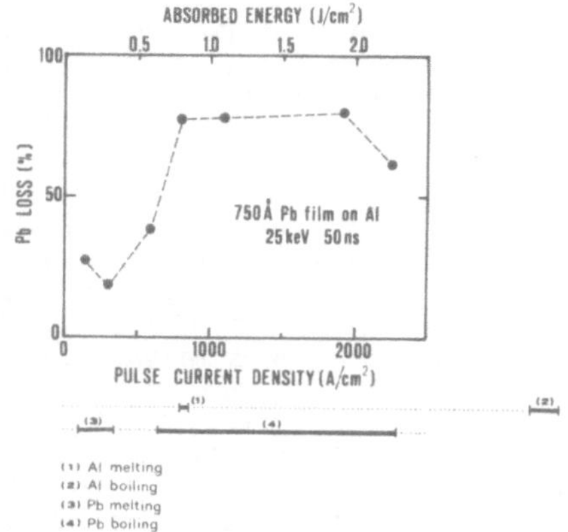

FIGURE 5. (a) Mass loss curves for Pb(750 Å)/Al. Thresholds for different phase transitions, obtained from heat flow calculations, are also shown. The ranges refer to a thermal contact resistance varying from zero (left) to infinity (right).

range, e-beam iradiating allows a magnification of the absorbed laser energy intervals, where significant phenomena occur. In this case, at the higher absorbed energy, the Al maximum temperature is still far from the Al ordinary boiling threshold, while at the lower fluence end, Al is certainly and Pb probably not yet molten. As a matter of fact, heat flow calculations show that, assuming a thermal contact resistance at the Pb-Al interface, (having a value 227 W/cm^2 °K (38A)), the "minimum" in the loss at 30 nm/cm^2 roughly corresponds to the Pb melting threshold, so that the loss at lower E_{abs} must be due to a mechanism in solid phase (e.g., ejection of solid Pb particles as a consequence of the violent emission of gases which are absorbed at the Al-Pb interface). With increasing current densities, liquid Pb coexists with solid Al (the signature of this fact being given by the appearance of Pb globules in the SEM pictures) and, when both metals are liquid, a slight mixing occurs. An estimate of the Pb maximum boiled-off thickness (on the basis of process (10b)) shows that at the higher absorbed energies, even in the extreme case of no thermal contact at the interface, an appreciable fraction of the Pb loss is still due to particle ejection in solid phase, or slipping off of the liquid globules, during the earlier part of the transient. Apparently, no clear evidence for convective motions comes either from surface SEM pictures or RBS spectra.

The loss from Pb films deposited over a Ni substrate under 16 ns ruby laser irradiation in air is reported in Fig. 5b for two film thicknesses (39). In both cases the Pb losses have a similar behavior consisting in a well-defined peak at lower fluences, followed by a minimum and by a new, rather milder, increase, which finally saturates at different values in the two cases. Heat flow calculations (perfect thermal contact) yield for the Pb melting threshold a value which is well below the lowest fluence value used in the experiment, while the Ni melting threshold is at 1.35 and 1.5 J/cm^2 for the 350 and 80 nm Pb film covered

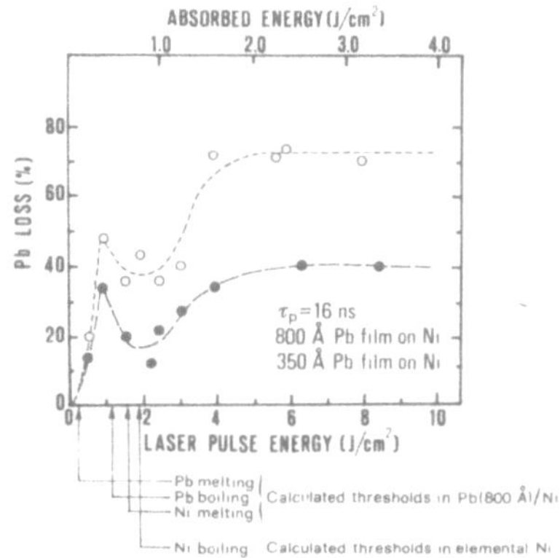

FIGURE 5. (b) Mass loss curves for Pb(350 Å)/- and Pb(800 Å)/Ni systems. Thresholds for different phase transitions obtained from heat flow calculations are also shown.

samples, respectively (assuming a Pb reflectivity equal to 0.67); the thresholds for Pb boiling are at 1.5 and 1.1 J/cm^2, respectively. Therefore, we may conclude that the loss curve trends observed in the Pb-Al system under e-beam irradiating are in the present case confined to the l.h.s. of the loss peak which shows up at 1-1.5 J/cm^2. We also conclude that the minima in the loss curves are due to Ni melting and to the subsequent coexistence of molten Pb and Ni during the transient; this fact reduces the rather uncontrolled loss mechanisms at work at the lower fluences. As a matter of fact, at fluences ≥ 3.9 J/cm^2 also Pb-Ni mixing occurs, depending both on the Ni molten phase duration and on the interface average temperature during the transient. As already remarked, at fluences greater than 1.1-1.5 J/cm^2, Pb may boil off quite consistently and this may explain the increase in the loss curves after the minimum, or alternatively, since in the mixing process the Ni atoms start in any case coming to the surface, we may imagine that both Ni boiling and convective motions of the Ni substrate set in, causing, at the same time, a consistent (measurable) Pb loss, and a good depth mixing. This is consistent with heat flow calculations on pure Ni sample, which yield ~1.8 J/cm^2 as the threshold for Ni boiling.

In the following we shall try a quantitative explanation for the saturated loss behavior at the higher fluences, on the basis of a model which takes into account convective motions. We shall at first try to characterize this phenomenon as occurring in ultrarapid laser heating.

3.2. Convective motions

Again, the evidence for convective motions during ultrarapid heating is widespread and goes back to the earlier experiments and it has been confirmed in the subsequent work (see (2,8) and references therein); this evidence is mainly based on: (a) the after transient metal surface, which shows quite a rough aspect as compared to the surface smoothness found after lower energy density transients; (b) the (implanted or deposited) impurity profile tails, which may be phenomenologically described by diffusion coefficients D having values much greater than 10^{-4} cm^2/s and which often extend well beyond the detection limit (matrix edge in the RBS spectra). In addition, these tails reach a depth which is often greater than the maximum molten depth as calculated on the basis of heat flow calculations, thus suggesting that convective motions may quite increase the depth over which a molten phase appears. A nice evidence for the existence of two different diffusion regimes, i.e., a simple liquid phase diffusion and a convective-type flat impurity redistribution, is found in Ref. 40, where the impurity (Sb) profiles in an Al matrix are measured by means of an RBS microbeam within the same laser ($\lambda = 1.06\ \mu m$) spot, which has a Gaussian intensity distribution. Probably because of radial thermal gradients, the peripheral circular region, which attains lower average temperatures, shows evidence for convective type motions, both because of the rough surface and of the Sb flat profile shape; the central region, which coresponds to the highest absorbed energy, is smooth and the related Sb profile is simply diffusion like. Finally, convection inhibits liquid phase epitaxy of irradiated single crystal samples, favoring a high residual damage (41).

The true nature of convective motions in thin molten pools as obtained under laser irradiating is a matter still open to discussion. In particular, the relationships between this very peculiar geometry and both the thermal gradients - either parallel or normal to the liquid surface - and the type and concentration of embedded impurities has to be described in detail. The main points which have to be understood seem to be: (1) conditions under which convection can occur and time necessary for its onset, (2) how long does it last and which is the need in energy supply, (3) relaxation of the liquid phase surface after that convective motions come to an end and before resolidification.

A recent experiment (42) has suggested answers to some of these points. Silicon samples (clean, or covered with SiO_2 layers of varying thickness - SiO_2 being formed with the isotope ^{18}O - or tailored in a sandwich system $Si/SiO_2/Si$ with the same marked oxide) were ruby laser (20 ns) irradiated under several different conditions, e.g., vacuum, O_2 (constituted of ^{16}O). N_2, CO_2,... atmospheres at several pressures, in order to study the oxygen and other species incorporation; the experimental data, among other things, show:

(a) An oxygen transport from the surface towards the bulk material or vice versa (sandwich experiments) leading to a uniform ^{16}O-^{18}O mixing in the after transient profiles. All data consistently suggest that this mixing has to occur already in the earlier part of the transient (e.g., in order to explain ^{18}O loss data in the sandwich samples) and that its characteristic time is shorter than the characteristic boiling off times ($\sim$10-15 ns on the basis of heat flow calculations within scheme (10b)), in order to explain the almost unappreciable ^{18}O loss in the thinnest oxide film samples. As it is well known, an ordinary diffusion mechanism requires times as long as $\sim$100 ns in order to cover appreciable lengths.

(b) A saturation of the final oxygen content both as a function of the laser fluence at a given O_2 pressure and as a function of pressure above the fluence threshold.

The authors can explain these and other data on the basis of a model which assumes convective motions to start at most in a few nanoseconds at the earlier stage of the liquid phase transient (when correspondingly the heat flow calculations show that the temperature gradient in the molten pool, along the normal to the surface, attains values as high as 8×10^7 °K/cm). The convective motions may be thought as due to a coupling of both natural (buoyant) and Marangoni (surface tension driven convection) (43), and ought to originate because of the occurrence of small surface perturbations, which may very well be induced by the oxidizing reactions or by the laser beam inhomogeneities. In order to explain the saturation behavior of the oxygen capture, the model requires a duration of the convective motions equal to 180 ns, i.e., ~2/5 of the total duration of the molten phase, as estimated on the basis of heat flow calculations (not including convection, of course).

As to the plausibility of a quick onset of the convective motions, the above authors notice that from the characteristic times needed to transfer a surface layer to a depth d, under natural or Marangoni convection, i.e., respectively (44):

$$\tau_c = d\,\frac{l_c}{(\eta/\varrho)}\,, \qquad \tau_c = d\left(\frac{\varrho\eta}{l_c}\right)^{1/3} \Big/ \left|\frac{d\sigma}{dT}\frac{\partial T}{\partial x}\right|^{2/3}, \qquad \text{(14a,b)}$$

where ℓ_c is the thickness of the layer where convection occurs, η the molten phase viscosity, and σ the surface tension, one may estimate for silicon (assuming $d = 10$ nm, $\ell_c = 100$ nm, and $|\partial T/\partial x| \sim 10^7$ °K/cm) values very near to 1 ns.

As a confirmation to the convective motion duration required by the above model, recall the work by Possin et al. (45), relating to a similar situation, where by solving approximately the Navier-Stokes equation, it is shown that the characteristic times for mass mixing are on the order of hundreds of ns.

Finally, it would be interesting to know the conditions under which convective motions die out and the molten pool freezes. We think that any discussion should be aware of the following two facts. First, the relative movement of the temperature pattern (which in this case would characterize the cooling process) and of the velocity pattern (which characterizes the penetration - by means of shear stresses - of the convective motion into the liquid) may be assessed (46) through the ratio between the lengths, covered by the two patterns in a given time t, i.e., by the quantity

$$\left(\frac{D_T t}{D_v t}\right)^{1/2} \equiv \frac{(K/\varrho c)^{1/2}}{(\eta/\varrho)^{1/2}} = \left(\frac{K}{\eta c}\right)^{1/2} \qquad \text{(15)}$$

Secondly, if a liquid freezing pool has time to relax quietly before solidfying (i.e., during the time interval which may run between the extinction of the convective motions and the actual resolidification), its surface tends to minimize its free energy by recovering a flat aspect as compared to the wavy and rough aspect proper of turbulent motions. As a consequence of these two facts, metals having a higher viscosity and a greater surface tension ought to exhibit smoother surfaces after thermal transients involving convection. This is, for instance, the case of Ni with respect to Al and Si*. Notice that the argument leading to (15) can be further refined and adapted to the present case by estimating the ratio of the molten pool (or resolidifying layer) thickness L_{max} to the length $(D_v \tau_{res})^{1/2}$, where $\tau_{res} = L_{max}/v_{res}$. It is easily found

$$\frac{L_{max}}{(D_v \tau_{res})^{1/2}} = \left(\frac{\varrho L_{max} v_{res}}{\eta} \right)^{1/2} , \tag{16}$$

which for comparable thermal transients (i.e., for a given absorbed energy) yields for Ni, Al and Si similar answers as Eq.(15) (L_{max} and v_{res} can be obtained from either heat flow calculations or "phenomenological" formulae, see Eq.(7) and Table III).

3.3. A quantitative example

An explanation for the saturation in the Pb loss curves of Fig. 5b may now be tried. We shall use an approach similar to that of Ref. 42. Assume that convective motions in the Ni molten pool effectively and quickly mix the Pb atoms over an effective depth ℓ_c, in such a way that at time t the Pb atom concentration is

$$n(t) = \frac{\xi(t)}{l_c} , \tag{17}$$

if $\xi(t)$ is the Pb content in at/cm^2 at time t. Then the amount of Pb atoms lost by the sample together with the boiling off Ni atoms is given by

$$d\xi = -n(t) \dot{S} dt , \tag{18}$$

where $\dot{S}$ is given by Eq.(10b) and in a first approximation may be put equal to S_b/τ_{boil}, i.e., to the ratio of the total boiled-off thickness over the boiling time. According to heat flow calculations, S_b varies strongly with E_{abs}, while τ_{boil} has a much weaker dependence on it (22). We then write

$$d\xi = -\xi(t) \frac{S_b}{l_c} \frac{dt}{\tau_{boil}} ,$$

which may be integrated to yield the evaporated amount as

$$\frac{\xi(t_b) - \xi(t)}{\xi(t_b)} = 1 - \exp\left[-\frac{S_b}{l_c} \frac{t - t_b}{\tau_{boil}} \right] \tag{19}$$

---

* Compare for instance Fig. 3 of Ref. 8 with Fig. 2b of Ref. 40.

where t_b is the time at which the Ni boiling off starts and $\xi(t_b)$ is the amount of Pb in at/cm^2, which is present at that time. In general, $\xi(t_b)$ is given by the initial Pb amount per cm^2 in the film - let it be ξ_o - minus the loss occurring either in solid or in liquid phase (see above). The loss (19) saturates to a constant value after the boiling off transient only if S_b/ℓ_c does not depend on the transient: Since we expect the length ℓ_c to be rather independent of it - it most probably scales as L_{max} and this in turn saturates under the boiling condition (10b) (see Ref. 7) - this cannot be the case and we are forced to assume that boiling off stops after a time $t_b + \tau^*$ such that $\tau^* = \Lambda/(Sb/\tau_{boil})$, where Λ represents a characteristic length of condensed phase material (either Ni or Ni-Pb solution). Λ may be interpreted as the amount of vaporized material that is able to decouple the laser beam from the liquid target, by means, e.g., of some kind of plasma formation. Another possible decoupling mechanism might consist in a rising of the boiling temperature and a parallel inhibition of boiling caused by the pressure increase which is associated with the recoil of the vaporizing atoms (47).

According to the above assumption the time τ^* is the shorter, as S_b/τ_{boil} is the larger. The boiled-off Pb loss then saturates to

$$\frac{\xi(t_b) - \xi(t_b + \tau^*)}{\xi(t_b)} = 1 - \exp\left[-\frac{\Lambda}{l_c}\right], \tag{20}$$

By introducing the experimentally measured quantity $(\xi_o - \xi(t_b + \tau^*))/\xi_o$ and by estimating the loss $\xi(t_b)$, which occurs earlier than t_b, as given by the amount at the minimum in the two experimental loss curves (see Fig. 5b), one gets for the parameter Λ/ℓ_c the values 0.29 and 0.69 in the case of a 35 and a 80 nm Pb film, respectively. This is reasonable since, whereas we expect Λ not to depend much on the Pb concentration in Ni, the effective length of the convective motions in Ni may well depend on the Pb atom concentration. Moreover, since ℓ_c may be estimated to be in the range 100-500 nm, a useful, even though rough, estimate may be obtained for Λ.

As a conclusion to this analysis we may say that thermal sputtering in the form given by Eq.(10b) exists and it is intimately connected to the appearance of convective motions. In addition, a strong thermal sputtering may have effects on the laser-metal coupling. In the above proposed explanation for the Pb loss in the Pb-Ni system, it is in fact at the basis of the saturation loss mechanism.

REFERENCES

1. See, e.g., Surface Modification and Alloying, edited by J. M. Poate, G. Foti, and D. C. Jacobson (Plenum Press, Trevi-Italy, 1983), NATO A.S.I.
2. C. W. Draper and J. M. Poate, Internat. Metal Reviews 30, 85 (1985).
3. See also the Proceedings of the Material Research Society held in Boston and dedicated to this subject since 1978. (Some of them are quoted below (5, 12, 35, 38, 44a).
4. H. S. Carslaw and J. C. Jaeger, Conduction of Heat in Solids, 2nd ed. (Oxford Press, 1959).
5. B. Baeri, in Laser and Electron Beam Interactions with Solids, edited by B. R. Appleton and G. K. Celler (Elsevier-North Holland, 1982), p. 151.
6. L. F. Dona dalle Rose and A. Miotello, Radiat. Eff. 53, 7 (1980).
7. A. K. Jain, V. N. Kulkarni, and D. K. Sood, Appl. Phys. 25, 127 (1981).
8. L. F. Dona dalle Rose, Journal de Physique C5, 469 (1983).
9. A. R. Ubbelohde, The Molten State of Matter (J. Wiley, New York, 1978), p. 317.
10. S. J. Peppiatt, Proc. R. Soc. Lond. A354, 413 (1975).
11. S. Williamson, G. Mourou, and J. C. M. Li, Phys. Rev. Lett 52, 2364 (1984).
12. F. Spaepen and D. Turbull, in Laser-Solid Interactions and Laser Processing (AIP, New York, 1979), p. 73.
13. S. R. Corriel and D. Turnbull, Acta Metall. 30, 2135 (1982).
14. Handbook of Chemistry and Physics, 55th ed. (CRC Press, 1974), p. E-47.
15. A. Chiozzi, Tesi di Laurea, Padua University, Italy, 1981.
16. L. F. Dona dalle Rose and A. Miotello, Radiat. Eff. 53, 19 (1980).

16a. L. F. Dona dalle Rose, A. Miotello, and R. Brotto, Radiat. Eff. 69, 1 (1983).

17. F. V. Bunkin and M. J. Tribel'skii, Sov. Phys. Uspekhi 23, 105 (1980).
18. R. Kelly and J. E. Rothenberg, Nucl. Instrum. Methods B7/8, 755 (1985).
19. V. A. Batanov, F. V. Bunkin, A. M. Prokhorov, and V. E. Federov, Sov. Phys. JETP 36, 311 (1973).
20. Thermophysical Properties of Matter, Vol. 10, Thermal Diffusivity, edited by Y. S. Touloukian, R. W. Powell, C. Y. Ho, and M. C. Nicolaov (IFI-Plenum, New York, 1973).
21. See, e.g., L. D. Landau and E. M. Lifshitz, Statistical Physics (Pergamon Press, Oxford, 1969), p. 272.
22. P. Meneghello, Tesi di Laurea, Padua University, Italy, 1981.
23. J. F. Ready, J. Appl. Phys. 36, 462 (1965).
24. F. W. Dabby and U. Paek, IEEE J. Quantum Electron. QE-8, 106 (1972).
25. S. J. Thomas, R. F. Harrison, and J. F. Figueira, Appl. Phys. Lett. 40, 200 (1982).
26. A. Miotello, L. F. Dona dalle Rose, and A. Desalvo, Appl. Phys. Lett. 40, 135 (1982).
27. A. Miotello and L. F. Dona dalle Rose, Phys. Lett. 87A, 317 (1982).
28. S. P. Murarka, T. Y. Kim, M. Y. Hsieh, and R. A. Swalin, Acta Metall. 22, 185 (1974).

29. See S. T. Picraus and D. M. Follstaedt, in Ref. 1, p. 300; see also P. S. Peercy, D. M. Follstaedt, S. T. Picraux, and W. R. Wampler, in Laser and Electron Beam Interactions with Solids, edited by B. R. Appleton and G. K. Celler (Elsevier-North Holland, 1982), p. 401.
30. W. W. Mullins and R. F. Sekerka, J. Appl. Phys. 35, 444 (1964).
31. C. W. Draper, E. N. Kaufmann, and L. Buene, Surface and Interface Analysis 4, 8 (1982).
32. G. Battaglin, A. Carnera, G. Della Mea, L. F. Dona dalle Rose, V. N. Kulkarni, P. Mazzoldi, A. Miotello, E. Jannitti, A. K. Jain, D. K. Sood, and J. Chaumont, J. Appl. Phys. 55, 3773 (1984).
33. J. E. Rothenberg and R. Kelly, Nucl. Instrum. Methods B1, 291 (1984).
34. B. Stritzker, A. Pospieszczyk, and J. A. Tagle, Phys. Rev. Lett. 47, 356 (1981).
35. A. M. Malvezzi, H. Kurz, and N. Bloembergen, in Energy Beam-Solid Interactions and Transient Thermal Processing, edited by J. C. C. Fan and N. M. Johnson (Elsevier-North Holland, 1984), p. 135; see also, by the same authors, "Picosecond Photoemission Studies of the Laser-Induced Phase Transition in Silicon," in press.
36. A. K. Jain, V. N. Kulkarni, D. K. Sood, M. Sundararaman, and R. D. S. Yadav, Nucl. Instrum. Methods 168, 275 (1980).
37. A. K. Jain, V. N. Kulkarni, K. B. Nambiar, D. K. Sood, S. C. L. Sharma, and P. Mazzoldi, Radiat. Eff. 63, 175 (1982).
38. G. Battaglin, A. Carnera, L. F. Dona dalle Rose, V. N. Kulkarni, P. Mazzoldi, E. D'Anna, G. Leggieri, and A. Luches, in Energy Beam-Solid Interactions and Transient Thermal Processing, edited by J. C. C. Fan and N. M. Johnson (Elsevier-North Holland, 1984), p. 769.
38a. L. E. Laghi, Tesi di Laurea, Padua University, Italy, 1984.
39. G. Battaglin, A. Carnera, G. Della Mea, L. F. Dona dalle Rose, V. N. Kulkarni, S. Lo Russo, and P. Mazzoldi, in Surface Engineering, edited by R. Kossowsky and S. C. Singhal (Nijhoff Publishers, Les Arcs, 1984), p. 330. NATO A.S.I.
40. A. K. Jain, V. N. Kulkarni, and D. K. Sood, Nucl. Instrum. Methods 191, 151 (1985).
41. G. Battaglin, A. Carnera, G. Della Mea, P. Mazzoldi, E. Jannitti, A. K. Jain and D. K. Sood, J. Appl. Phys. 53, 3224 (1982).
42. M. Berti, L. F. Dona dalle Rose, A. V. Drigo, G. G. Bentini, C. Cohen, J. Siejka, E. Jannitti, to be published; see also, M. Berti et al., in Proceedings of the MRS-Europe meeting of Strasbourg, 1985, to be published in J. de physique.
43. F. Rosenberger, Fundamentals of Crystal Growth I (Springer-Verlag, New York, 1979), Chap. V, p. 387.
44. D. Schwabe and A. Scharmann, J. Cryst. Growth 52, 435 (1981).
45. G. E. Possin, H. G. Parks, and S. W. Chiang, In Laser and Electron Beam Solid Interactions and Materials Processing, edited by S. F. Gibbons, L. D. Hess and T. W. Sigmon (Elsevier-North Holland, 1981), p. 73.
46. T. R. Anthony and H. E. Cline, J. Appl. Phys. 48, 3888 (1977).
47. G. A. Askar'yan and E. M. Moroz, Sov. Phys. JETP 16, 1638 (1963).

NUMERICAL RESULTS OF THERMAL ACTIONS INDUCED BY HIGH-FREQUENCY SHORT-PULSED LASER TRAINS ON METALS

CLAIRE GIRARDEAU-MONTAUT AND JEAN-PIERRE GIRARDEAU-MONTAUT

Université Claude Bernard - Lyon 1, Groupe de Physique des Interactions Laser-Materiaux, 43 Bd du 11 Novembre 1918, 69622 Villeurbanne Cedex, France

Key Words: heating efficiency, heat flow calculation: one-dimensional, three-dimensional, pulsed laser (picosecond), pulse trains

1. INTRODUCTION

We present here numerical evaluation of thermal and thermo-mechanical actions induced by high-frequency (> GHz), high-intensity (> MW/cm²) and very short pulsed (< 100 psec) laser trains on material.

This new type of problem appears, for instance, in the future realization of very high energy electron accelerators (> 1 TeV) with new electron source, as Lasertron. Such an accelerator requires the production of very high electron densities during a very short time, with a high repetition rate. The characteristics of this new system must be very high: yield ≥ 75% and maximum emitted RF-power ≤ 1 GW. A solution was proposed recently by Takeda (1), using efficient interaction of a laser on a cathode: The laser beam whose intensity is modulated at the RF frequency illuminates a photocathode; the photo-emitted electron beam is accelerated by a DC voltage towards the output cavity from which the RF power is extracted (Figure 1).

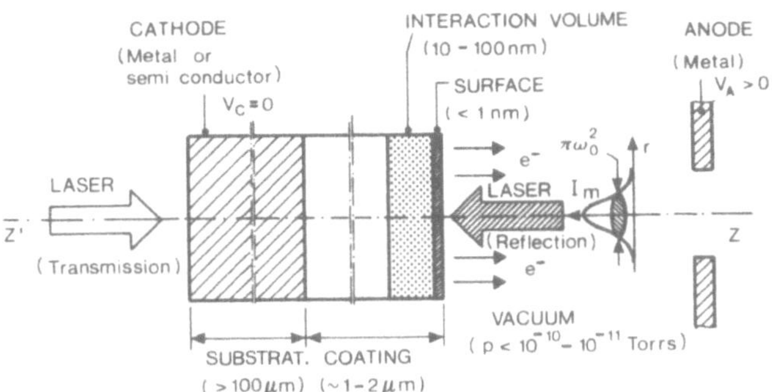

FIGURE 1. Schematic diagram of lasertron.

From preliminary analysis (2) it seems that an advantageous solution could be the production of these electrons in 1 μs bursts, consisting of a train of very short pulses (≃35 ps) with an internal repetition rate ≃3 or 6 GHz, the repetition rate of the trains being on the order of 10^3 Hz. Supposing a quasi-instantaneous electronic response when the laser interacts with the material, we choose to make evaluation of thermal effects at the surface in the case of laser pulse trains with such values.

2. CONDITIONS OF LASER-MATERIAL INTERACTION

The important parameters of the required laser are the photon wavelength λ or its frequency ω, the maximum intensity I_m and the pulse duration τ_p. Depending on the value of the material work function Φ (typically 1.5 eV to 5 eV), the efficient λ corresponds to near IR, visible and near UV. The photoelectric quantum efficiency and the reflectivity R of the surface of material are both functions of λ. The polarization and coherence of laser light are also important in the interaction, but their roles deserve to be studied more precisely. Last, the beam cross section and the spatial energy distribution have to be adjusted to the surface of material; it is always possible to transform the typical Gaussian energy distribution into a rectangular one by an appropriate optical system (3).

To remove from the target a charge estimated to be 0.5 μCb/cm^2, a calculation shows that the maximum power for each incident 35 ps pulse must be greater than 0.5 MW/cm^2, and probably more when all possible losses of energy are considered. All calculations were done supposing a Nd:YAG laser with single (1.06 μm) and doubled (0.53 μm) frequencies, and intensities from 1 MW/cm^2 to 1 GW/cm^2.

The interaction of the laser beam with the cathode not only directly controls the electron production, but also the resistance to damage and the lifetime of the cathode. Figure 2 presents a diagram of all processes induced in laser-material interaction and their connections. The first problem to be solved is the realization of the higher possible coupling between incident laser energy and the material. This coupling depends on the roughness of the surface and its chemical composition. According to the nature (crystalline or amorphous) of the material, the inclincation of incident laser beam introduces a variation of the absorptivity A. In the visible and UV range, A is generally < 50%, and consequently, total conversion efficiency cannot be more than 0.5, even after mechanical or chemical treatment of the surface. Note that it is not possible in our application to cover the surface with an absorbing layer such as carbon to increase A, because chemical reactivity induced by laser would limit the photoelectric yield and maximize target damage. Of course, the laser-induced temperature change in the target is of great importance because it determines much of the processes of electron production, and because it leads to thermomechanical stresses, changes in surface state, and even to irreversible damage. A very important problem is that, even if the mean temperature rise is very small when only one pulse interacts with the material, the high repetition rate will multiply this effect, so the study of cooling is one of our major purposes. Our analysis of temperature changes is done with a view to avoid melting or vaporization. This is the first reason that controls the choice of the cathode material: We can choose between metals (tungsten or cold alkalides for instance), semi-metals (as LaB_6 used in thermionic gun), and semiconductors (doped Si, or GaAs which offers a very high quantum yield of ~10%). Considering damage thresholds and electrical conductivity, metals are certainly better than semiconductors which offer, however, higher quantum yields. So, we present here numerical results corresponding to metals, principally tungsten, W.

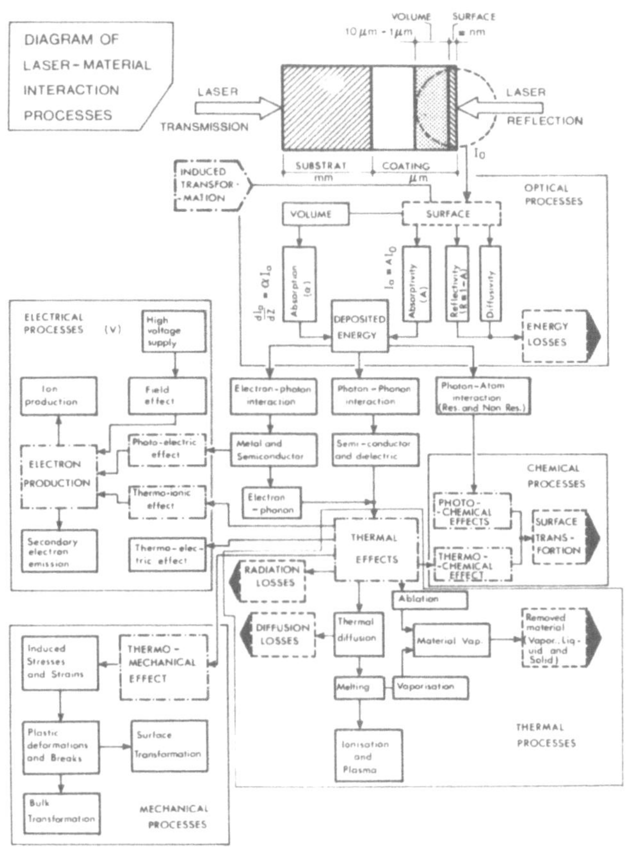

FIGURE 2. Diagram of processes in laser-material interaction.

3. THERMAL ANALYSIS

The first process that we cannot avoid is the thermal one. A part of incident energy, absorbed in surface, is converted into heat which diffuses progressively in the bulk of material. The thermal diffusion is characterized by the length:

$$d \propto 2(\kappa \tau_p)^{1/2} \qquad (1)$$

where κ is the thermal diffusivity (in metals, typically 0.5-1 cm^2/s). If $\tau_p \sim 10^{-11}s - 10^{-10}s$, for W($\kappa = 0.7\ cm^2/s$), d varies from 50 to

150 nm, which is comparable to the absorption depth α^{-1} of the light in the metal. Note that in semiconductors this situation is less critical, but there are other problems such as non-linear absorption.

3.1. Evaluation of the temperature rise induced by a pulsed laser train

At each instant or for each very small time interval, we suppose material parameters independent of temperature. Then, we can use the general heat equation (4):

$$\nabla^2 T - \frac{1}{\kappa}\frac{\partial T}{\partial t} = -\frac{A(\bar{r},t)}{K} \tag{2}$$

K is the thermal conductivity and the diffusivity $\kappa = K/\rho C$ where ρ is the density of the material and C its specific heat. T is the temperature at time t. $A(\bar{r},t)$ is the heat source term corresponding here to the laser pulsed train r being the space component (x,y are in the plane of the surface, z is perpendicular to it):

$$A(\bar{r},t) = q(\bar{r}) \cdot f(t) \tag{3}$$

If we consider a very short interval of time ($\Delta t < 10$ psec), a term of the form $\frac{1}{v^2}\frac{\partial^2 T}{\partial t^2}$ (v velocity of sound in material) would have to be introduced in Eq.(2) because heat diffusion cannot be considered instantaneously the same everywhere (5).

General solution of Eq.(2) gives the variation of temperature T above the initial one.

$$\Delta T = \int_R \frac{q(\bar{r}')}{\rho C}\, d\bar{r}' \int_0^t f(t')g(\bar{r},t/\bar{r}',t')dt' \tag{4}$$

where $g(\bar{r},t/\bar{r}',t')$ is the Green function.

Now, we suppose a Gaussian spatial distribution of laser energy:

$$q(\bar{r}) = \frac{\alpha P}{\pi\delta^2}(1 - R)\exp - \frac{x^2 + y^2}{\delta^2} \exp(-\alpha z) \tag{5}$$

where P is the peak power of laser pulse, $I_M = P/\pi\delta^2$ is its maximum intensity, δ being the laser beam radius at e^{-1} of the power. α (cm^{-1}) is the absorption coefficient of the surface (typically in metals $\sim 10^5\ cm^{-1}$) depending on λ. Also, depending on is the surface reflectivity of material $R = 1\text{-}A$. Then, the maximum temperature rise, at the spot center (x=y=z=0), at the time t, is given by equation:

$$\Delta T = \frac{\alpha I_M(1 - R)}{2\rho C} \int_0^t \frac{f(t')dt'}{1 + a^2/\delta^2} \; 2 \exp \frac{\alpha^2 a^2}{4} \; \text{erfc} \; \frac{a\alpha}{2} \tag{6}$$

with
$$a = 2[\kappa(t - t')]^{1/2} \tag{7}$$

is related to the diffusion length.

Now we suppose identical periodic pulses with the following train characteristics: FWHM pulse duration = τ_p, repetition pulse frequency = $1/T_p = 2\pi/\omega$, train duration = τ_{tr} and repetition train frequency = $1/T_{tr}$. The temporary function $f(t)$ depends on the form of each individual laser pulse. Thus, if we consider a Gaussian pulse:

$$f(t) = \exp(- t^2/\tau^2) \tag{8}$$

with time constant
$$\tau = \tau_p/2 \sqrt{\log 2} \tag{9}$$

From supposed qualities of the pulse train, when $\tau_p << T_p$, we can use Fourier analysis to express $f(t)$ as a sum of cosine terms. Making a hypothesis that the first pulse maximum in the train corresponds to the time t_o:

$$f(t) = R_o \left\{ a + 2 \sum_{n=a}^{\infty} X \cos n\omega \, (t - t_o) \right\} \tag{10}$$

$R_o = \tau_p/T_p$ is the pulse repetition rate and values of a and X depend directly on the form of pulses. Their expressions for three typical forms are given in Table 1.

Then in the general case, ΔT can be expressed as a sum of two terms

$$\Delta T = \Delta T_n + \Delta T_{o\Delta c} \tag{11}$$

the first term corresponding to a non-periodic temperature rise while the second term is periodic. Solutions for these two terms, in the particular case of a Gaussian beam, are, respectively:

$$\Delta T_n = \frac{T_o}{2} \int_0^t \frac{d\Theta}{1 + \frac{4\Theta\kappa}{\delta^2}} \; F(A) \tag{12}$$

$$\Delta T_{o\Delta c} = T_o \sum_{n=1}^{\infty} \left\{ \exp \left\{ - \left\{ \frac{n\pi\tau}{T_p} \right\}^2 \int_0^t \frac{d\Theta}{1 + \frac{4\kappa\Theta}{\delta^2}} \; F(A) \cos n\omega(\Theta - (t - t_o)) \right\} \right\} \tag{13}$$

with

$$\begin{aligned} T_o &= \frac{\alpha I_M(1 - R)}{\rho c} \; R_o \sqrt{\frac{\pi}{\log 2}} && \text{(a)} \\ \Theta &= t - t' && \text{(b)} \\ A &= \kappa\Theta\delta^2 && \text{(c)} \\ F(A) &= 2 \exp(A) \int_{\sqrt{A}}^{\infty} e^{-\xi^2} d\xi && \text{(d)} \end{aligned} \qquad (14)$$

TABLE 1. Expression of parameters a and X related to Eq.(10).

Temporal Pulsed Form $f(t)$	a	X	Limit of X when $R \ll 1$
Rectangular	1	$\frac{\sin n\pi R_o}{n\pi R_o}$	1
Triangular	1/2	$\frac{1 - \cos n\pi R_o}{(n\pi R_o)^2}$	1
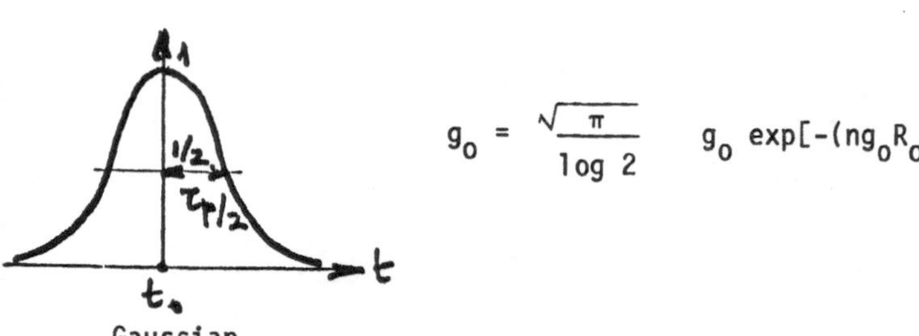 Gaussian	$g_o = \sqrt{\frac{\pi}{\log 2}}$	$g_o \exp[-(n g_o R_o)^2]$	g_o

To integrate the rapidly oscillating terms, we use a numerical method which considers the sine and cosine terms as weighting functions of the remaining term which presents a regular and a slow variation. We have also included the variation of thermal and optical coefficients with T, when tabulated values or formulas were available (6), introducing their values at each step of the numerical integration. Principal results for tungsten are shown in Figures 3 to 6.

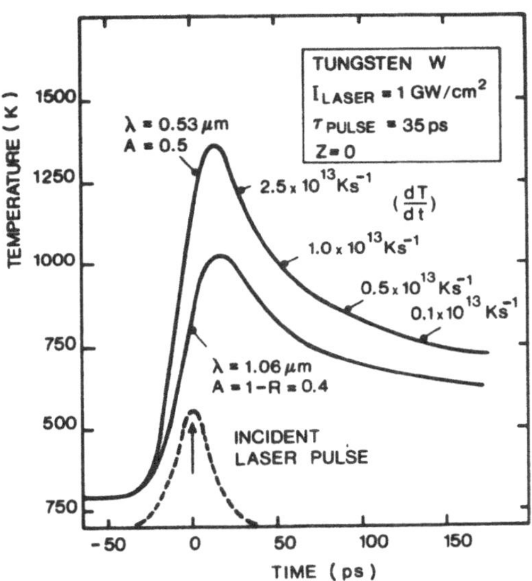

FIGURE 3. Variation of the tungsten surface temperature versus time for two wavelengths of incident laser pulse.

Figure 3 presents the variation of the surface temperature for two different laser wavelengths, when the first pulse of a train is only considered. For identical conditions, we verify that our method of calculation gives results consistent with those reported previously by Bechtel (7). When incident laser intensity $I_{//} = 1$ GW/cm^2 and the pulse duration is also shorter than 35 ps, we observe an amplitude of heating and cooling gradients $>10^{13}$ Ks^{-1}. The influence of surface absorptivity A, which greatly varies with λ, on amplitude of temperature also appears clearly. The direct proportionality between the incident laser intensity and the surface temperature is illustrated in Figure 4. When successive pulses are considered (Figure 5), successive heating and cooling of the surface appears distinctly (full lines), while the mean temperature of the surface, corresponding to a cw incident equivalent energy on material, is slowly increased (dotted lines). At last, for incident maximum laser intensity ~ 1 GW/cm^2 (certainly an upper limit compared to the damage threshold of tungsten), the time needed to reach the melting temperature at the surface is less than 20 ns (Figure 6), corresponding to less than 60 consecutive pulses, but a total energy $\simeq 2$ J/cm^2.

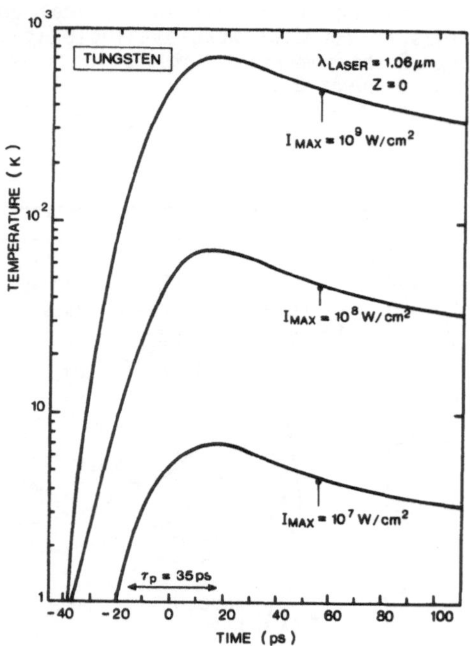

FIGURE 4. Variation of surface temperature versus time for different laser intensities I_{max} at 1.06 μm on tungsten.

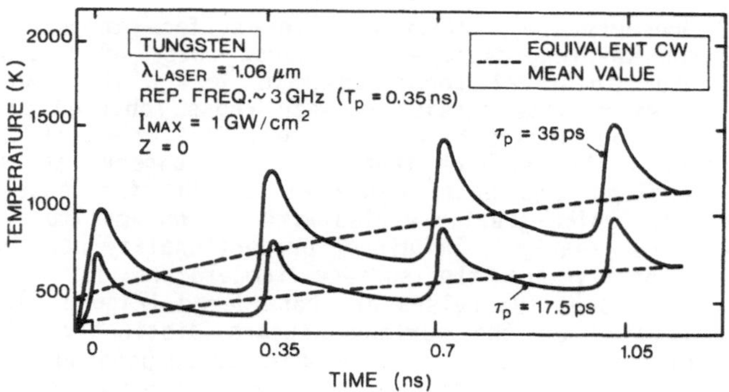

FIGURE 5. Maximum temperature and equivalent cw mean value versus time for different τ_p at λ = 1.06 μm on tungsten.

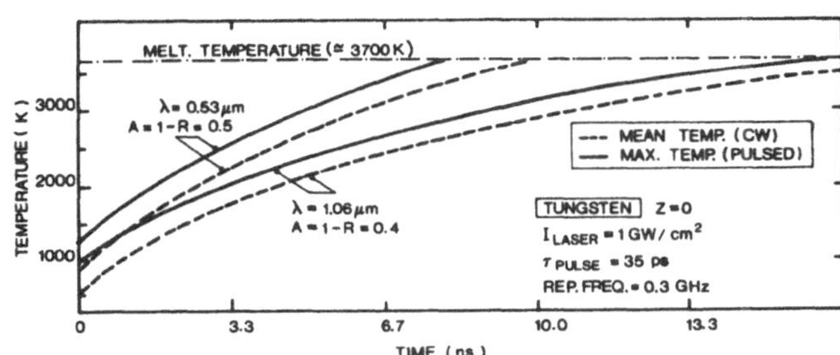

FIGURE 6. Comparison between temperature variations of tungsten surface versus time for two different wavelengths and max intensity $\simeq 1$ GW/cm^2.

The results can be generalized to all the other metals. Effectively, for the same absorbed laser intensity it is possible to show that the heating of the metal surface depends on the product $(K\rho C)^{1/2}$ as it appears in the simplified Equation (15). Including the temperature variations of parameters K and C, variations of this factor for different metals versus the temperature are given in Figure 7. The heating times necessary to reach the melting temperature at the surface of metals, when absorbed intensity is I = 1 MW/cm^2 and a unique train

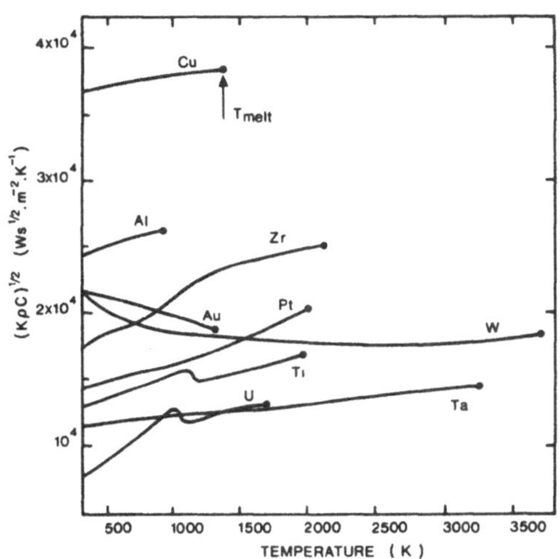

FIGURE 7. Dependence of $(K\rho C)^{1/2}$ versus temperature for various metals.

of pulses, are reported in Figure 8. From these data a simple rule can be applied to determine the best adapted train duration τ_{tr} corresponding to any absorbed intensity I_{abs}. If y is an algebraic coefficient, and $I_{abs} = Ixy$, then $\tau_{tr} = t/y^2$, i.e., τ_{tr} varies as the inverse of squared intensity I_{abs}, and thermal conversion is increased when τ_{tr} is decreased. So, the use of pulsed laser trains can be very interesting to control the thermal conversion efficiency of incident energy.

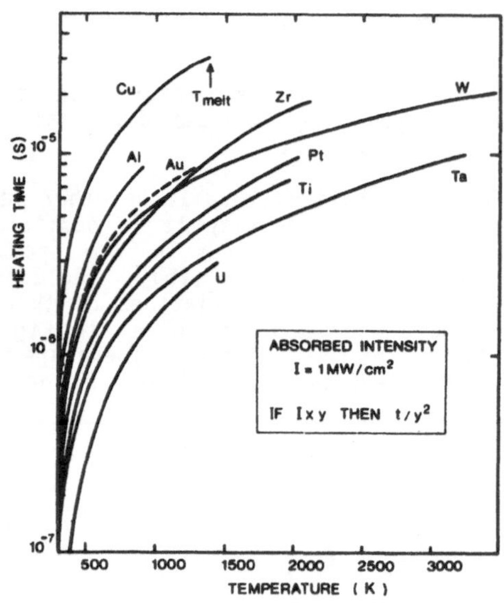

FIGURE 8. Heating time until melting versus T for various metals when absorbed energy $I_{abs} = 1$ MW/cm^2.

3.2. Surface Cooling

As it appears from Figures 5 and 9, though between two consecutive pulses there is a rapid cooling of the surface, at the time scale of a train, we observe a net increase of the mean temperature. But our application forbids any damage at the cathode surface, and consequently, its temperature must always be less than the melting point. Then it is important to study also the cooling of the surface; although repetition frequency of trains is high (~1 kHz), there is a relatively long time (ms compared to μs) between two consecutive trains. However, total cooling would require a very long time (>1 min), as there is a residual temperature which accumulates, depending directly on the repetition rate frequency of trains.

It is possible to evaluate the cooling due to conduction energy loss (8). Note that losses due to radiation are negligible and that convection is impossible because the cathode is in vacuum. Now, suppose that the preceding heating was due to a rectangular laser pulse with maximum intensity I_0 and duration t_0, equivalent to a train. Then, at the point (x=y=z=0) of the surface, the temperature rise above the ambient, for $t=t_0$, is given by a simplified formula:

$$\Delta T(0,t_0) = \frac{I_0(1-R)}{(K\rho C)^{1/2}} \frac{2}{\sqrt{\pi}} \sqrt{t_0} \tag{15}$$

Results given by Eq.(15) are consistent within 20% to our previous more precise calculations, when $t_0 >> \tau_p$ and in choosing for maximum intensity:

$$I_0 = I_M \frac{\sqrt{\pi}}{2\sqrt{\log 2}} \cdot \frac{\tau_p}{T_p} \tag{16}$$

i.e., the mean intensity of the laser pulses on the interval of time T_p. If $t_0 = \tau_{tr}$, the first condition is satisfied.

Due to the cooling term, at time $t > t_0$, the surface temperature becomes:

$$T(0,t > t_0) = \frac{I_0(1-R)}{(K\rho C)^{1/2}} \cdot \frac{2}{\sqrt{\pi}} \{\sqrt{t} - \sqrt{t-t_0}\} \tag{17}$$

Then, with $n = t/t_0$ (for example: $t = T_{tr}, t_0 = \tau_{tr}$), we show that the ratio of the residual temperature at time t to the maximum temperature at t_0, is given by:

$$a = \frac{T_{res}}{T_{max}} \simeq \sqrt{n} - \sqrt{n-1} \tag{18}$$

For $n >> 1$, $a \simeq \dfrac{1}{2\sqrt{n}}$ and $n \simeq \dfrac{1}{4a^2}$.

From these formulae we can evaluate the residual temperature due to N consecutive trains. A calculation with the total quantities of heat given to and by the material at each cycle gives the minimum residual temperature corresponding to the N-th train relative to that of the first:

$$\frac{T_{res,N}}{T_{res,1}} \geq 1 + \frac{N}{2}\sqrt{\frac{\tau_{tr}}{T_{tr}}} \tag{19}$$

For example, if $\tau_{tr} = 1\ \mu s$ and $T_{tr} = 1$ ms corresponding to a train repetition of 1 kHz, formula (19) gives:

$$\tau_{res,N} \geq T_{res,1}\ [1 + 0.016\ N] \qquad (20)$$

Supposing $T_{res,1} \sim 10^{-2}$°C, $T_{res,N} \sim 100$°C after only 10 minutes and $T_{res,N} \sim 1000$°C after 1 hour and 45 min. Consequently, a forced cooling of the cathode is absolutely necessary.

Figure 9 shows surface temperature rise versus the number of consecutive trains N, for different repetition rate frequency of trains and two absorbed intensities. These data correspond to a numerical calculation done pulse per pulse, including the variation with temperature of K and C. We have verified that formula (20) gives results consistent with this more refined evaluation.

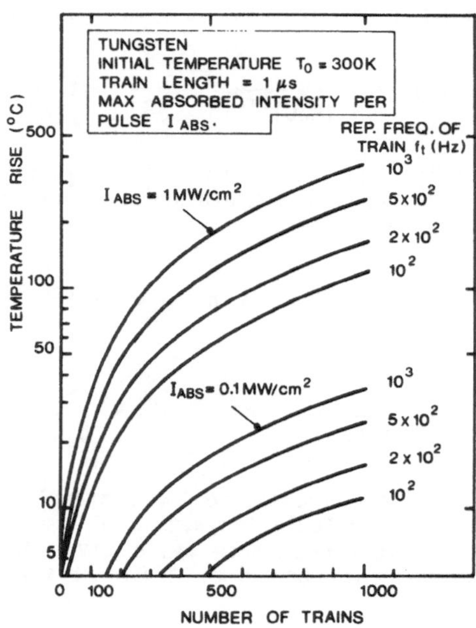

FIGURE 9. Influence of trains frequency on temperature rise of the surface of tungsten at $\lambda = 1.06\ \mu$m.

4. STRESS AND DAMAGE

A consequence of the excessively high repetition rate of the pulses in a burst (3 or 6 GHz) is the very rapid thermal variations of the surface, as shown in Figure 10. Then, thermal stresses are probably developed in the material. These will be unimportant in the normal direction but very high in the two directions parallel to the surface (9). When these stresses (estimated as ~ GPa) exceed the elastic limit of the material, the surface suffers plastic deformation, and though its analysis is complex (10), this problem is important enough to be studied in much more detail.

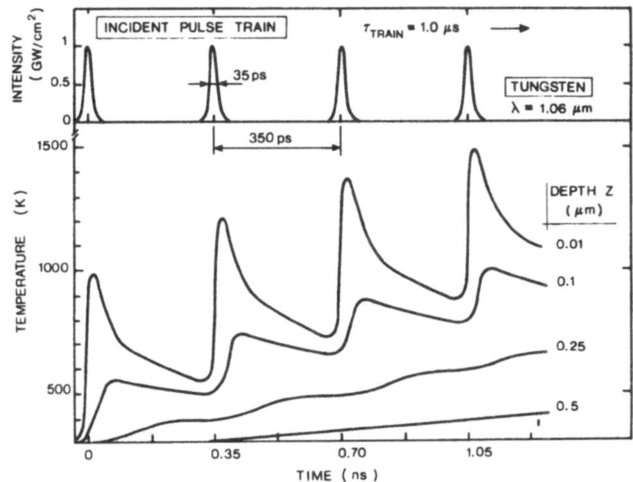

FIGURE 10. Variations of temperature at different depths for 1 GW/cm^2 incident laser pulse train on tungsten at $\lambda = 1.06\ \mu m$.

The occurrence of damage at the surface is a very limiting process because any transformation will induce a variation of the electron distribution and influence directly the coupling between the laser and the surface. Note that semiconductors are mechanically more brittle than metals, and it is clear that conditions of work of a lasertron forbid any damage of any kind to the cathode. Note also that the threshold of laser-induced damage is lowered when the laser pulse repetition frequency is increased (11). Certainly this would be another limitation of the possible maximum incident laser intensity.

5. CONCLUSION

We have presented a study of thermal effects induced by successive high-intensity and high-repetition psec laser pulse trains on materials and principally on metals. Numerical applications give results consistent with the one-pulse case and are successfully extended to the situation of a large number of successive laser pulses. Thus, rapid variations of the temperature versus time at the surface of material are clearly demonstrated, and in spite of the natural cooling of the target, we note an increase of the mean temperature at the surface. Consequently, the surface temperature can rapidly reach the melting point. Influence of this permanent heating on stress and damage will require a forced cooling of the cathode and a reduction of the maximum laser intensity below 10 MW/cm^2 (case of tungsten for instance). These data are consistent with the observation of an important lowering of the damage threshold for large values of pulsed laser repetition rate.

Finally, this study leads us to believe that repetitive laser pulse trains can be used efficiently in controlled thermal applications of laser on materials.

REFERENCES

1. M. Takeda et al., "Lasertron Mark I, a Prototype of Laser-Triggered RF-Source for LINAC in the TeV Region," Institute for Nuclear Study, University of Tokyo, INS-Rep-490, March (1984) and LINAC - Stanford 84 Conference.
2. E. L. Garwin et al., "An Experimental Program to Build a Multimegawatt Lasertron for Super Linear Colliders," SLAC Rep. (1985); and National French Group Project on "Very High Energies Particle Production and Acceleration" (1985).
3. J. P. Girardeau-Montaut, J. C. Li, and C. Girardeau-Montaut, "Optical Device Analysis for Uniform Intensity Irradiation from High-Energy Gaussian Beam," to be published.
4. H. S. Carslaw and J. C. Jaeger, Conduction of Heat in Solids, 2nd ed. (Oxford Univ. Press, London, 1959).
5. B. Boley, in High-Temperature Structures and Materials, edited by A. M. Freudenthal et al. (Pergamon Press, 1964), p. 263.
6. Physics Data: Optical Properties of Metals, Fach-Informations Zentrum, Karlsruhe, No. 18, Vol. 1 and Vol. 2 (Springer-Verlag, 1981).
7. J. H. Bechtel, J. Appl. Phys. 46, 1585-1593 (1975).
8. E. M. Breinan and B. H. Kearin, Laser Material Processing, edited by M. Bass (North Holland, 1981), Chap. 9, pp. 239-245.
9. H. M. Musal, Jr., "Thermomechanical Stress Degradation of Metal Mirror Surfaces under Pulsed Laser Irradiation," N.B.S. Special Pub. on Laser-Induced Damage in Optical Materials (1979), p. 159.
10. V. V. Apollonov et al., "Thermoelastic Action of the Powerful High Repetition Rate Laser Radiations on the Solid State Surface," NBS Special Pub. on Laser-Induced Damage (1981), p. 313.
11. R. M. Wood et al., "Variation of Laser-Induced Damage Threshold with Laser Pulse Repetition Frequency," NBS Special Pub. on Laser-Induced Damage (1982), p. 44.; P. M. Faucket and A. E. Siegman, "Surface Damage Mechanisms in Non-Transparent Media," Damage Conference (USA), Oct. 1984.

NUMERICAL DESCRIPTION OF THE INTERACTION OF LASER BEAMS WITH LIVING TISSUE

ELIAHU ARMON AND GABRIEL LAUFER
Faculty of Mechanical Engineering, Technion Haifa, 32000 Israel

Key words: evaporation, heat flow calculation: three dimensional, laser-living tissue interaction, thermochemical damage, tissue cutting

ABSTRACT

The interaction of cutting lasers with matter consists normally of absorption of the radiation, rapid thermalization of the energy, evaporation and the removal of the vapors from the interaction site. A general theoretical model which describes this interaction has to account for heat dissipation via conduction, non-linearities associated with phase changes, propagation of the laser-matter interaction front, thermal damage at the vicinity of the interaction site and absorption of radiation by vapor and plasma in the beam path.

A three-dimensional numerical model which describes all these effects has been developed. Although this model may be easily adapted for industrial applications such as metal cutting or heat treatment, we focused our attention on the interaction with living tissue. The thermal damage at the vicinity of the interaction site was modeled by a semi-empirical Arrhenius-type function while tissue removal was modeled as water evaporation. Exposure conditions which optimize the ratio between the extent of removed tissue and the thermal damage were identified. Techniques which may further improve this ratio will be presented and discussed.

1. INTRODUCTION

The number of applications for high-intensity CO_2 lasers in surgery is increasing rapidly. In many of these applications the beam replaces the conventional mechanical scalpel in cutting and removing excessive tissue (1,2). The cutting is accomplished by rapid absorption and thermalization of the beam energy, thereby causing a local temperature rise and evaporation. At the incidence point a crater is formed. This is the desired effect of the interaction with the laser beam (3,4). On the other hand, heat absorption and dissipation at the carter walls induce undesired thermochemical damage due to denaturization of protein and enzyme molecules. This effect is secondary to the desired effect of evaporation. An estimate of this damage, of its shape and its dependence on beam parameters, is required.

Most theoretical work on the interaction of laser beams with biological tissue (5-7) does not consider the possibility of a phase transition, i.e., interface propagation and crater formation are ignored. A comparison (8) between the extent of the evaporated tissue and the denaturized tissue was done using a one-dimensional model which ignored variations in surface topography. Another analysis (9) modeled the absorption of the laser beam by a surface heat flux. The phase transition was modeled by an artificial pyrolysis energy. This was intended to describe the phase front propagation. However, the pyrolysis energy exceeds the evaporation latent heat and therefore its application is questionable.

The purpose of our work was to present a theoretical investigation of the interaction of a single laser pulse with living tissue. A two-dimensional mathematical model which considered phase transition, front propagtion due to material removal and tissue denaturization due to a temperature rise has been developed and solved numerically. The model yielded the shape of the crater, the damaged zone around the crater and their dependence on pulse duration, beam radius and pulse intensity. Results of this model were used for the optimization of the surgical process and to identify new techniques for damage control.

The mathematical model is described in detail elsewhere (10). The analysis assumes exposure to a Gaussian axisymmetric CO_2 laser beam with a beam waist of R_o. The beam is absorbed within a depth of $1/\beta$ by a homogeneous water-like medium. The absorbed energy is thermalized instantaneously and dissipated in the medium by heat conduction. Tissue is assumed to be removed by an evaporation process which takes place at the boiling point of water $T_E = 100°C$.

The damage created in the unevaporated tissue is estimated by using an equation which describes the decomposition rates of enzyme and protein molecules at elevated temperatures (11). A local damage parameter, Ω, is defined. when $\Omega \geq 1$, the model considers that spot as permanently damaged.

The problem was solved numerically. At each time step the temperature field was evaluated and grid cells in which the enthalpy exceeded the evaporation enthalpy were identified. In order to account for the screening and attenuation of the laser beam by water vapors which remain in the beam path, the residence time, τ , of evaporated tissue in the beam path was estimated. Evaporated grid cells were removed by the algorithm and a new free surface was exposed only when this residence time had elapsed. The residence time was obtained from the ratio between an estimated escape velocity, v_{es}, and the beam radius. In all calculations the laser was kept at a constant intensity throughout the exposure time, t_p, and was subsequently turned off.

The secondary damage was calculated following each time step by applying the trapezoidal method to the equation of Ω (11). This calculation was performed during exposure and following it until full decay of the temperature disturbance had been obtained.

The numerical model was tested against previously known analytical and numerical results. The comparison was within the resolution limits of the numerical grid.

2. RESULTS

The objective of the analysis was to determine the beam parameters which yield the most extensive cut with the least secondary damage. The crater boundary and the boundary of the thermochemically damaged envelope were outlined.

The absorption coefficient of water at wavelength of 10 μm, $\beta = 767\ cm^{-1}$ (12), has been selected as a representative absorption coefficient of the tissue. Similarly, the latent heat of water and the specific heat of water vapor $L = 2.257 \times 10^6 J/kg$ and

$c_2 = 2.014 \times 10^3$ J/kg°K were taken (13). From a comprehensive list of parameters describing tissue thermal behavior (14), the following values were selected: $\rho_1 = 1050$ kg/m^3, $c_1 = 3.77 \times 10^3$ J/kg°K. The heat conductivity of well perfused tissue in vivo is $k = 0.7$ W/m°K (15).

An insight on the effect of pulse duration on tissue cutting can be obtained by comparing the craters and damage envelopes of similar pulses at different durations. Figure 1a presents two craters formed by two separate 1J pulses at a radius of 0.5 mm. The left crater was formed by a $t_p = 10^{-3}$ sec pulse while the other was formed by a $t_p = 1$ sec pulse.

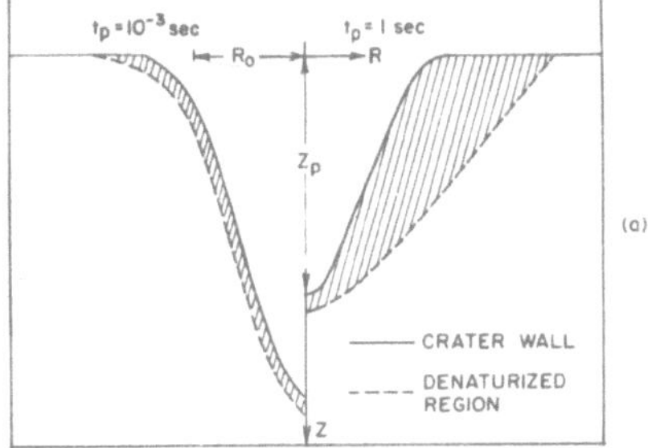

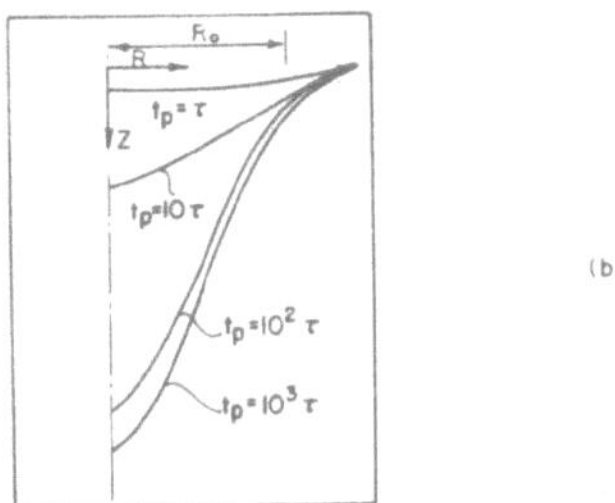

FIGURE 1. The effect of thermal conduction and beam attenuation by tissue vapors on crater formation.

It is evident that the longer pulse is less effective. The crater maximum depth, Z_e, and the evaporated volume, V_e, are decreasing as exposure duration increases. This is due to conductive dissipation of energy which accumulates to a substantial loss as time evolves. This dissipated energy increases the temperature around the crater, thereby increasing the volume of the damaged envelope, V_Ω.

When the pulse is short, the crater radius matches approximately the beam waist. The intensity at the wings of the beam profile is insufficient to induce tissue evaporation. Nevertheless, it contributes to the tissue heating. Therefore, most of the secondary damage is induced at the crater circumference. The depth of the secondary damage along the centerline beyond the crater bottom is almost independent of pulse duration and is controlled by the absorption of the laser radiation at the end of the pulse.

Before identifying the optimal exposure parameters, the effect of beam attenuation by tissue vapors must be determined. Since the literature does not quote a well-established value of the excape velocity of tissue vapors following a laser pulse, calculations were made for a range of escape velocities. Some of the results are presented in Figure 1b in terms of the ratio t_p/τ. The deepest crater is obtained when attenuation is minimal, i.e., when the residence time of the vapor within the beam path is short, relative to pulse duration. Decreasing pulse duration below the residence time reduces the beam effectivity. Normally, residence times cannot be selected; pulse durations, however, are controllable and must be selected such that beam attentuation as well as losses due to conduction are kept at a minimum.

Figure 2 presents the cutting efficiency, V_e/V_Ω, following a single laser pulse vs. pulse duration. Throughout these calculations the beam diameter was 0.5 mm and pulse energy was 1 J. In the absence of attenuation by tissue vapors ($\tau = 0$), short pulses yield the highest cutting efficiency, which due to heat conduction decrease with increasing pulse duration.

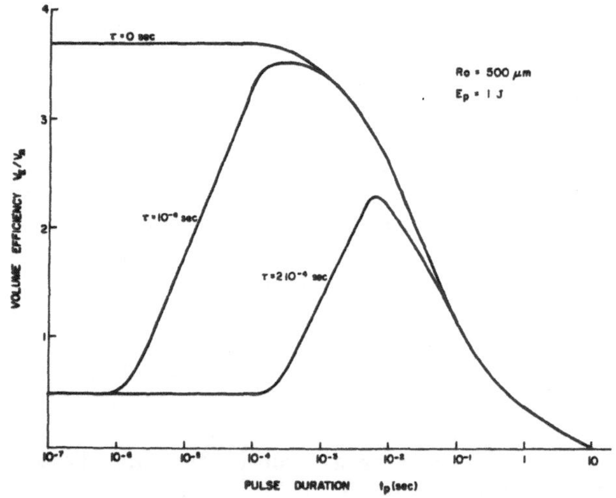

FIGURE 2. The cutting efficiency (V_e/V_Ω) vs. pulse duration. Exposure to a single pulse $E_p = 1$ J, $R_o = 0.5$ mm.

At longer residence times, which represent a more realistic situation, decreasing pulse length beyond a certain optimum results in a drop-off in cutting efficiency. Pronounced maxima in volume efficiency are observed both for $\tau = 10^{-6}$ sec and $\tau = 2 \times 10^{-4}$ sec. While the first represents a microexplosion-controlled tissue vapor removal, the second represents a suction-controlled process. Though the correct escape mechanism and the velocity are yet to be determined, operation at exposure durations of 10^{-2} to 10^{-3} sec is likely to result in maximum tissue extraction. This conclusion suggests that the application of a Q-switched or a TEA laser is likely to be inefficient.

In order to generalize the above analysis and include other beam parameters such as beam waist and energy and allow for a variety of tissue thermophysical constants, the computation was made dimensionless. Details of this analysis are presented elsewhere (16).

The expression for the thermochemical damage (11) demonstrates clearly that irreversible damage is induced even at a slight temperature increase. Optimal exposure conditions which minimize this damage cannot be obtained by the commercial surgical lasers. Thus, any attempt to decrease the thermochemical damage must concentrate on new, laser-independent parameters.

3. TISSUE PRECOOLING

One such attempt was made by Wakaki et al. (4). They used dry nitrogen to cool the tissue. The cooling was synchronized with the exposure and was sustained for a while following it. They reported that the original body temperature, at a depth of 1 mm, has been recovered within 5 sec. This, however, is likely to be too late, since the thermochemical damage, at temperatures beyond 60°C, develops within less than 1 sec. Such a competition between the heat and the cooling fronts favors the heat front which is propelled by the direct absorption and by a much steeper temperature gradient. Thus, if cooling is to succeed as a technique for thermochemical damage control, the cooling must be given a good head start, i.e., the tissue must be prepared, prior to laser exposure, at a low temperature.

In order to estimate the effect the precooling may have on the thermochemical damage, the numerical code was applied (17). A dimensionless damaged volume $\bar{V}_\Omega = V_\Omega/\pi R_p^2/\beta$ was computed as a function of a dimensionless exposure time for damage, $\bar{t}_\Omega = t_p \cdot \alpha \cdot \beta / R_p$, and for different initial temperatures T_0 where $R_p = R_0[1/2\ \ell n(I_0 t_p \beta / h_e)]^{1/2}$ is the maximum crater radius, α is the thermal diffusivity and h_e is the evaporation enthalpy. The results are presented in Figure 3 where four curves with T_0 as a parameter are presented. It is apparent that lowering T_0 decreases the extent of the minimal damage and also extends the range of $\bar{t}_\Omega$ within which this minimum can be obtained. Thus, operating with a beam of 0.1 mm radius 0.1 sec pulse duration and 50 W power on a water-like tissue where $\alpha = 10^{-7}$ m^2/sec, $\beta = 76{,}700$ m^{-1} and $h_e = 2.619 \times 10^9$ J/m^3 yields $\bar{t}_\Omega = 3.59$. If the tissue is precooled to $T_0 = 0$°C, the thermal damage is reduced by about a factor of two and is now close to the otherwise minimal damage.

It should be noted that precooling, which appears to be an efficient technique for damage control, has only a slight effect on the extent of tissue removal. This stems from the high non-linearity of the damage function which makes it more sensitive to temperature than the evaporation process.

Finally, recent experiments which were conducted on feline skins indicated very dramatically the improvement associated with tissue precooling. Cuts induced by laser were sutured and were allowed to heal. Cuts which were performed on precooled tissue left only a minute scar unlike the ordinary cuts which tended to leave a relatively thick scar.

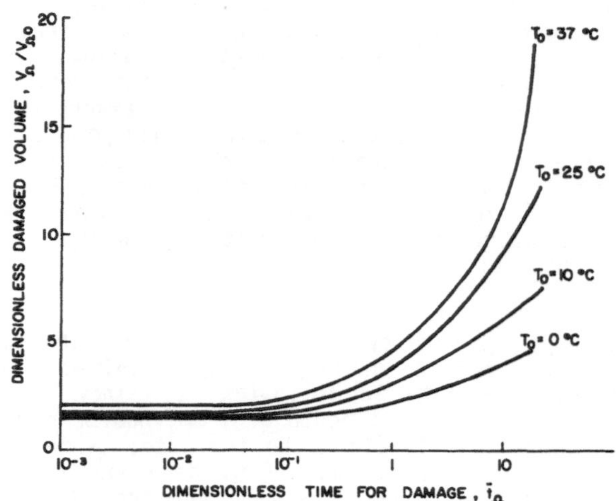

FIGURE 3. Dimensionless damaged volume, $\overline{V}_\Omega$, vs. the dimensionless time for damage, $\overline{t}_\Omega$, for several precooling temperatures.

4. CONCLUSION

A numerical model has been developed and applied for the analysis of tissue removal by laser radiation. The shape of the crater formed by a single pulse and the denaturization damage were drawn. Two physical effects control the process: thermal conduction and beam attentuation by tissue vapors. The extent of the removed tissue depends on both mechanisms, and exposure conditions for maximum tissue removal may be defined.

New techniques for reducing the thermal damage were proposed. Out of these techniques, precooling was closely examined and was proven theoretically and experimentally as a viable technique.

REFERENCES

1. J. A. Dixon, Proc. IEEE 70, 579-588 (1982).
2. M. W. Berns, Laser Focus 19, 66-81 (1983).
3. S. Mihashi et al., in Laser Surgery, edited by I. Kaplan (Academic Press, Jerusalem, 1979), pp. 17-16.
4. M. Wakaki et al., in Laser Surgery, edited by I. Kaplan (Academic Press, Jerusalem, 1979), pp. 27-41.
5. M. A. Mainster et al. J. Opt. Soc. Am. 60, 264-270 (1970).
6. L. A. Priebe and A. J. Welch, ASME J. Biomechanical Eng. 100, 49-54 (1978).
7. J. Langerholc, Appl. Opt. 18, 2286-2293 (1979).
8. G. Laufer, Appl. Opt. 22, 676-681 (1983).
9. F. O. Incropera et al. Med. and Bio. Eng., 199-206 (1974).
10. E. Armon and G. Laufer, J. Biomechanical Eng. 107, 286 (1985).
11. F. C. Henriques, Arch. Pathol. 43, 489-502 (1947).
12. J. G. Bayley, V. B. Kartha, and W. H. Stevens, in Infrared Physics (Pergamon Press, Britain, 1963), Vol. 3, pp. 211-223.
13. Handbook of Chemistry and Physics, 60th edition (CRC Press).
14. J. C. Chato, in Advanced Heat Transfer, edited by B. T. Chao (Univ. of Illinois Press, 1969), pp. 395-414.
15. A. Shitzer, personal communication.
16. E. Armon and G. Laufer, "Asymptotic and Dimensionless Analysis of the Response of Living Tissue to Surgical Laser," submitted to J. Biomechanical Eng.
17. E. Armon and G. Laufer, "New Techniques for Reducing the Thermochemical Damage in the Course of Laser Surgery," submitted to J. Biomechanical Eng.

SUMMARY AND DISCUSSION - CHAPTER 3

L. G. DONA DALLE ROSE

The above papers show that at all time domains the heat diffusion equation is the basic tool on which not only the heat flow but also the mass transport, either diffusive of convective, can be modeled. In the case of mass transport other tools are also needed, such as the particle diffusion equation, in several versions according to the physical phenomenon to be depicted, or such as the hydrodynamical momentum equations. The degree of complexity and sophistication has attained quite unequal levels in the different areas of interest; the modeling of convective motions seems by far to be the most difficult (according to Mazumder, writing a computer code which models three-dimensional convective motions means to graduate in supercomputing!).

Most of the modeling comes through the boundary conditions and the way by which the possible phase transitions (melting, vaporization,...) are accounted for. Often there are several possibilities even for a single modeling step, like, for instance, the inclusion of the latent heat of melting: Mazumder introduces a step increase in the specific heat vs. temperature curve, when describing his three-dimensional heat flow model; Gay, in his Fig. 6, adopts a singular-like behavior for the same curve, and Dona dalle Rose relates the latent heat to a boundary condition at the liquid-solid interface.

Many concepts are common to different areas. For instance, the thermal histories under transient irradiating, like those including melting, see Fig. 8 in Gay and Fig. 4 (schematic) in the Dona dalle Rose paper, are substantially similar, in quite different time domains. When comparing, care must be taken in recognizing the melting and vaporization thresholds, since at longer times plasma formation and keyholing can alter (and increase) the coupling of the laser beam to the processed material - see Ref. 5 in Mazumder paper or Rochstroh contribution in this book - thus lowering the average power density needed to produce a given effect. Nevertheless, there exist conditions under which vaporization can be avoided in all time domains: Examples were given in the papers above, relating to pulsed laser irradiating (Dona dalle Rose, part 2), to pulsed laser trains in a case where even melting is to be avoided (Girardeau-Montaut), and to steels processing with a scanning continuous laser (Gay); notice that the change (reduction) in absorption coefficient measured by Gay is clearly due to phenomena other than plasma formation and such as a surface alloying process, which makes the surface to recover a metal-like reflectance. In the transient reported by Gay, when compared to those calculated for Q-switched lasers, no kinks or plateau due to latent heat of fusion/resolidification appear; among other things, this fact can be related both to the rather low amount of absorbed energy transformed into latent heat during that transient (about 8%) and to the rather short time needed for the resolidification of 0.3 mm of nodular cast iron (about 30 ms, if Eq.(7) of Dona dalle Rose is used), as compared to the overall transient time scale.

At the Institute of S. Miniato, the discussions after the presentation of the above papers raised several interesting points. Some of them were concerned with the applicability of the model calculations and their testing.

Mazumder stated clearly that his two-dimensional model for convection holds only for a molten pool having a flat surface; therefore, the model only works when the laser scanning velocity is high and the keyhole is not forming. The temperature and velocity profiles, the cooling rates, etc. - that were shown during his presentation for a given plane transverse to the surface of the molten pool (see Ref.(13) in his paper), refer to the instant at which the laser scanning beam has just passed it. Of course, the model allows following the whole thermal cycle and also, in principle, to calculate the percentage of the absorbed energy going into kinetic energy of convection. Testing of the model through comparison with experiment is at present limited to the experiments performed at Urbana, on the mass transport and redistribution of surface-alloyed species in the molten pool. In this context surface segregation effects or dendritic growth are only minor events which do not affect the convection modeling in an (almost) homogeneous liquid.

Gay pointed out that a criterion for the practical applicability of a one-dimensional heat flow model in the time regime on the order of one second is that the heat penetration (or diffusion) length be about one half of the laser beam diameter and of the sample thickness.

During the presentation of Dona dalle Rose, a discussion arose concerning the ways which detect or characterize convective motions in the nanosecond regime. In particular, the criterion relying on the observation of long flat tails in the impurity profile RBS spectra was questioned, since, it was said, it might be due to some artifacts caused by the accompanying very rough sample surface, as seen, e.g., with SEM (Scanning Electron Microscopy); supporters of the criterion said that the artifacts ought not to be there, even in the presence of rough surfaces, if the RBS profile is invariant under changes in the inclination of the sample with respect to the analyzing beam. Several remarks in the discussion, mainly coming from metallurgists, concerned the actual possibility of having convective motions in a molten pool, about 1,000 nm thick and having a duration of some hundreds of nanoseconds, but it was finally agreed that they could exist. Later it was also stressed that a somewhat related, but very important in itself, problem is to investigate the nucleation time necessary for the onset of a boiling process in a molten metallic pool.

The discussions following the other two papers were somewhat more technical; in particular, Girardeau-Montaut underlined the fact that the main purpose of making a lasertron is to produce a high-frequency pulsed current; therefore, only photoemitted electrons are useful, since they are supposed to be closely related with the incident light pulses; the thermal electrons, on the other hand, would yield a current which is modulated but not pulsed, since he showed that the mean temperature of the metal irradiated by the pulsed laser trains is continuously increasing, even in the presence a good cooling facility.

Laufer, finally, pointed out that the use in tissue irradiating of an excimer laser (i.e., with a wavelength shorter than a CO_2 laser) might provoke an additional photochemical effect.

As already remarked in the introduction, the above papers on modeling of heat and mass transport present a varying degree of comparison with experiment. In any case, this comparison has been pursued in a relevant manner by many other papers presented at this Institute and collected in this book, from both the metallurgists and the physicists point of view. In particular, I would like to mention here the results presented independently by MacDonald and by Peercy, about the first measurements in metals of a resolidification velocity in the nanoor subnanosecond regime. This comes after some years of a similar, but perhaps conceptually and experimentally simpler, work done on silicon; silicon in the past years has offered a great laboratory for testing heat flow calculations in the shorter time domains (see the related chapter in the present book), the attention paid to it being probably due to the more complex and maybe appealing physical mechanisms involved, e.g., light absorption, undercooling during resolidification,... and to the possibilities of technological and applicative developments. Nevertheless, this Institute has shown that something new is occurring also for metals and that much work in modeling is still needed.

CHAPTER 4. PROPERTIES OF LASER-PROCESSED METALLIC SURFACES

CHAPTER INTRODUCTION - B. STRITZKER, E. MC CAFFERTY

This chapter summarizes the prospects for the application of laser processing in different fields of research for the improvement of both mechanical, chemical and electronic properties of metallic surfaces. The different areas covered in this chapter by review articles are wear, corrosion, telecommunications, and superconductivity. In addition, the modifications of electrical and optical properties of Ge-Al alloys by laser processing are discussed in detail.

It is shown that laser processing is advantageous in special areas of each field, but also that the different authors have varying opinions about the importance of laser processing in the future.

For the area of telecommunications, C. W. Draper gives the most advanced examples for real applications of laser processing producing new materials like "stainless Cu" or diffused Au/PdAg contacts. These alloys not only show improved electrical and mechanical properties, but also the savings of precious metals are quite substantial. In conclusion, laser processing has a great future in modern telecommunications.

E. McCafferty gives quite a variety of examples for laser-processed surfaces showing improved corrosion and pitting behavior. For the future he favors the production of advanced alloys, amorphous surface alloys and the use of powder injection techniques to make improved coatings. Quite a number of applications with exciting results in wear and corrosion were shown by J. Mazumder. He reported an improvement of at least a factor of three in wear properties after laser processing.

In superconductivity, B. Stritzker pointed out the great potential of pulsed laser techniques for the production of amorphous superconducting alloys. They not only show interesting superconducting properties, but they can also lead to a basic understanding of the rapid quenching mechanism, since an intense knowledge of other non-equilibrium processes has been gathered through the last 20 years. However, the situation is not so promising for the production of high-T_c materials, where the essential long-range ordering of a rather complicated crystal structure has not yet been achieved. The potential of laser processing Ge-Al alloys, which are possible candidates for contact materials to semiconductors and for optical storage materials, is discussed by C. Alfonso.

In general, the following papers show that laser processing is quite a useful tool for the modification of electrical, chemical, and mechanical properties.

ELECTROCHEMICAL BEHAVIOR OF LASER-PROCESSED METAL SURFACES

E. McCAFFERTY AND P. G. MOORE
Naval Research Laboratory, Washington, DC 20375

Key Words: corrosion, pitting, passivity, surface alloying, surface melting

ABSTRACT

Laser processing of a metal surface can modify its corrosion behavior by altering the surface composition, microstructure, or distribution of impurities and second phases. Examples considered include: anodic behavior of Fe-Cr binary alloys, effect of laser surface melting on the pitting of type 304 stainless steel, preparation and pitting behavior of Mo-bearing surface stainless steel alloys, the effect of laser melting on the corrosion of aluminum and aluminum bronzes, laser-formed amorphous surface alloys, and the use of laser processing for consolidation of metallic coatings. Suggestions for further research are also given.

1. INTRODUCTION

The attainment of high-power densities with laser beams has provided new opportunities for the modification of metallic surfaces to improve their corrosion behavior. Laser processing uses a high-power laser beam to rapidly heat a thin surface region, with the underlying bulk providing self-quenching. For surface modification regarding corrosion applications, the surface is usually melted, so that processing entails rapid surface melting followed by rapid solidification at cooling rates as high as 10^7 deg/sec. Laser procesing can modify the corrosion behavior by altering the surface compositon, microstructure, and the distribution of major components, impurities, or second phases. This paper will briefly describe the types of laser processing techniques useful for corrosion applications and will give examples of recent research on the corrosion electrochemistry of laser-processed surfaces. Finally, suggestions for further research will be given.

2. LASER PROCESSING TECHNIQUES

The following techniques (1,2) are useful for corrosion applications:

2.1. Laser-surface melting

In laser-surface melting a laser beam melts a thin surface layer, and the underlying bulk provides self-quenching, with cooling rates of up to 10^7 K/sec. The melting and rapid solidification can improve the corrosion resistance of some alloys by eliminating or minimizing phase separations so as to produce a more chemically homogeneous surface.

2.2. Laser-surface alloying

Laser-surface alloying consists of melting the surface of a metal workpiece, adding known amounts of other metals, mixing these components, and allowing them to resolidify. This process produces a surface layer with a chemical composition and properties which are different from the substrate material. This technique allows the surface properties of a structure to be tailored to the surface requirements without sacrificing the bulk characteristics. The surface layer is also metallurgically bonded to the substrate and provides a high degree of adhesion. During the last decade there has been much concern with the supply and availability of certain technologically important metals (3,4). Laser-surface alloying provides a method of conserving such scarce, expensive, or critical materials by concentrating them in the surface where they are required for applications such as corrosion protection, wear resistance, or catalytic performance. One possible disadvantage to laser-surface alloying is that there is a certain amount of roughness introduced by the melting process and, although conditions can be chosen to minimize the roughness, either the application must be tolerant of the roughness or the surface must be refinished after laser processing.

2.3. Laser melt/particle injection

Laser melt/particle injection consists of melting a shallow pool on the surface of a sample which is translated under a focused laser beam, and of blowing particles into the melt pool from a fine nozzle positioned about 10 mm away. There are several variations to this technique: (a) The powder may dissolve to only a limited extent in the melt, as with the injection of carbide particles to produce wear-resisting surfaces. (b) Complete dissolution of metallic particles can produce surface alloys. (c) Processing conditions can be adjusted so that the beam melts just enough of the surface to weld down a coating, which is built up from powder blown into the melt pool.

2.4. Consolidation of coatings

In consolidation of coatings, a coating previously applied by a process such as flame spraying or plasma spraying is laser-melted to remove residual porosity or to improve its adherence to the base metal.

A typical experimental apparatus used for surface melting, alloying, or consolidation of coatings using kilowatt class continuous lasers is shown schematically in Figure 1. The only focusing element is a single, spherical mirror which is used to obtain a sharply focused beam. Test specimens are mounted on a rotating turntable, swept through the focused beam at speeds ranging up to 2 m/sec, and protected during the processing by a flowing helium gas shield. The laser beam rapidly melts a small volume of metal, which subsequently rapidly solidifies by conduction of heat to the bulk specimen. Each pass results in the processing of a ribbon of material, typically 0.25 mm wide and 0.1 mm deep. The width and depth of such a ribbon can be varied by changing the processing conditions such as sweep speed, laser power or spot diameter. The complete coverage of a large surface is obtained by using successive passes spaced a fraction of a pass width from one another. Table 1 lists typical processing conditions for surface modification for corrosion applications.

The procedure for laser melt/particle injection, as illustrated in Figure 2, is similar to that above except that a nozzle is used to blow powder particles into the melt pool as decribed by Ayers, Schaefer and Robey (5). The flow of the powder stream is sensitive to air currents so that such processing is generally performed in a vacuum of 0.1 to 1 torr. The processing can also be done at atmospheric pressure as long as the powder stream from the nozzle remains collimated and there is no adverse atmospheric contamination of the melted material.

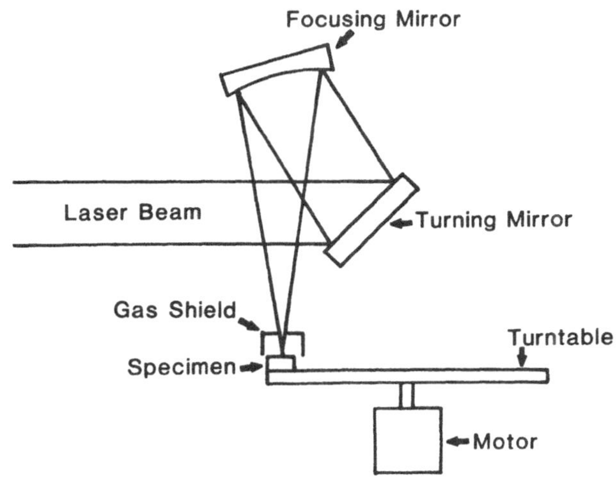

FIGURE 1. Schematic diagram of the laser processing apparatus.

TABLE 1. Typical laser processing conditions for surface modification for corrosion applications.

Output power:	7.5 kW
Spot diameter:	0.15 mm
Average power density:	4×10^7 W/cm^2
Sweep speed:	50 cm/sec
Interaction time:	0.6 msec
Time metal is molten:	1 msec
Melt depth:	50 μm
Melt width:	260 μm
Cooling rate:	10^7 K/sec

3. RECENT CORROSION RESEARCH

The use of laser processing to improve surface properties is still in the formative stage. However, there have been a number of recent research studies which point to promising applications. The following survey is intended to be illustrative rather than exhaustive.

3.1. Fe-Cr binary surface alloys

One of the earliest electrochemical studies on laser surface alloys was on the passivation of binary Fe-Cr surface alloys (6) for comparison with their bulk counterparts. Preparation of the laser surface alloys has been described before (7), but in brief, specimens of AISI 1018 were

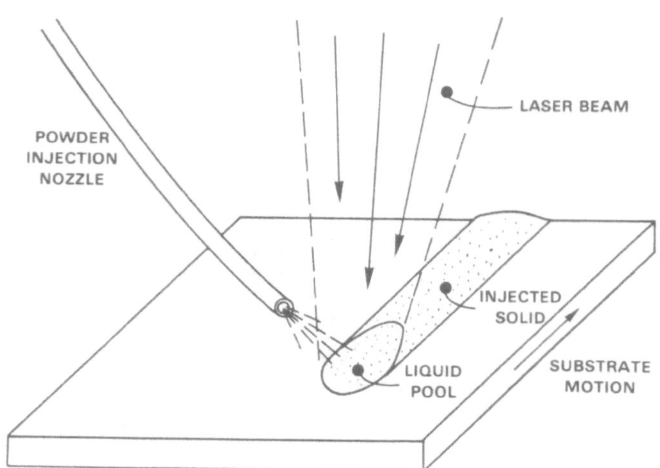

FIGURE 2. Injection of particles into a melt zone established by a high-power laser.

first coated with sputtered deposited chromium layers ranging in thickness from 10 to 20 μm. As usual, the depth of melting, and hence the alloy composition, was controlled by varying the sweep velocity of the turntable. Figure 3 shows a micrograph of a cross section through a typical Fe-Cr surface alloy produced by a single pass of the laser, and Figure 4 shows a set of microprobe traces across the surface alloy shown in Figure 3. Figure 4 shows that the average Cr content is about 20% throughout the melt. There is some local fluctuation in composition, but the overall dispersion of Cr is essentially uniform.

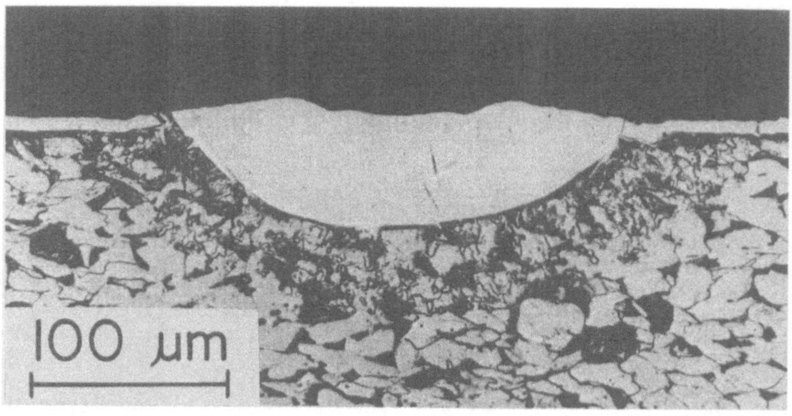

FIGURE 3. Transverse cross section of an Fe-Cr laser surface alloy with average Cr content of 20%.

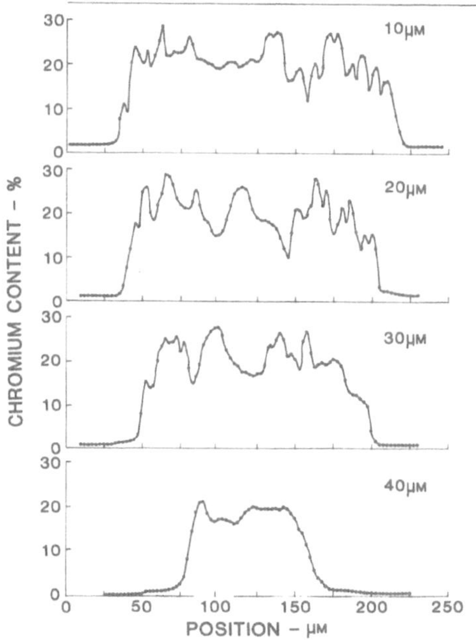

FIGURE 4. Electron microprobe traces taken across the Fe-Cr surface alloy in Fig. 3 at different depths into the melt.

To produce a surface alloy over an extensive area, successive laser passes, spaced a fraction of a melt width apart, were employed. A cross section of such a surface alloy is shown in Figure 5. Electron microprobe analysis indicated that the distribution of components was similar to that observed for individual melts.

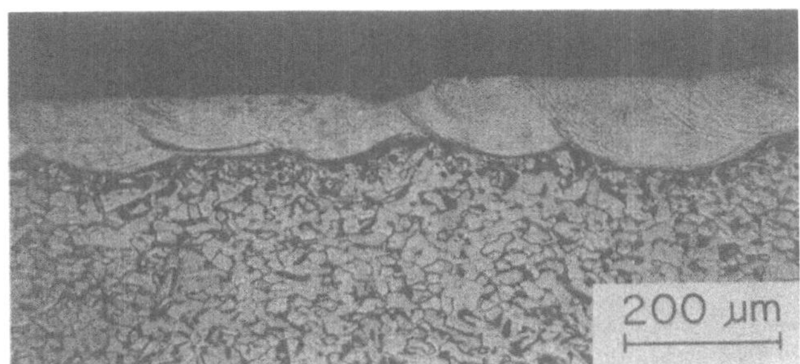

FIGURE 5. Transverse cross section of a laser surface alloy, with average Cr content of 16%, produced by successive, overlapping laser passes.

The anodic behavior of the Fe-Cr surface alloys was studied in de-aerated 0.1 M Na_2SO_4 at 25°C. Each sample was immersed for 30 minutes and then held cathodically at -1.0 V vs. S.C.E. for 5 minutes. Following this cathodic treatment, steady-state open-circuit corrosion potentials were attained by each sample after an additional 30-minute immersion period as shown in Figure 6. Anodic polarization curves were determined potentiodynamically at a scan rate of 10 mV/min.

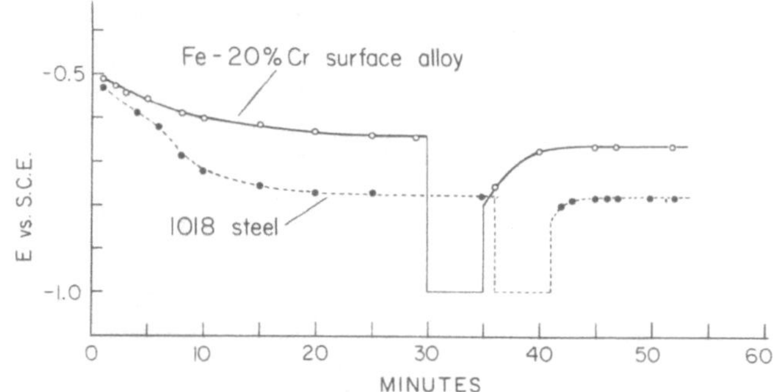

FIGURE 6. Open circuit potentials in 0.1 M Na_2SO_4. Both samples were cathodically pulsed for 5 minutes at -1.0 V, as indicated.

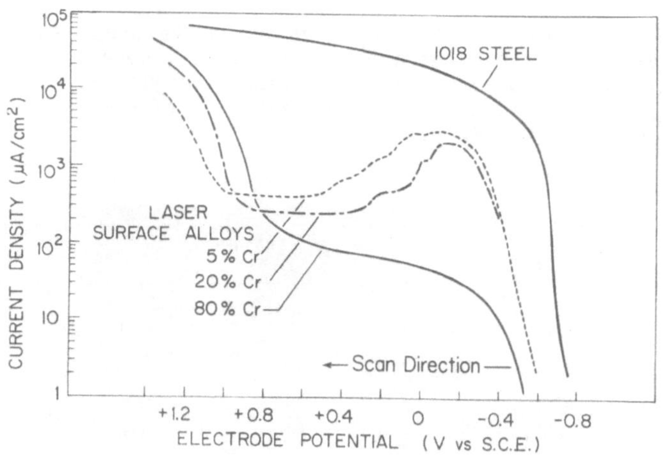

FIGURE 7. Anodic polarization curves in de-aerated 0.1 M Na_2SO_4 at 25°C.

Figure 7 shows anodic polarization curves for the 1018 steel substrate and for three Fe-Cr laser surface alloys in de-aerated 0.1 M Na_2SO_4. The 1018 steel undergoes extensive dissolution at all anodic potentials, whereas all three Fe-Cr surface alloys passivate. (The increases in current density above +0.8 V are not indicative of increased corrosion, but of the onset of a new anodic reaction, i.e., oxygen evolution.) As seen in Figure 7, with increasing Cr content, there are decreases in both the critical current density for passivation and the current density in the passive region, as is the case for bulk Fe-Cr alloys (8,9).

However, the current densities in Figure 7 in the passive region are about 100 times that for type 430 stainless steel (16% Cr, 0.4% Mn, 0.3% Si, 0.05% C, balance Fe) in the same solution and 5-50 times that of comparable Fe-Cr binary alloys in 1 N H_2SO_4 (10,11). Two reasons can be given to explain the higher passive current densities for the Fe-Cr laser surface alloys. First there are local chemical inhomogeneities in the laser surface alloy, as shown in Figure 4, which can promote dissolution. Second, rapid solidification of the Fe-Cr surface alloys results in the formation of small surface cracks on the high Cr alloys. These surface cracks are much shallower than the thickness of the surface alloy, but indicate that there are local residual strains in the surface which can also assist dissolution. Annealing of the surface alloys would probably relieve these strains as well as reduce local composition fluctuations.

Cottrell and co-workers (12) have studied the effect of laser surface melting on the breakdown of the passive film on an Fe-19% Cr binary alloy and have also suggested that laser melting introduces strains and defects in the melt layer. These investigators found that laser melting enriched the surface oxide film in chromium, but yet degraded the electrochemical behavior. For the LSM sample, there was premature breakdown of the passive film and subsequent pitting when the electrode potential was swept from the passive region into the active region in 1 N H_2SO_4. This breakdown is believed to initiate at points of stress arising at sites exposed to multiple melt events. As a result, pitting occured at a faster rate and with a different morphology in the melt layer than in the annealed bulk. This effect is similar to that observed previously where the surface layer was deformed and stressed by mechanical polishing (13).

The existence of residual stresses in laser-melted surfaces has been verified recently by Lamb, Steen, and West (14) for two stainless steels and by James, Gnanamuthu, and Moores (15) for two plain carbon steels. Both groups used X-ray techniques to calculate the surface stress from the measured strain.

3.2. Laser-surface melted stainless steels

Type 304 stainless steel (18% Cr - 8% Ni - balance Fe) is used in many applications because its passive film provides resistance to general corrosion in a variety of electrolytes. However, 304 stainless steel is often susceptible to localized attack, such as pitting or crevice corrosion. Recent work at the Naval Research Laboratory (16,17) and at Rockwell International (18) has shown that laser surface melting improved the resistance of 304 stainless to pitting corrosion in chloride solutions.

Figure 8 shows a cross section through a 304 stainless steel specimen which was laser-surface melted at the Naval Research Laboratory. It is

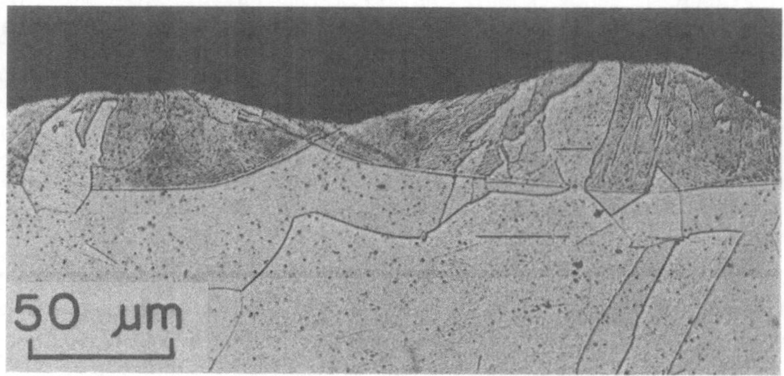

FIGURE 8. Cross section of a laser-surface melted 304 stainless steel.

clearly seen that the rapidly solidified melt region is not amorphous or microcrystalline and that the growth in the resolidified melt is epitaxial, extending from grains in the base metal. The grain size is slightly larger than in the base material, and there is a refinement in the sub-grain microstructure, as discussed elsewhere, due to the formation of regularly spaced dendrites (7,19).

Figure 9 shows the effect of laser surface melting on the anodic behavior of 304 stainless steel in 0.1 M NaCl. These polarization curves were determined by sweeping the electrode potential at a moderate scan rate (10 mV/min). The important characteristic of each curve is the pitting potential, i.e., the electrode potential at which there is a

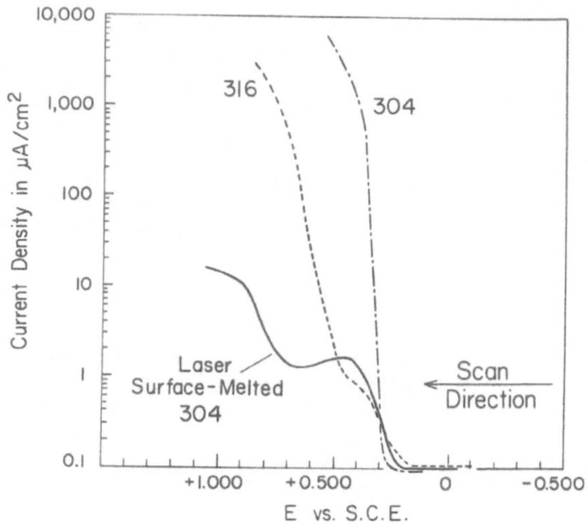

FIGURE 9. Effect of laser surface melting on the anodic behavior of 304 stainless steel in 0.1 M NaCl (sweep rate 10 mV/min).

sudden increase in current density due to the initiation of corrosion pits. At potentials below (less positive than) the pitting potential, pits do not initiate; but above the pitting potential, pits initiate and grow. A higher (more positive) pitting potential represents an increased resistance to pit initiation. Thus, the effect of laser surface melting is to increse the resistance of 304 stainless steel to pitting. Note that the laser surface treatment is more effective than is the usual practice of using a Mo-containing stainless steel (316 instead of 304).

The improvement in pitting potential as a result of laser surface melting is independent of the anodic sweep rate as seen in Figure 10. Although a range of pitting potentials was observed for the laser-surface melted 304, all were at least 200 mV more positive than the pitting potential for 304. Pitting potentials were also determined for a few samples using the potentiostatic technique, in which the specimen is held at a constant potential until the current becomes steady. The potential is then stepped to a more positive value and the procedure repeated until pitting initiates. Pitting potentials determined potentiostatically were: -0.725 V for laser-melted 304 having surface ripples intact, and -0.500 V for a laser-melted 304 sample polished past the surface ripples but only partially through the melt zone. These two values for E_{pit} lie within the envelope of data determined potentiodynamically for laser-surface melted 304.

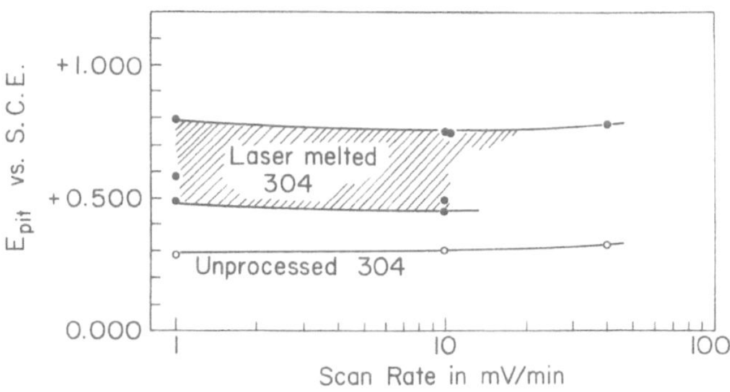

FIGURE 10. Effect of anodic sweep rate on the pitting potentials in 0.1 M NaCl.

This observation indicates that physical heterogeneities produced in the textured outer surface by rapid solidification of the melt pool are not preferred sites for pit initiation compared to incipient physical heterogeneities in the laser-melted planar surface which was polished down through the surface ripples. If surface roughness had affected the pitting potential of the laser-melted free surface, E_{pit} would have been shifted to more negative potentials, as is the case for iron and mild steel (20).

The improved resistance to pitting upon laser surface melting of 304 stainless steel is believed to be caused by the removal or redistribution of large-scale sulfide inclusions, which are known to be preferred sites for pit initiation in stainless steels (21-23). The redistribution of these inclusions upon rapid solidification processing, such as laser surface melting, could result in a larger number of total possible sites for pitting than in the unprocessed material; but the amount of segregated impurities at a given site may be less than that necessary to allow for breakdown of the film. In addition, the high temperatures obtained during laser processing may cause evaporation of sulfides and carbides so as to reduce the amount of inclusions.

Figure 11 shows an SEM micrograph and the corresponding EDAX display for a typical manganese sulfide inclusion present in the bulk stainless steel. The approximate size of a typical sulfide inclusion is 1 μm by 10 μm, and the planar concentration is about 1 inclusion per 10,000 square micrometers. Extensive examination of the laser-melted region with the scanning electron microscope showed that such sulfides were not present in the laser-melted region.

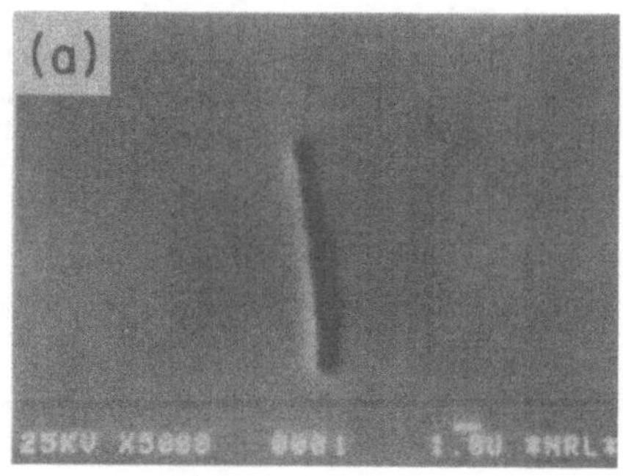

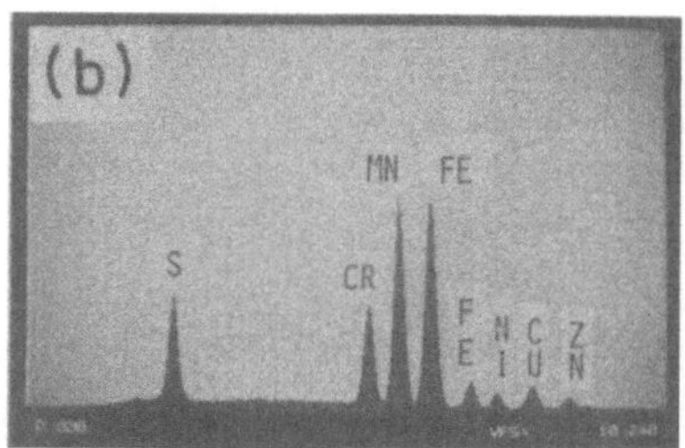

FIGURE 11. (a) SEM photograph and (b) corresponding EDAX display (0 to 10.240 keV) of a sulfide inclusion in bulk 304 stainless steel.

However, electron microprobe results suggest that some sulfur is retained in the laser-melted region (presumably melted and resolidified as smaller sulfides). Figure 12 shows the sampling scheme followed to analyze the laser-melted region for S using the microprobe. Individual square areas of 15 μm by 15 μm were sampled for 100 seconds; counts were taken for 30 such squares extending over adjacent overlapping melt passes. For each of the 30 individual squares, 100 second background counts off the sulfur peak were also taken.

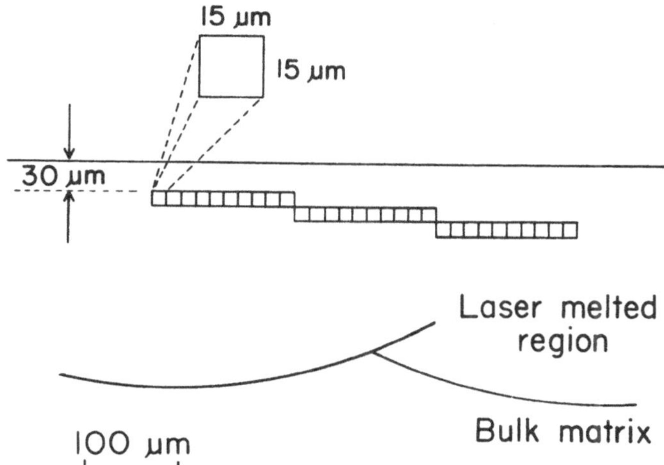

FIGURE 12. Sampling scheme used for microprobe analysis of S in the laser-melted region of 304 stainless steel.

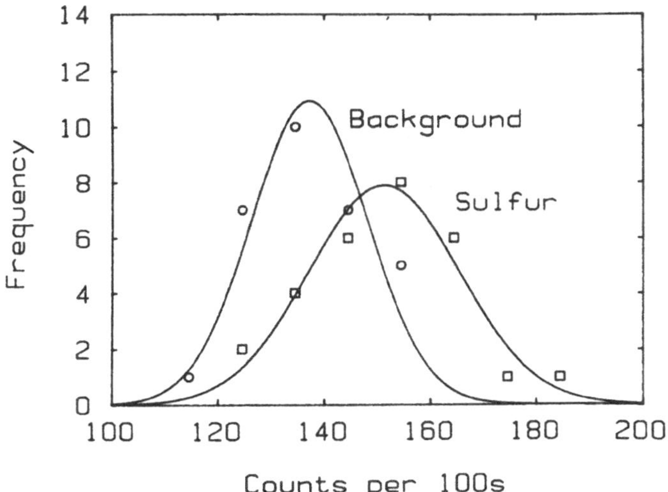

FIGURE 13. Electron microprobe results for sulfur in the laser-melted region of 304 stainless steel. Values for the abscissa are plotted at the midpoint of histograms taken at intervals of 10 counts/100 sec.

As shown in Figure 13, both the sulfur and background counts follow a normal distribution, with the sulfur distribution shifted about 20 counts/100 sec above background. For a MnS inclusion in the bulk, the S count in the point mode gave 44,450 counts/100 sec. Based on this value, the expected S count in the laser-melted region should be 45 counts/100 sec above background if the sulfur present in the steel (~0.05 atomic percent) was remelted and totally retained upon laser processing. As a first estimate, the microprobe data in Figure 13 suggest that about half the sulfur originally present is retained with the other half eliminated by evaporation during laser processing.

Auger analysis indicated no differences in the surface composition of the untreated and laser-melted 304 stainless steels. Thus, the improvement in pitting resistance cannot be attributed to compositional changes resulting from melting and rapid solidification.

Lumsden and co-workers (18) have also found that laser surface melting of 304 stainless steel raised the pitting potential in 0.1 N NaCl, in agreement with the results described above. Laser surface melting also facilitated passivation in 1 N H_2SO_4 by decreasing the critical current density for passivation. Lumsden et al. also suggest that the mechanism of improvement involves the elimination or dispersion of second-phase inclusions such as sulfides.

However, Bonora (24) has recently reported that surface melting of 304 stainless steel with a 5.6 J/cm^2 laser pulse promoted anodic dissolution and pit nucleation in Cl^- containing 0.5 N Na_2SO_4. In this case, laser melting produced an unfavorable surface finish consisting of craters and thermal fatigue striations, so as to enhance pit nucleation. In related work on pure iron, Bonora and co-workers (25) found that pulsed laser melting at 2 Jcm^2 decreased the corrosion rate in 0.1% Na_2SO_4, but that pulsed laser melting at 3 J/cm^2 was ineffective due to the larger number of active sites produced by the higher irradiation energy. In a borate buffer (a very mild solution), irradiation at either 2 J/cm^2 or 3 J/cm^2 was effective in reducing the passive current density.

Similarly, Lumsden et al. (18) found that laser melting and rapid solidification had differing effects on the pitting behavior of a series of ferritic steels of compositon Fe-13 Cr-x Mo, where x varies from 0 to 5%. As shown in Table 2, unless the Mo content was at least 3.5%, laser melting had either a deleterious effect or no effect on the pitting potential. An increase in pitting potential was obtained only for the 5% Mo alloy.

TABLE 2. Effect of laser surface melting on the pitting potential of ferritic stainless steels in 0.1 N NaCl (18).

Composition	E_{pit} (mV vs. SCE)		Effect of Laser Melting on Pitting
	Untreated	Laser Melted	
Fe-13 Cr	115	- 100 ± 40	harmful
Fe-13 Cr-2 Mo	200	- 5 ± 5	harmful
Fe-13 Cr-3.5 Mo	230	280 ± 20	none
Fe-13 Cr-5 Mo	280	420 ± 40	beneficial

These varying results with ferrous alloys indicate that the effect of laser melting on corrosion behavior depends on the details of the specific system, including the effect of laser melting on surface morphology and surface composition and on the aggressiveness of the aqueous solution.

The first application of laser processing for improving the corrosion resistance of metals appears to be the work of Anthony and Cline on the surface normalization (de-sensitization) of type 304 stainless steel (26). Under certain heat treatments or welding practices, 304 stainless steel becomes "sensitized" and susceptible to catastrophic intergranular corrosion. Within the sensitization temperature range, carbon rapidly diffuses to grain boundaries where it combines with chromium to form chromium carbides ($Cr_{23}C_6$), thus depleting the grain boundary regions of chromium. Not only do the grain boundaries contain less than the amount of Cr required for passivity, but a galvanic cell is set up between the grain boundary region (small anodic area) and the unaffected grain (large cathodic area). The result is rapid electrochemical attack along the grain boundaries and deep penetration into the bulk (27).

It is well known that sensitization can be avoided by rapid cooling through the sensitization temperature range. Anthony and Cline (26) used a scanning laser to melt and rapidly self quench a surface layer of sensitized 304 stainless steel. Specimens processed in this manner were resistant to intergranular corrosion when subjected for 72 hours to a standard Strauss test (a boiling solution of 10% H_2SO_4 and 10% $CuSO_4$), whereas there was severe intergranluar corrosion of the unprocessed (sensitized) surfaces.

Nakao and Nishimoto (28) have recently used laser surface melting to desensitize the heat-affected zone near welds on type 304 stainless steel. After laser melting, specimens were corrosion tested by a standard 10% oxalic acid electrolytic etch test, and the HAZ, which otherwise suffers "weld decay," was found to be immune to intergranular attack.

3.3. Laser-surface alloyed stainless steels

The preparation and electrochemical characterization of laser-alloyed surface stainless steels has been carried out by groups at Rockwell International (29) and at the Naval Research Laboratory (17,30). Both groups used a high-power (~10 kW), continuous-wave CO_2 laser.

Lumsden, Gnanamuthu, and Moore (29) at Rockwell International laser-alloyed Cr and Ni powder mixtures into a plain carbon steel (AISI 4140) substrate and studied the behavior of the resulting surface alloy in 1 N H_2SO_4. The corrosion resistance of all three surface alloys was found to be superior to that of the 4140 steel, with the critical current density for passivation decreasing in the order: 4140 > Fe-11 Cr-4Ni > Fe-19 Cr-8 Ni > Fe-29 Cr-13 Ni. The passivation behavior of Fe-11 Cr-4 Ni was found to be inferior to 304 stainless steel, the Fe-19 Cr-8 Ni comparable, and the Fe-29 Cr-13 Ni superior. However, these authors have presented no results on the pitting behavior of these surface alloys in chloride solutions, although it is an area of much practical interest.

McCafferty and Moore (17,30) took a slightly different approach and laser-alloyed Mo into a 304 stainless steel substrate to produce Fe-Cr-Ni-Mo surface alloys. Two types of surface alloys were prepared: Fe-18 Cr-10 Ni-3 Mo, which is within the specifications for bulk 316 stainless steel (which is often used instead of type 304 stainless when improved resistance to localized corrosion is needed), and Fe-19 Cr-12 Ni-9 Mo.

Wrought 304 stainless steel was used as a substrate to retain its formability and to promote good adhesion between the surface and bulk. In the alloys of interest, it was desired to maintain a chromium content of 18-20%, to increase the nickel content to about 10%, and to produce molybdenum contents ranging up to 10%. To achieve these compositions from the compositions of wrought 304 required the addition of chromium, nickel, and molybdenum. Up to thirty alternating layers of pure molybdenum, a 56% Cr-46% Ni alloy, and a 90% Ni-10% Cr alloy were applied by sputter deposition. Table 3 shows one sequence which was used to coat the 304 substrate before laser processing. The number and thickness of the coatings were adjusted to produce the equivalent of elemental coatings of 4.5 μm Mo-3 μm Ni-0.5 μm Cr, 5 μm Mo-3.5 μm Ni-1 μm Cr, and 10 μm Mo-4.5 μm Ni-2.5 μm Cr. The alloying of these specimens to a depth of 150 μm resulted in the desired compositions. The specimens were processed at a shallower depth of 100 μm two more times to further homogenize the composition of the surface alloy produced by the first set of passes.

TABLE 3. Sequence for coating 304 stainless steel prior to laser alloying.

	Mo	$Ni_{46}Cr_{54}$	$Ni_{90}Cr_{10}$
Sequence	1	2	3
	4	5	6
	7	8	9
	10	11	12
	13	14	15
	16	17	18
	19	20	21
	22	22	24
	25	26	27
	28	29	30
Total Thickness	5 μm	1.25 μm	3.25 μm
Equivalent Thickness		Mo 5 μm Ni 3.5 μm Cr 1.0 μm	

Figure 14 shows a cross section through the 3% Mo surface alloy. The outlines of the melt passes for the two sets of processing conditions (initial alloying followed by shallower homogenization) can be seen in

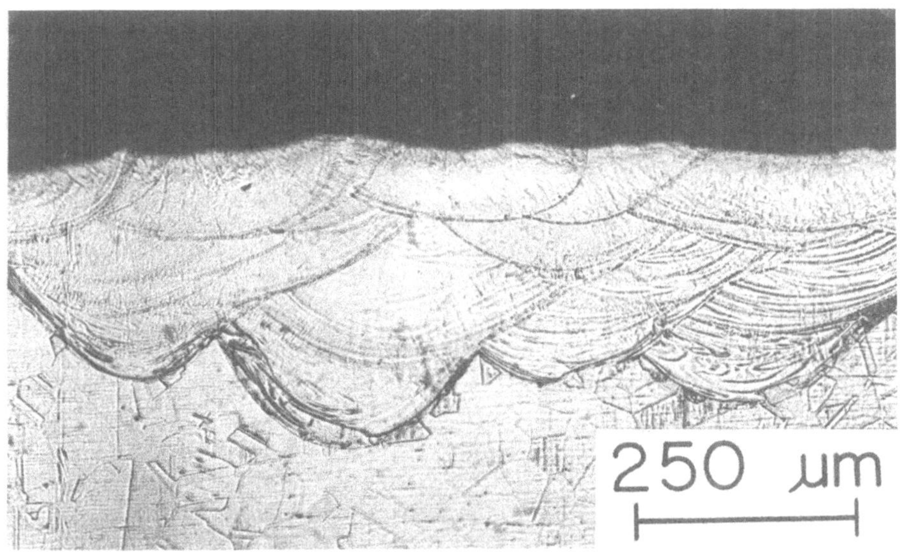

FIGURE 14. Optical micrograph of a cross section of a 3% Mo laser surface alloy.

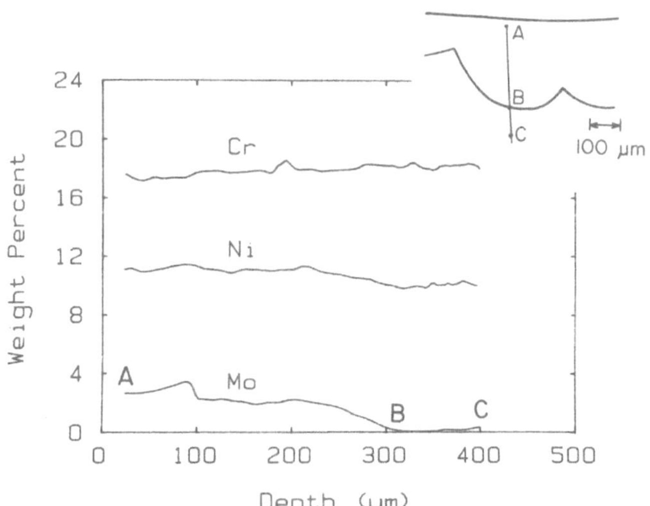

FIGURE 15. Microprobe traces across the 3% Mo surface alloy. The inset to the right shows the outline of the laser surface alloy.

Figure 14. Figure 15 shows electron microprobe traces taken across the 3% Mo surface alloy. It can be seen that Mo is distributed evenly throughout the surface alloy, except at the bottom of the laser-melted region. The more uniform composition near the free surface is an indication of the effectiveness of the homogenization that results from additional sets of passes which process to a shallower melt depth. The 9% Mo surface alloy was similar to the 3% Mo surface alloy, both in its microstructure and in the effectiveness of mixing and dispersion of the alloying additions.

The anodic behavior of the two Mo surface alloys in 0.1 M NaCl is shown in Figure 16. More detail on procedures is given elsewhere (17,30), but in brief, the test samples were first cathodically cleaned in 1 N H_2SO_4 prior to immersion in order to remove surface oxides which result from redeposition of oxidized metal vapors during laser processing. The samples were immersed in 0.1 N NaCl for 24 hours and the anodic polarization curves determined by standard potentiostatic techniques.

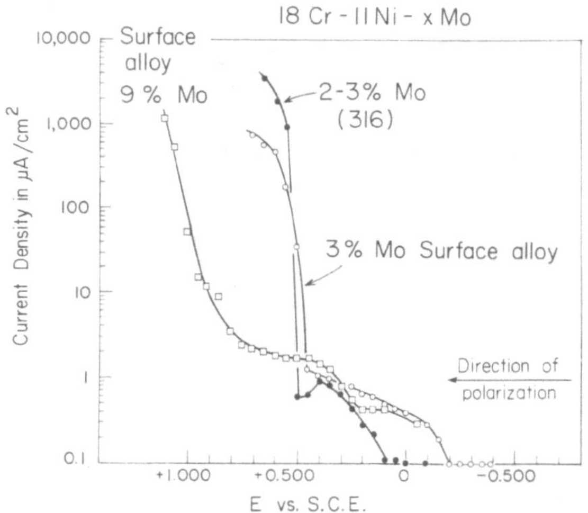

FIGURE 16. Anodic polarization curves of Fe-Cr-Ni-Mo alloys in de-aerated 0.1 M NaCl at 25°C.

As seen in Figure 16, the pitting potential of the 3% Mo surface alloy is similar to that of bulk 316 stainless steel. The 9% Mo surface alloy did not undergo pitting up to potentials of oxygen evolution. The compositions and the pitting potentials are summarized in Table 4. The compositions of the surface alloys were detemined by X-ray fluorescence analysis, and composition ranges for wrought 304 and 316 alloys are given for comparison.

Thus the 3% Mo surface alloy prepared by laser surface alloying exhibits both a surface composition and a pitting resistance equivalent to type 316 stainless steel, but conserves the amount of Mo required by restricting its presence to the near-surface region. The rapid solidification feature of the laser-alloying process enables production of a

TABLE 4. Summary of composition of Fe-Cr-Ni-Mo alloys and pitting potentials in 0.1 M NaCl.

Sample	Cr	Ni	Mo	E_{pit} (V vs. SCE)
304 stainless steel	18-20	8-10	0	+ 0.300
316 stainless steel	16-18	10-14	2-3	+ 0.550
3% Mo surface alloy	18.9	9.1	3.7	+ 0.500
9% Mo surface alloy	19.2	11.7	9.6	did not pit

300-series type surface stainless steel containing 9% Mo, an amount in excess of that possible by conventional alloying techniques. The improved pitting resistance of the 9% Mo surface alloy is comparable to that normally otained with higher alloys containing larger amounts of Ni and/or Cr, so that use of the 9% Mo surface alloy minimizes the amount of Ni and Cr required to achieve the equivalent corrosion performance, as well as the amount of Mo required by virtue of the surface alloying.

3.4. Laser-melted aluminum

The electrochemical and corrosion behavior of laser-melted aluminum surfaces has beeen studied by groups in the United States (31) and Italy (32,33).

McCafferty and co-workers (31) showed that laser surface melting improved the resistance of 3003* aluminum to general corrosion, but had no effect on the pitting potential or on anodization behavior. The 3003 aluminum was laser processed in a low vacuum using a single pulse 10.6 μm CO_2 laser at a 50 J output for 1 μsec duration (34). The irradiated area was slightly less than 1 cm diameter, so that the power density ($\sim 10^8$ W/cm^2) for this pulsed laser was about the same as that used with high-power continuous-wave CO_2 lasers.

The interaction of the micro-second duration laser pulse with the 3003 aluminum alloy modifies its near surface microstructure, surface topography, and surface chemistry. Figure 17 shows an optical micrograph of a cross section through the laser-melted region and the underlying bulk metals. As seen in Figure 17, there is an abrupt and dramatic change in the microstructure in the laser-melted region. In the bulk alloy the alloying elements are contained in the phases (Mn,Fe)Al_6 (i.e., $MnAl_6$ containing some dissolved iron substituted for manganese), the solid solutions α-Al(Mn,Fe)Si, and silicon. These second phases appear in the bulk alloy as dispersed particles as shown in Figure 17. X-ray mapping of the bulk alloy showed that manganese, iron and silicon are present in both the large and the small second phases show in in Figure 17. The effect of laser melting is to transform the microstructure in the solidified melt pool into a system of striated bands parallel to the free surface.

* Major alloying elements: 1.2% Mn, 0.6% Si, 0.7% Fe

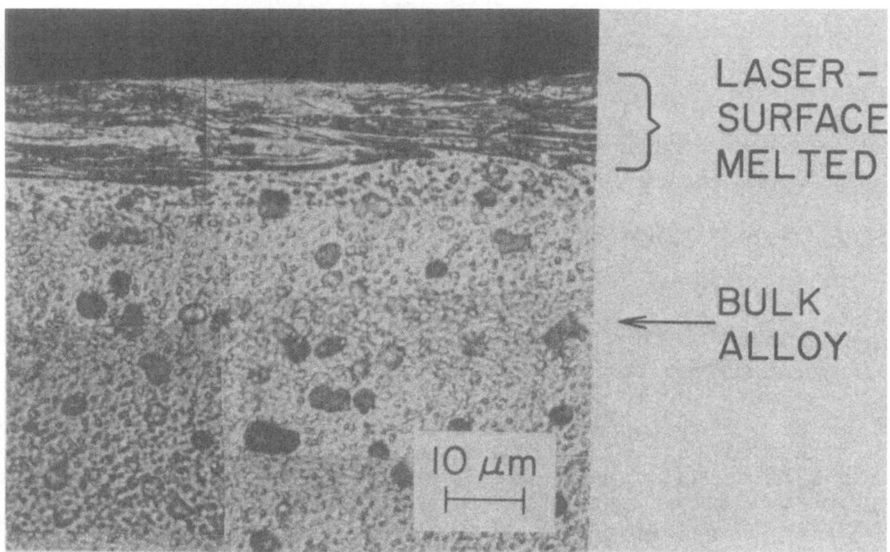

FIGURE 17. Optical micrograph showing a cross section through laser-melted 3003 aluminum (etched with Keller's reagent).

The rapid melt-solidification process also modifies the chemical composition of the outermost surface. Auger spectroscopy has shown that laser melting produces a surface that is essentially unalloyed aluminum, being depleted of manganese, iron and silicon. The depletion of these alloying elements in the rapidly solidified surface is not surprising inasmuch as surface tension data for pure liquid metals (35) show that manganese, iron and silicon are not surface active relative to aluminum. See Figure 18. The actual temperature of the melt pool is not known, but must lie somewhere between the melting point of aluminum (660°C) and its boiling point (2500°C). When all the metallic components are melted (at approximately 1550°C), aluminum is the constituent with the lowest surface tension and hence is surface active. The outermost surface of the laser-melted sample also contains a network of surface ripples, although the surface is macroscopically smooth (31).

Figure 19 shows the effect of laser surface melting on the uniform corrosion of 3003 aluminum in de-aerated 0.5 N HCl. The corrosion rate of the laser-modified surface was about half that of the untreated surface (152 uA/cm^2 and 314 uA/cm^2, respectively). However, the lifetime of the laser-modified region is limited by its 10 μm thickness to be approximately 50 hours in that particular environment. For 0.1 N HCl, the effect of pulsed laser melting was again to reduce the corrosion rate in half (from 31 to 19 uA/cm^2). In this weaker acid, the expected lifetime of the laser-modified region is increased to 18 days, but is again limited by the thickness of the modified surface before the normal corrosion rate of the underlying bulk alloy is realized.

The laser-modified surface also reduced the corrosion rate in de-aerated 0.1 M sodium citrate. Figure 20 shows anodic polarization

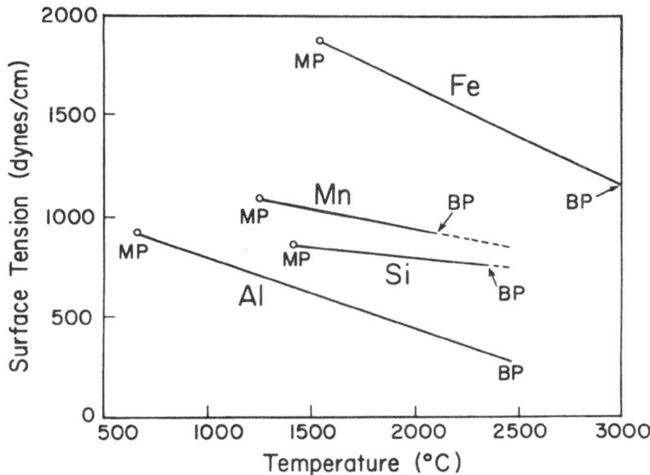

FIGURE 18. Surface tension of various alloying elements in 3003 aluminum. MP and BP refer to the melting point and boiling point, respectively.

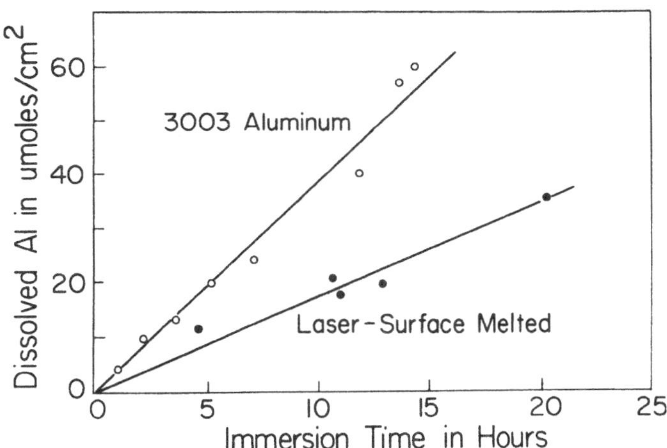

FIGURE 19. Corrosion-time curves for 3003 aluminum in de-aerated 0.5 N HCl.

curves in 0.1 M sodium citrate after 8 hours immersion at open-circuit potential. The rate of anodic dissolution of the laser-surface melted alloy is less than the rate for the conventional alloy at all anodic potentials. Both curves display an active-passive type of behavior, but there was considerable corrosion of the conventional alloy surface. Figure 20 also shows anodic polarization curves after 24 hours immersion at open-circuit potential. The laser-treated sample has a lower dissolution rate at potentials below -1.0 V S.C.E., but at higher anodic potentials both types of surfaces have essentially the same corrosion rate.

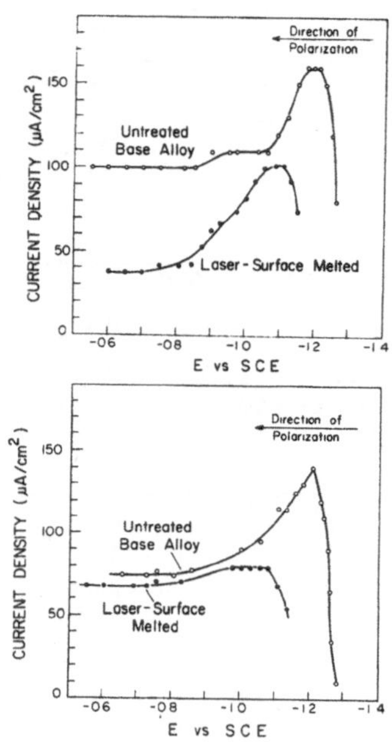

FIGURE 20. Anodic polarization of 3003 aluminum in de-aerated 0.1 M sodium citrate. Top - after 8 hrs immersion; bottom - after 24 hrs immersion.

Surface melting with the pulsed laser had no effect on the pitting potential of the 3003 aluminum alloy in 0.1 M NaCl, in agreement with the results of Bonora and co-workers (32), who have reported that pure aluminum and its laser-modified surface have the same pitting potential in 0.5 M NaCl. However, Bonora et al. report that the pitting corrosion rate (expressed as the anodic current density at potentials more positive than the pitting potential) is noticeably lower for irradiated specimens. However, whether this represents an improvement in pitting resistance would depend on how the anodic current density is related to the number of pits and the pit depth distribution.

The effect of laser surface melting on the anodizing of aluminum has been studied in some detail (31), both in sulfuric acid (which produces thick, porous films) and in ammonium tartrate (which produces thinner, compact films). Figure 21 shows anodic charging curves for galvanostatic anodizing of the laser-surface melted alloy in 1.5 M sulfuric acid at various current densities. Similar curves were obtained for the untreated alloy. Each charging curve displays a region wherein the cell voltage rises linearly with time up to a plateau or equilibrium voltage. These observed curves are similar to those previously reported for the anodization of pure aluminum in a variety of electrolytes (36,37).

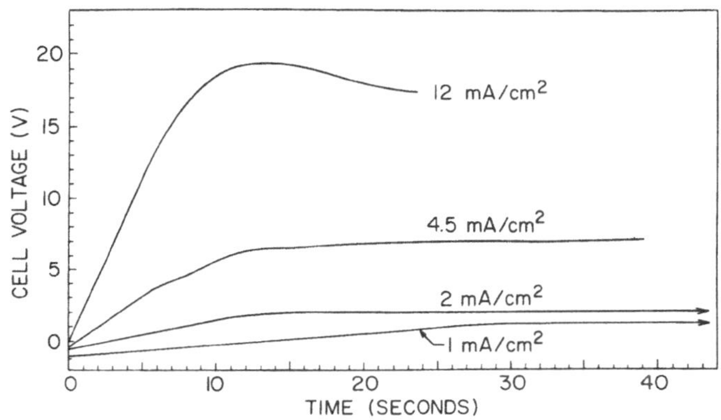

FIGURE 21. Anodic charging curves for galvanostatic anodizing of laser-surface melted 3003 aluminum in 1.5 M H_2SO_4.

The linear rise in cell voltage with time is due to oxide film formation under a constant electric field. The current density is related to the electric field H by (37,38)

$$i = Ae^{BH} \tag{1}$$

where A and B are constants, and $H = dE_f/d\delta$ where E_f is the potential difference across the oxide film of thickness δ. The potential difference E across the cell is the sum of E_f and a constant term ϕ which includes all interface potentials, so that H is given by $H = dE/d\delta$. Under a constant anodizing current applied for t sec, the oxide film thickens by the amount $\delta_a = rit$, where $r = 5.16 \times 10^{-5}$ cm^3/C for aluminum. The total oxide film thickness δ is $\delta = \delta_o + \delta_a$, where δ_o is the thickness of the prepolarized air-formed film, with usually $\delta_a >> \delta_o$. These considerations give

$$\log i = \log A + \frac{B}{2.303\ r} R_i \tag{2}$$

where R_i is the unitary formation rate R_i defined by (39)

$$R_i = \frac{1}{i} \left\{\frac{dE}{dt}\right\}_i \tag{3}$$

Figure 22 shows a plot of R_i vs. log i for both the 3003 base alloy and the laser-modified surface. Both types of surfaces can be described by the same plot. Figure 23 compares anodization characteristics for the 3003 base alloy and the laser-surface melted 3003 in 1.5 M sulfuric acid. The observed range of values for the charge pased before reaching the maximum cell voltage and the calculated film thicknesses to that point are in good agreement with the values reported by Yahalom and Hoar for pure aluminum in 15% sulfuric acid (36). As shown in Figure 23, there is no difference in film thicknesses for the 3003 base alloy and the laser-surface melted sample. Thus, laser surface melting has no effect on the growth of porous oxide films formed by anodization in sulfuric acid.

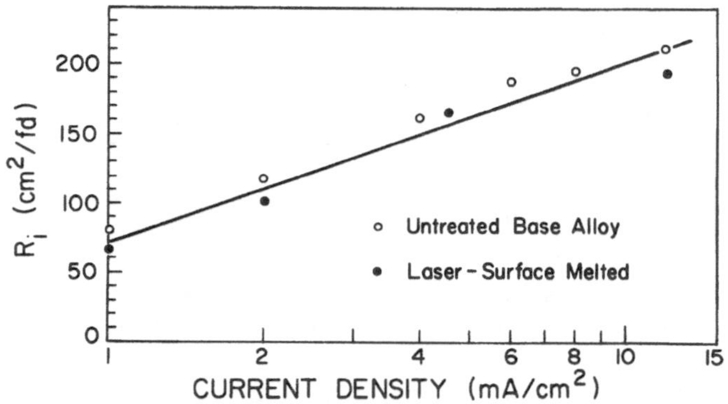

FIGURE 22. Plots of R_i vs. log current density for both types of 3003 aluminum in 1.5 M H_2SO_4.

For the anodic films formed in ammonium tartrate, the galvanostatic charging curves display a pronounced curvature with only an initial region, so that Eq.(2) does not apply throughout the entire period of film growth. Figure 24 compares equilibrium cell voltages for the laser-surface melted and untreated specimens. Within experimental limits, the anodization behavior is the same for both types of surfaces.

Bonora and co-workers (32,33) have reported somewhat different results on the anodization behavior of laser-treated pure aluminum. These investigators used a nanosecond laser pulse (rather than a microsecond pulse, as in the work described above) and have presented evidence which suggests that an amorphous surface is formed (40). The effect of laser treatment prior to anodizing was to reduce the thickness of the anodic films formed in ammonium tartrate and to increase the thickness of the films formed in sulfuric acid. However, Bonora et al. used only a single polarizing potential of 6 V for their work in ammonium tartrate and the corresponding anodic current densities were much less than in the NRL work. Thus, because of the differences in the conditions in both laser processing and in anodizing, it would appear that more work is required to better understand the effect of laser treatment on the anodization of aluminum.

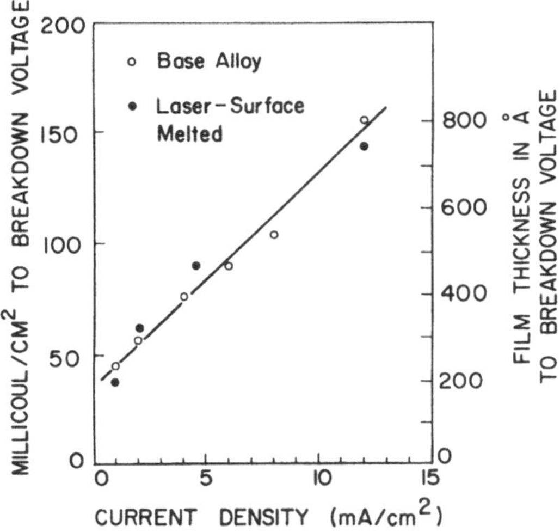

FIGURE 23. Anodizing characteristics of both types of 3003 aluminum surfaces in 1.5 M H_2SO_4.

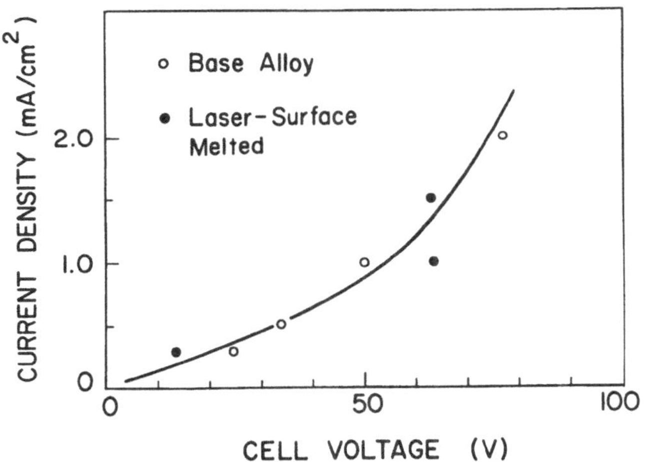

FIGURE 24. Comparison of equilibrium cell voltages for both types of 3003 aluminum surfaces in 3% ammonium tartrate.

3.5. Laser surface melting of copper alloys

Draper and co-workers (41-45) have demonstrated that laser surface melting improves the corrosion resistance of a series of aluminum bronzes (Cu-Al-Fe) by modifying their microstructure. This finding is significant because the most important factor governing the corrosion rate of the aluminum bronzes is their microstructure (46). For Cu-Al alloys with less than 8.5% Al, the alloys consist of a single phase (α); but above 8.5% Al a duplex structure (α+β) is formed. Slow cooling or reheating above 300°C may allow the β to decompose partially to an (α+γ_2) eutectoid. The aluminum-rich γ_2 phase is more anodic than α or β phases (47), so that aluminum bronzes often undergo galvanic attack by de-alloying of aluminum ("de-aluminumification").

For the Fe-containing aluminum bronzes studied by Draper et al. (41-45), the microstructure also contains iron-rich δ precipitates dispersed throughout both the matrix and grain boundaries. See Figure 25, which shows the two-phase microstructure of alloy C61400. Figure 25

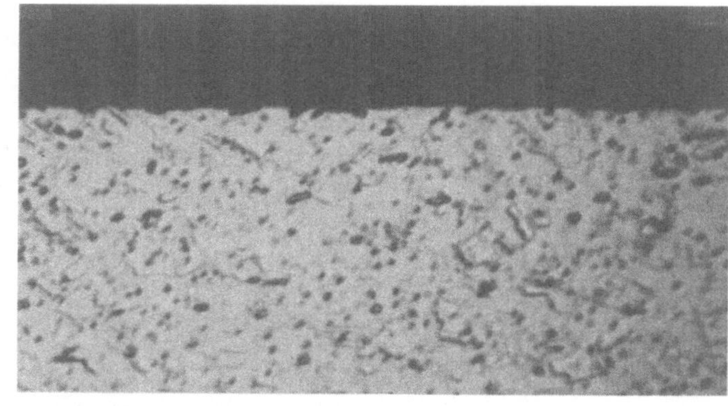

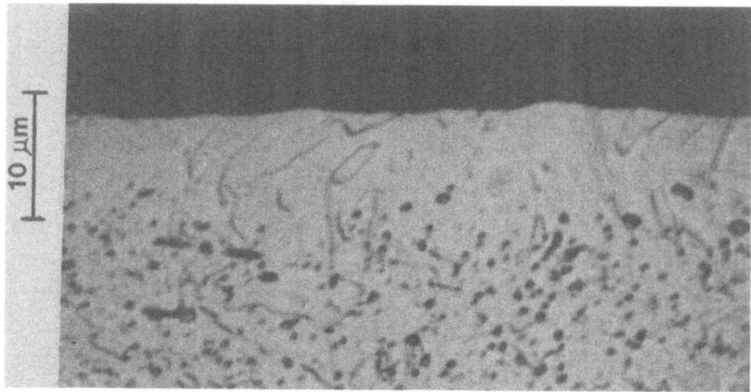

FIGURE 25. Effect of laser surface melting on the microstructure of C61400 Fe-aluminum bronze (90.0% Cu, 6.3% Al, 3.7% Fe). Top - untreated; bottom - laser melted. Note the elimination of the Fe-rich phase in the laser-melted region.

also shows that the effect of laser surface melting is to homogenize the two-phase microstructure into a single phase devoid of iron-rich precipitates, as verified by scanning Auger analysis (43,45). EDAX analysis of corrosion films formed in acidified 3% NaCl showed that selective dealloying of aluminum was retarded as a result of the laser surface melting and homogenization (41). Laser surface melting also reduced the rate of anodic dissolution in 0.5 M H_2SO_4 from the open circuit potential up to anodic potentials where there was selective dissolution of Cu (44).

The effect of laser surface melting on two additional aluminum bronzes was similar in terms of homogenization of the multiple phase structure and anodic dissolution in 0.5 M H_2SO_4. In addition, laser surface melting also increased the resistance to cavitation erosion in distilled water (42,45) as shown in Figure 26.

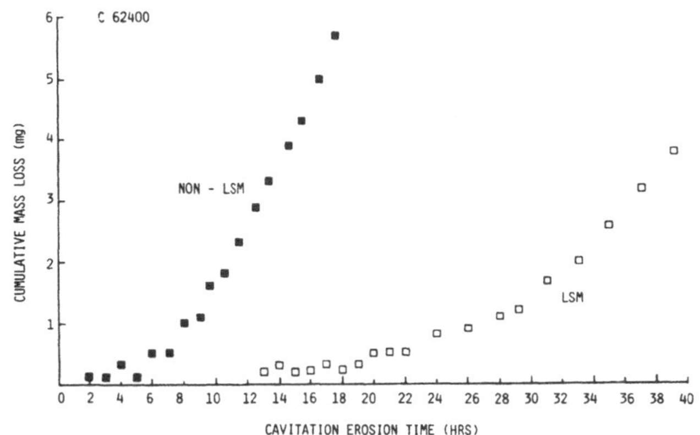

FIGURE 26. Effect of laser surface melting on the cavitation erosion in water of alloy C62400 (85.6% Cu, 10.4% Al, 3.6% Fe).

Draper et al. (48) have also investigated the effect of laser melting on the corrosion behavior of tin-modified copper-nickel alloy (C 72500: 88.2% Cu, 9.5% Ni, 2.3% Sn) in humid atmospheres containing H_2S or Cl_2 pollutants. In both cases, the effect of laser surface melting was to significantly decrease the thickness of the corrosion film. In preliminary results on copper which was laser alloyed with Cr or Cr + Ni, it has been reported that the surface alloys are more inert than conventional copper alloys in moist air containing H_2S (49).

3.6. Other metal systems

Draper and co-workers (50) have laser-surface alloyed Pd into a titanium substrate to produce a noble metal enriched surface which provides corrosion protection in boiling HCl. This result is similar to that for bulk Pd-Ti alloys, where it is well known that small additions of Pd produce a dramatic reduction in the corrosion rate of titanium in hot, concentrated acids (51,52). See Figure 27. The work of Draper et al. is of added interest because comparisons can be made with Pd-Ti surface alloys prepared by ion implantation (53). For these two surface modification techniques, which can be considered complementary techniques, the

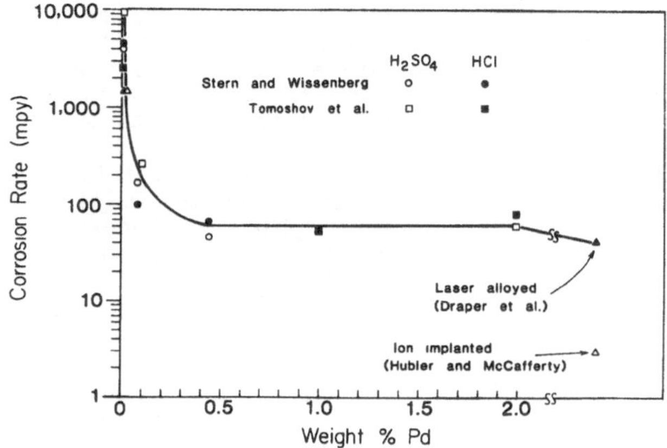

FIGURE 27. Corrosion rate of bulk and surface Pd-Ti alloys in 2-3 N H_2SO_4 or HCl at 100°C.

surface alloys become enriched in Pd (to about 20 atomic percent) and galvanic effects between cathodic sites (Pd) and anodic sites (Ti) drive the resulting mixed corrosion potential into a region where titanium is passive. Both laser processing and ion implantation are useful here in conserving the total amount of Pd required by restricting its location to the near surface region.

There has been much recent interest in the use of metallic glasses as corrosion resistant materials (54,55). Some amorphous alloys owe their corrosion resistance to the lack of defects associated with the solid state, such as grain boundaries, dislocations, and stacking faults, and to the chemical homogeneity resulting from rapid quenching, such as the absence of second phases, precipitates, and segregates. Amorphous metals are thermodynamically unstable and provide corrosion protection by spontaneous dissolution to form passive films (56). Not all amorphous alloys are corrosion resistant (57).

There has been considerable work on the preparation of metallic glasses by rapid solidification of the liquid into ribbons or powders, but only recently has laser processing been attempted as a means of producing metallic glass surface alloys (58-62). In addition, there have been but a few reports on the corrosion behavior of laser-formed metallic glasses (59,62).

Sepold (58) and Hashimoto (59) found that amorphous layers could be produced by laser melting Ni-Nb and Fe-Si-B alloys, respectively, but a complication arose in that partial recrystallization occurred in the next overlapping melt pass. By decreasing the time of laser irradiation and selecting surface alloy compositions having a longer time for conversion of the amorphous phase to the crystalline phase, Hashimoto was able to prepare amorphous surface alloys of Pd-Cu-Si, Fe-Cr-P-C, and Fe-Cr-Mo-P-C by laser processing (59-62).

Figure 28 shows the effect of laser surface treatment on the anodic behavior of a Fe-10 Cr-14.5 P-9.5 C alloy in 1 N HCl (59). The passive current density before laser processing is of the same order as that of the crystalline alloy. The passive current density after treatment has been reduced by an order of magnitude, but is, however, higher than that of the melt spun ribbon, which passivates spontaneously. The presence of some microcrystallinity and of cracks in the laser-melted alloy prevented a drastic decrease in the passive current density.

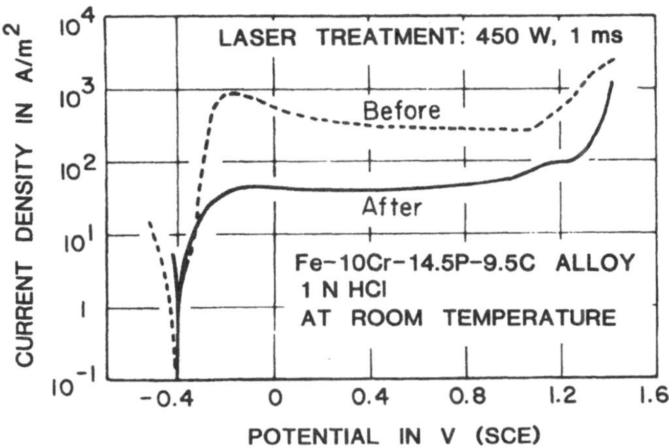

FIGURE 28. Anodic polarization curves of Fe-10 Cr-14.5 P-9.5 C in 1 N HCl at room temperature before and after laser treatment (from Ref. 59).

In more recent work, Hashimoto and co-workers (62) have produced laser-formed Pd-based surface alloys which passivate similarly to the melt spun alloy, as shown in Figure 29. A crystalline Pd-25 Rh-10 P-9 Si surface alloy on a nickel substrate is seen to exhibit a high current density in the active region, whereas both the laser-processed and melt spun amorphous specimens spontaneously passivate up about + 1.0 V where chlorine evolution occurs on all specimens.

3.7. Laser-processed coatings

Laser processing can improve the corrosion resistance of metallic coatings by removal of residual porosity. Although plasma spraying is a versatile technique for applying many different metallic and inorganic coatings to a variety of substrate metals, a major deficiency of plasma-sprayed coatings is their residual porosity, which can cause problems if corrosive liquids can penetrate the pores and attack the substrate metal. The following two examples show how laser treatment can improve the corrosion behavior of porous metallic coatings.

In work at the Naval Research Laboratory, a high-energy laser was used to remelt and consolidate the pores in a plasma-sprayed titanium coating on steel. Details have been given elsewhere (63); but in brief, 2 x 2 x 1/4 inch samples were plasma sprayed with commercial purity titanium powder in a pre-evacuated chamber maintained at 30 torr during the spraying. The sprayed coatings were laser-surface melted in vacuum to a depth of approximately one-third of the coating thickness.

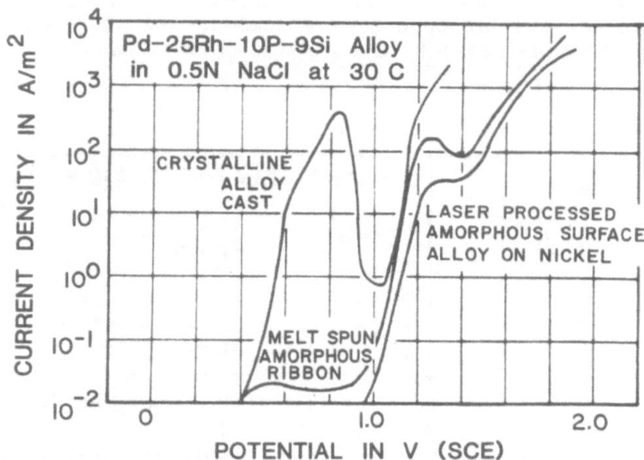

FIGURE 29. Anodic polarization curves of amorphous and crystalline alloys of Pd-25 Rh-10 P-9 Si in 0.5 N NaCl at 30°C (from Ref. 62).

Figure 30 shows electrode potential data for a 15-day immersion in natural seawater. After 15 days, the electrode potential of the laser consolidated titanium coating was similar to that of pure titanium, as shown in Figure 30. In contrast, the electrode potential of the porous as-sprayed coating was much closer to the potential of the steel base than to that of pure titanium. This mixed potential resulted from localized corrosion at the steel base beneath the porous plasma-sprayed coating.

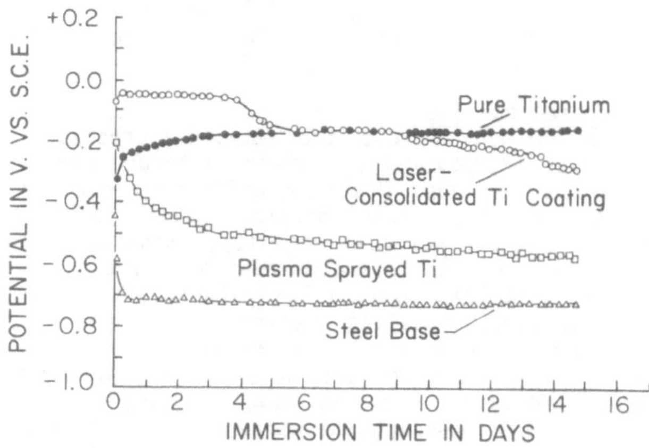

FIGURE 30. Electrode potential data in natural seawater for titanium, steel, and titanium-coated steel.

Figure 31 shows typical cross sections through the two types of titanium coatings after the 15-day immersion period. As seen in the figure, corrosion pitting occurred at the steel substrate beneath the porous plasma-sprayed titanium coating. Laser remelt consolidation of this porosity prevented the occurrence of such pitting, as shown in Figure 31.

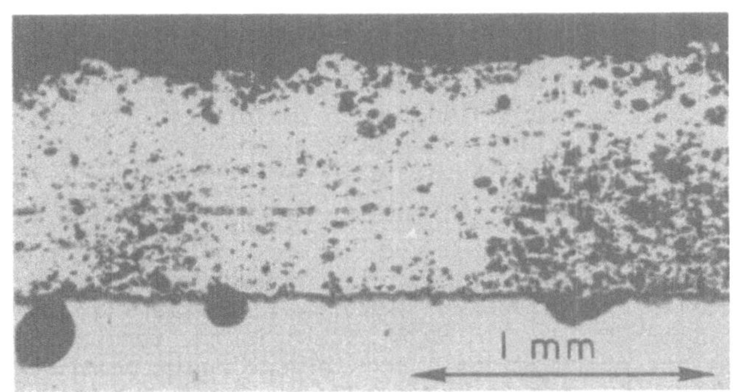

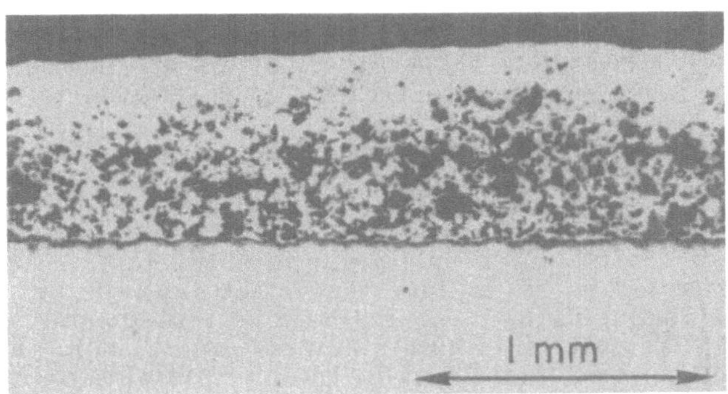

FIGURE 31. Cross-sectional views through titanium coatings on steel after 15 days immersion in seawater. The unconsolidated sample (above) shows pitting attack of the steel substrate. The sample below was consolidated by laser melting one third of the coating thickness and shows no evidence of corrosion.

Bhat, Herman, and Coyle (64) have demonstrated that laser processing improves the corrosion resistance of porous Ni-Cr coatings. Bhat et al. prepared plasma-sprayed Ni-20 Cr coatings ($\sim$300 μm thick) on low carbon steel substrates and then closed the pores in the top 25 μm by laser surface melting. Short-term tests in various HCl solutions showed that laser consolidation of pores prevented dissolution of the substrate.

Consolidation of pores in both examples decribed above is of critical importance, because both coatings are more noble than the substrate so that penetration of the corrodent to the base metal leads to its accelerated galvanic attack.

4. SUGGESTIONS FOR FURTHER WORK

As noted earlier, the use of laser processing techniques to improve corrosion resistance is still relatively new. Most of the examples reviewed above deal with short-term laboratory studies on small samples, rather than with more practical tests performed over a longer period of time on larger samples. There are several promising approaches which warrant increased activity. These are: (1) laser alloying to produce high-performance surface alloys, (2) laser alloying to produce amorphous surface alloys, (3) laser melt/particle injection techniques to produce corrosion-resistant coatings of substantial (1-3 mm) thickness.

There are many commercially available alloys which provide excellent corrosion resistance in given environments. For example, Ni-Cr-Mo alloys or stainless steels containing large amounts of these three alloying elements provide protection in seawater. It should be possible to produce the surface equivalents of such corrosion-resistant bulk alloys by laser alloying overcoats of the alloying elements directly into suitable substrates, as described earlier. The benefits of surface alloying in such cases are conservation of scarce, expensive, or critical materials as well as retention of mechanical properties of the bulk.

By laser alloying overcoats into the substrate, it may also be possible to produce amorphous surface alloys if the required metalloids are contained in the overcoatings. This effect would be somewhat analogous to ion implantation of a selected alloying element plus a metalloid to produce amorphous surface alloys on crystalline substrates (65). If successful, laser alloying would obviate the usual need for subsequent consolidation of amorphous ribbons or powders into bulk materials. As noted earlier, however, not all amorphous alloys are inherently corrosion resistant and there also may be problems with recrystalization in overlapping melt passes.

The laser melt/particle injection technique (5) offers an alternate way to produce the general types of surface alloys mentioned above. If powders of the desired compositions of the crystalline or amorphous alloys are available, then the powders may be blown into the melt pool to build up a coating layer by layer. Here the laser operating conditions are adjusted so as to fuse the injected powder to the previous layer with minimal melting. For a 100 μm melt width, the required particle size of the powders is about 140 mesh, a size which has been handled before using this approach (5). Where crystalline powders are used, the coating could be laser remelted through a portion of its thickness to consolidate any existing porosity. This technique offers the possibility of producing large-area samples which can be corrosion tested in service environments for extended periods of time.

5. SUMMARY

Laser surface melting of a metal surface can modify the corrosion behavior by altering the surface composition, microstructure, or distribution of impurities and second phases. Laser surface alloying of overcoats into the substrate permits production of corrosion resistant surface alloys, which in some cases may be unattainable by bulk alloying techniques.

Some examples of the successful use of laser melting to improve corrosion behavior are as follows. Laser melting of type 304 austenitic stainless (Fe-18 Cr-8 Ni-balance Fe) and certain ferritic stainless steels (Fe-13 Cr-5 Mo) improves the resistance to pitting by evaporation and/or redistribution of sulfide inclusions. Laser melting of sensitized

304 stainless steel redistributes Cr in otherwise Cr-depleted grain boundaries and restores resistance to intergranular corrosion. Laser melting of aluminum bronzes improves the resistance to corrosion and cavitation erosion by homogenization of multiple phases. Laser melting of 3003 aluminum (Al-1% Mn) with a microsecond laser pulse improves the resistance to uniform corrosion (but not pitting), while laser melting with a nanosecond pulse produces a surface which improves the properties of anodized films. Laser remelting partially through the thickness of plasma-sprayed metallic coatings removes residual porosity so as to isolate the underlying substrate fom the environment.

Laser surface alloying has been used to produce Fe-Cr binary alloys, and Fe-Cr-Ni and Fe-Cr-Ni-Mo surface stainless steels which have good passivation behavior or increased resistance to localized attack by pitting corrosion. Promising directions for further study include laser alloying to produce high-performance surface alloys and amorphous surface alloys, and the use of laser melt/particle injection techniques to form corrosion-resistant coatings from metallic powders.

REFERENCES

1. D. S. Gnanamuthu in "Applications of Lasers in Materials Processing," edited by E. A. Metzbower (American Society for Metals, Metals Park, Ohio, 1979), p. 177.
2. L. R. Hettche, E. A. Metzbower, J. D. Ayers, and P. G. Moore, Nav. Res. Rev. 33, 3 (1981).
3. J. J. Harwood, ASTM Standardization News 3, 12 (1975).
4. A. B. Gray, Metal Progress 117, 32 (1980).
5. J. D. Ayers, R. J. Schaefer, and W. P. Robey, J. Metals 33, 19 (1981).
6. P. G. Moore and E. McCafferty, J. Electrochem. Soc. 128, 1391 (1981).
7. L. S. Weinman, J. N. DeVault, and P. Moore, in Ref. 1, p. 259.
8. H. H. Uhlig and G. E. Woodside, J. Phys. Chem. 57, 280 (1953).
9. G. C. Wood and G. F. Cammack, Corros. Sci. 8, 159 (1968).
10. J. B. Lumsden, in Passivity of Metals, edited by R. P. Frankenthal and J. Kruger (The Electrochemical Society, Princeton, NJ, 1978), p. 730.
11. E. A. Lizlovs and A. P. Bond, J. Electrochem. Soc. 118, 22 (1971).
12. P. T. Cottrell, R. P. Frankenthal, G. W. Kammlott, D. J. Siconolfi, and C. W. Draper, J. Electrochem. Soc. 130, 998 (1983).
13. R. P. Frankenthal, Corros. Sci. 8, 491 (1968).
14. M. Lamb, W. M. Steen, and D. R. F. West, in Stainless Steels '84 (Institute of Metals, London, 1985), p. 295.
15. M. R. James, D. S. Gnanamuthu, and R. J. Moores, Scr. Metall. 18, 357 (1984).
16. E. McCafferty, P. G. Moore, J. D. Ayers, and G. K. Hubler, in Corrosion of Metals Processed by Directed Energy Beams, edited by C. R. Clayton and C. M. Preece (A.I.M.E., Warrandale, PA, 1982), p. 1.
17. E. McCafferty and P. G. Moore, in Fundamental Aspects of Corrosion Protection by Surface Modification, edited by E. McCafferty, C. R. Clayton, and J. Oudar (The Electrochemical Society, Pennington, NJ, 1984), p. 114.
18. J. B. Lumsden, D. S. Gnanamuthu, and R. J. Moores, in Ref. 17, p. 122.

19. P. G. Moore in Ref. 17, p. 102.
20. J. N. DeFranq, Br. Corrosion J. 1, 29 (1974).
21. G. Wrangler, in Sulfide Inclusions in Steel, edited by J. J. deBarbadillo and E. Snipe (A.S.M., Metals Park, Ohio, 1975), p. 361.
22. Z. Szklarska-Smialowska in Ref. 21, p. 380.
23. A. J. Sedriks, International Met. Revs. 28, 295 (1983).
24. P. L. Bonora, Mater. Sci. Eng. 69, 253 (1985).
25. P. L. Bonora, M. Bassoli, P. L. DeAnna, C. Battaglin, G. Della Mea, P. Mazzoldi, and E. Jannitti, Mater. Chem. 5, 73 (1980).
26. T. R. Anthony and H. R. Cline, J. Appl. Phys. 49, 1248 (1978).
27. H. H. Uhlig, Corrosion and Corrosion Control (John Wiley, New York, 1971), p. 300.
28. Y. Nakao and K. Nishimoto, "Desensitization of Stainless Steels by Laser Surface Heat Treatment," Osaka University (September, 1985), IIW Doc. IX-1348-85.
29. J. B. Lumsden, D. S. Gnanamuthu, and R. J. Moores in Ref. 16, p. 129.
30. P.G. Moore and E. McCafferty, "Proceedings of the 9th International Congress on Metallic Corrosion," Vol. 2, p. 636 (1984).
31. E. McCafferty, P. G. Moore, and G. T. Peace, J. Electrochem. Soc. 129, 9 (1982).
32. P. L. Bonora, M. Bassoli, P. L. DeAnna, G. Battaglin, G. Della Mea, P. Mazzoldi, and A. Miotello, Electrochim. Acta 25, 1497 (1980).
33. P. L. Bonora, M. Bassoli, G. Cerisola, P. L. DeAnna, G. Battaglin, G. Della Mea, and P. Mazzoldi, Thin Solid Films 81, 339 (1981).
34. J. A. McKay and J. T. Schriempf, Appl. Phys. Lett. 35, 433 (1979).
35. B. C. Allen, in Liquid Metals: Chemistry and Physics, edited by S. Z. Beer (Marcel Dekker, New York, 1972), p. 161.
36. J. Yahalom and T. P. Hoar, Electrochim. Acta 15, 877 (1970).
37. E. A. Ammar, Corros. Prevention Control 19 (2), 8 (1972).
38. A. Charlesby, Proc. Phys. Soc. B66, 317 (1953).
39. H. A. Johansen, G. B. Adams, Jr., and P. Van Ryselberghe, J. Electrochem. Soc. 104, 339 (1957).
40. P. Mazzoldi, G. Della Mea, G. Battaglin, A. Miotello, M. Servidori, D. Bacci, and E. Jannitti, Phys. Rev. Lett. 44, 88 (1980).
41. C. W. Draper, R. E. Woods, and L. S. Meyer, Corrosion 36, 405 (1980).
42. M. W. Gabriel, C. M. Preece, A. Staudinger, and C. W. Draper, IEEE J. Quantum Electron. 17, 2000 (1981).
43. C. W. Draper, J. Mater. Sci. 16, 2774 (1981).
44. J. Javadpour, C. R. Clayton, and C. W. Draper, in Ref. 16, p. 135.
45. C. W. Draper, J. M. Vandenberg, C. M. Preece, and C. R. Clayton, in Rapidly Solidified Amorphous and Crystalline Alloys, edited by B. H. Kear, B. C. Giessen, and M. Cohen (Elsevier, 1982), p. 529.
46. A. A. Smith, Corrosion Prevention and Control 19, 29 (1963).
47. J. C. Rowlands, Corros. Sci. 2, 89 (1962).
48. C. W. Draper and S. P. Sharma, Thin Solid Films 84, 333 (1981).
49. C. W. Draper, D. C. Jacobson, J. M. Gibson, J. M. Poate, J. M. Vandenberg, and A. G. Cullis, in Laser and Electron-Beam Interactions with Solids, edited by B. R. Appleton and G. K. Celler (Elsevier, 1982), p. 413.
50. C. W. Draper, L. S. Meyer, D. C. Jacobson, L. Buene, and J. M. Poate, Thin Solid Films 75, 237 (1981).
51. M. Stern and H. Wissenberg, J. Electrochem. Soc. 106, 759 (1959).

52. N. D. Tomashov, R. M. Altovsky, and G. P. Chernova, J. Electrochem. Soc. 108, 113 (1961); Russ. J. Phys. Chem. 35, 523 (1961).
53. G. K. Hubler and E. McCafferty, Corros. Sci. 20, 103 (1980).
54. Y. Waseda and K. T. Aust, J. Mater. Sci. 16, 2337 (1981).
55. K. Hashimoto, in Amorphous Metallic Alloys, edited by F. E. Luborsky (Butterworths, London, 1983), p. 471.
56. K. Hashimoto, K. Osada, T. Masumoto, and S. Shimodaira, Corros. Sci. 16, 71 (1976).
57. See, for example, M. Wislawska and M. Janik-Czachor, Werk. U. Korros. 20, 36 (1985).
58. R. Becker, G. Sepold, and P. L. Ryder, in Chemistry and Physics of Rapidly Solidified Materials, edited by B. J. Berkowitz and R. O. Scattergood (A.I.M.E., 1983), p. 235.
59. K. Asami, T. Sato, and K. Hashimoto, J. Non-Cryst. Solids 68, 261 (1984).
60. H. Yoshioka, K. Asami, and K. Hashimoto, Scr. Metall. 18, 1215 (1984).
61. H. Yoshioka, K. Asami, A. Kawashima, and K. Hashimoto, in "Fifth International Conference on Rapidly Quenched Metals," Wurzburg, 1984.
62. K. Hashimoto, K. Asami, and A. Kawashima, in "Critical Issues in Reducing the Corrosion of Steels - Proceedings of USA-Japan Seminar," edited by H. Leidheiser, Jr., and S. Haruyama, p. 214 (1985).
63. J. D. Ayers, R. J. Schaefer, F. D. Bogar, and E. McCafferty, Corrosion 37, 55 (1981).
64. H. Bhat, H. Herman, and R. J. Coyle, in Laser in Materials Processing, edited by E. A. Metzbower (A.S.M., Metals Park, Ohio, 1983), p. 176.
65. C. R. Clayton, W. K. Chan, J. K. Hirvonen, G. K. Hubler, and J. R. Reed, in Ref. 17, p. 17.

LASER SURFACE ALLOYING AND CLADDING FOR CORROSION AND WEAR

J. MAZUMDER, J. SINGH
Department of Mechanical and Industrial Engineering, University of Illinois at Urbana-Champaign, Urbana, IL 61801

Key Words: corrosion, friction, wear, ferrous alloys

In order to develop corrosion- and wear-resistant surfaces, two processes, laser surface alloying and laser surface cladding, were used. They are discussed in turn.

1. LASER SURFACE ALLOYING (LSA)

Laser surface alloying is a process in which the surface of a workpiece is melted to a desired depth using the laser beam with the simultaneous addition of powdered alloying elements. This leads to a rapid method of localized alloy synthesis. In this process, since alloying elements diffuse in a thin liquid layer by convection, it is feasible to obtain the required depth of alloying in small time intervals (typically 0.1 to 10 ms). Thus, a desired alloy composition can be generated <u>in situ</u> on given substrate surfaces. The alloy composition will govern microstructure, and laser-processing conditions (cooling rates) will govern the degree of microstructural refinement. Depending upon the choice of alloy design or development at the surface, a less expensive base material such as AISI 1016 steel can be locally modified to increase the resistance to wear, erosion, corrosion, and high-temperature oxidation. Only those surfaces locally modified will possess properties characteristic of high-performance alloys. Using this technique, Fe-Cr-Ni surface alloys have been developed for corrosion resistance and Fe-Cr-Mn-C alloys for wear resistance. The experimental procedures, the surface properties, and microstructure developed during laser surface alloying are discussed below.

1.1. Experimental Procedure

The experimental apparatus for laser surface alloying and cladding consists of two units working simultaneously, the laser and powder delivery. The laser system, first unit, produces a beam that interacts with the substrate and powder to form an alloy. The LSA was carried out using an AVCO HPL 10 kW continuous-wave CO_2 laser with F7 casegrain optics as shown in Fig. 1. The laser was operated at a TEM_{01}^{*} mode. The beam produced by the casegrain optics was focused downward towards the substrate by a flat mirror. The LSA was done with typically a 2 mm beam diameter. Powder delivery system, the second unit, delivers powders to the substrate.

Commercially available Cr and Ni powder (2 μm diameter) in the different ratios was used as mixed powder feed for laser surface alloying. The powder was delivered at the point of laser material interaction. The powder flow was regulated by varying the speed and changing the size of the feed screw. Argon gas with a flow rate of 0.017 lb/s was used to maintain a steady powder flow through the copper tubing leading to the

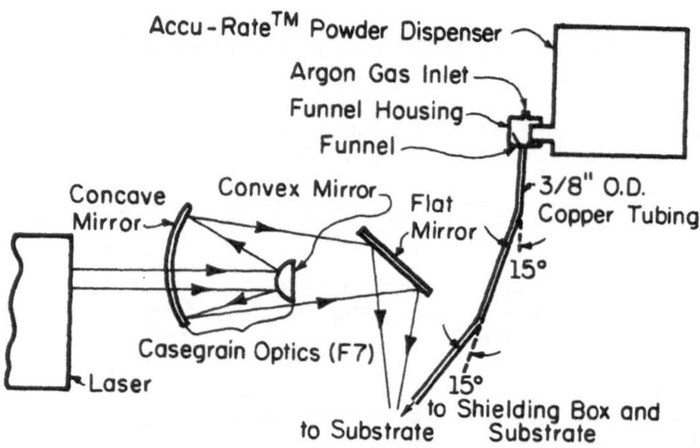

FIGURE 1. Laser optics and powder delivery system.

substrate. A shielding of argon or helium gas with a shielding box was used to minimize surface contamination during laser processing.

The laser was operated at power densities up to 10^6 W/cm^2. The substrate was traversed relative to the laser beam at speeds up to 3 cm/sec. The final composition of the LSA region depends upon the processing conditions such as laser power, size and shape of the laser beam, scan velocity, composition of the premixed powder and powder feed rate. The average composition of the Fe-Ni-Cr alloy as the function of laser power speed and feed rate is given in Table 1. The corrosion samples

TABLE 1. Averaged composition of Fe + Cr + Ni alloys by EPMA

Laser Power (kW)	Speed (mm/s)	Feed Rate (g/s)	Cr (wt-pct)	Ni (wt-pct)
6	16.5	0.25	22.1	17.2
5	16.5	0.25	35.1	25.5
5	16.5	0.25	38.3	23.7
6	20.7	0.18	13.1	10.1
6	20.7	0.19	16.3	12.3
6	24.9	0.2	28.4	19.5
6	29.5	0.2	34.8	23.3
5	24.8	0.2	37.6	21.8

were made from the LSA region. TEM samples were also made from the alloyed zone adjacent to the corrosion sample. Corrosion tests were carried out using standard potentiostate/galvanostate technique using 3.5 percent sodium chloride solution in distilled water.

2.2. Results and Discussion

The laser-alloyed samples passivated spontaneously (Figs. 2 and 3) in 3.5 percent NaCl solution and had a current density in the passive state about the same or less than that recorded for 304 grade stainless steel (0.12 mA/cm^2). The corrosion potential and pitting potential for some samples were more active than that recorded for 304 stainless steel (see Fig. 2). However, some samples have better corrosion resistance than 304 stainless (see Fig. 3).

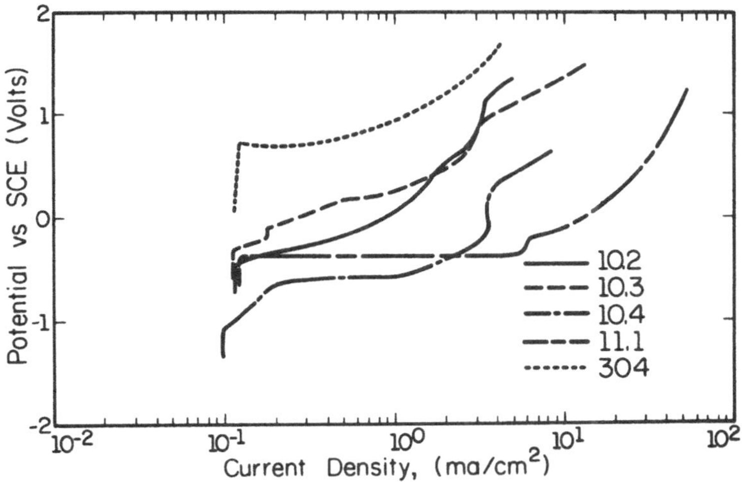

FIGURE 2. Anodic potentiodynamic scans for laser-processed samples and bulk 304 stainless steel in 3.5 percent salt solution. (Average compositions in weight percent are: 10.2 = 16 Cr, 12 Ni; 10.3 = 28 Cr, 26 Ni; 10.4 = 35 Cr, 23 Ni; 11.1 = 37 Cr, 22 Ni).

Corrosion results imply that the alloys were mechanically and metallurgically sound and the process was reproducible. There were no cracks through which the salt solution could corrode the base material directly. Also, the alloys had sufficient amounts of Cr and Ni in solution for them to spontaneously passivate and show good corrosion resistance. The samples were tested in the as-processed condition. As most samples had surface irregularities and some even had shallow grooves, these could have produced locally severe crevice corrosion conditions. This may explain the observed fact that pitting potentials for these samples were generally more active than the pitting potential recorded for bulk 304

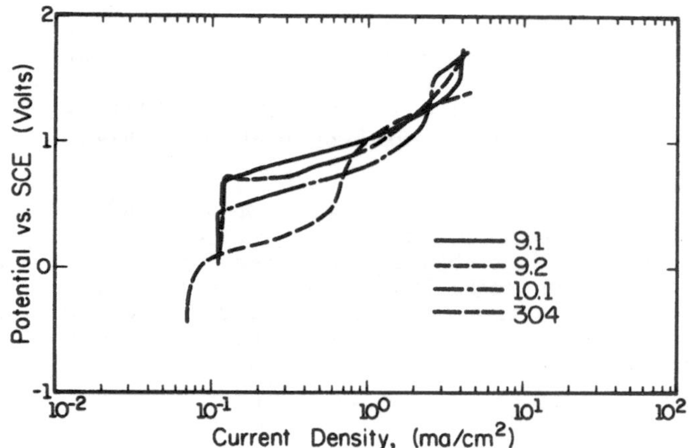

FIGURE 3. Anodic potentiodynamic scans for laser-processed samples and bulk 304 stainless steel in 3.5 percent salt solution. (Average compositions in weight percent are: 9.1 = 22 Cr, 17 Ni; 9.2 = 35 Cr, 26 Ni; 10.1 = 13 Cr, 10 Ni).

stainless steel which had a flat flow free surface. Results from Lamb (1) suggest that residual tensile stress in laser processed material may also contribute to corrosion. However, present data are insufficient to make a definite conclusion regarding corrosion and pitting potentials.

The corrosion current density in the passive state for all laser-alloyed samples was about the same as that measured for bulk 304 stainless steel. This implies that even with surface imperfections, the corrosion resistance performance of the present laser surface alloys is comparable to that of 304 stainless steel. The corrosion properties basically depend on the overall composition and microstructure of the LSA region which is discussed below.

Optical examination of the Laser-Alloyed Zones (LAZ) showed that the highly alloyed Fe-Cr alloys had a grain size about 11 times greater than that seen in the Fe-Cr-Ni alloys. A high degree of refinement was observed in some of the Fe+Ni alloys, showing structures on the scale of 5 nm. Transmission electron microscopic investigation of the LAZ was also carried out. Cr-rich blocky precipitates were observed at grain boundaries (Fig. 4). A BCC structure with a highly dislocated lath microstructure was commonly seen (Fig. 5). Diffraction patterns for these foils did not show any orientation relationships between the laths. These observations are generally characteristic of low carbon steel quenched structures. The presence of preferred orientation was seen in another foil, while several other foils also showed the presence of microcrystalline areas. In addition to this, featureless amorphous regions were also seen in a LAZ made at 8 x 10^5 W/cm^2 and a traverse of 50 mm/s.

---

(1) M. Lamb, CISFEL, 1984.

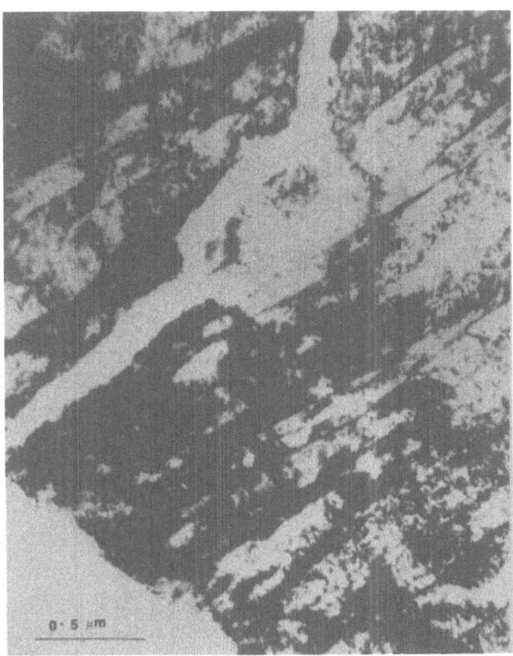

FIGURE 4. Cr-rich grain boundary precipitates at a depth below 375 μm from the surface in sample made at 6 kW laser power, 3 mm beam diameter and 12.7 mm/s traverse speed with Cr powder feed.

The observed microstructures are a function of both composition and cooling rate. With a suitable composition, amorphous materials can be made at fairly modest cooling rates (up to a few million degrees per second). Cooling rates increase as solidification proceeds towards the surface and, as seen here, amorphous material is expected at the top rather than the bottom of the pool. With the large amounts of Cr in solution and the 0.16 percent carbon in the base materials, precipitation of Cr-rich precipitates is possible at grain boundaries. The sample showing lath structure but lack of orientation relationship between laths had about 12 percent by weight of Cr (Fig. 5). It must have passed through the $\gamma \rightarrow \alpha$ region, and the lack of orientation relationship probably means the laths were separated by low-angle boundaries. The commonly seen large dislocation density in the foils is to be expected in rapidly solidified steels. Large grains high in Cr, Fe-Cr alloys could occur if they formed at high temperature during solidification. There are no solid-state transformations that could occur at high cooling rates to refine the microstructure and the large grains would be retained at room temperature. This would also explain the lack of segregation and the resultant difficulty in developing the microstructure during etching.

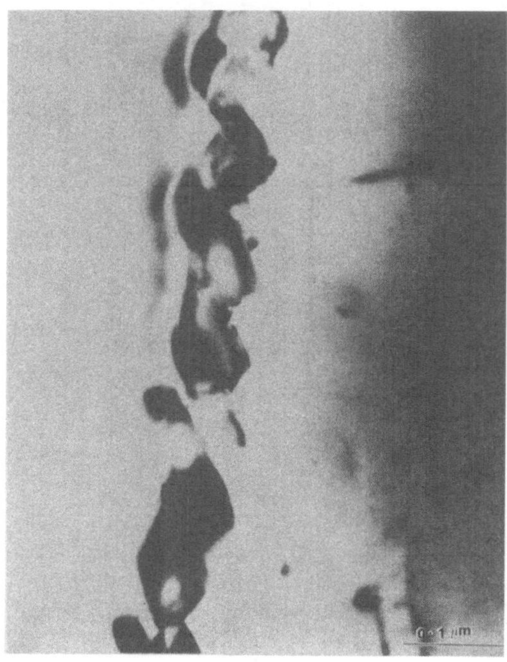

FIGURE 5. Dislocated lath structure from a laser alloy with 12.5 percent Cr and 1.5 percent Ni that showed BCC single-crystal diffraction pattern and no orientation relationships between laths.

It is worth noting that alloys with 58 percent Cr, 26 percent Ni were produced. Not only would such alloys have good oxidation resistance at elevated temperatures, but their susceptibility to Cr depletion at grain boundaries would be lower, as there is plenty of Cr within the bulk of the grain to diffuse to the grain boundary and compensate for Cr depletion.

2. LASER SURFACE CLADDING (LSC)

Laser surface cladding is a process where the powders of different compositions are delivered into the laser-generated thin melt pool of the substrate and the powders are also melted by the laser. A thin layer of cladded alloy is formed with a different chemistry from the substrate. The main objective of the laser cladding process is to clad a substrate with another material with a different chemistry by melting a thin interfacial layer to produce a metallurgical bond with minimum dilution of the clad layer and to provide good surface wear and the corrosion properties.

There is continuous demand and challenging opportunities towards the development of wear, friction, and corrosion-resistant coatings for many industries. In response to this challenge, laser-cladding process was exploited. To achieve better wear and friction properties, the laser cladding was focused on the development of Fe-Cr-Mn-C systems. The wear and friction properties and microstructure development during laser surface cladding are discussed below.

2.1. Experimental Procedure

AISI 1016 steel was used as a substrate. Cr, Mn, and C powders in the ratio of 10:1:1 were used as mixed powder for cladding. Cladding was carried out by AVCO HPL 10 kW cw CO_2 laser with F7 casegrain optics. The laser was operated at approximately 3 and 5 kW with a defocused beam of 2 mm diameter. Specimens were traversed relative to the laser beam at a speed of approximately 0.6 and 5 cm/s.

2.2. Results and Discussion

The preliminary friction and wear results for LSC are averaged and plotted in Fig. 6 as a function of the table speed and laser power. For comparison purposes, two additional values of both friction and wear are shown. One was obtained from the base material of the block (AISI 1016 steel) and the other from Stellite 6. The wear data indicate that the LSC has superior tribological characteristics when compared to the Stellite 6 for the operating conditions considered. By using laser alloying and cladding, surfaces with the same or superior wear characteristics were produced more economically and without cobalt. This avoids cobalt contamination problems associated with Stellite cladding. It should be noted that the wear data given in Fig. 6 are in terms of "width of the wear scar." If these data were plotted in terms of wear volume, a more dramatic difference could be seen between the laser-alloyed surfaces and Stellite 6.

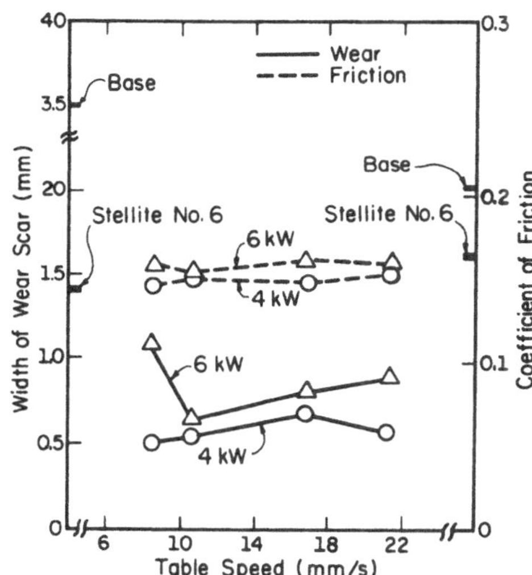

FIGURE 6. Friction and wear of laser-cladded surfaces as a function of table speed and laser power.

The wear data presented in Fig. 6 indicate that better results are obtained with the laser power at 4 kW than at 6 kW. These findings are not surprising considering the more rapid solidification rates obtained when using 4 kW. This is because at 4 kW a smaller volume is melted compared to a power of 6 kW and, therefore, the substrate can self quench the melted zone at a faster rate. Also, smaller volume means higher concentration of alloying elements leading to a higher proportion of alloy carbides which in turn produces better wear resistance.

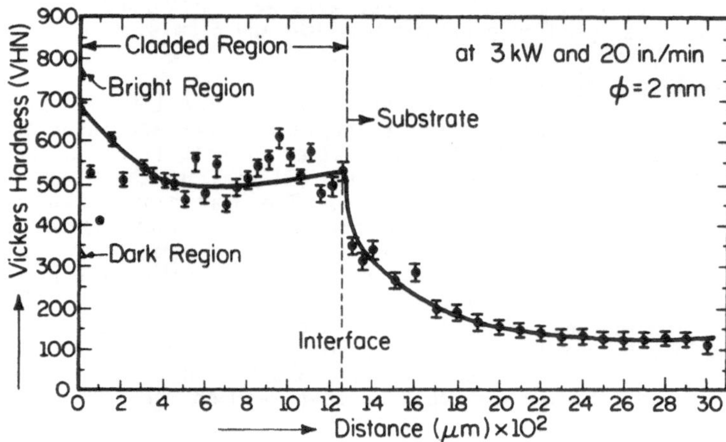

FIGURE 7. Hardness profile across the laser-cladded and substrate region.

Figure 7 shows the variation in hardness (VHN) across the laser-cladded region and the substrate. The scattering and fluctuation in hardness was due to the presence of fine and uniform distributions of the second phases in the matrix. The degree of uniformity and fine microstructure depends upon the laser processing connditions. Subsequently, the final microstructure has also an influence on the wear and friction properties. The best wear and friction properties were achieved at the lower laser power (3 kW) and high traverse speed (1 cm/s). The wear and friction properties are also governed by the presence of different phases in the cladded region and solid solubility of alloying elements in matrix. A general microstructural survey of the sample shows the presence of M_7C_3 and M_6 type carbides in the ferrite matrix (Figs. 8b,c, respectively). The solid solibility of Cr in ferrite was increased up to 50 percent and it also depends upon the laser processing conditions (Fig. 9). The volume fraction of these phases could be further controlled by the laser processing conditions as well as the initial composition of the powder which eventually control the wear and friction properties.

In order to improve the wear, friction, and corrosion-resistant properties, the Fe-Cr-Mn-C surface alloy was also developed. It has been observed that the wear properties of the laser surface alloys are much superior to the Stellite 6 (Fig. 10). The coefficient of friction for Stellite and the laser surface alloyed is approximately the same. An interesting observation is that both friction and wear are not significantly affected by table speed for the range of alloys considered. The microstructure for laser surface alloyed materials is similar to laser-cladded Fe-Cr-Mn-C alloy. Therefore, microstructure is discussed in detail in the section on cladding.

3. CONCLUDING REMARKS

It is evident from the above discussion on laser alloying and cladding that novel alloys can be synthesized on metal surfaces with relative ease. These alloys are not confined by equilibrium thermodynamics. Thus, this provides an enormous opportunity to engineer the microstructure to specific needs.

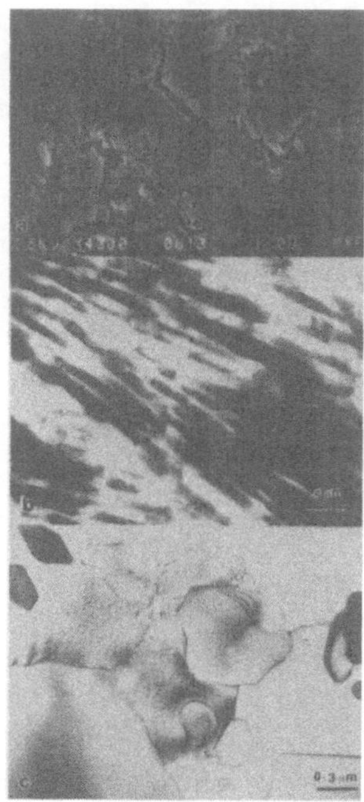

FIGURE 8. Representative SEM (a) and TEM (b and c) micrographs of laser-cladded region showing the aligned M_7C_3 type carbide and M_6C type carbide precipitates in ferrite matrix, respectively.

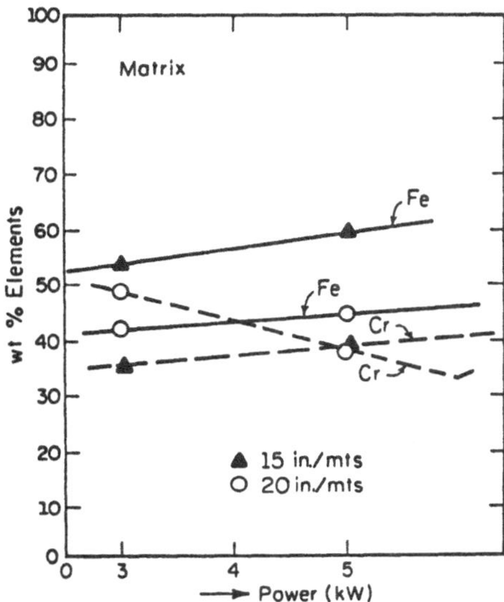

FIGURE 9. Effect of alloying elements in matrix with function of laser power and traverse speed.

LASER PREPARATION OF METAL SURFACES FOR TELECOMMUNICATION NEEDS

CLIFTON W. DRAPER
AT&T Engineering Research Center, Princeton, USA

Key Words: gold alloys, stainless coppers, contact finishes

1. INTRODUCTION

The requirements placed on metal surface finishes for use as connector contacts, switches and relays are quite stringent. The contact surfaces must be conductive and maintain stable contact resistance for long periods, even in polluted gas-phase type environments. In addition, open-close and multiple insertion mechanical actions result in the need for wear resistance.

Laser surface treatment offers a means to achieve these objectives. In this article three examples from our own research activity will be reviewed. Two of the examples fall into the category of laser surface alloying or mixing, while the other is an example of laser surface melting as a superior surface finishing method.

Laser alloying is a material processing method which utilizes the high power density available from focused laser sources to melt metal coatings and a portion of the underlying substrate (1,2). Since the melting occurs in a very short time and only at the surface, the bulk of the material remains cool, thus serving as an intimate heat sink. Large temperature gradients exist across the boundary between the melted surface region and the underlying solid substrate. The result is rapid self-quenching and resolidification. Quench rates as great as 10^{11}K sec^{-1} and concomitant resolidification velocities of 20 m sec^{-1} have already been realized.

What makes laser surface alloying both attractive and interesting is the wide variety of chemical and microstructural states that can be retained because of the rapid quench from the liquid phase. These include chemical profiles where the "alloyed" element is highly concentrated near the atomic surface and decreases in concentration over shallow depths (hundereds of nanometers). The types of microstructures observed include extended solid solutions, metastable crystalline phases, and metallic glasses. The technique is quite unique for tailoring surfaces and thereby surface properties.

2. PROCEDURE

There are presently a large number of commercially available laser sources used to induce the melting needed. Of these a relatively small number, including the carbon dioxide (CO_2), neodymium doped yittrium-aluminum garnet group, (Nd:YAG), neodymium doped glass (Nd:glass) and chromium doped aluminum oxide (Ruby), account for nearly all surface alloying work. The laser characteristics - wavelength, output power, beam diameter, output mode, pulse length and repetition rate - are important processing factors that come into play when considering the choice of laser source. In addition, the laser source may be modified as in the use of harmonic generators to frequency double Nd-YAG and Ruby lasers into the green and ultraviolet respectively, or the use of acousto-optical modulation to "Q-switch" a solid state laser source.

Figure 1 presents the normal spectral reflectance of Au (3). Annotated on the abscissa are four laser wavelengths. Of these laser sources the optimum choice is the frequency doubled Nd-YAG.

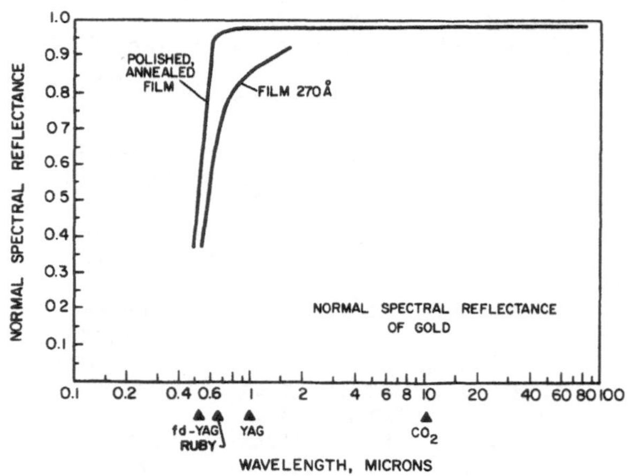

FIGURE 1. Normal spectral reflectance of Au.

For a Q-switched laser (high-power, short-pulse laser) source, the "pulse length" is the time of exposure. The laser pulses are emitted in a train of pulses characterized by a repetition rate. This train of pulses is raster-scanned across the metal surface to produce area coverage. For these lasers, the effective spot size, degree of overlap, and repetition rate determine the area per unit time which can be produced.

For all laser sources (continuous-wave, pulsed and Q-switched), the exposure time (dwell time or pulse length) strongly influences the depth that will be melted. Longer exposure times result in deeper melting. Since deeper melting means a longer total time in the molten state, that means more time available for diffusion of the one or more alloying elements into the molten portion of the substrate. Deeper melting and longer melt times therefore result in more dilute surface alloys, while shallow melting and shorter melt times result in more concentrated surface alloys.

An appreciation of the order of the melt depth and the scale of the melt time is necessary to determine mass transfer. Consider, as an example, a thin deposited film A on metal B. Q-switched laser sources, with pulse lengths (t_p) of 10's to 100's of nanoseconds, will produce melt times (t_L) on the order of 50 to 500 nanoseconds. Liquid phase diffusion coefficients (D_L) for metal solutes in metal melts are nearly all in the range of 10^{-4} to 10^{-5} cm^2 sec^{-1}. Thus the diffusion length or mixing range ($\sqrt{D_L t_L}$) for this short melt time-simple diffusion case will be on the order of 7 to 70 nm, which is significantly less than the calculated melt depth. Thus we would expect that the solute depth profile

(A_xB_{1-x}) would be: concentration peaked at the surface, sharp drop off over a depth on the scale of the diffusion length, a low (near zero value) out to the melt depth, and a zero value beyond the melt depth.

3. EXAMPLES

Such a profile appears in Fig. 2 for the case of Au surface alloyed into Ni following irradiation by a Q-switched laser source (4). These profiles have been successfully reproduced with straightforward models incorporating little more than known liquid state diffusion coefficients and heat flow estimates of the melt time (5).

For comparison we also look at the case of relatively thin films and deeper melting illustrated by the Au in Ni depth profiles (4) in Fig. 2 for a melt time greater than 50 μsec (CW-CO_2 laser). The melt depth and melt time are much greater than those for the Q-switched lasers. The greatly increased melt time allows diffusion of the Au over much greater depths. Over the depth range analyzed the Au profile in Fig. 2 is completely flat.

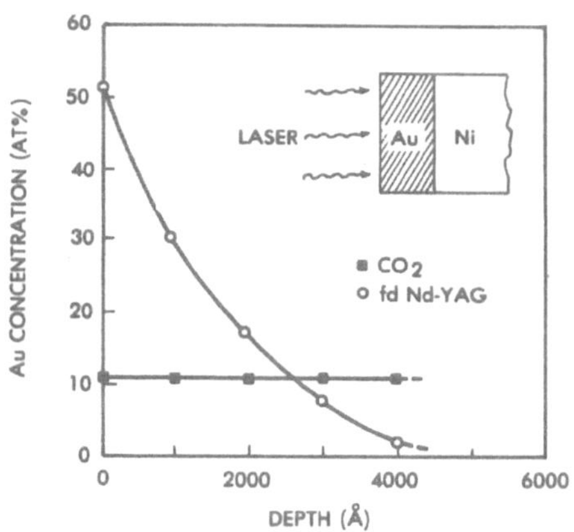

FIGURE 2. Surface alloys introduced by laser alloying (CW-CO_2 or Q-fd-Nd:YAG) Au films on Ni (4). t_L for the Nd:YAG is about 500 nsec, for the CW-CO_2 greater than 50 sec. Polycrystalline samples (10 x 20 mm) are prepared from strip stock (0.64 mm thick) of commercial grade nickel 200. Thin Au films (150 nm, ○ ; 350 nm, ■) are vacuum deposited onto room-temperature substrates at pressures of 1 x 10^{-5} torr. The surface alloys produced by the various laser systems were analyzed using Rutherford backscattering spectroscopy.

The structural relationship of the Au-Ni surface alloy to the parent base metal, was examined with Rutherford backscattering and channeling (4). The fact that the Au (110) and random yields are in the same ratio as the Ni (110) and random yields indicates that the Au atoms are substitutional. The measured ratio of 60% is a measure of the high degree of disorder in the Au-Ni lattice.

The highly competitive forces in the electronics and telecommunications market place great pressure on the R&D sector to produce reliable contact finishes that reduce or eliminate the need for gold. One of the more recently introduced contact finishes in AT&T is the so called "diffused gold" surface (6). Very thin films of gold are diffused into palladium or palladium-silver inlays, or into palladium electrodeposits. In 1985 the savings realized in AT&T on a few components finished with gold-flashed palladium electrodeposits instead of electroplated gold was more than $12 million dollars (7). "Diffused gold" surfaces can be prepared by two different methods. In the first method the thin Au layer and a portion of the Pd underlayer are melted on a nanosecond timescale with Q-switched laser radiation (8). The intermixing is quenched by the resolidification process such that a graded distribution of Au in Pd results. In the second method the thin Au layer is diffused into the underlying Pd or PdAg alloys during an elevated temperature inlaying process (6). Here the solid state interdiffusion of the metals occurs over times that are long compared to the laser liquid state method, but sufficiently rapid to make it a viable production method. This is possible in the case of Au and Pd because interdiffusion is measurable even at room temperature and is quite extensive at only 550K (9). In either method the Au distribution in the Pd or PdAg layer is much like that of Au in Ni (open circles) presented in Fig. 2 above.

Another family of surface alloys produced by laser mixing of predeposited layers has come to be known as "stainless coppers". In these laser surface alloys the substate is copper or a copper alloy and the thin film elements are Cr/Ni or Cr/Cu.

Consider the binary Cr-Cu system. There is a limited region of liquid immiscibility, a two-phase regime below the liquidus that spans nearly the entire diagram, and a sharply decreasing solid solubility for Cr in Cu with decreasing temperture (see Fig. 3). It is not possible, therefore, by conventional bulk metallurgical manufacturing methods to produce single-phase alloys of Cr in Cu at concentrations greater than a fraction of an atomic percent.

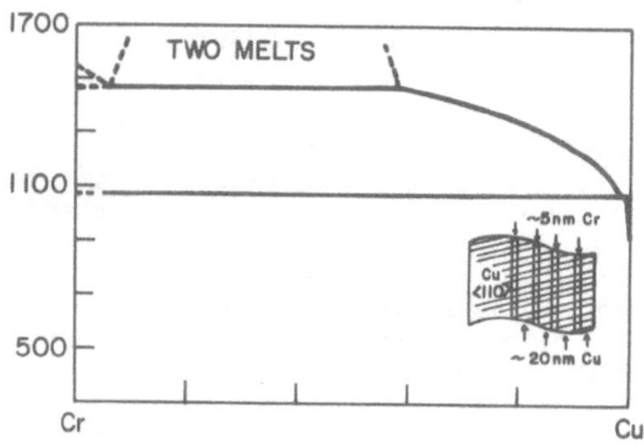

FIGURE 3. Cr-Cu Phase Diagram With Multilayer Sample Configuration Insert

We have prepared (10) single-crystal (110) Cu with a multilayer Cr-Cu film structure (See Fig. 3) which has been laser alloyed using

Q-switched fd Nd-YAG laser pulses. Following laser alloying the Cr diffuses over 240 nm with a peak concentration of 18 at.-% at 70 nm and the surface layer is epitaxial as confirmed by both TEM and He^+ channeling.

An example (11) from the ternary Cu/Cr/Ni case is given in Fig. 4. In this case polycrystalline substrates of a copper alloy containing 2-3 at % Sn were sequentially deposited with thin films of Cr and Ni-8at% V. Laser mixing was accomplished with a raster scanned, frequency doubled Q-switched Nd-YAG laser. The laser incident power density used was 95 MW cm^{-2}. Surface alloyed samples were examined for lateral uniformity with scanning electron microscopy - energy dispersive X-ray element mapping and with scanning Auger microscopy. Within the recognized limitations of both of these methods, the surfaces appear to be laterally uniform.

The Auger sputter depth profile of the as-deposited sample in Fig. 4a shows the clearly defined interfaces that result from discrete layers. It is evident that the interface boundaries loose resolution as the sputtering proceeds deeper into the material. The interface that is closer to the surface, separating the outermost Ni layer and the underlying Cr, appears to be substantially sharper than the Cr/Cu interface that is some 120 nm from the surface.

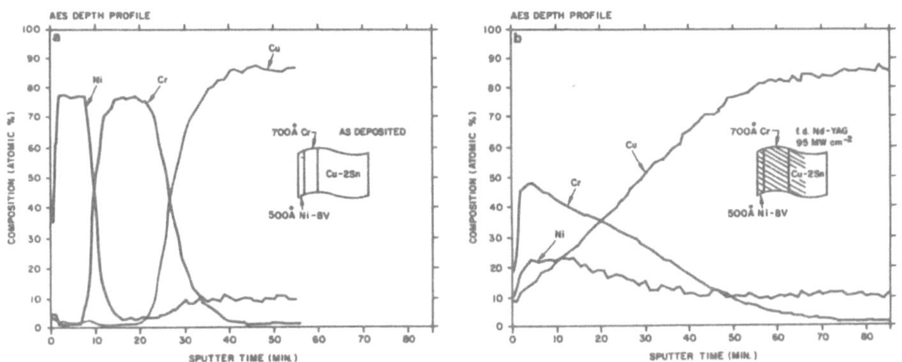

FIGURE 4. AES sputter profiles for the as-deposited and 95 MW cm^{-2} frequency doubled, Q-switched Nd-YAG laser mixed sample. (a) AES sputter profile, as deposited; (b) AES sputter profile, 95 MW cm^{-2}. The insert in each figure is a schematic cross sectional representation. Solid hatch marks indicate the extent of the melt front.

Auger sputter depth profile characterization of the 95 MW cm^{-2} laser mixed sample is shown in Fig. 4b. Both the Ni/Cr and Cr/Cu interfaces have been obliterated by the effect of the laser mixing. It is apparent that not only have the layered elements been mixed and penetrated somewhat into the Cu substrate, but that sufficient time in the liquid state has allowed Cu and Sn (not shown) to diffuse to the surface.

If one accounts for the overlap of Cu in the Ni window, then one can see that the Cr and Ni maintain a roughly 2:1 ratio form the surface to a depth of at least 200 nm.

The microstructure of this laser mixed surface has been investigated by glancing angle x-ray diffraction and by transmission electron microscopy. Microstructural anlaysis on the same sample in Fig. 4 confirms that in the case of thin multilayers of Ni and Cr laser alloyed into Cu-2Sn the resulting near surface region is a metallic glass.

High relative humidity, elevated temperature gaseous Cl_2 and H_2S environments are frequently used to test precious metal overlayers and precious metal substitutes for device applications. Such a gaseous test facility was used to study some stainless copper surfaces in a H_2S accelerated corrosion environment. After prolonged exposure (equivalent to more than 30 years) there was no detectable film growth on the stainless copper surfaces. These experiments suggested that the name "stainless" may in fact be appropriate.

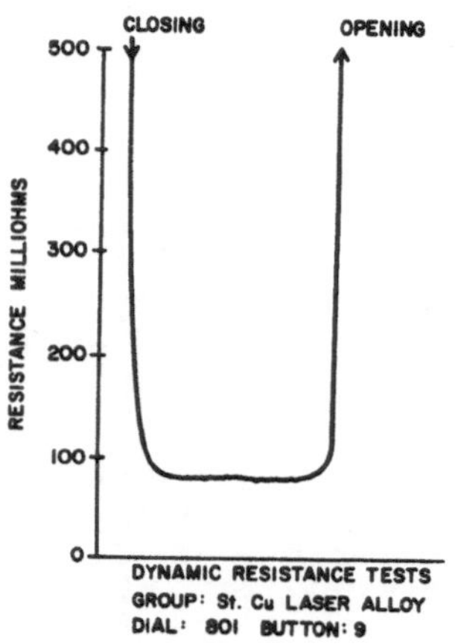

FIGURE 5. Dynamic circuit resistance test data on stainless Cu laser alloy. The abscissa is time for open-close-open clicking action for dial button.

A low, stable contact resistance is required of any finish used in telecommunication applications such as switches, relays, and connectors. Controlled load plungers that simulate the opening and closing clicking actions of switches are frequently used to evaluate material finishes for suitability. Dials were assembled from laser alloyed material that was punched out from surface alloyed strip stock. Each dial contained 12 buttons. The buttons were tested under a controlled load plunger. Data were automatically stored on each button of each dial through multiples of 50,000 cycles. Fig. 5 presents one such open-close cycle. The desired behavior is a flat well bottom below 300 mΩ (package circuit resistance) that does not drift over the duration of the cycle testing. Those requirements were easily met by the stainless coppers.

The focus of this article to this point has been on laser alloying, however, there are two other ways that lasers have been used in relation to gold coating methods. The first is laser enhanced electroplating wherein the laser beam defines the track of gold deposited from the electrolyte. The use of lasers for spatial definition of Au deposition from solution has been receiving considerable attention since it was first reported by von Gutfeld (12). Those interested in details of the process and the mechanisms should consult a review article by von Gutfeld in the IBM journal (13), or see the article by Celis, et al. in this NATO book. It has been reported at CLEO meetings in 1984 and 1985 that the process is being used to make products in IBM's Endicott, New York plant.

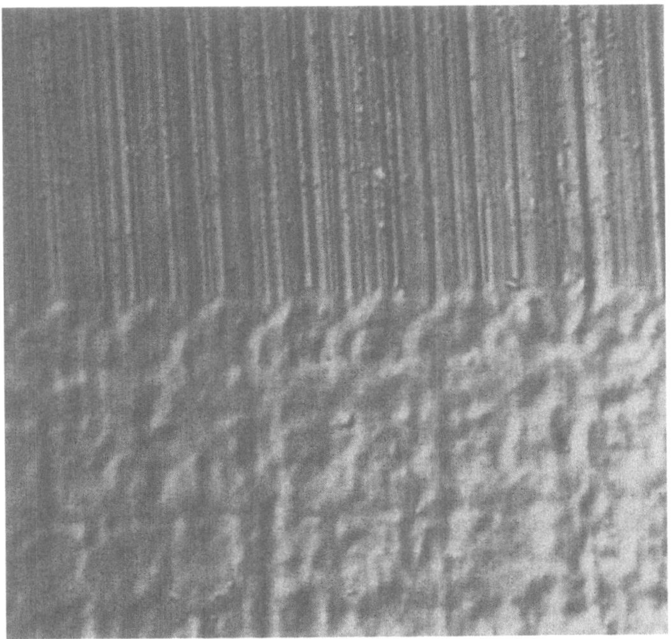

FIGURE 6. Surface micrograph of laser surface melted Cu alloy.

The second other area is laser surface finishing of copper alloys prior to conventional electroplating of gold. Laser surface melting of copper alloys has been demonstarted (14,15) to produce an ultrasmooth finish on a microscopic scale. The photomicrograph in Fig. 6 shows a before (top) and after (bottom) surface finish on a copper alloy that has been laser surface melted with a Q-switched frequency doubled Nd:YAG laser. The before surface finish is that of a high quality cold rolled surface. The rolling marks stand out at this magnification because of the use of Nomarski interference constrast microscopy. The after laser melting finish literally converts the surface finish to mirror like.

These surfaces were found to result in superior quality gold electroplates with significantly reduced porosity (14). Since the pore count (N cm^{-2}) (porosity) of a gold electroplate is inversely related to the thickness of the plating required, a reduction in porosity means less gold may be used. In addition, it was found that these surfaces themselves (uncoated with Au) exhibited improved resistance to both sulfur and chlorine corrosive atmospheres (15).

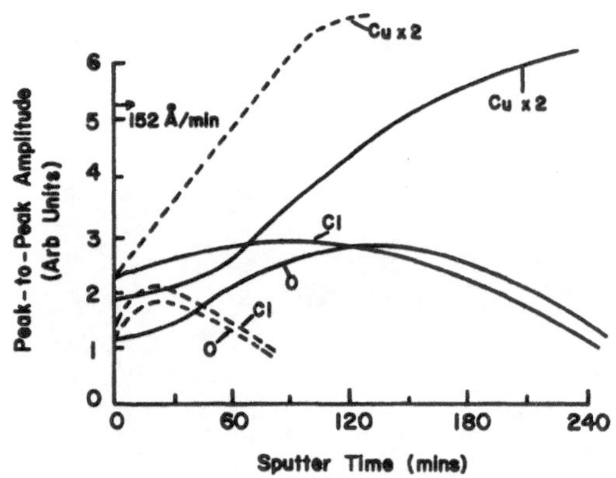

FIGURE 7. Auger depth profile of the C72500 sample exposed to 1.8 ppm Cl_2 at 80% RH for 4 days. Solid curves are for untreated Cu alloy surfaces; dashed curves are for laser surface melted surfaces.

Figure 7 presents an example of this result for a laser surface melted Cu-Ni-Sn alloy (UNS designation C72500). The solid curves in Fig. 7 show Auger depth profiles for the non-LSM C72500 surface exposed for 4 days to 1.8 ppm Cl_2 at 80% relative humidity. The estimated film thickness on this coupon is about 3,600 nm. In comparison, the dashed curves in Fig. 7show the depth profiles from the LSM surface exposed to equivalent conditions. It is estimated that the film thickness is about 900 nm. This shows a fourfold reduction in the corrosion film thickness. Thus, a significant improvement in corrosion behavior is observed in a very aggressive Cl_2 environment test. It should be noted that the corrosion film thickness found on the non-LSM portion of these samples was comparable with the results routinely obtained on copper and its alloys, which have been studied in AT&T laboratories for many years.

4. SUMMARY

A number of examples of how laser processing of metal surfaces can be used to meet the surface finishing needs of the telecommunication industry have been briefly discussed. Work in AT&T and other companies has shown that laser surface processing holds great promise for being an effective method of reducing precious metal usage.

REFERENCES

1. C. W. Draper and J. M. Poate, International Metals Review 30, 85-108 (1985).
2. C. W. Draper, Journal of Metals 34, 24-32 (1982).
3 Y. S. Touloukian and D. P. DeWitt, Thermophysical Properties of Matter (IFI/Plenum, New York, 1970), Vol. 7, p. 258.
4. C. W. Draper, L. S. Meyer, L. Buene, D. C. Jacobson, and J. M. Poate, Appl. Surf. Sci. 7, 276-280 (1981).
5. K. Rozniakowski and A. Dolny, Thin Solid Films 121, 121-126 (1984).
6. F. E. Bader, Diffused Gold R156-A New Inlay Contact Material for Bell System Connectors, Proceedings 11th Intern. Conf. Electrical Contact Phenomena, West Berlin, 7 June 1982.
7. J. A. Abys and H. S. Trop, AT&T Bell Laboratories Record, pp. 4-8, January 1985.
8. C. W. Draper and J. M. Poate, "Laser Surface Alloying" US Patent 4,495,255, Jan. 22, 1985.
9. H. D. Shih, E. Bauer, and H. Poppa, Thin Solid Films 88, L21 (1982).
10. C. W. Draper et al., in Laser and Electron Beam Interactions with Solids, edited by P. R. Appleton, and G. K. Celler (North-Holland, Amsterdam, 1982), pp. 413-418.
11. I. Sawchyn and C. W. Draper, Appl. Surf. Sci. 18, 86-105 (1984).
12. R. J. von Gutfeld, E. E. Tynan, R. L. Melcher, and S. E. Blum, Appl. Phys. Lett. 35, 651 (1979).
13. R. J. von Gutfeld, R. E. Acosta, and L. T. Romankiw, IBM Journal of Research and Development 26, 136 (1982).
14. C. W. Draper and S. P. Sharma, "Surface Melting of a Substrate Prior to Plating," US Patent 4,348,263, Sept. 7, 1983.
15. C. W. Draper and S. P. Sharma, Thin Solid Films 84, 333-340 (1981).

LASER ANNEALING AND LASER QUENCHING: PRODUCTION OF SUPERCONDUCTING ALLOYS

BERND STRITZKER
Institut für Festkörperforschung der Kernforschungsanlage, Jülich, West Germany

Key Words: Superconductivity, pulsed laser annealing, high T_c materials, amorphous superconductors

ABSTRACT

The effects of pulsed laser processing on the stoichiometry, microstructure and superconducting properties of high-T_c materials are reviewed. These materials require a perfect long-range order to show high-T_c values. The short annealing times of pulsed laser annealing limit the perfection of the long-range order.

In contrast, laser processing is perfectly suited for the production of metastable, superconducting alloys. Various laser-quenching experiments of targets at different temperatures are reviewed. Special emphasis is made on the comparison of this highly non-equilibrium method with other techniques like ion irradiation, vapor and liquid quenching. The comparison is mainly based on electrical and superconducting properties.

X-ray diffraction, electron microscopy and Rutherford backscattering yield additional information in some of the systems under investigation.

1. INTRODUCTION

Starting with the discovery of superconductivity in 1904, i.e., the disappearance of any electrical DC-resistance of a metal below a certain temperature, T_c, physicists and metallurgists managed during the course of this century to find new alloys with higher and higher T_c values (1). In 1973 the present best superconductor, Nb_3Ge, was found with a T_c of 23.2 K (2). The reason for the steady increase of T_c was always based on the application of the newest production techniques in order to stabilize the high-T_c phases, which unfortunately have a strong tendency not to crystallize in structures which one can readily obtain by equilibrium production techniques. That is the reason that laser processing was used immediately after its availability for the formation of superconductors (3). In the following paper a review is given of the modification of superconducting alloys by many different kinds of laser processing. Two main attempts can be distinguished:

(1) Lasers are used to form and to anneal well-ordered, high-T_c materials.
(2) Pulsed lasers are used for the production of amorphous superconductors and for the comparison with other non-equilibrium techniques, well known in superconductivity for many years.

A very brief introduction to superconductivity should help the reader to understand the basic problems. A more detailed discussion can be found in numerous textbooks (4,5). Superconductivity is caused by the formation of Cooper pairs, i.e., two electrons with opposite spins and opposite moments. The two electrons attract each other via an electron-phonon interaction. This attractive interaction can be increased in two ways:

(1) A high electron density of states at the Fermi level. This can be achieved in superconducting materials with a high degree of long-range order.
(2) A weak phonon density of states, i.e., many phonons with low energies support superconductivity. This can be achieved by disorder in a superconductor. For example, there are many atoms without a close-by neighbor in an amorphous alloy. Thus these atoms are only loosely bound to the others, i.e., they weaken the phonon spectrum.

Unfortunately, these requirements contradict each other. The first one can be fulfilled best in ordered transition metal alloys, whereas the second one can be achieved in non-transition metal systems. In the first case, T_c = 23 K can be reached, whereas T_c values ≤ 12 K are typical for the second one. The interesting fact in the latter case is that many non-superconducting, non-transition metals can be transformed only by disorder into superconductors at all.

Besides T_c, other parameters are equally important for the real application of superconductivity, i.e., the critical magnetic field, B_c, and the critical current density, j_c. Each of the three parameters - temperature, magnetic field and current density - can destroy superconductivity when the critical values are surpassed. In the following experiments only T_c and j_c will be discussed. j_c can be increased if one is able to stop the movement of magnetic flux lines inside the superconductor. The magnetic flux due to an outer applied field or to the current itself penetrates a superconductor of technical interest in flux quanta. The interaction between magnetic field and the current leads to a force perpendicular to B and j, and thus the flux lines start to move, leading to an energy dissipation, i.e., resistance. This can be hindered if the flux lines are pinned to grain boundaries or fine-dispersed precipitations. Thus the occurrence of electrical resistance can be hindered and j_c can be enhanced.

In the following the results of laser processing will be discussed with respect to the different classes of materials involved:

(1) High-T_c superconductors
(2) Pure superconducting elements
(3) Metastable and disordered superconductors

It will be seen that most of the different kinds of laser processing used for semiconducting materials have been applied to superconductors as well. A lot of different starting materials were used, i.e., thin films prepared by sputtering or evaporation, single crystals, both as-grown and ion-damaged. A large variety of lasers and to a lesser extent electron beams have been applied, i.e., ns pulses to cw lasers, single-cycle or multicycle treatment and also reactive processing. Besides the results discussed in each of the following parts, a complete listing of papers dealing with this subject is given.

2. HIGH T_c MATERIALS

Nearly all high T_c materials ($T_c > 16$ K) belong to either one of the following two crystal structures:

A 15 (or β-W structure): cubic structure with Nb or V chains in all three directions. High electronic density of states along the chains due to the large overlap of the electron orbits of the transition metals (TM). A large variety of non-transition metals (NTM) can occupy the corners of the cube, ratio TM/NTM = 3/1.

B 1 (or NaCl structure): simple cubic structure with TM atoms intermittent with N or C atoms. For the A 15 materials a perfect long-range order is essential for a high T_c. This is not so important for B 1 superconductors, where perfect stoichiometry is more important.

2.1. Laser processing of A 15 Materials

V_3Si

Among these superconductors V_3Si with a $T_c = 17$ K can be easily produced by conventional metallurgical methods, since it forms an A 15 phase stable at room temperature. Therefore, this easy material was chosen for a thorough investigation of laser processing.

In a first experiment (6) a multilayer sample (4 V, 4 Si layers on Al_2O_3, ratio V/Si = 3) was used as starting material. Besides measurements of the superconducting transition temperature, Rutherford-Backscattering (RBS), transmission electron microscopy (TEM) and X-ray diffraction (glancing incidence) were used to characterize the sample during the different treatments. These include both thermal annealing and laser zapping with a ~20 ns ruby laser pulse.

The results are summarized in Fig. 1. Besides the obtained T_c values the dominant crystal structures are plotted as a function of laser energy density. The lower curve shows the results after laser treatment. The as-evaporated multilayer has both T_c and crystal structure of the V layers. . At about 0.6 J/cm^2 the superconducting transition width ΔT_c broadens, indicating an increasing inhomogeneity in agreement with a broadening of the bcc diffraction peaks. Si starts to mix into the V layer, resulting in the observed decrease of T_c and the increase of ΔT_c. TEM and RBS reveal that 0.9 J/cm^2 pulses result in complete melting and mixing of the sample. Annealing with higher energy density of 1.5 J/cm^2 yields disordered bcc besides the formation of A 15. However, T_c decreases below the detection limit of 1.5 K. In a second step these samples have been heat treated in a furnace at 775 K for one hour. The as-evaporated sample shows a slight decrease in T_c, probably due to diffusion of Si, i.e,, dilution of the superconducting V layers with the non-superconducting Si. The samples which had been laser-zapped with energy densities above 0.9 J/cm^2 show only A 15 diffraction lines. It is important to note that T_c is higher for the sample 0.9 J/cm^2 compared to 1.5 J/cm^2. This is the first hint that it is difficult to obtain perfect A 15 from a disordered A 15 produced by laser processing. This trend becomes much clearer after a subsequent 925 K annealing for one hour (upper curve). All samples reveal A 15 lines. However, the as-evaporated sample has the highest T_c of 14.5 K. Increasing the energy density of the laser, which had initially produced A 15, has a deteriorating effect on T_c. The interpretation, which is in agreement

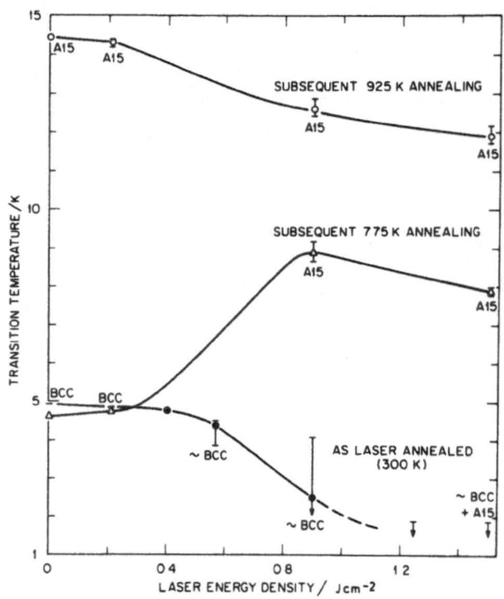

FIGURE 1. Effects of T_c on the structure of single-pulse laser annealing and subsequent thermal annealing of V-Si multilayer samples (6).

with further experiments, assumes that the rapid solidification due to the laser treatment produces very small grains of A 15. Subsequent thermal annealing improves the quality rather than the size of the microcrystallites. In contrast, thermal annealing of bcc V in a Si surrounding results in polycrystalline V_3Si with large grains and thus high T_c values. From this result one can conclude that laser annealing with a pulsed ruby laser has no obvious advantage to more conventional thermal annealing.

In another experiment V_3Si films with an initially high T_c of 15.5 K had been heavily damaged with $\sim 10^{16}/cm^{-2}$ (300 keV B) to a T_c of 2.4 K. Then pulsed ruby laser annealing was used to remove the ion damage (7). Figure 2 shows the recovery of T_c as a function of the cumulative energy density for films with different thicknesses. For values exceeding 2 J/cm^2 both T_c and ΔT_c saturate at 10 K and 1.5 K. The initial sharp transition of the ion-damaged film broadens quite remarkably.. The initial T_c value can never be reached. Pulsed laser annealing (20 ns ruby) cannot restore the undamaged T_c. This is again in agreement with the assumption that pulsed laser "annealing" introduces a laser damage of its own due to the high regrowth velocity of the solid-liquid interface, resulting in microcrystallized V_3Si.

This laser damage can actually be proven by channeling measurements of a V_3Si-single crystal before and after pulsed laser annealing (6). Figure 3 shows the result. The backscattering yield of 2.5 MeV He^+ is plotted as a function of channel number (He^+ energy). Besides a random RBS spectrum, three spectra are shown for the aligned V_3Si <100>

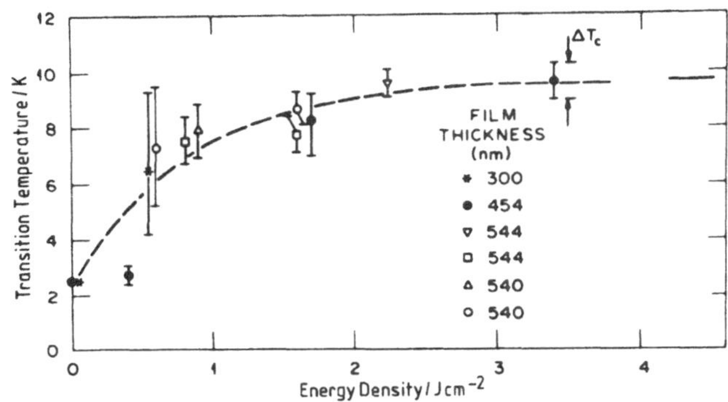

FIGURE 2. T_c of ion-damaged V_3Si versus cumulative laser energy density (7).

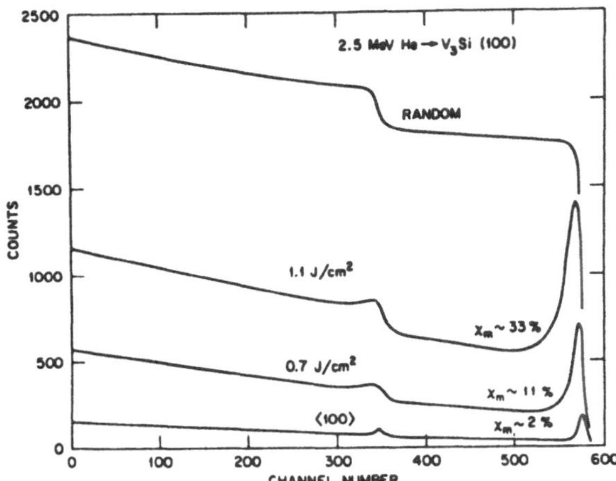

FIGURE 3. Channeling analysis of the <100> direction of a (100) V_3Si single crystal before and after annealing with laser pulses of 0.7 and 1.1 J/cm^2 (6).

crystal. The lower curve shows the result for the virgin crystal. The minimum backscattering yield $X_m \approx 2\%$ proves the high quality of the crystal. Laser pulses of 0.7 J/cm^2 and 1.1 J/cm^2 increase X_m to 11% and 33%. In addition, the surface peak is substantially enhanced and broadened. This result demonstrates that laser annealing introduces a substantial damage into the surface of a single crystal.

At these energy densities surface cracking can also be observed in SEM (6). This can be explained by the substantial thermal expansion of the heat-treated layer with respect to the cold crystalline substrate.

Nb_3Sn, Nb_3Ge

In a very interesting set of experiments the influence of both pulsed laser (PLA, 20 ns) and pulsed electron beam annealing (PEBA, 300 ns) on the critical current densities j_c of Nb_3Sn and Nb_3Ge films on top of Hastelloy B has been studied (8,9). PLA was found to increase j_c by 10 to 40% for understiochiometric Nb_3Ge due to nucleation of Nb_5Ge_3 precipitates (≈ 3 nm) in the heat-affected zone and not in the molten region. These precipitates act as pinning centers - unfortunately they are not homogeneously distributed over the entire volume. PEBA, which influences a larger volume of the films, had no positive effect on j_c of Nb_3Ge (Fig. 4). Above the melting threshold j_c deteriorates rapidly before the films crack and "explode" due to the different thermal expansion of A 15 and substrate. However, a 40% increase of j_c was observed in one case for Nb_3Sn near the melting threshold. Subsequent PEBA destroys this positive effect. In addition, the authors investigated different substrates and showed that their observations agreed very well with computer simulations and the various coefficients of thermal expansion.

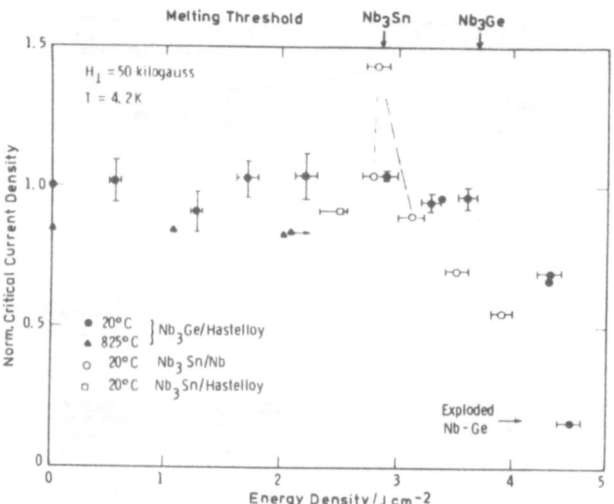

FIGURE 4. Critical current denity (normalized to the value of the untreated sample) of Nb_3Sn and Nb_3Ge versus energy density of the pulsed electron beam (9).

In summary, the experiments on A 15 materials provide no convincing evidence that lasaer treatment (including cw laser) is a very promising way to increase T_c and j_c further. The high regrowth velocity of the solid-liquid interface hinders the formation of the essential long-range order. Perhaps subsequent laser treatment with different annealing parameters is a way to go. The first pulse is used to quench the A 15 phase from the melt to room temperature (in the case of the unstable Nb_3Ge and Nb_3Al), whereas the following pulses initiate ordering in the solid phase (10). The reader is referred to Refs. 11-14 for additional papers on laser treatment of A 15 materials.

2.2. Laser processing of B 1 materials

The experiments have been performed dominantly on NbN and Nb-C-N (11). Sputtering of these materials onto alumina results in films with different superconducting properties dependent on the substrate temperature T_s. The effect of PLA is also quite different.

T_s = 500°C: Optimum values for $T_c \approx 17$ K and $\Delta T_c \approx 1$ K, PLA has no effect.

T_s = 700°C: Non optimum films: $T_c = 11$ K, $\Delta T_c \approx 3$ K, PLA increases T_c to 16 K, but no change in ΔT_c.

T_s = 25°C: Amorphous films, $T_c = 6$ K, PLA increases T_c to 13 K, but $\Delta T_c \approx 8$ K.

These results show that PLA is much more favorable for the annealing of B 1 materials than for the complicated A 15 structure. However, also for B 1 materials, PLA deteriorates the surface of single crystals. This was demonstrated by channeling and SEM. Figure 5 shows a SEM micrograph of a flaking NbN single crystal. Further experiments on B 1 superconductors, including reactive laser processing, are described in Ref. 15.

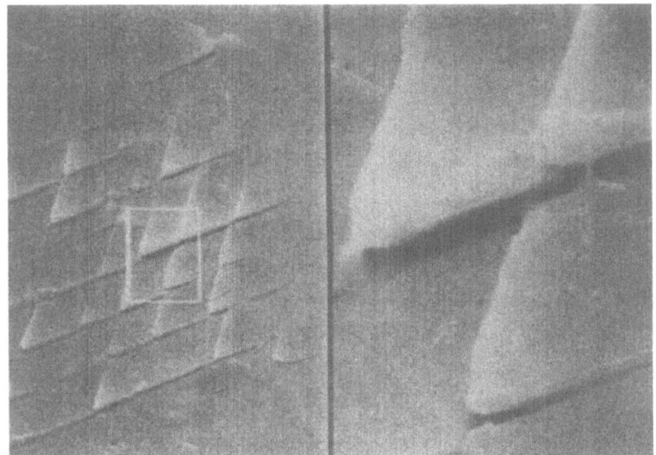

FIGURE 5. SEM analysis (the height of the inset box is 15 um) of a NbN single crystal after a single laser pulse of 1.5 J/cm^2 (6).

3. PURE SUPERCONDUCTING ELEMENTS

V single crystals have been used to study the influence of PEBA (16). Figure 6 shows the yield of backscattering He^+ as a function of channel number (He^+ energy). The upper and the lower curves show the RBS spectra of the virgin crystal in a random and an aligned <111> direction. Curves A through D have been obtained after PEBA with the energy densities plotted in the insert of Fig. 6. The melting threshold was determined by the redistribution of implanted Bi atoms (5×10^{14} cm^{-2}, 350 keV). They appear on the high energy side of the spectra.

Redistribution, i.e., epitaxial regrowth and surface segregation, is seen for treatment D. Below the melting threshold an increasing surface disorder is introduced by PEBA (curves A B C). Melting (D) results in epitaxial regrowth with a large amount of defects.

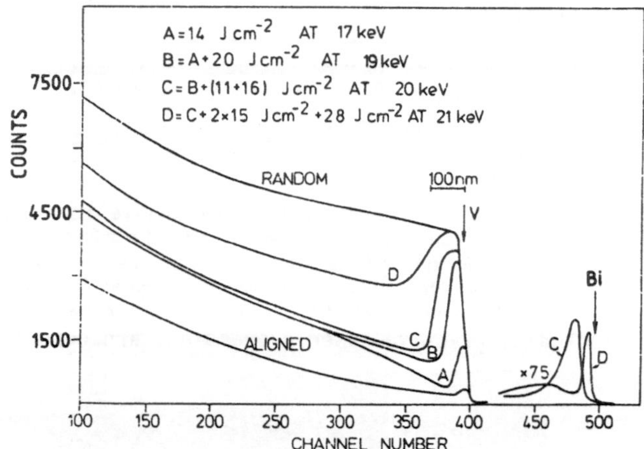

FIGURE 6. Channeling spectra using 2 MeV He^+ ions scattered from a (111) V crystal before and after treatment with different electron energy depositions. The low dose (5×10^{14} cm^{-2}, 350 keV) Bi implant was used for the determination of the melting threshold (16).

In summary, PEBA cannot be applied for the improvement of V crystals. However, PLA can be used to improve the superconducting properties of Nb films consisting of bad starting material (17). In this case, it is more probable that gaseous impurities have been removed from the Nb. Thus T_c approaches more the value of bulk Nb.

4. METASTABLE AND DISORDERED SUPERCONDUCTORS

In this part it is shown that PLA and PEBA are promising techniques for the production of metastable (TaZr, Mo-C-N) and amorphous (AuBi) superconductors.

4.1. Ta-Zr system

The composition range of the TaZr system is limited to very small Zr concentrations (<4.5 at % Zr at 450°C and substantially smaller at 25°C). In order to extend the Zr content in the bcc phase, non-equilibrium techniques like splat-cooling and co-sputtering have been applied. Thus the superconducting transition temperature could be raised from 4.5 K of pure Ta to nearly 8 K at the maximum content of 25 at % Zr. However, these methods are restricted to very special preparation conditions. These restrictions could be overcome by the application of PEBA to amorphous Ta-Zr alloys. Thus bcc Ta-Zr alloys could be produced over a wide composition range (18). The Ta-Zr alloys have been investigated with respect to their possible application as alternative tunnel junctions for use in Josephson circuits. PEBA has the advantage that heating of the substrate, e.g., organic materials, is avoided. Figure 7a shows the X-ray diffraction of an as-evaporated $Ta_{73}Zr_{27}$ film. The coevaporation of Ta and Zr was performed onto sapphire substrates at room temperature. It can be seen that the resulting films are amorphous. This film is crystallized with PEBA at 2.3 J/cm^2 (300 ns pulse length). Figure 7b shows the resulting metastable bcc phase. This method results in single-phase bcc TaZr alloys with Zr concentrations up to x = 54 at %. These metastable films decompose totally at >1100°C during furnace annealing. With respect to superconductivity, a maximum T_c = 7.7 K ($\Delta T_c \approx 0.1$ K) has been obtained for the highest Zr content.

Summarizing, PEBA has been successfully applied for the extension of the composition range of bcc Ta-Zr alloys to Zr concentrations of 5 K at % with T_c values of nearly 8 K.

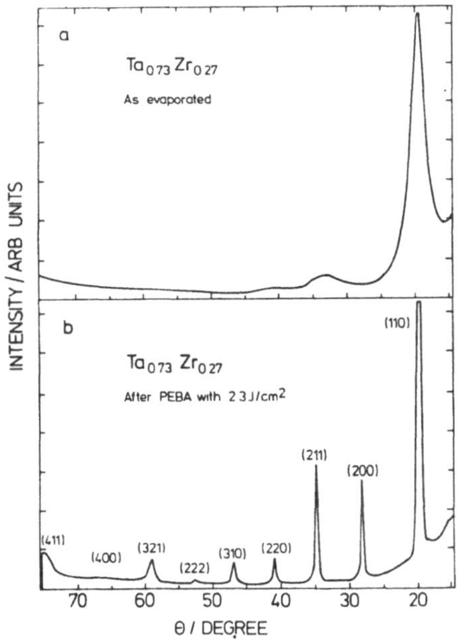

FIGURE 7. X-ray spectra from a $Ta_{73}Zr_{27}$ film (18). (a) as-evaporated, revealing an amorphous structure, (b) after PEBA, showing bcc structure and supersaturated alloy formation.

4.2. Mo-C alloys

In the following experiment a combination of ion implantation and PLA was used to produce concentrated Mo-C alloys (19). The main interest of the authors was the comparison of superconducting material produced by these two highly non-equilibrium methods.

Either foils or films of Mo were used as starting materials. Then the C was introduced via C implantation at about 600 K, resulting in a Gaussian type concentration profile. The resulting values for T_c are plotted in Fig. 8 as a function of C concentration (averaged concentration of the implanted C peak). T_c increases with increasing C content from ≈1 K to ≈5 K. For comparison, earlier data (20) for C implantation into Mo at low temperatures (4 K) are included (solid line). There the T_c values are always higher, the reason being that low-temperature implantation results in a higher degree of lattice disorder due to a higher quench rate involved. Thus higher T_c values in these highly disordered or even amorphous Mo-C alloys had been obtained. Subsequently, the implanted alloys were rapidly heated and "laser quenched" while affixed to a substrate at 5 K. The laser quenching was performed with a

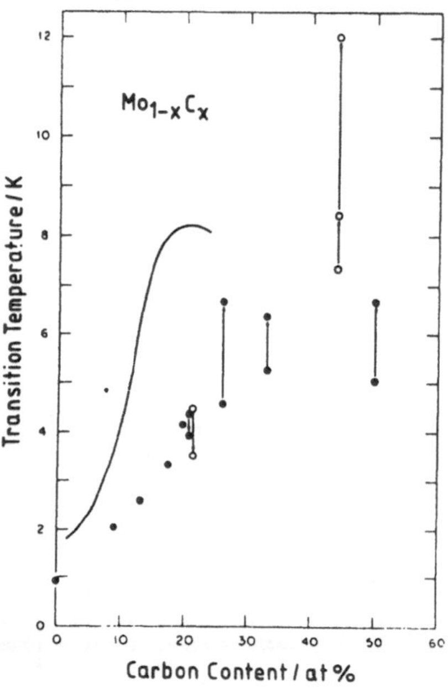

FIGURE 8. T_c of Mo foils (filled circles) and Mo films (open circles) versus implanted C concentration. Vertical arrows show the influence of laser quenching (19). The solid line indicates T_c values obtained by C implantation into Mo at 4 K (20).

Q-switched ruby laser. The arrows in Fig. 8 show the resulting influence on T_c of the implanted Mo-C alloys. An increase of T_c to ≈6.5 K is observed for all alloys with C concentrations above 30 at %. From these results it can be concluded that laser quenching has a quench-rate between that of ion implantation at substrate temperatures of 600 K and 5 K. The situation is different for the $Mo_{57}C_{43}$ film, which was homogeneously implanted. After PLA two superconducting transitions at 12 K and 8.5 K indicate that no disordered alloy had been formed, but a B 1 and a hcp phase. It seems that for this nearly stoichiometric composition it is more favorable for the system to form an ordered compound instead of a disordered alloy. Future X-ray measurements will give a better insight in the different phases in comparison to those obtained by other preparation techniques.

Besides the Mo-C system Mo-B alloys have also been studied (19). In both cases, PLA leads to an improvement of T_c owing to the high quench rate involved which favors the formation of highly disordered systems.

4.3. Au-Bi system

The Au-Bi system was chosen for PLA experiments (21) because it was known that the system can be made amorphous both by vapor-quenching and ion irradiation at low temperatures. The amorphous phase has a $T_c \approx 6$ K. Thus it can be very well distinguished from the equilibrium phase, which always contains Au_2Bi with a T_c of only 1.9 K among other non-superconducting phases. In Fig. 9 T_c of $Au_{35}Bi_{65}$ is plotted as a function of energy density of an excimer laser (20 ns pulse length, 249 nm wavelength). The temperature of the substrate remains at ≈ 4 K. With increasing energy density of the laser pulse, three different regions can be distinguished. Up to ≈ 40 mJ/cm^2 there is no change of T_c ($T_c = 1.9$ K, Au_2Bi). Then T_c increases steeply and saturates at a high value of 5.4 K for energy densities ≥ 80 mJ/cm^2. This result can be explained unambiguously in the following way. In the first region the energy density of the laser beam is not high enough to melt the surface of the sample. Above 40 mJ/cm^2 the melting threshold is exceeded and the surface starts to melt. The molten surface layer solidifies very rapidly after the laser pulse due to the cold substrate. This rapid solidification yields a "high" T_c material at the surface. With increasing energy density the molten surface layer, and thus the resulting layer of "high" T_c material, becomes thicker until the proximity effect from the underlying material, can be neglected and T_c saturates at the high value.

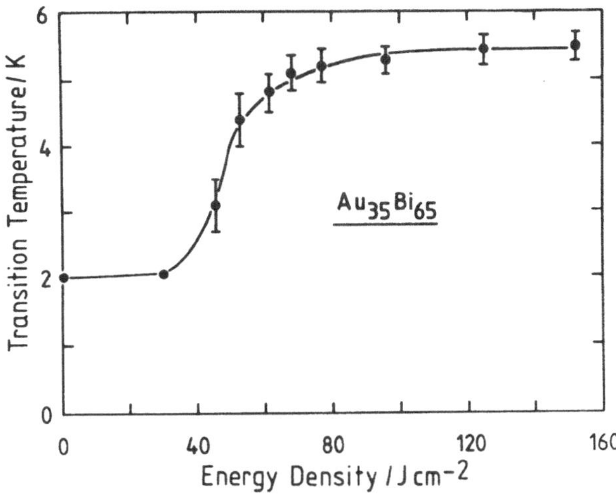

FIGURE 9. T_c of a $Au_{35}Bi_{65}$ film versus energy density of the laser pulse (21).

The resulting "high" T_c material has a considerably higher resistivity in comparison to the starting material. Thus not only the melting threshold but also the thickness of the molten and resolidified layer can be simply determined by measuring the resistivity of the sample. From this measurement it could be shown that the whole $Au_{35}Bi_{65}$ film (46 nm thick) has been molten for energy densities >80 mJ/cm^2.

Besides determination of the melting threshold and layer thickness, the measurement of resistance, R(T), can be used for the determination of phase transitions during annealing of the "high" T_c phase. A transformation into another phase can be determined by the following observations during annealing:

(1) A sudden, irreversible change of the resistance
(2) A different reversible R(T) behavior of the new phase
(3) A different T_c value of the new phase.

The annealing experiments show three or four different phases for Bi contents above or below 33 at %. The experiment shows that for the AuBi system the quenching rate involved in PLA is sufficient to produce amorphous Au-Bi. This is different from the Au-Te system (22). There the amorphous phase could only be obtained by vapor quenching and ion irradiation at 5 K, but not with laser quenching. The different abilities of laser quenching in Te-Au and Bi-Au to produce an amorphous phase may be the result of different quenching rates, due to different absorption coefficients and thermal conductivities, and different glass-forming potentials of Te and Bi.

5. CONCLUSIONS

A wide variety of laser techniques have been applied for the production of superconducting alloys on a large number of different starting materials with respect to crystallinity, phases, purity, composition and so on. Thus a widespread metallurgical knowledge has been obtained for many metallic systems, which is of interest for other applications of lasers on metals like hardening etc. It was shown that laser techniques are not very well suited for the production of complicated crystal structures with long-range order. They are better for the production of transition metal-carbides and -nitrides. Moreover, pulsed laser and electron methods are very well suited for the amorphization of metallic systems.

With respect to superconductivity, it was shown that laser treatment is not very promising for high-T_c materials, where long-range order is essential. On the other hand, pulsed laser and electron techniques yield interesting amorphous superconductors. However, the quenching rates for ns pulses are not as high as for vapor quenching and ion irradiation.

The investigation of the production of superconducting alloys by laser and electron beam treatment resulted in a better understanding of these techniques applied to metallic alloys. The investigation of superconductors is especially informative since a lot of other non-conventional production techniques have been applied in the past. Thus a comparison to these methods can be readily made. In addition, the different crystallographic phases can be easily detected by their different electrical and superconducting properties just by measuring the electrical resistance.

REFERENCES

1. B. W. Roberts: "Survey of Superconductive Materials and Critical Evaluation of Selected Properties," J. Phys. Chem., Ref. Data 5, 581 (1976) and NBS Technical Note 983 (1978).
2. L. R. Testardi, J. H. Wernick. and W. A. Royer, Solid State Comm. 15, 1 (1974); J. R. Gavaler, M. H. Janoko, and C. K. Jones, J. Appl. Phys. 47, 7 (1974).
3. I. Ya. Lekhtyar, L. I. Ivanov, N. V. Karlov, G. P. Kuz'min, M. M. Nishchenko, A. M. Prokhorov, N. N. Rykalin, and V. A. Yanushkevich, Sov. J. Quant. Electron. 6, 460 (1976).
4. C. Kittel, Introduction to Solid State Physics (J. Wiley, New York), Chap. 11.
5. P. G. DeGennes, Superconductivity of Metals and Alloys (W. A. Benjamin, New York, 1966).
6. B. R. Appleton, B. Stritzker, C. W. White, J. Narayan, J. Fletcher, O. Meyer, and S. S. Lau, Laser and Electron-Beam Solid Interactions and Materials Processing, edited by J. F. Gibbons, L. D. Hess, and T. W. Sigmod (North Holland, 1981), p. 607.
7. J. R. Thompson, B. R. Appleton, O. Meyer, S. T. Sekula, and C. W. White, Solid State Div. Progress Report, ORNL-5640, 110 (1980).
8. A. I. Braginski, J. R. Gavaler, R. C. Kuznicki, B. R. Appleton, and C. W. White, Appl. Phys. Lett. 39, 277 (1981).
9. A. I. Braginski, J. Greggi, M. A. Janocko, T. Kleiser, and O. Meyer, Nucl. Instr. Meth. B5, 525 (1984).
10. T. Shibata, J. F. Gibbons, J. Kwo, R. D. Feldman, and T. H. Geballe, J. Appl. Phys. 52, 1537 (1981).
11. B. R. Appleton, C. W. White, B. Stritzker, O. Meyer, J. R. Gavaler, A. I. Braginski, and M. Ashkin, Laser and Electron Beam Processing of Materials, edited by C. W. White and P. S. Peercy (Academic Press, New York, 1980), p. 714.
12. B. Pànnetier, T. H. Geballe, R. H. Hammond, and J. F. Gibbons, Physica 107B, 471 (1981).
13. B. Stritzker, B. R. Appleton, C. W. White, and S. S. Lau, Solid State Commun. 41, 321. (1982).
14. H. Asano, K. Nakamura, and A. Terada, Jpn. J. Appl. Phys. 22, 429 (1983).
15. K. Nakamura, M. Hikita, H. Asano, and A. Terada, Jpn. J. Appl. Phys. 21, 672 (1982).
16. J. M. Lombaard, O. Meyer, Radiation Effects 69, 239 (1983).
17. K. Takei, K. Nagai, and T. Inamura, Jpn. J. Appl. Phys. 19, 2392 (1980).
18. G. Linker and J. Geerk, Solid State Commun. 48, 1089 (1983).
19. S. T. Sekula, J. R. Thompson, G. M. Beardsley, and D. H. Lowndes, J. Appl. Phys. 54, 6517 (1983).
20. O. Meyer, Inst. Phys. Conf. Ser. 28, 168 (1976).
21. A. Wolthius and B. Stritzker, Energy Beam-Solid Interactions and Transient Thermal Processing, edited by J. C. C. Fan and N. M. Johnson (Elsevier, 1984), p. 757 and references therein.
22. B. Stritzker, Amorphous Metals and Non-Equilibrium Processing, edited by M. von Allmen (Editions de Physique, 1984), p. 14.

LASER PROCESSING OF Al-Ge MULTILAYER THIN FILMS

C. N. AFONSO AND C. ORTIZ
Instituto de Optica, C.S.I.C., Serrano 121, 28006 Madrid, Spain

Key Words: Al-Ge thin films, laser alloying, metal-semiconductor alloys, optical materials, metastable alloys, pulsed lasers

ABSTRACT

A comparative study on nanoand microsecond laser processing in the Al-Ge system is presented. The samples are multilayer films either as-grown or preprocessed with an excimer laser. When the films are irradiated in the low-power microsecond regime, the results suggest a layer mixing process. When increasing the laser power, there is a distinct difference in the damage or ablation process for the Ge-rich preprocessed film due probably to the existence of Ge crystals segregated at the surface.

1. INTRODUCTION

Laser alloying is a technique with a continuously growing field of application (1,2). One of the reasons for its interest lies in the very rapid quenching velocities from the liquid phase which can favor the formation of metastable phases or new compounds (3). One way to promote alloy formation is to process material with a multilayer configuration. The two materials to be alloyed are grown in the form of alternating layers and the relative thicknesses are chosen to achieve the desired film composition.

In our work we have selected the study of the Al-Ge system because, on one hand, it has a simple phase diagram with a single eutectic and no equilibrium phases and, on the other hand, the local formation of metal-semiconductor alloys is an important subject in the field of semiconducting devices. Silicide formation by conventional methods has been extensively studied (4) and laser processing has proven to be a successful method to obtain new silicides (5). Although the Ge-metal alloys have been proposed as a good contact element for IR detectors (6) and GaAs devices (7), no laser-induced germanide formation has yet been reported and we would like to investigate this point further.

There is another technological field in which we are primarily interested: optical storage. For many years the base material for write-once memories has been Te (8). Due to its corrosion and stability problems, many alloying elements have been considered, among which Ge has been one with good complementary characteristics. Several attempts with alternative materials have been made. Among the metal-semiconducting alloys, aluminum alloys have received special attention (9,10). Nevertheless, the threshold power for hole opening in the Si/Al system is still nearly one order of magnitude higher than that reported for GeTe alloys (11).

In recent years much effort has been devoted to induce reversible phase transitions, in the search for a physical mechanism which operates as a reversible process (12). Since the incubation time for phase transitions in many chalcogenide compounds (13) is in the microsecond regime, alternative materials need to be found. Metallic alloys might be the answer since phase transformation processes would presumably be faster in them.

This paper will describe the comparative study of two kinds of laser processing in the Al-Ge system: the nanosecond regime, which is performed by means of an excimer laser over broad areas of material ($\sim cm^2$), and the microsecond regime which is performed by means of an Ar laser focused on a small area ($\sim \mu m^2$). In the nanosecond regime we attempt to generate metastable alloys. In the microsecond regime we will analyze the role in the hole-opening process of a metastable alloy being the surface material as compared to pure Ge. The possible structural changes or mixing induced mechanisms at low-power irradiation will be discussed.

2. EXPERIMENTAL

The thin films were grown in a DC-triode sputtering system, the Al and Ge targets being independently polarized. The experimental details are similar to those described previously for the Te/Ge system (14). The films had a six-layer configuration (three of Ge alternating with three of Al). Total thicknesses were either 100 nm or 200 nm. The former thickness was chosen in order to be able to analyze the light transmitted by the films and the latter one to optimize the RBS analysis. The substrate was Corning glass. Two compositions were studied: that corresponding to the Al-Ge eutectic mixture (referred to as 7/3) and that corresponding to equal atomic percent of the two components (referred to as 1/1). In all cases, the Ge layer was deposited last, since it is more stable to surface oxidation than Al.

In the nanosecond regime, an excimer laser was used for laser processing (15) with an energy density in the 24-160 mJ/cm^2 range. The pulse length was 12 ns and the cumulative irradiation time was changed by using a different number of exposures (1-64) with a repetition rate of 10 Hz. The exposed area was in the cm^2 range. Two different wavelengths have been used (193, 248 nm), but this factor did not induce any striking effect on the degree of alloying. The alloying depth was studied by RBS, the surface morphology by SEM, and the possible material segregation at the surface by AES. The material structure was analyzed by X-ray diffraction and cross-sectional TEM.

The second type of laser processing was performed by means of an argon laser tuned to its 488 nm line. The laser beam was focused onto the films by means of a 0.4 numerical aperture objective and the exposed area was in the μm^2 range. The irradiation time was controlled by means of an acousto-optic modulator and the selected values were 5, 50 and 500 microseconds. The irradiation power was in the 5-80 mW range. The laser-induced process was studied by means of the changes in the optical properties (transmitted or reflected light). The laser exposures were done in static conditions, while the optical properties were recorded by scanning the films at a typical sweeping rate of 1 µm/s. The morphology of the exposed area was finally analyzed by SEM.

3. RESULTS

3.1. The nanosecond regime

The first parameter to be determined is the energy density threshold for mixing. For energy densities higher than 42 mJ/cm^2, we found mixing in all the material configurations studied. The energy density needed to produce surface damage and evaporation was higher than 150 mJ/cm^2. If we compare these values to those determined for the Te/Ge system (14), the mixing interval is slightly shifted to higher energy densities.

The cumulative shot effect and energy density dependence have been studied and the detailed results will be reported elsewhere (15). Figure 1 illustrates the results on the achieved mixing process in (a) 200 nm thick films, and (b) 100 nm films. The penetration depth of the laser mixing is plotted versus the energy density (for a fixed number of shots) or versus the number of shots (for a fixed energy density). In both figures the full line curves correspond to 1/1 films and the dashed line curves to 7/3 films. There is a saturation of the mixing depth as the number of shots (that is, the cumulative irradiation time) is increased. Upon increasing the energy density, a fast increase in the penetration depth is observed; however, the damage threshold is achieved before the six layers are fully mixed. In most of the conditions investigated, energy density saturation was not observed. Another important result which can also be deduced from Fig. 1 is that a non-eutectic composition (1/1) mixes faster than the eutectic one (7/3). This is a surprising result since it is expected that the eutectic composition, having a lower melting point, would require lower energy density for the mixing process.

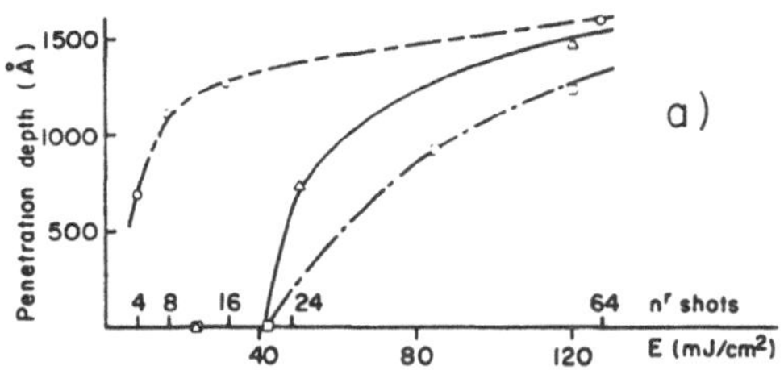

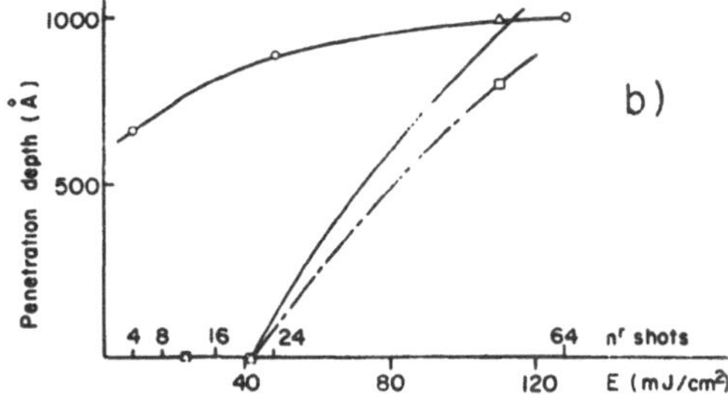

FIGURE 1. Penetration depth versus the number of shots (o) (the energy density is 70 mJ/cm^2 for 2000 Å thick films (a) and 80 mJ/cm^2 for 1000 Å films (b)) and versus the energy density (Δ,□) (the number of shots is 8). The dashed lines correspond to 7/3 films and the full lines to 1/1 films.

In order to analyze the structure of the mixed layer, we selected a 200 nm film with those irradiation conditions which induce the mixing of the four first layers as evidenced by RBS. The composition was a 1/1 film. The cross-sectional TEM micrograph is shown in Fig. 2, and it can be seen that the uppermost four layers are mixed and there remains an amorphous Ge and crystalline Al layer unmixed. This is a dark field image where the light contrast crystals, mainly nucleated at the interfaces, are Ge. The surface layer matrix where these Ge crystals are segregated has also been analyzed by electron diffraction and it is amorphous, presumably with the eutectic composition. In all the different laser-processed samples, X-ray diffraction analysis has never revealed evidence of new crystalline phases and only crystalline Ge was found. These results allow us to conclude that the processing of layers with eutectic composition induces the formation of an amorphous alloy. In the case where the composition is richer in Ge than the eutectic one, an amorphous eutectic layer with Ge-segregated crystals is observed. As a general but surprising result, we may say that the nanosecond regime induces a mixing process which behaves as expected from the equilibrium phase diagram.

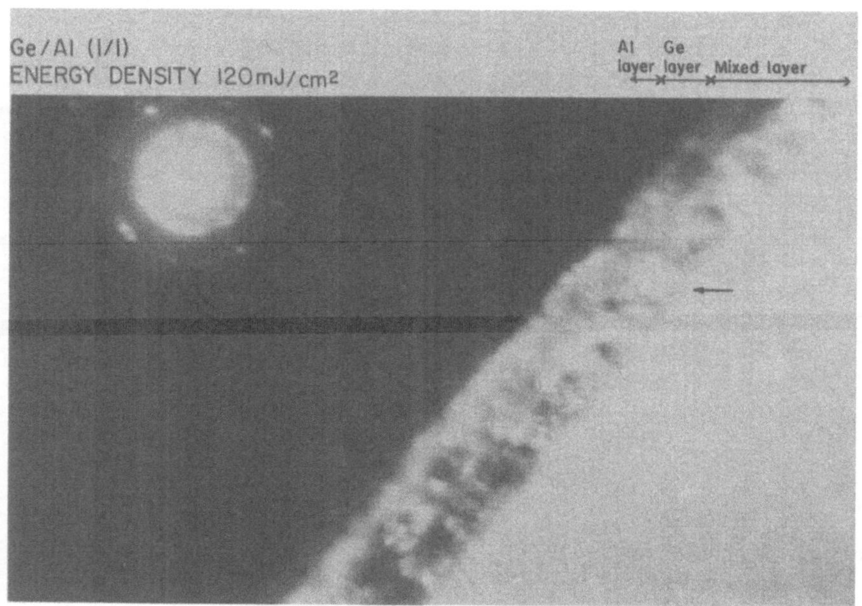

FIGURE 2. Cross-sectional TEM dark field micrograph of a 2000 Å, 1/1 film laser processed with a 120 mJ/cm^2 energy density. The diffraction pattern corresponds to the white crystals segregated in the mixed layer, which are identified as Ge.

3.2. The microsecond regime

In this regime we have studied mainly two kinds of 100 nm samples. The as-grown films and those films which were previously treated with the excimer laser (referred to as preprocessed films). We have selected a 1/1 film processed with eight shots of 110 mJ/cm^2 in which the six layers were mixed, resulting in an amorphous eutectic alloy with Ge-segregated crystals. The other selected film was a 7/3 composition processed with eight shots of 110 mJ/cm^2 where the mixing of the four first layers was produced resulting in an amorphous eutectic alloy.

As the irradiation power is increased, two types of laser-material interaction take place. The first evaporation does not take place and we will refer to it as low-power regime. The second behavior starts when the damage power threshold is reached, ablation with evaporation takes place, and a hole is opened. The threshold for the hole regime is easily detected from the optical curves since the light transmitted through the films changes drastically. The measured changes in the light transmitted are expected to be very abrupt while smooth changes in the reflected light are expected.

We defined the contrast ratio as the normalized changes observed in the transmitted (T) or reflected (R) intensity (14):

$$CR(T) = + \frac{(I_i - I_o)}{(I_i + I_o)} \quad ; \quad CR(R) = - \frac{(I_i - I_o)}{(I_i + I_o)}$$

where o refers to the original intensity values and i to those observed following laser irradiation. The signs have been chosen so both contrast ratios are positive in the hole regime. Figure 3 shows the contrast ratio versus the irradiation power measured in the 1/1 films for an exposure time of 500 microseconds. Both results for the as-grown and preprocessed films are included. We have selected this composition and exposure parameters since the low power and hole regimes previously mentioned are well illustrated. A more complete study can be found elsewhere (16).

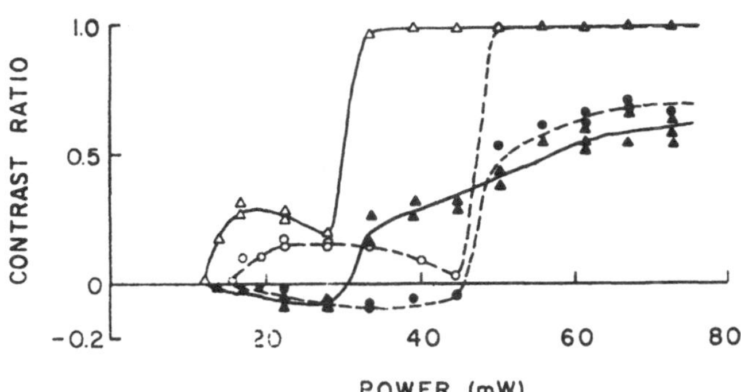

FIGURE 3. Optical contrast ratio measured for a 1/1 film versus the irradiation power. (O,Δ) correspond to that measured in the transmitted light and (●,▲) to that measured in the reflected light. The results obtained in the as-grown film are the full line curves and those in the preprocessed film are the dashed line curves.

It is a general result for all the as-grown films and exposures studied that the threshold power to induce optical changes is similar to that shown in Fig. 3. The 7/3 films present a slight increase in this threshold as the exposure time is decreased. All the preprocessed films present a 2-4 mW shift of the power threshold towards high powers.

The hole regime threshold is determined from the optical contrast ratio through the high increase in the transmitted light and the sign change of the reflected contrast ratio. For 1/1 films, it can be seen that the preprocessed films present damage resistance in the sense that the power threshold for the hole opening is considerably higher than in the as-grown films. In the case of 7/3 films, no striking differences between the as-grown and preprocessed films are observed.

The 50 and 5 microsecond regimes present similar features, but as the time decreases, the hole formation threshold is highly increased.

Figures 4 and 5 show the morphology of the damage areas in 1/1 and 7/3 films, respectively, as seen by SEM. In both cases, we include two micrographs of the as-grown films processed with powers below and above the hole threshold power and a micrograph corresponding to the preprocessed films with an irradiation power above the threshold power. The images support our results deduced from the optical curves, in the sense that for 7/3 films no special differences are observed, while for 1/1 films the morphology looks different.

4. DISCUSSION

For samples exposed to the microsecond pulses, it is of interest to understand the similarities observed in the 7/3 films and the differences in the 1/1 ones. In the eutectuc films, both as-grown and preprocessed, we have studied the optical properties of the exposed area for low-power exposures, and a similar dependence was observed, which is also similar to that observed in the as-grown film processed with nanosecond pulses. The same surface contrast is also observed in SEM. These results allow us to conclude that the processes induced in the 7/3 films for irradiation energies below the damage threshold, both in the nanosecond and microsecond regimes, are the same; that is, the mixing of the multilayer structure by means of a eutectic liquid. When increasing the laser power, similar ablation properties were encountered, as expected.

In the case of the as-grown 1/1 films, the process begins in a similar way to that of the eutectic composition, and a Ge-rich eutectic liquid is formed when the heat wave reaches the interface. The resolidified material is similar to that generated by the excimer laser. As the irradiation power is increased, ablation is the dominant process and the hole regime is reached.

When the non-eutectic, preprocessed films are studied, one has to keep in mind that the surface layer is an amorphous eutectic layer with Ge crystals segregated at the surface. The laser energy required to induce full melt is higher this time since the melting temperature of crystalline Ge is higher than that of the amorphous one (17). Before the Ge crystals at the surface layer melt, a liquid underlayer will be formed, producing pressure-induced blisters. When the irradiation power is increased, these blisters explode in agreement with the pictures observed in Fig. 4 for the preprocessed film.

A further, more dramatic result is seen in the as-grown films in Fig. 4: There is a remarkable inhomogeneity induced in the film that manifests itself as patterns irradiating out beyond the initial laser spot. These patterns are somehow related to an inhomogeneous heat

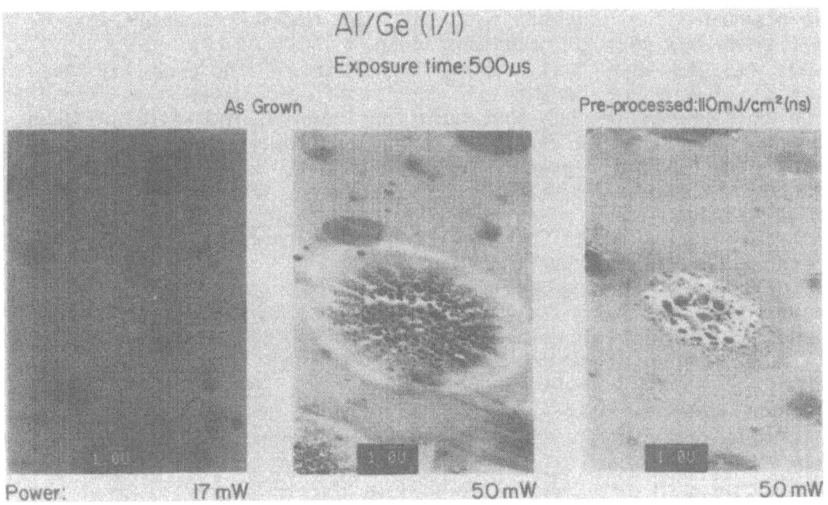

FIGURE 4. SEM micrographs of the laser-induced damage in the 1/1 as-grown film for 17 and 50 mW irradiation power and in the preprocessed film (see text) for a 50 mW irradiation power.

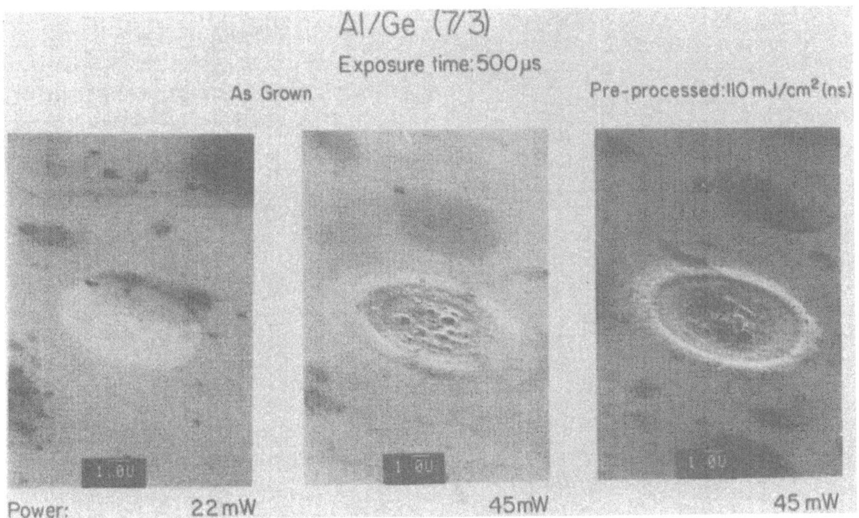

FIGURE 5. SEM micrographs of the laser-induced changes in 7/3 as-grown film for 22 and 45 mW irradiation power and the preprocessed film (see text) for a 45 mW irradiation power.

conduction parallel to the surface. The comparison between as-grown and preprocessed films suggests that the high thermal conductivity of the Al underlayers may play an important role.

Our results show that taking into account the area of the exposed material, the pulse length and the irradiation power, we find that the calculated energy density threshold for laser mixing with a focused laser (Ar-processing) is an order of magnitude lower than that with a non-focused one (excimer processing). Our conclusion is, therefore, that reducing the exposed area dimensions decreases the energy density threshold for mixing. This conclusion is consistent with the result that in the laser processing of Ge, the presence of thermal gradients lowers the threshold for crystallization of Ge (18).

Finally, and as a general conclusion from our comparative study, we can say that the laser processing of the Al/Ge multilayer films in the nanosecond and microsecond regimes induces similar processes with different laser energy density thresholds. In the first stage (low-power regime) of the interaction, a mixing of the layers is observed and an amorphous eutectic material (with or without crystalline Ge segregation) is formed. For higher energy density exposures, ablation or evaporation takes place.

ACKNOWLEDGMENTS

The present work was partially supported by CAYCIT (Spain). We would like to thank C. Grovenor (Metallurgy Department, Oxford) for the cross-sectional TEM analysis and J. E. E. Baglin and G. J. Clark (IBM, Yorktown Heights) for the helpful discussion on RBS.

REFERENCES

1. Laser Annealing of Semiconductors, edited by J. M. Poate and J. W. Mayer (Academic Press, New York, 1982).
2. C. W. Draper and J. M. Poate, Int. Met. Rev. 30, 85 (1985).
3. M. Von Allmen, "Glassy Metals II," edited by H. J. Gunthrodt and H. Beck, in Topics in Applied Physics (Springer Verlag, Berlin, 1983).
4. S. P. Munarka, Ann. Rev. Mater. Sci. 13, 117 (1983).
5. W. W. Duley, Laser Processing and Analysis of Materials (Plenum Press, 1984), Chap. 3.
6. S. S. Lau and W. F. van der Weg, Thin Films Interdiffusion and Reactions, edited by J. M. Poate, K. N. Tu, and J. W. Mayer (John Wiley, 1978).
7. R. T. Young and R. F. Wood, Ann. Rev. Mater. Sci 12, 323 (1982).
8. See, for instance, Proceedings of "Optical Data STorage," O.S.A., Monterey, USA (1984).
9. H. G. Parks and C. G. Kirkpatrick, AIP Conf. Proc. 50, 515 (1978).
10. K. Yoshii, M. Umeno, S. Murata, H. Kawabe, K. Yamda, I. Watanabe, and T. Kubo, J. Appl. Phys. 55, 223 (1984).
11. M. Chen, V. Marrello, and U. G. Gerber, Appl. Phys. Lett. 41, 894 (1982).
12. See, for instance, SPIE 420 "Optical Storage Media" (1983).
13. M. Chen, K. A. Rubin, V. Marrello, U. G. Gerber, and V. B. Jipson, Appl. Phys. Lett. 46, 734 (1985).
14. C. Ortiz, C. N. Afonso, and E. Acosta, Optica Acta, 32 (1985).
15. C. Ortiz, G. C. Clark, C. N. Afonso, J. E. E. Baglin, C. Grovenor, and J. Rothenberg, to be published.
16. C. N. Afonso, C. Ortiz, and L. Caballero, to be published.
17. P. Baeri and S. U. Campisano, Chap. 4 of Reference 1.
18. U. Zammit, M. Marinelli, G. Vitali, and F. Scudieri, J. Phys. 44, 313 (1983).

EDITED QUESTIONS - CHAPTER 4

MC CAFFERTY, MAZUMDER, DRAPER, STRITZKER, AFONSO

MC CAFFERTY

Q. On laser surface alloying of Fe/Cr alloys, did you plate the Cr directly or was there an intermediate layer?
A. The Cr was directly electroplated or sputter deposited onto the substrate.

Q. Once you reach the passivation region and reverse the potential, how does the current density behave?
A. We didn't do those experiments, but the higher Cr content alloys would remain passive and display no hysteresis.

Q. Does the rate at which you vary the potential vary the current density?
A. Yes, the rate changes the shape of the curve. A better experiment would be to apply discrete potential steps, although slow scan rates provide an approach to the steady state.

Q. If you pulsed (potential steps) up into the passive region, would not the initial current be greater?
A. Yes, it will be greater as the double layer is charged and before the current assumes the steady-state value.

Q. Were the experiments done in aerated solutions?
A. The solutions were de-aerated sodium sulfate solutions. The samples were first immersed in the electrolyte for 30 min until a steady-state potential was reached. They were then given a cathodic pulse for five minutes. The oxide films were not reduced, but a reproducible sample surface was produced. Electrode potentials were swept at 10 mV/minute.

Q. Did you see Cr break through?
A. No, the pure Cr undergoes transpassive dissolution, not the Fe-Cr alloys.

Q. Is the potential always the independent variable (in current density vs. potential)?
A. Almost always. In the early days before potentiostats, current density was usually the independent variable. However, for constant current sources one can miss active/passive transitions in the anodic polarization curve.

Q. For laser-melted stainless steel, might inter-dendritic corrosion be an important mechanism, or from the tight spacing and segregation is corrosion resistance improved?

A. We initially thought that segregation of Cr or Ni to the edges of the dendrites would improve the corrosion resistance, especially for the top of the melt pool where dendrites are aligned parallel to the surface. Although Auger analysis showed no surface enrichment of Cr or Ni, the pitting potential was increased so that inter-dendritic corrision was not a problem.

Q. What are the typical processes that go on at the interface and does changing the composition of solution have an effect?

A. Detailed electrode kinetic steps are not well known for pitting reactions but involve adsorption of the chloride ion at the oxide surface, penetration through the oxide film, and reaction with the underlying metal. Decreasing the chloride ion concentration decreases the pitting potential.

Q. Does pit morphology verify the reduction in sulfur?

A. We found no difference in pit morphology for the laser-melted and untreated surfaces. Pit morphology also depends in part on the aqueous solution one uses to allow pitting to occur.

Q. For high Mo content surface alloys, how do you measure the effects of pitting?

A. The pitting potential is higher than the untreated material.

Q. Why did you use 30 layers of alloying constituents?

A. We wanted to insure complete mixing but probably could have used fewer layers.

Q. For laser surface melting of aluminum, did you find any Mn after melting?

A. Not at the surface. The alloying elements were all depleted at the surface, which was essentially pure aluminum.

Q. You mentioned that ion implantation improves corrosion resistance. Which ions improve pitting resistance of Al?

A. Niobium, zirconium, molybdenum, and possibly tantalum.

Q. On the improved corrosion resistance in the active region which you attribute to microstructural modification, could it be due to oxide formation?

A. No, the oxides dissolve rapidly in the acidic solutions used.

BERGMANN - COMMENT

You described the use of laser processing to improve the corrosion resistance of initially porous coatings. I would like to mention that in some of our work we were not able to achieve this effect when laser-processed corrosion-resistant coatings were subjected to high-pressure cycling of acids. The service conditions were too severe.

MC CAFFERTY (continued)

Q. Is the magnitude of your surface melt ripple enough to form runaway pitting?
A. It is difficult to say whether pits initiate at ripples until more SEM is done. Gross roughness is only 10% and microscopic roughness is not great.

Q. Is it better to insure you have a microcrystalline layer on the surface?
A. Yes, if the structure is corrosion resistant.

Q. Is there a minimum size of Mn-S particle which no longer affects corrosion resistance?
A. We don't know the answer yet.

Q. From your presentation it appears that there are no current advantages over conventional plating techniques.
A. Adhesion problems with conventional coatings are avoided with laser surface alloys which provide a gradation in composition across the interface. In addition, laser processing has other advantages such as the possibility of producing novel alloy compositions or useful microstructures.

Q. Does the surface roughness increase after corrosion testing?
A. There is usually no measurable difference, especially for the case of pitting corrosion where most of the surface is unaffected.

Q. In our experiments on laser processing of coatings, large pores collected in the free volume. Did you see this effect?
A. No, this one case (titanium) worked out nicely. I see how it could become a problem, analogous to the formation of Xe bubbles during ion beam mixing of a coating into a substrate using Xe ions.

MAZUMDER

Q. Can you control the amount of the various carbides?
A. So far we cannot control the volume fraction. We suspect it is a function of cooling rate and are attempting to empirically determine the relation.

Q. Where were your convergent beam measurements made?
A. All the microanalysis was done at the University of Illinois.

Q. What plane did you get streaking on in the particular carbide electron diffraction pattern?
A. (1000) plane or direction.

DRAPER

Q. Were the frequency-doubled and fundamental Nd:YAG beams homogenized?
A. No, they were Gaussian.

Q. A frequency-doubled YAG is your preferred laser - why not a ruby?
A. The ruby pulse rate is too slow to be of practical industrial use.

Q. Why not an excimer?
A. Because our early model (#002) Lambda Physik laser has never been reliable. I understand from others here that many of the early "bugs" are being worked out however.

The following table and two figures were presented by Clif Draper to quiz the graduate students at the ASI during his talk. These are experimental results on Metglas 2605 SC. The object was to see if the students could correctly predict whether the amorphous (a) ribbon would remain amorphous or nucleate the crystalline (c) phase upon irradiation as a function of laser pulse length. The same question was asked for 2605 Metglas which had been oven crystallized prior to laser irradiation. During the quiz the boxes were empty.

Allied Chemical Metglas™ Ribbons 0.5 mm Thick		10 ns Ruby	150 ns fd Nd:YAG	10 μs CO_2	1 ms CO_2
Starts out amorphous	a	a → [a]	a → [a]	a → [a]	a → [a]
Starts out crystalline	c	c → [a]	c → [a]	c → [a]	c → [c]

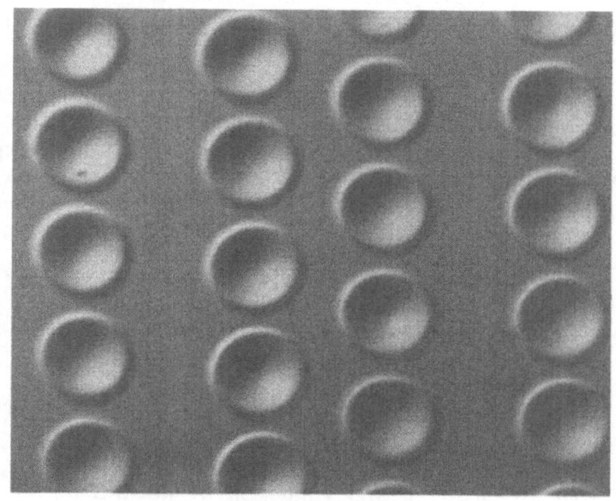

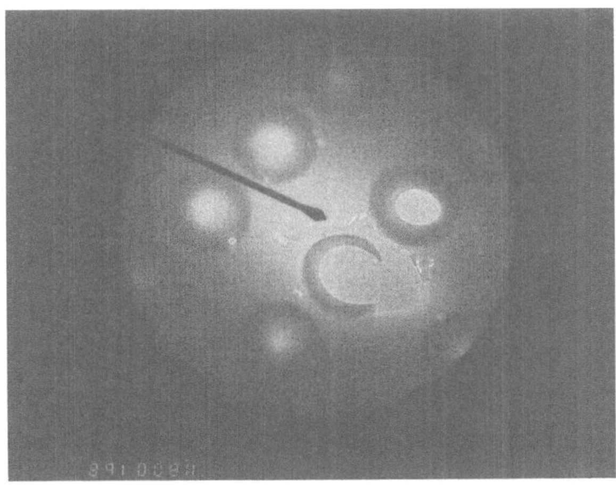

Ribbon samples were laser patterned as shown in figures, then thinned from the backside for TEM and electron diffraction analysis of laser-irradiated versus virgin areas. All laser pulse lengths were sufficient to retain the amorphous phase, even at the long 1 ms CO_2 laser pulse. For the oven-crystallized ribbon the glass phase was formed in the laser melt puddles for all pulse lengths except 1 ms. The difference lies in the "seed" below (around) the melt. For the amorphous case, homogeneous nucleation of the crystallites would be required. For the crystalline case, only heterogeneous, as the crystalline seed is present at the liquid-solid interface.

STRITZKER

Q. Why is 30°K the magic number for the superconductor transition temperature target?
A. A superconductor can be used with nearly all its advantageous properties with respect to j_c, H_c at about 2/3 T_c. Thus cooling at 20°K would be sufficient, and the less expensive cooling with liquid hydrogen could be used.

Q. What about the magnetic field induced by the current flow in the superconductor?
A. This magnetic field is added to the external field. The superconductor becomes normal conducting if the sum of these fields exceeds the critical value H_c.

Q. Are the equilibrium diagrams simple?
A. No, they are quite complex.

Q. What does the 2.9 eV activation energy correspond to?
A. Diffusion only.

Q. Is there a pressure dependence of stability since the compounds are unstable at room temperature?
A. To my knowledge, this has not been studied. In general, the effect of pressure is a reduction in T_c with <u>increasing</u> pressure due to a stiffening of the phonons.

Q. Is A15 more dense or less dense with pressure?
A. It is more dense. But A15 behaves normally, i.e., T_c decreases with increasing pressure.

Q. Are these reactions stoichiometric or N_2 deficient?
A. Stoichiometric, but N_2 deficient after laser annealing.

Q. Why did you use $Ta_{0.7}Zr_{0.3}$ instead of Nb-Zr since Ta-Zr seems to be an extreme?
A. Due to the thermal stability of the layers with regard to their possible application in Josephson computers.

Q. Pulsed current annealing - does it also work in drawn samples such as wire?
A. To my knowledge no attempts have been made in this direction.

Q. Approximately ten years ago Bell Labs noted the "universal disorder theory" in which T_c is optimal for a well-ordered superconductor, whereas T_c goes down in a universal manner with decreasing resistance ratio, independently from the kind of disorder introduced?
A. This is true for A15 materials only. Generally, one finds that a well-ordered high T_c material becomes worse with disorder, whereas a low T_c material becomes better with disorder. Thus values up to 17K in PdCuH (disordered) have been obtained.

Q. Have any of these alloys been melt spun?
A. Yes, many of these alloys have, but the resulting T_c's were always lower compared to the ion irradiation case, due to the lower quench rate involved.

<u>AFONSO</u>

Q. Were the films premixed?
A. They were processed with a nanosecond Nd:YAG laser, resulting in amorphous Al with Ge crystals.

Q. What was the initial reflectivity of the amorphous premixed films? Was it different from the unprocessed material?
A. The relative reflectance (defined in paper) changes by less than 10%, meaning the absolute reflectance changes were less. Therefore, the damage is probably not due to reduced reflectance.

Q. What was the thickness of the amorphous films?
A. 350 angstroms.

Q. Could you tell what the Ge and Al phases were for the damaged samples?
A. They were amorphous from the TEM measurements.

CHAPTER 5. RECENT DEVELOPMENTS IN LASER SURFACE TECHNIQUES FOR ENGINEERING APPLICATIONS

CHAPTER INTRODUCTION - H. W. BERGMANN, B. L. MORDIKE AND W. M. STEEN

High-power, continuous-wave CO_2 lasers are finding increasing use in engineering applications for improving the surface properties of hardness, wear, corrosion and fatigue by transformation hardening, surface melting, surface alloying and surface cladding. The beneficial effects are achieved by modifying the microstructures and surface composition using this uniquely localized and flexible energy source. In the following ten papers it will be seen that the laser is capable of generating ultrafine to amorphous microstructures, sometimes involving metastable phases due to the rapid solidification possible. Furthermore, due to the steep thermal gradients resulting in considerable convection, homogeneous surface layers can be obtained. Clad layers can be formed by feeding an appropriate material into the laser melt pool. These layers can be made with a fusion bond and low dilution and offer advantages over present techniques. A characteristic of laser treatment is the production of residual stresses which can be compressive or tensile. Sufficient work has now been done to identify the associated problems in many cases. The laser currently offers to industry one of the most flexible energy sources, and all of the processes described in this chapter could be coupled for full automation.

LASER SURFACE MELTING OF IRON-BASE ALLOYS

H. W. BERGMANN
Institut für Werkstoffkunde und Werkstofftechnik, TU Clausthal,
Agricolastrasse 2, D-3392 Clausthal-Zellerfeld, FRG

Key Words: cast iron, fatigue, wear, corrosion, rapid solidification

1. INTRODUCTION

Laser surface melting of cast iron is, apart from laser cutting and welding, a major area of industrial interest. There are a number of technical reasons which justify the use of lasers in this area. First of all, cast iron is a cheap starting material with a lower melting point compared to iron. On the other hand, casting is still the cheapest way of metal forming. For this reason it is suitable for the production of automobile car parts. Such parts are manufactured in large numbers, and therefore the advantage of lasers is the high degree of possible automation. On the other hand, the high flexibility of laser manufacturing allows small variations in components of the various models in one type of car. The metallurgical reason why laser surface melting of cast iron is an interesting process is the almost ideal combination of strength and ductility of the core and the wear resistance of the melted surface. Favorable compared to classical methods is the fact that also relatively thin surface layers can be produced (1). In the following the metallurgical and technical aspects of laser surface melting of cast iron are discussed.

In gray cast iron the important effect of hardness increase arises from the solidification in the metastable $Fe-Fe_3C$ system. Gray cast irons can be characterized by the structure of the matrix and the morphology, size and distribution of the graphite phase. In laser melting, the major influence is the structure of the matrix. Variations occur in the case depth, the microstructure and depth of the HAZ. The differences in case depth depend upon the thermal conductivity of the matrix, and differences in HAZ depend upon the different thermal responses of the matrices, including incomplete transformations. For bainitic and martensitic matrices the complicated structure in the HAZ can be eliminated by suitable choice of processing parameters. Laser melting can be applied to various graphite morphologies, lamellar, flaky and spheriodal graphite. Differences in size and distribution of the graphite may require adaption of the interaction time for a homogeneous melt.

The hardness of ledeburitic structures results from the eutectic cementite, and therefore ledeburitic structures are not too sensitive to annealing effects which occur on subsequent processing due to self annealing. In Figure 1 the different response on self annealing for a plain carbon steel and cast iron is demonstrated. Technological advantages arise when one stage of the production line can be eliminated. For laser processing of cast iron car parts, two possible concepts can be applied:

Concept 1: precision casting, grinding, laser melting, finishing.
Concept 2: conventional casting, deep welding, deep grinding, finishing.

Draper, C.W. and Mazzoldi, P. (eds.), Laser Surface Treatment of Metals. ISBN 90-247-3405-3.

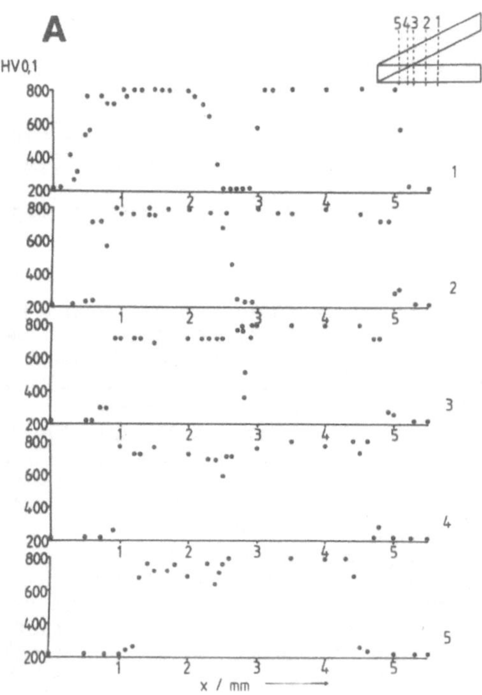

FIGURE 1. The effect of self-annealing of successive paths: (a) cast iron substrate.

Concept 1 was realized for a rocker arm shown in Figure 2a-c. The roughness of 1 to 1.5 µm was removed by a final 10 µm grinding process. The second one was realized by melting a camshaft, see Figure 3. In any case, it is necessary to melt the surface and produce a crack-free, porous-free layer. To this end, special arrangements for the treatment gas are necessary which allow changes in the gas flow rate, angle of impingement and the shape of the gas jet.

Together with a higher power density, this allows an increased feed rate, and on the other hand, avoids massive plasma formation. Often the massive plasma is responsible for crack formation and oxidation. This is demonstrated in Figure 4.

An important influence on the melting behavior results from the graphite arrangement. For the same composition, graphite morphology and cell size, only hardening or melting is observed, see Figure 5, for A or E graphite quality, respectively (graphite arangements due to German standards). The melting quality is further influenced by the casting line, molds and painting.

Examples are given in Tables 1 and 2. The quality decreases from green sand to β-set, croning, oil sand, OBB and sodium silicate bound sand. The painting has only a minor influence. The above demonstrates that suitable choice of laser parameters, composition and casting line allows reproducible melting of shot blast cast iron with a resulting smooth, crack-free, shiny and porous-free surface.

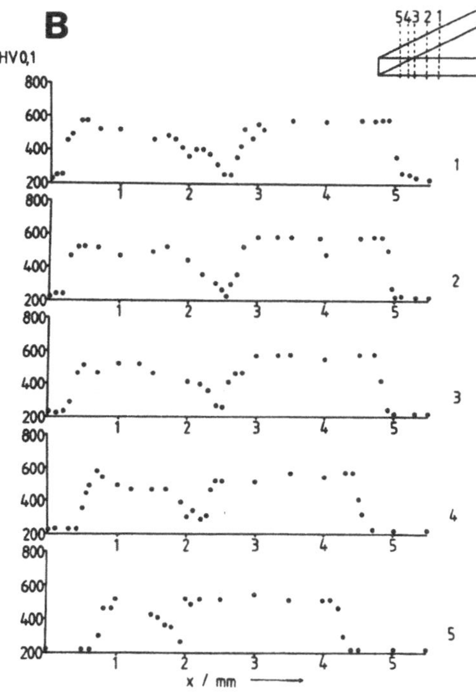

FIGURE 1. (b) carbon steel C45.

2. RESULTS AND DISCUSSION

2.1. Mechanical properties of laser-melted gray cast iron

The properties of laser-melted cast irons have not been fully investigated as yet, but the few results available are quite encouraging, especially in the case of S.G. iron. The mechanical properties of laser-melted S.G. irons depend on both the area ratio of melt depth to substrate and HAZ to substrate. For S.G. iron the HAZ is small when compared to the melt depth and may be neglected in a first approximation. The stress-strain curves of the lasered tensile test specimens are similar to those of untreated specimens, except that above the yield point, the case cracks circumferentially, giving a feature on the curve not dissimilar to discontinuous yielding, and this is accompanied by an acoustic emission. At least 1% elongation occurs before the case cracks.

The case is more brittle than the core, though still surprisingly tough. A unique feature of this material after tensile testing is the occurrence of equidistant circumferential cracks along the gauge length. These cracks do not penetrate further than the case core interface because of workhardening of the ductile core. This effect is not

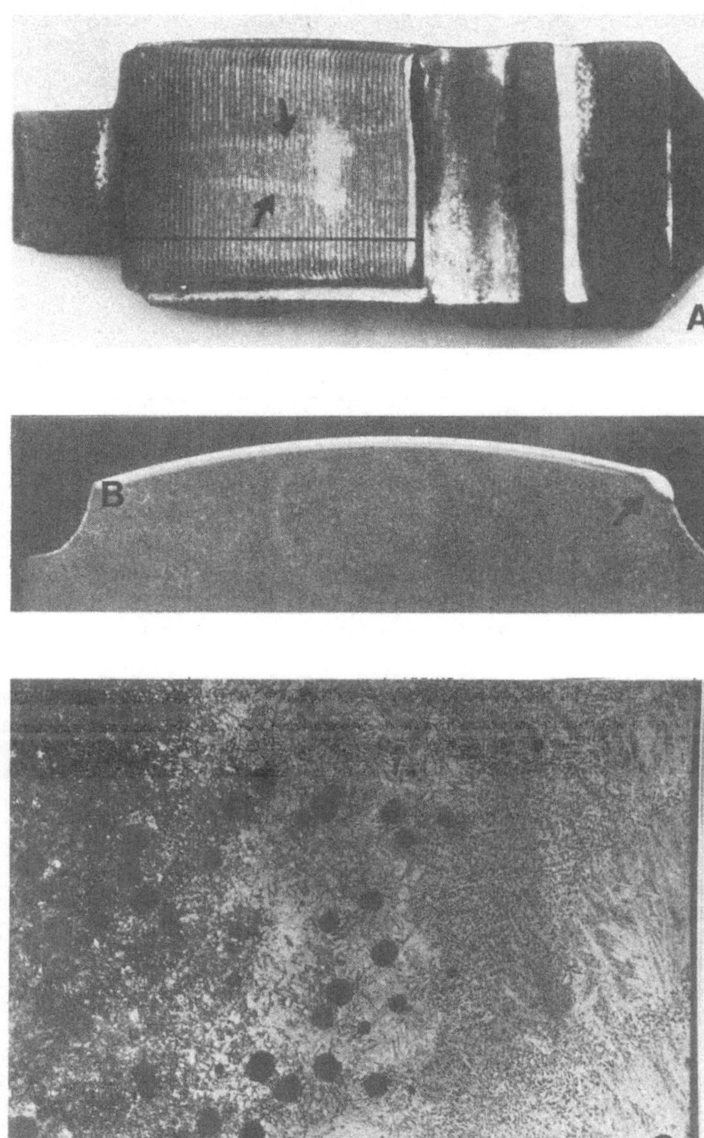

FIGURE 2. Laser-melted cast iron rocker arm: (a) top view, (b) longitudinal section, (c) enlargement of (b).

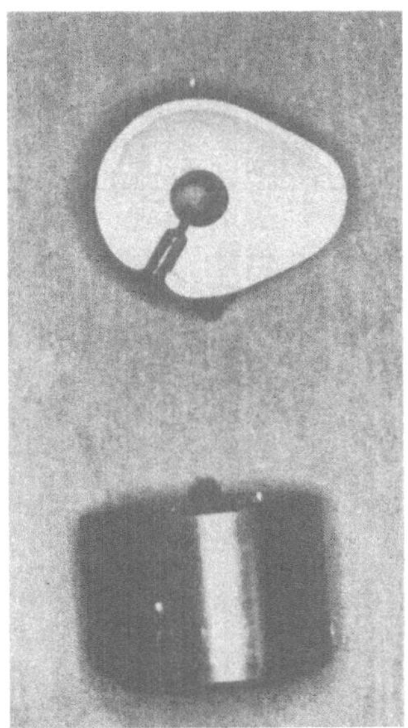

FIGURE 3. Laser-melted camshaft.

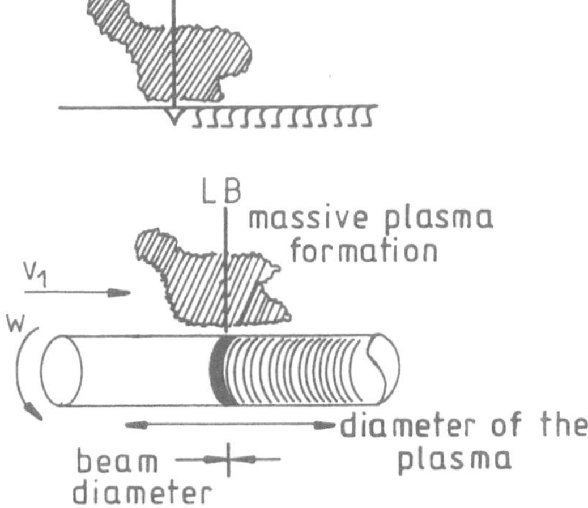

FIGURE 4. Schematic drawing of the influence of massive plasma formation on the quality of the melted cast iron components.

TABLE 1. Influence of composition and initial surface treatment on the laser surface melting of gray cast iron, which was cast in green sand without mold wash.

Substrate Quality	Pre-Heating	Feed Rate m/min	Surface Condition	Roughness	Color	Cracks	Quantity of Pores
TI6	RT	1	as cast	small	blue	no	few
Chill cast	RT	1	as cast	medium	blue	no	medium
GGG40	RT	1	as cast	smooth	bright	no	few
TI6	400°C	1	as cast	small	blue	no	few
Chill cast	400°C	1	as cast	medium	blue	no	none
GGG40	400°C	1	as cast	smooth	bright	no	few
TI6	RT	0,5	sand-blasted	small	blue	no	few
Chill cast	RT	0,5	sand-blasted	medium	blue	no	none
GGG40	RT	0,5	sand-blasted	smooth	bright	no	none
TI6	RT	1	machined	smooth	bright	no	few
Chill cast	RT	1	machined	smooth	bright	few	medium
GGG40	RT	1	machined	smooth	bright	no	few
TI6	400°C	0,5	machined	smooth	bright	no	few
Chill cast	400°C	0,5	machined	smooth	bright	no	few
GGG40	400°C	0,5	machined	smooth	bright	no	few
TI6	RT	1	ground	smooth	bright	no	none
Chill cast	RT	1	ground	smooth	bright	few	few
GGG40	RT	1	ground	smooth	bright	no	none
TI6	400°C	0,5	ground	smooth	bright	no	none
Chill cast	400°C	0,5	ground	smooth	bright	no	none
GGG40	400°C	0,5	ground	smooth	bright	no	none

influenced by metallurgical inhomogeneities between laser tracks, as there are none, and it occurs with longitudinal tracks as well as for spiral melting. This behavior occurs for ferritic, pearlitic and bainitic core structures which have a higher toughness than the case. When a martensitic matrix is used, the initial case crack continues through the brittle core.

Tensile test results for different matrix structures show no major differences compared with untreated material, providing that the laser-melted regions were small when compared with the untreated area. For a deeper case, e.g., 1/3 to 1/2 of the total cross section, an increase in strength, a decrease in elongation and a detectable increase in Young's modulus can be observed. It should be noted that even when the case is that deep, the mechanical properties obtained are still superior to those of the corresponding white castings.

TABLE 2. Influence of molding sand and mold wash on the laser surface melting of gray cast iron.

Substrate Quality	Sand	Mold Wash	Pre-Heating	Feed Rate m/min	Surface Condi-tion	Rough-ness	Color	Cracks	Quantity of Pores
TIG	CO_2	-	400°C	1	as cast	medium	bright	no	some
TIG	CO_2	varnish	400°C	1	as cast	small	bright/ blue	no	medium
TIG	CO_2	alcohol	400°C	1	as cast	small	blue	no	some
TIG	green sand	-	400°C	1	as cast	medium	blue	no	medium, many
TIG	ß-set	-	400°C	1	as cast	rough/ medium	blue	no	medium
TIG	croming	-	400°C	1	as cast	medium	blue/ bright	no	medium
TIG	OBB	-	400°C	1	as cast	small	blue	no	few
TIG	oil	-	400°C	1	as cast	medium	blue	no	few

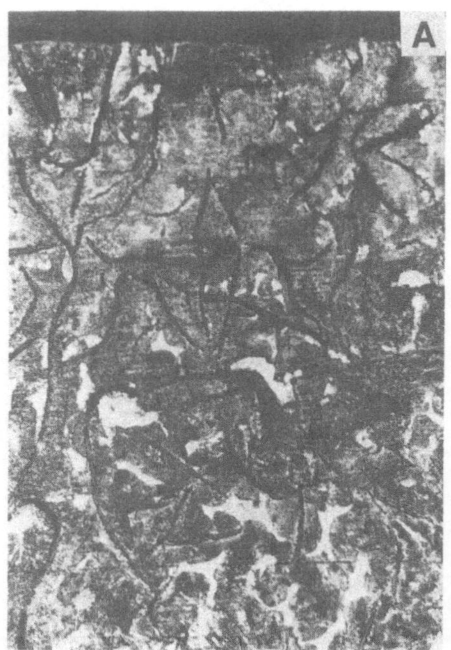

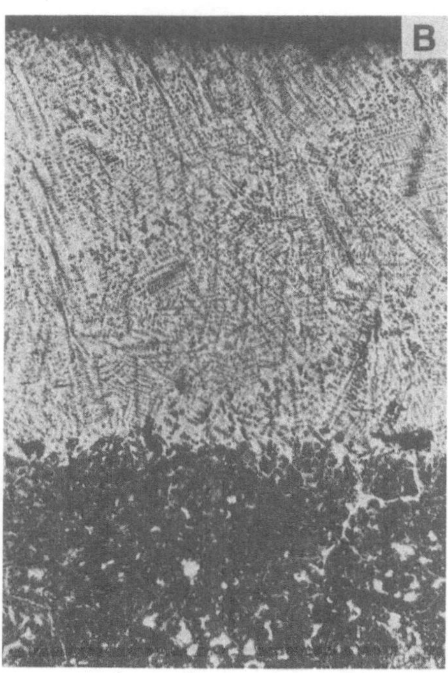

FIGURE 5. Micrograph of laser-treated cast iron. Both samples have the same nominal composition and have been treated with identical laser parameters. (a), (b) different graphite arrangements.

The tensile properties were also investigated for bainitic and martensitic structures after laser melting. For the martensitic matrix remelting does not deteriorate or possibly benefit the mechanical properties. Remelting of the bainitic SG-iron results in higher values of elongation to fracture because of the high amount of retained austenite, which transforms under load and stops the propagating cracks. A laser treatment may cause here an additional amount of transformation and therefore reduces the plasticity. However, the obtained values are still good compared to steels with equivalent strength and hardness. From what has been said above, it is apparent that impact strength is reduced with an increasing amount of transformed cross section. Although no proper impact tests have been carried out so far, preliminary tests do confirm this. The fractographs demonstrate the difference between the brittle case and ductile core and show no delamination of the lasered cases. The observed impact strength lies between the two limiting cases of gray and white cast irons.

2.2. Internal stresses introduced by laser melting and the influence of subsequent heat treatment

Laser surface melting results in internal stresses on solidification. Several factors contribute to the final stress situations, for example, the volume difference on solidification, differences in shrinkage in the solid state for core and surface due to both temperature differences and different coefficients of thermal expansion. However, the various transformations in both case and core have an effect. For cast iron with pearlitic matrix and flaky graphite (1), it was found that in the surface, compressive stresses were present which change to tensile stresses at a certain distance below the surface. Depending on the case depth, the sign of the stress changes in either the core or the surface layer. S.G. iron contains compressive stresses in the as-lasered surface (3). Tensile stresses at the surface were found in white cast iron in the as-lasered condition (4). They gradually change to compressive stresses on further heat treatment.

2.3. Fatigue properties

The fatigue properties of ferritic S.G. iron were studied with the pull-pull test. The mean tensile stress was ~50% of the yield point, that is, ≃150 Nmm^{-2}. A 10 Hz frequency of various amplitudes was then applied to the specimens and the fatigue limit determined. Untreated specimens were ground after machining. As no relevant data is available in the literature, optimized processing parameters for laser treatment had to be defined. This was done by keeping the case depth constant at about 10% of the cross section. Compared to the untreated S.G. iron, a decrease in fatigue limit was found in the as-lasered condition. This was more pronounced when N_2, CO_2 or Ar was used as the protective gas, but less with He. In addition, a spiral laser track gives better results than a longitudinal series of tracks. Grinding the surface, i.e., smoothing small amounts of roughness produced by the laser treatment, leads to a small decrease in fatigue limit as compared with untreated value.

The most favorable values, see Fig. 6, were found when the specimens were annealed at 240°C for two hrs after laser treatment with helium and subsequently ground. In a second series the influence of a deeper case was studied. Here the mean stress was chosen as 340 N/mm^2 because of the higher yield point, see Fig. 6. It can be seen that the untreated material for a medium mean load can carry a higher amplitude. However, with increasing load the advantage of strengthening due to laser melting allows working at mean loads over the yield point of the untreated material.

It was already mentioned for the tensile tests that the plasticity of bainitic SG-iron is reduced by laser treatment. The fatigue behavior of laser-melted bainitic SG-iron is given in Fig. 7, where Wöhler diagrams for two mean loads are shown. In Fig. 8 the corresponding Smith diagram gives the fatigue life as a function of the mean load. Pure fatigue behavior was found in the as-lasered specimen, which may partly depend on the surface finish and partly on internal stresses. Grinding at the surface improves the fatigue behavior but is not able to give properties equivalent to the untreated material.

2.4. Wear properties

The excellent wear properties of ledeburitic surface layers on cast iron have been demonstrated by various authors (5-8). Most of the work has been carried out on TIG melted surfaces (6,8), while for the new technique of laser melting, only a limited amount of data is available (5,7). From References 6,8 it is known that surface-melted layers produced by the TIG technique can be run under higher applied loads than for hardened steels. The tests were performed employing various

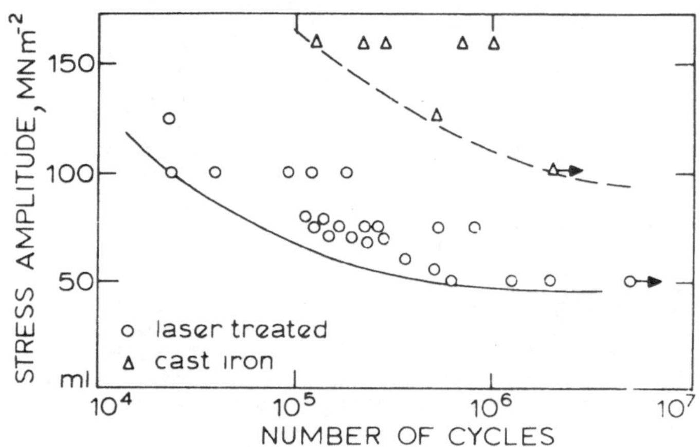

FIGURE 6. Fatigue behavior of laser-melted S.G. iron with ferrite matrix.

lubricants. The optimized combinations are surface-melted cast irons running against surface-melted and nitrided cast irons. The tests were carried out with camshafts and rocker arms. For lasered gray iron with pearlitic matrix and flaky graphite, Bell and co-workers demonstrated that the wear properties in dry pin on disc tests are improved by laser melting by one order of magnitude. There was still a significant increase compared to fully martensitic microstructures.

The advantage of laser-melted S.G. iron was demonstrated for rolls which run dry against each other with a fixed relative slip (9), one wheel being driven and the other partially braked (Fig. 9). Various stresses were applied (e.g., 500 and 1000 Nmm^{-2}) and the humidity was controlled. For a slip of approximately 3-5% and the higher load, melting occurred after a couple of minutes when steel rolls were used, but the cast irons showed no evidence of any deformation. For comparison, ~1% slip was used (Figs. 9-11). It is obvious that the wear properties of lasered cast iron are superior to those of hardened, conventional steels. Combinations of lasered irons and steels must be avoided, as massive deformation of the steel occurs. When laser treatments were carried out under He, better results were found than with other gases. Excellent results were obtained when laser-melted S.G. irons were used in combination with TiN- or TiC-coated, hardened steels, the TiN/TiC surface suffering the wear. After the tests, no deformation is visible on the ledeburitic surface. Good wear properties are obtained in combinations of lasered S.G. iron with nitrided or borided steels. A comparison between lasered and TIG-melted ledeburitic surfaces favors the laser process. The fine microstructure may be the reason for this. For extremely high loads $\simeq$4000 N/mm^2 it was found that the ledeburitic case has to be about 1 mm thick to avoid fracture as a result of the Hertzian stresses. If a case of this thickness is required, the laser-melted or TIG-welded microstructures are almost equivalent and so are the wear properties.

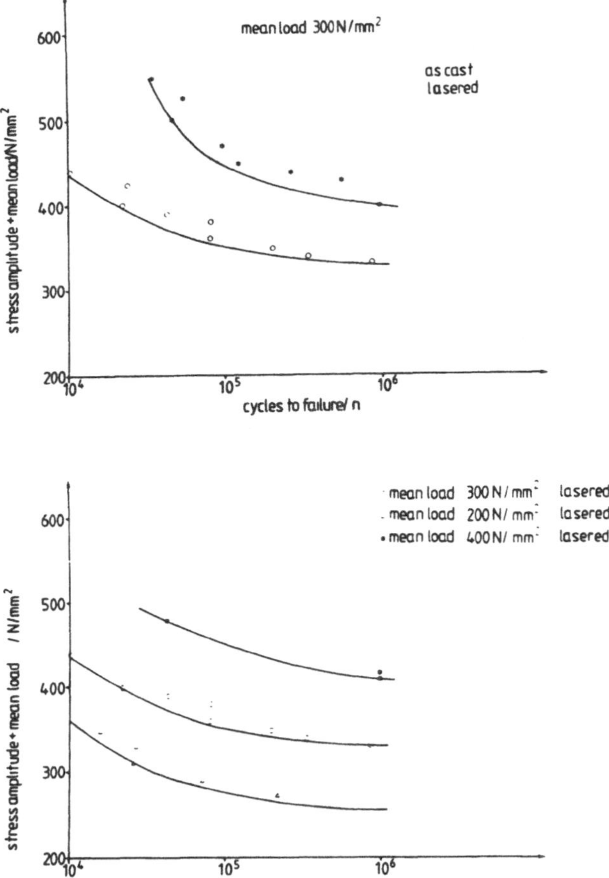

FIGURE 7. Fatigue behavior of laser-melted S.G. iron with bainitic matrix.

Better wear resistance of laser-melted S.G. iron compared with steels does not imply a change in the coefficient of friction, as is demonstrated in Fig. 10. The coefficient of friction was determined for various loads and velocities as a function of the slip (9). In all combinations the same curves were obtained (Fig. 10b). The wear behavior, however, does show differences, as can be seen in Fig. 10a.

Laser-melted S.G. iron also exhibits superior wear properties if tested under lubrication. The machine used is shown schematically in Fig. 11a and the test results in Fig. 11b. Tests of real components used in the car industry on a testing machine as well as after running in a test car are in progress.

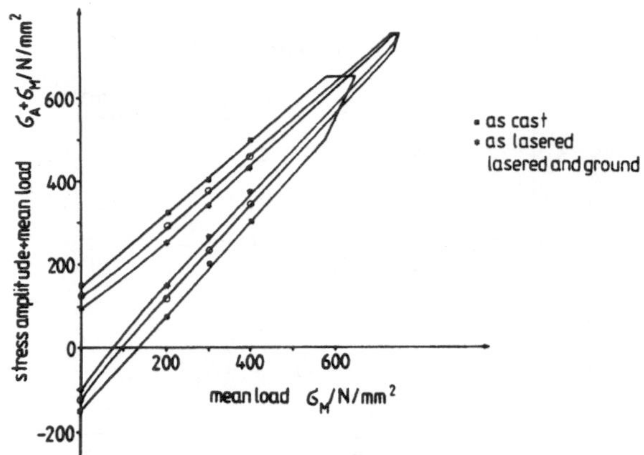

FIGURE 8. Smith diagram of Figure 7.

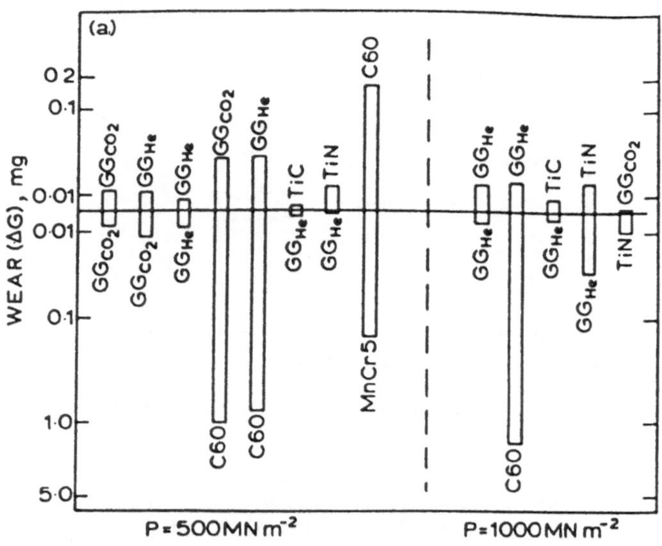

FIGURE 9. Comparison of wear properties of laser and TIG surface melted SG iron with those of various steels, with and without surface treatments: P=load on rolls during test, S=roll slip during test.

(a) C60 represents 0.6% carbon steel, GG laser-melted SG cast iron, MnCr5 case-hardened 16 MnCr5 steel (64HRC), and TiC and TiN case-hardened 16 MnCr5 steel coated with TiC and TiN, respectively.

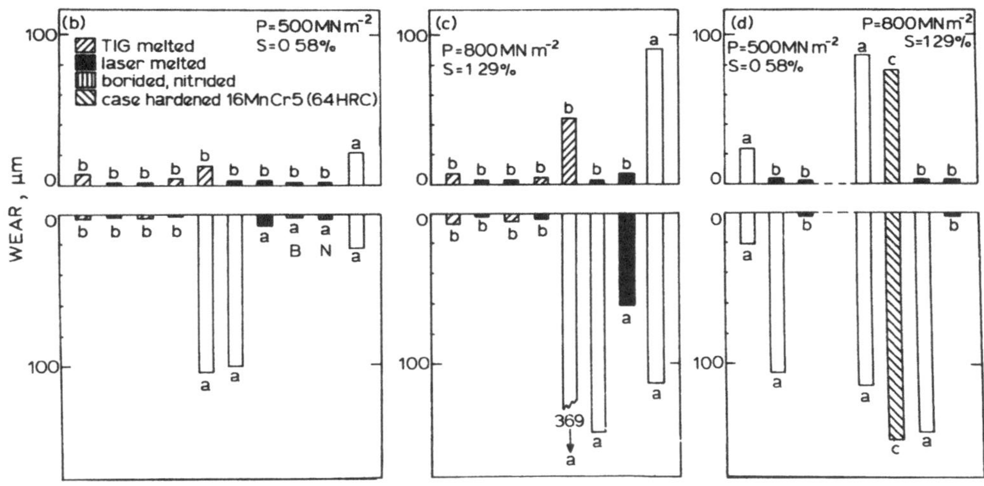

FIGURE 9. Comparison of wear properties of laser and TIG surface melted SG iron with those of various steels, with and without surface treatments: P=load on rolls during test, S=roll slip during test.
(b-d) (a) represents 0.6% carbon steel, (b) surface-melted SG iron, and (c) case-hardened 16 MnCr5 steel (64 HRC).

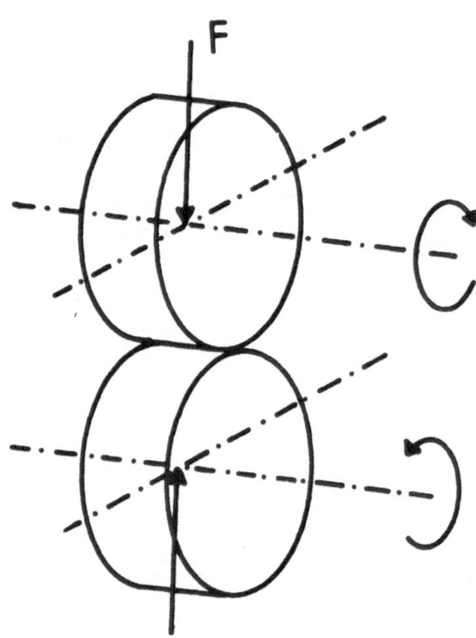

FIGURE 10. Wear properties and coefficient of friction between rolls measured using equipment illustrated, P=load on rolls during test.

2.5. Corrosion properties

During metallographical preparation it is a common feature that laser-melted iron in the as-quenched condition etches less than the substrate, and it is easy to etch mm steps between treated and untreated materials by deep etching. This indicates that the remelted material exhibits better corrosion properties.

From the current-density-potential curves one can derive that the remelted as-quenched material shows a higher value of the corrosion potential. This means that the remelted material is more noble than the unmelted one. The fact that this is true even for white cast substrates can only be interpreted by the fact that the higher supersaturation and small grain size prevents the $\gamma \rightarrow \alpha$-transformation almost completely so that the difference in the potential corresponds to the difference in γ- and α-iron. This would explain the etching behavior in the as-quenched condition and is consistent with the fact that the corrosion behavior does change when the lasered material is annealed. The second thing which is obvious is that for all potentials the current density is about a factor 3-6 smaller than for the untreated material.

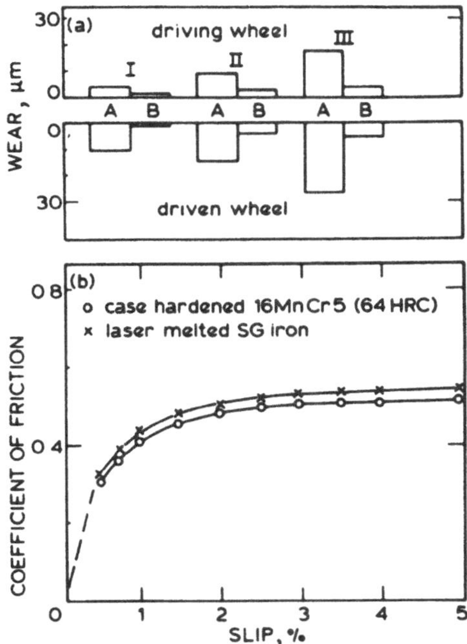

FIGURE 10. Wear properties and coefficient of friction between rolls measured using equipment illustrated, P=load on rolls during test. (a) Comparative wear: I, P=500 MNm^{-2} at 200 rev min^{-1}; II, P=500 MNm^{-2} at 1000 rev min^{-1}; III, P=1000 MNm^{-2} at 200 rev min^{-1}, A, case-hardened 16 MnCr5 steel (64 HRC); B, laser-melted GGG40 SG cast iron. (b) Variation of coefficient of friction with roll slip.

3. GENERAL COMMENTS AND POSSIBLE APPLICATIONS

Apart from the fact that laser melting enhances certain desirable properties mentioned above, there are additional beneficial features obtained with this technique. The melting process can be carried out on an almost finished component, as the distortion associated with the process is negligible and surface roughness is in the order or 1.4 μm, which can easily be improved by grinding if necessary.

There is no need for a sophisticated handling system, as a uniform and homogeneous case can be achieved if lasered within the focal distance, i.e., + 1.5 cm for a 25.4 cm focal length lens.

Laser melting is a hardening process which can be fully automated. It is also a fast and cheap process. The laser-melted component shown in Fig. 2 achieved a four times better test lifetime when compared to TIG melting. Figure 12 shows a micrograph after 40,000 km.

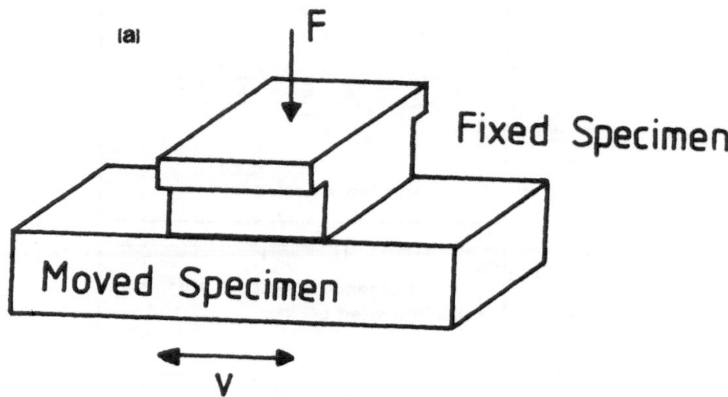

FIGURE 11. Comparison of properties in lubricated wear test of laser-melted SG cast iron and case-hardened steel: v = 80 mms^{-1}
(a) Schematic diagram of testing machine.

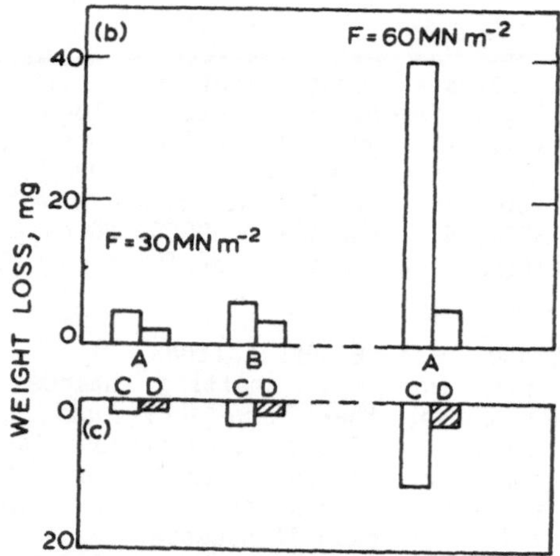

FIGURE 11. (b) Results of test for fixed specimen: A, case-hardened 16CrNi6 steel; B, laser-melted SG cast iron;
(c) Results of test for moving specimen: C and D represent two copper-based alloys.

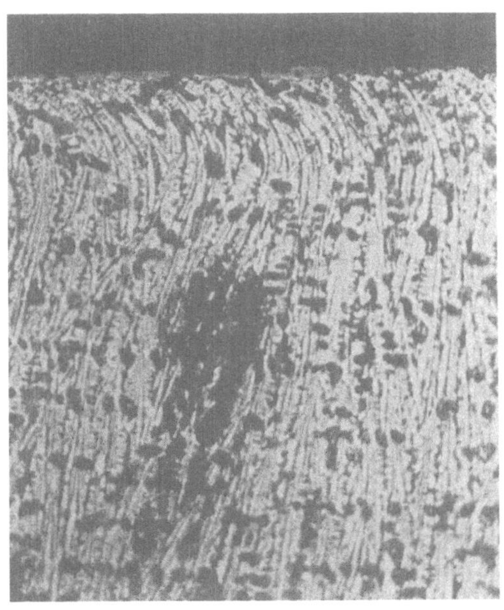

FIGURE 12. Micrograph of laser-melted cast iron rock arm after testing.

REFERENCES

1. H. W. Bergmann, Surface Engineering 1, 137 (1985).
2. H. W. Bergmann, B. L. Mordike, and T. Bell, in Optoelectronics in Engineering, edited by W. Waidelich (Springer-Verlag, Berlin, 1984), p. 335.
3. H. Krause et al., Technische Hochschule Aachen, unpublished work.
4. H. W. Bergmann, G. Barton, and J. Betz, Z. Werkstofftechnik 14, 244 (1983).
5. F. H. Reinke, "Local Electric Arc Remelting Process for the Generation of Wear-Resistant White Iron Layers on Workpieces of Grey Cast Iron, especially Camshafts and Cam Followers," AEG Elotherm, Remscheid, FRG, 1983.
6. "Cams and Tappets: A Survey of Information," British Technical Council of the Motor and Petroleum Industries, 1972.
7. J. Emde, Elektrowärme Int. 37B, 3 (1979).
8. K. Heck, Doktorarbeit, Technische Universität München, 1983.
9. H. Krause, H. Schröllkamp, and H. W. Bergmann, Technische Hochschule Aachen/Technische Universität Clausthal, unpublished work.

LASER SURFACE CLADDING

W. M. STEEN
Metallurgy and Materials Science Department, Imperial College,
London SW7 2BP, UK

Key Words: cladding, powder feed, steel reflectance

1. DESCRIPTION OF THE PROCESS

The objective in laser cladding is to fuse an alloy on to the surface of a substrate with a minimum of dilution from the substrate. Areas are clad by overlapping single-clad tracks.

The process can be performed by either preplacing a powder on the substrate or blowing the powder into the laser-generated melt pool. It can also be done by applying the clad material as a wire sheet or plasma spraycoat or electroplate coat.

In preplaced powder cladding decribed by Powell (1), the laser sends a melt wave through the powder bed. Since the powder bed has a low thermal conductivity, the pool is almost thermally insulated until it reaches the substrate surface. At that moment it will freeze back, forming only a solid/liquid bond which is relatively weak compared to a full fusion bond. Continued heating will remelt the resolidified material and then cause a fusion bond to form. However, it will be seen that this allows a relatively small operating region in which there is a fusion bond with low dilution. The process is illustrated in Fig. 1. One of the principal problems with this process is the difficulty in keeping the powder in place while it is melted by the beam.

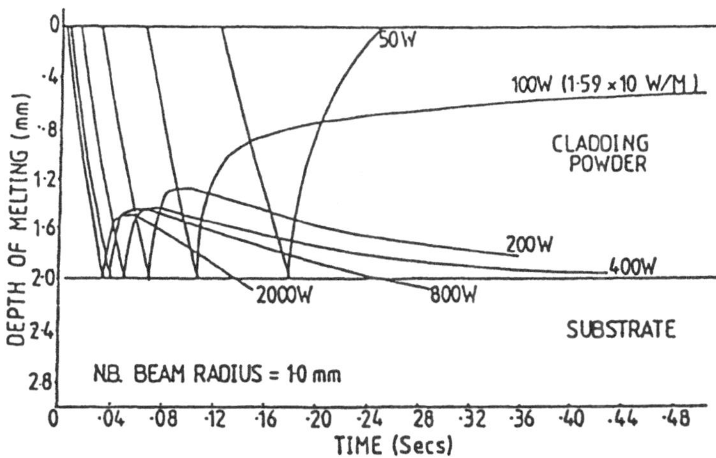

FIGURE 1. Movement of molten front with time at different laser powers.

In blown powder cladding (2,3) the powder is blown by an inert gas stream into the laser-generated melt pool, as illustrated in Figs. 2 and 3. The leading edge of the melt pool will incorporate the substrate.

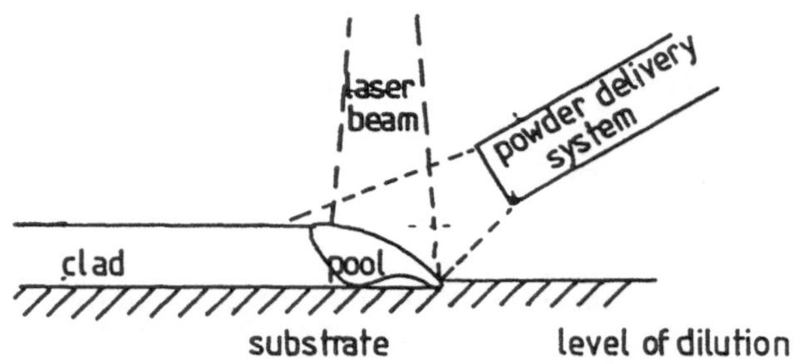

FIGURE 2. Laser cladding with blown powder.

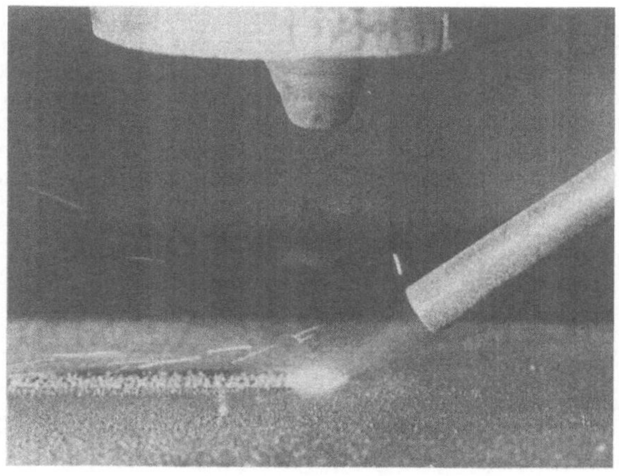

FIGURE 3. Laser cladding by powder injection.

Particles arriving in this area will be solid. If the leading edge of the substrate is also solid, then the particle will not stick and cladding will not occur. If, however, the leading edge is molten, then the particles will stick and will melt almost instantly under the power from the beam, thus forming a fusion bond. The level of dilution is controlled by the powder feed rate determining the size of the substrate's molten leading edge. Uniform clad layers are formed by overlapping single tracks, as illustrated in Fig. 4(a,b). The process cricitally depends upon a uniform powder feed rate. Such a feeder was developed. Its performance is illustrated in Fig. 5.

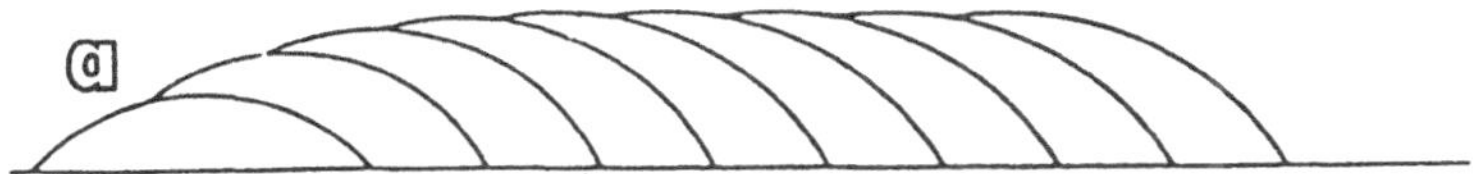

FIGURE 4. (a) Development of a uniform clad layer by overlapping.

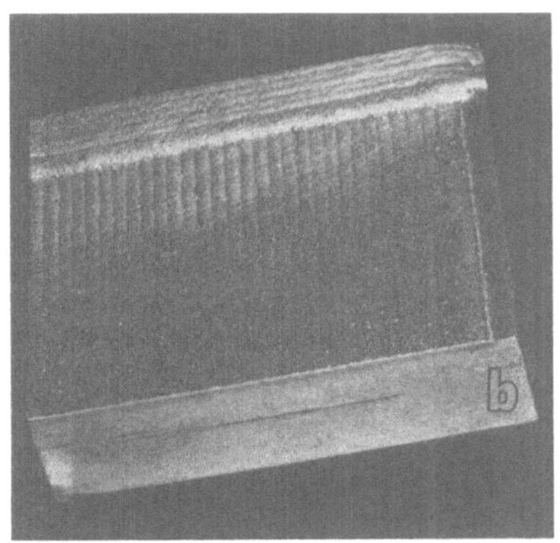

FIGURE 4. (b) a laser-clad plate. Plate thickness 12.5 mm. Single layer is 0.3 mm thick, double layer 1.5 mm thick.

If the clad material is fed as either wire or sheet, there is a problem with reflectivity and so the process is less efficient but still possible.

Consolidation of surfaces by laser remelting of plasma spray-coated or electroplated surfaces is also practiced (4,5).

The main characteristics of the blown powder process are:

- Controlled levels of dilution
- Localized heating which reduces thermal distortion and the size of the heat affected zone (HAZ)
- Controlled shape of clad within certain limits
- Smooth surface finish (≈ 25 μm)
- Good fusion bonding
- Fine quench microstructures
- Non-contact method of application
- Easily automated
- Omnidirectional
- Near isotropic mechanical properties
- Thin clad layers are possible (>0.3 mm)
- Minimum surface preparation is required for many applications
- Process is flexible

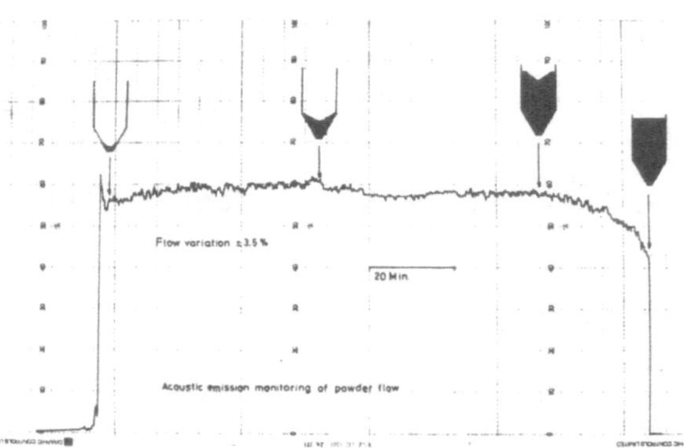

FIGURE 5. In-process monitoring of powder feed rate using an acoustic emission technique (11).

1.2. Process variations

Mixed powder feed (6): By this method alloys can be formed *in situ* or non-homogeneous deposits formed.

Optical feedback systems (2,3) have been developed which increase the efficiency of utilization of the beam power by around 40%.

Vibro laser cladding (7): By this method the substrate is vibrated ultrasonically while cladding proceeds. There is considerably less cracking and porosity observed.

1.3. Applications

The first industrial use of lasers in cladding was done by Rolls Royce (8) in 1981. They clad turbine blade shroud interlocks on the RG 211 engine.

Since then many companies have applied or are considering applying this process.

Eboo (9) lists the activity reported in Table 1.

1.4. Comparison with alternative processes

One reason for the great industrial interest in this process is that it is one of the very few surfacing processes which cause little thermal damage to the substrate, and relatively slight distortion (10). It is also the only fusion-cladding process which allows a patterned clad to be laid down.

Alternative processes are listed in Table 2.

2. PROCESS MECHANICS OF THE BLOWN-POWDER PROCESS

2.1. Characteristic process phenomena

The powder injection technique is fundamentally more flexible and superior to the pre-placed powder technique (11) in that localized areas of components of complex geometry can be clad with better control on dilution and clad thickness.

The use of the cladding material in the form of a powder has an added attraction due to the increased efficiency obtained in coupling the laser energy. Powder particles in or near the surface appear to enhance the absorption of laser energy. A molten pool is generated on the ground surface when powder is injected whereas no melting is observed without powder. Metallurgically, the use of powder may reduce macro-segregation effects during solidification.

TABLE 1. Representative laser cladding efforts.

Company	Component	Comment
Production Stage		
Rolls Royce	Turbine blade shroud interlock	Cobalt base alloy powder feed
Pratt & Whitney	Turbine blade	PWA 694/nimonic preplaced chips
G.E.	Proprietary	Reverse machining with Ti powder feed
Pilot Demonstration Stage		
Combustion Eng.	Offshore drilling & production parts	Stellites, colmonoys and other alloys including carbides
	Valve components boiler firewall	Powder feed
FIAT	Valve stem valve seat aluminum block	Cr, C, Cr, Ni, Mo/cast Fe preplaced powder
GM	Automotive	Cast-iron systems
Rockwell	Aerospace	T-800, stellites, powder feed
Westinghouse	Turbine blades	Stellites, colmonoys preplaced beds and gravity
NRL	Proprietary	Multiple alloy, powder feed

Superficial melting of the substrate surface is required so that a fusion bond takes place. The particles need not necessarily arrive at the melt pool surface in a molten state. In fact, theoretical calculations and high-speed photography show that an average size particle hardly gets red hot while traveling through the beam (12).

Solid particles are often observed in plasma-sprayed coatings. In powder injection laser cladding, no embedded solid particles were observed in the cast structures. It has been shown theoretically that the melting time of a particle is much lower than its time of residence

TABLE 2.

Process	Interface Bond S = Solid L= Liquid Clad	Subs	Dilution %	Deposition Rate 16/hr	Min. Thickness In.	Heat Spot Size In.	Appl. to Automa-tions	Appl. to Internal L = Large only	Surface Finish
Flame Spray	L	S	1-10	1-6	1/32	1			S
Fuseweld	S/L	S	1-30						S
Oxyacet +Rod	L	L	15-25			1			
MMA	L	L	15-25	5-25	1/8	1/2			
MIG	L	L		1-6	1/8	1/2	x	L	
GTA,TIG	L	L	10-20	1-8	1/32	1/2	x	L	
Plasma TR Arc	L	L	5-25	1-15	1/16		x	L	
Plasma Spray	L	S	5-30	1-15	1/32	1/2	x	L	S
Plasma Spray	L	L	5-30				x	L	S
Saw	L	L	10-50	10-60	1/8-5/16	2	x		
Plasma + FNC	L	S/L	1-30						S
Roll bonding	S	S	0						(S)
Explosion	S	S	0		1/8			L*	(S)
Detonation	S	S	0		1/64				S
Electroplate	S	S	0		10^{-5}		x	x	S
PVD	S	S	0		0			x	S
CVD	S	S	0		0			x	S
Ion Plating	S	S	0		0			x	S
5 kW Laser	S/L	L	0-90 Control-lable	1-10	1/64	1/100 Control-lable	-1/2 x	x	S if correct

within the superheated melt pool (10). Also, theoretical calculations show that particles may penetrate the melt pool surface only to a shallow depth before melting completely or may ricochet from the melt surface if the impact angle becomes smaller than a critical angle for ricochet.

Particles falling on the "mushy" region leave a "crater" and, as a result, the surface of the clad bead appears to be "pock-marked," Fig. 6. Normally, as much as 80% of the powder falling on the molten pool is utilized to create the clad bead. However, the overall powder utilization will be much lower if the particles falling on the area surrounding the melt pool are also accounted. Recycling of powder is possible if there is efficient shrouding.

The process parameters are listed in Table 3, categorized into three systems: laser, powder injection and substrate handling.

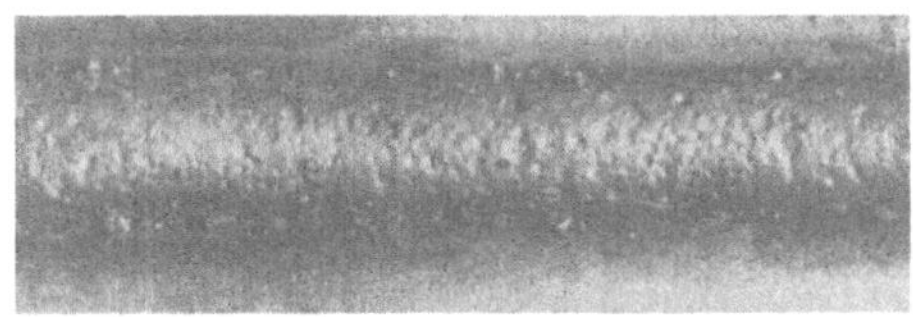

FIGURE 6. Characteristic "pock-marked" surface finish of a clad bead.

3. EVALUATION OF CLADDING RATES

From numerous experiments, Weerasinghe (10,3) was able to draw up the following equations relating the geometry of the deposit tracks to the cladding rate:

$$S = a - bW$$
$$K = \exp(-T/1.8H)$$
$$SH = d$$
$$C = KWS = xS$$

where

S = cladding speed mm/s
W = single-track width mm
H = single-track height mm
T = uniform clad thickness mm
K = overlap factor defined as (x/W)
x = transverse traverse mm
C = cladding rate mm^2/s
a,b,d = constants

For a laser power of 3 kW and beam diameter of 5 mm the constants are:

$$a = 57.36, \quad b = 10.81, \quad d = 5.17$$

It is seen that there is an optimum overlap factor "K" for a given clad thickness "T," since the same clad thickness can be obtained with a low "K" and a high "S" or a high "K" and a low "S." The optimum "K" is that which gives the maximum "C" and is found by differentiation of $C = f(K,T)$. Such calculations are presented in Fig. 7, showing the maximum cladding rate for a particular clad thickness.

TABLE 3. Main operating variables for laser cladding by powder injection (typical values are given in brackets).

System Variable	Method of Monitoring
LASER - cw, CO_2	
Power (up to 3 kW)	Flowing cone calorimeter
Beam diameter (1-5 mm)	Rotating rod ((LBA) 14,15)
Mode structure	Prints, optical geometry, fluorescent screens, LBA
POWDER INJECTION	Load cell on feed hopper
Mass flow rate (0.04-0.35 g/s inside diameter of injector tube 3 mm)	Acoustic emission sensor on feed line
Particle velocity (1.4 m/s for conveying gas velocity of 5.8 m/s	Rotameters, fast-action cinephotography, photographic tracer technique
Particles shape and size (-100 mesh, avg. size 60 um)	Microscopy, sieve analysis
SUBSTRATE MOVEMENT	
Traverse speed 5-50 mm/s	Electronic timer
Traverse index (manual 0.3-2.0 mm)	Scale calibrated to 0.1 mm

* Other monitoring methods available for some aspects.

It is noted that the graphs in Fig. 7 go through the origin (0,0). However, it must be stated that there is a definite region within which satisfactory cladding is obtained. Although the graphs can be extrapolated to high power levels, they cannot be safely extended to power levels below about 1.0 kW if using a 5 mm spot. There is a low and a high speed limit, both depending on the laser power or rather the power density (i.e., power/spot area) and the powder mass flow. The high speed limit is where cladding ceases due to insufficient heat input to melt the substrate surface. The low speed limit is where the high specific energy input distorts the substrate plate to unacceptable levels and/or the process becomes uneconomical.

The cladding rates shown in Fig. 7 can be greatly enhanced by using a hemispherical reflector to recycle the reflected energy losses, Figs. 8 and 9, and shot-blasting the substrate surface, Fig. 10.

By offsetting the axis of the beam to the axis of the dome, the reflected beam could be positioned away from the main beam and so be

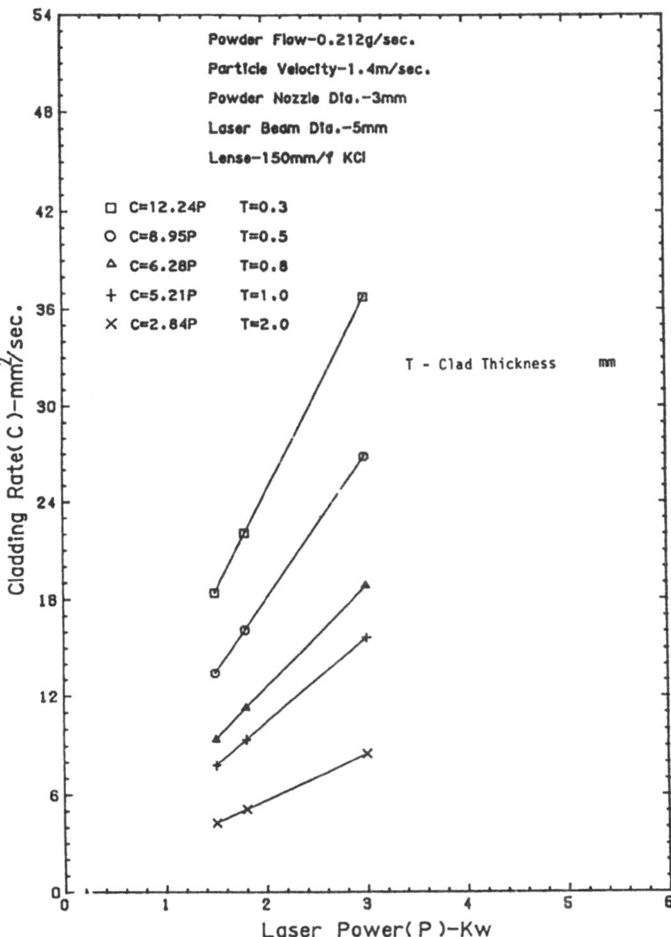

FIGURE 7. Cladding coverage rates calculated from relationship in Section 3, not experimental data.

used for either pre or post heat, Fig. 11. It also allows an experimental determination of the reflected energy by collecting the reflected radiation in a calorimeter. Thus this device, when clean, recycles some 40% of the incident beam energy.

Referring to Fig. 9, it can be seen that the advantage of using the reflecting dome is greater for thinner clad thicknesses, i.e., at higher cladding speeds. This is because at high cladding speeds, a small area is heated to high temperatures compared to the total area on which the laser beam is incident. Since reflectivity reduces at high temperatures, then at high cladding speeds with reduced temperatures, a higher proportion of the incident laser power will be reflected.

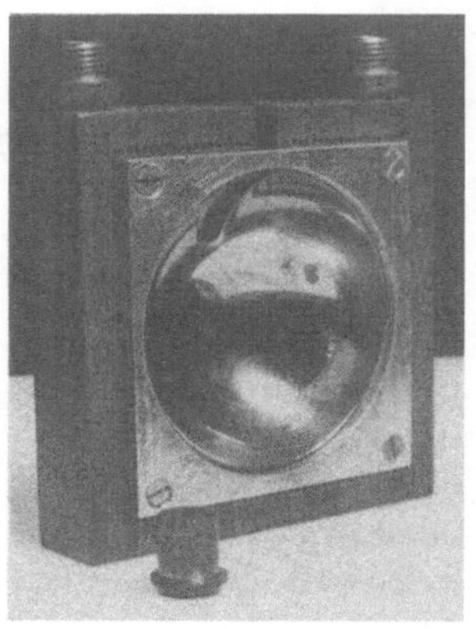

FIGURE 8. Spherical reflecting dome.

4. THREE BASIC BEAD PROFILES

Three basic single-track bead profiles emerged from the numerous section profiles which were examined, Fig. 12.

Profile "c" with an obtuse contact angle is the preferred section for low-dilution cladding. At higher powder feed rates or slower speeds, profile "a" is produced, while at lower powder feed rates and/or higher power densities, profile "b" is produced.

Multiple-track clad layers produced by overlapping of profile "c" will be of good surface finish, minimum or no porosity, and of no dilution. Profile "a" will produce multiple-track clad layers of poor surface finish, greater thickness, no dilution and heavy porosity, especially at the root in between runs. Clad layers produced by profile "b" will be of good surface finish, no porosity, high dilution and generally of lesser thickness than "c". Further, the penetration pattern shown in Fig. 12 is characteristic of a Gaussian beam where there is a peak power intensity at the center. (With a "doughnut" beam, the penetration is more pronounced at the bead edges and is generally of less severity.)

5. EFFECT OF POWDER INJECTION PARAMETERS

The extent of dilution is controlled by the injected powder mass flow or rather the powder flux (g/smm^2), Fig. 13. The optimum powder flux is that which gives the minimum dilution and maximum depositon. It is dependent on the power density (W/mm^2) and mode structure of the laser beam but is independent of the cladding speed. For a lower powder flux the dilution will increase and mass depositon decrease. For a higher powder flux, the effect is reversed.

The optimum powder mass flow was found to be directly proportional to (P/D x n) where "P" is the laser power, "D" the spot diameter, and "n" is a beam shape factor depending on the power intensity distribution.

The optimum stainless powder (-100 mesh size) flux was found to be 10 $mg/S\ mm^2$ for a laser power of 1800 W, spot diameter of 5 mm, and a "doughnut" intensity distribution TEM 01*. A 10% higher flux was required for a Gaussian beam due to its more centalized power distribution.

A 10% increase in the cladding rate was obtained when the average particle size was reduced from 77 microns to 58 microns (3).

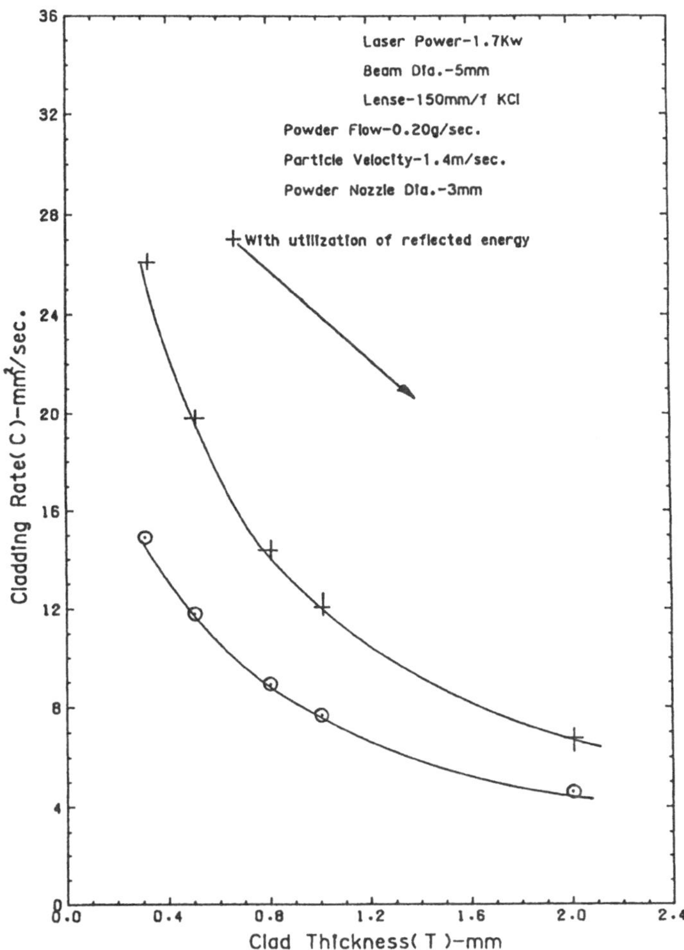

FIGURE 9. Effect of recycling the reflected energy on cladding rate.

A low particle velocity (1.4 m/s) is desirable to minimize ejection and ricochet losses from the molten pool. Since there is a minimum gas velocity required for efficient conveying (2.8 m/s), a limit is imposed. However, some amount of gas can be purged through fine holes near the injector tube exit and so reduce the particle velocity (3).

The major effect of the powder injection angle is due to the variation of the powder flux (g/smm^2) input to the molten pool. The distance from the molten pool to the injector tube has a similar effect due to divergence of the powder clad.

The powder jet is positioned in relation to the beam so that the whole of the molten pool is flooded with powder. Normally, only about

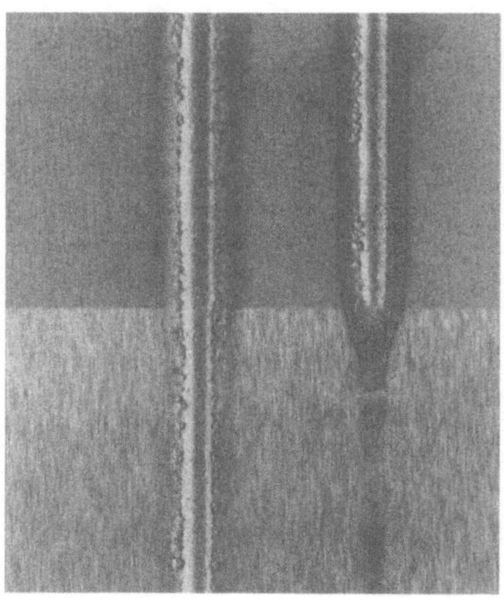

FIGURE 10. Effect of shot blasting the substrate surface. The top half of the substrate surface is shot blasted. The bottom was masked to retain the original ground finish. The track on the left was produced with the "dome" and continues on both sections, since the reflected energy is recycled.

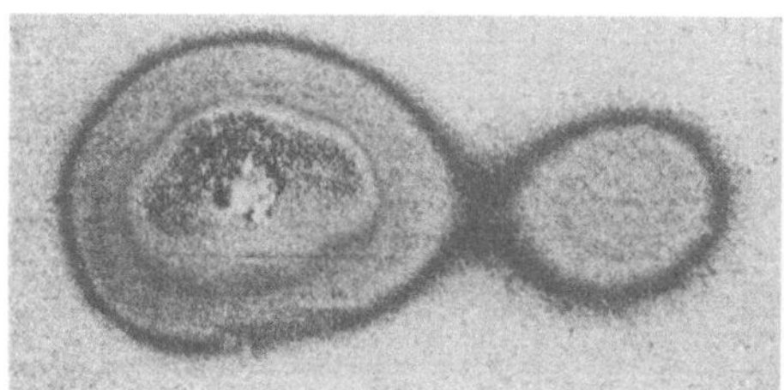

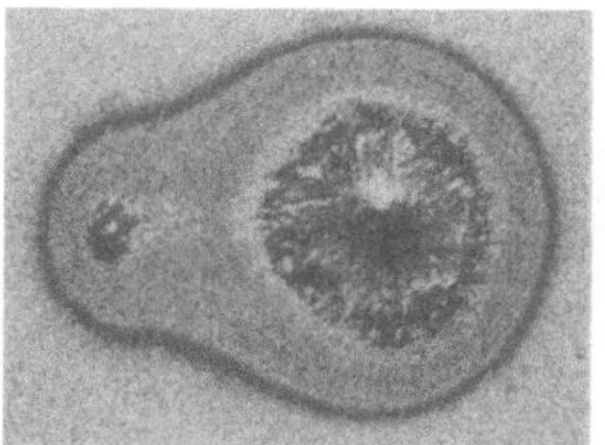

FIGURE 11. Reflected beam (right), positioned away from the main beam (left).

10% of the laser power is absorbed by the powder cloud. This was verified by theoretical calculation and by experiment (3).

In practice, an injection angle of 45-38° (defined from the horizontal) was used with a distance to the molten pool around 10-12 mm from the injector tube end.

6. EFFECT OF LASER BEAM PARAMETERS

Power, spot diameter and mode structure are the beam parameters. Effects due to beam polarization are well known in cutting (16), namely, preferential absorption at a certain orientation of the cut leading edge. See the paper by Keilmann in Chapter 1 of this book. A similar situation

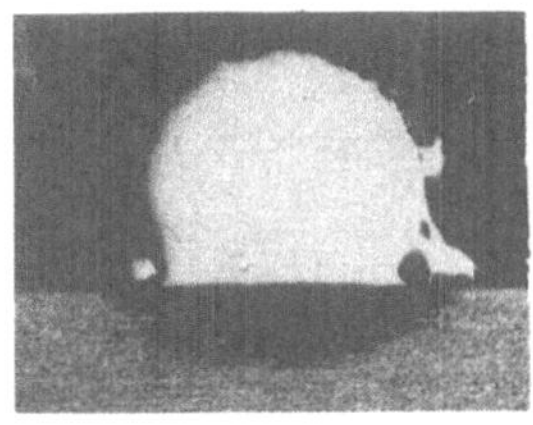 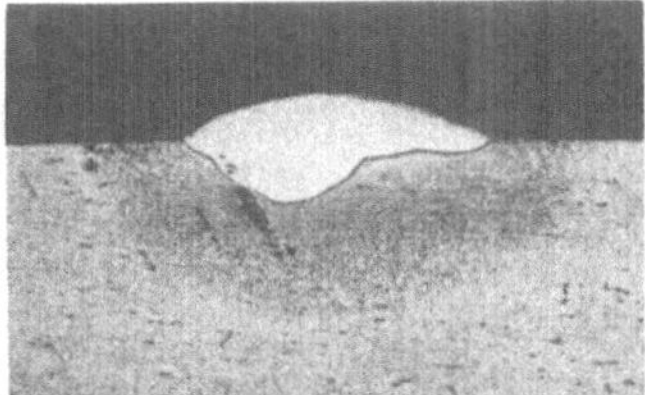 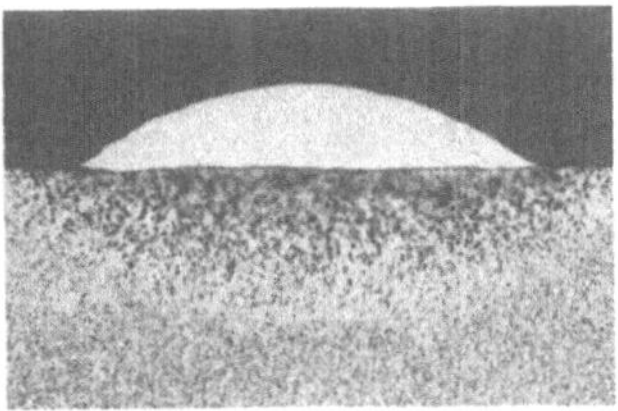

FIGURE 12. Three basic single-track bead profiles.

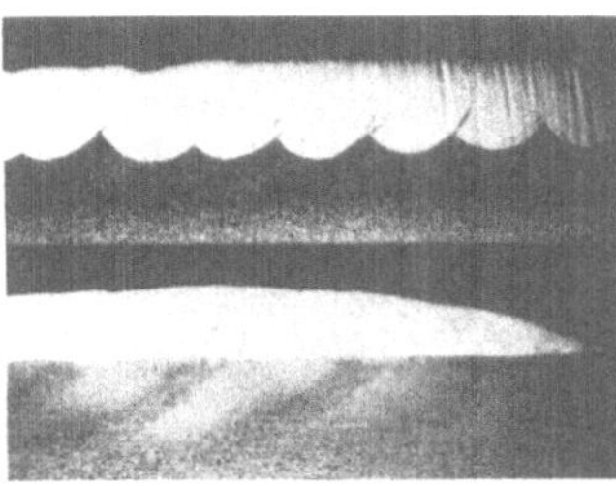

FIGURE 13. Control of dilution by powder mass flow. Powder flow 0.090 g/s top, 0.212 g/s bottom.

exists in cladding where the molten pool leading edge is inclined at an angle and also when overlapping. These polarization effects were not investigated in the present study, but are certainly not as marked as in cutting.

The spatial power intensity distribution of a laser beam is not uniform. In fact, it can be a complex distribution depending on the beam mode. Two distribution patterns commonly found in gas lasers are the Gaussian and the "doughnut," known as TEM 00 and TEM 01*, respectively.

The Gaussian beam is superior for cutting and welding applications, whereas for surface treatment the "doughnut" mode is preferred because of its more uniform heating effect. In cladding this effect is utilized to minimize dilution and obtain a desirable bead profile. Beam symmetry is also important.

An inherent advantage of using a laser as a heat source is that the source input can be localized to a small area. However, such localized heating causes rapid self-quenching and steep temperature gradients. In melting, these effects often cause solidification cracking.

In the present study a low power density, i.e., a large spot diameter of 5 mm, is used, coupled with slow speeds, to produce crack-free clad layers. Many other factors can affect this too.

7. METALLURGICAL AND PHYSICAL ASPECTS OF A LASER-CLAD AUSTENITIC STAINLESS 316 LAYER

A detailed evaluation (including corrosion properties) is the subject of a future paper. A summary is presented here in order to illustrate many aspects which may not be peculiar to stainless steel.

7.1. Surface finish

The surface finish of a clad layer produced by overlapping of single-clad beads is characterized by the "peak and valley" effect (see Fig. 4(a)). A typical "peak to valley" distance of 40 μm can be obtained with a bead of obtuse contact angle (see Fig. 12(c)) and a 60% overlap (as compared to 0.15 mm typically with weld overlay). The surface finish can be evaluated further from the amount of material which needs to be removed to obtain a clear surface (after the plate is mangled flat). A typical value per unit area is 0.6 Kg/m^2.

7.2. Porosity

Porosity in laser-clad layers may be caused by one or a combination of the following: cavities between two overlapped beads (usually formed near the root and will be referred to as inter-run porosity), solidification cavities and/or gas evolution.

Solidification cavities occur as porosity at or near the interface. If the clad layer has a significantly higher melting point than the substrate, the solidification front may finish at the interface, thus causing shrinkage cavities (e.g., stainless steels - aluminum).

In conventional welding, porosity attributed to gas evolution by way of dissolved gases and oxidation reactions is well known, and such phenomena are also applicable in laser cladding.

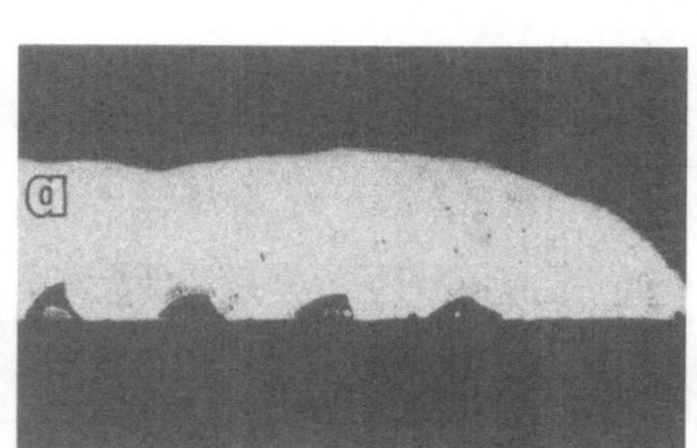

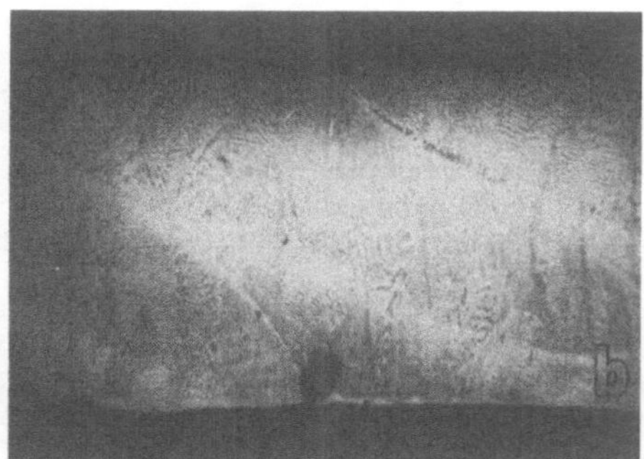

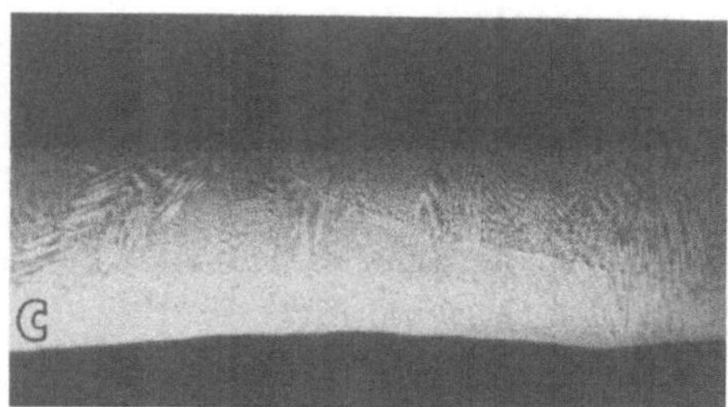

FIGURE 14. (a) Inter-run porosity, (b) location of pore in relation to interfaces shown by etching. The substrate appears totally blackened; (c) a clad layer with no porosity produced with beds of low contact angle.

In cladding stainless steel to mild steel, use of a good shrouding technique and use of dried powder limit the problem to inter-run porosity.

The formation of inter-run porosity is due to a purely "physical" effect, i.e., the contact angle of a single bead or the leading contact angle of an overlapped bead, Fig. 14(a,b,c).

In general, a bead width/height ratio of greater than five (i.e., contact angle 43°) and a percentage overlap of less than 70% will produce clad layers of no inter-run porosity.

7.3. Residual stress/plate distortion

Distortion of laser-clad plates is very small, typically a 5 m radius for a 1.4 mm clad on a 12.5 mm plate. There is minimal thermal penetration of the substrate, the heat-affected zone being of the order 1-2 mm.

Surface residual stresses were measured using the X-ray diffraction method. High tensile stresses of the order 285MPa were found on the clad surfaces. Using a pre-tensioning technique, it was possible to reduce the residual stress dramatically to compressive 8MPa (3).

7.4. Mechanical properties

Satisfactory results were obtained from tensile, bend and shear tests carried out in accordance to ASTM 264, Fig. 15(a,b).

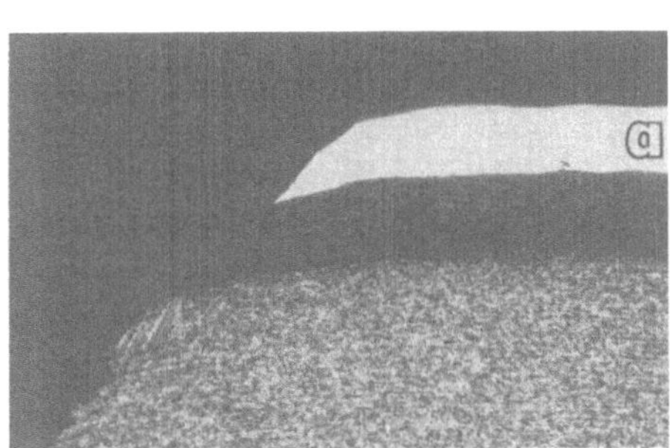

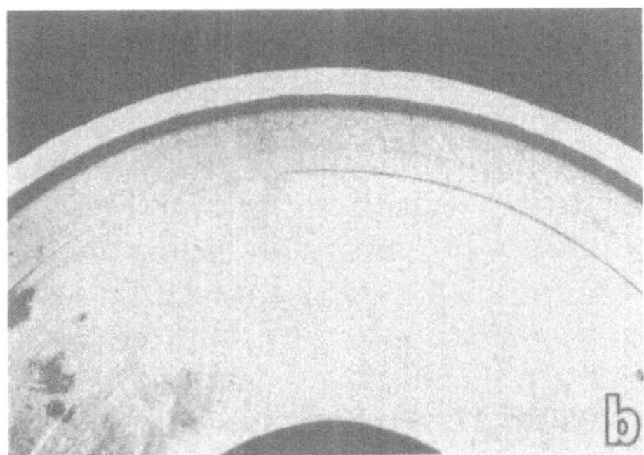

FIGURE 15. (a) Section of fracture surface of tensile specimen showing no delamination of the clad layer. Clad thickness 1.5 mm. (b) Bend test specimen - 12.5 mm thick mild steel clad with 1.5 mm thick stainless.

7.5. Microstructure

The dendritic microstructure of the laser-clad stainless 316L layer was observed to be basically similar to that of a conventional weld bead or a submerged arc strip clad, i.e., austenitic matrix with residual delta ferrite. The dendrite size is much finer due to the higher cooling rate, Fig. 16(a,b).

7.6. Cracking

In hardfacing, cracking is related to the hardness of the clad layer and can be eliminated by substrate pre-heat, Fig. 17. In austenitic stainless steels, cracking is known to take place at high temperatures (1200°C), and as such, preheating has proved to be ineffective (17).

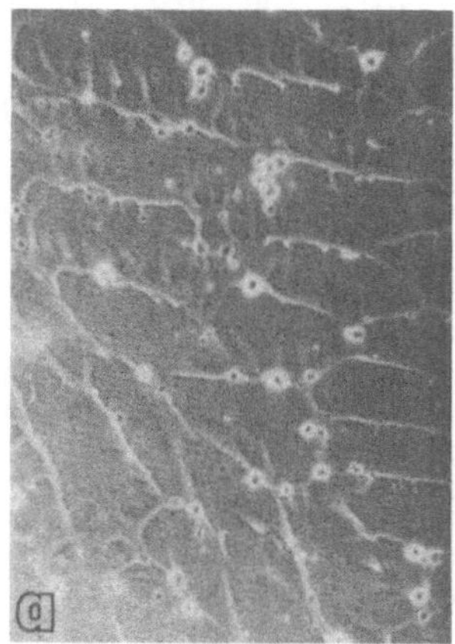

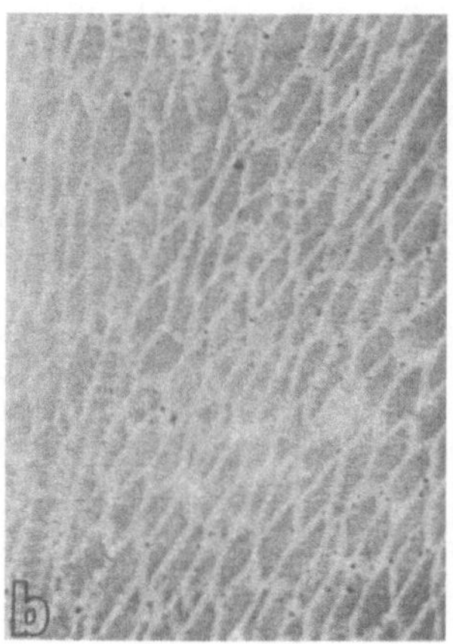

FIGURE 16. Effect of cooling rate on dendrite size - SEM micrographs. (a) cladding speed 7 mm/sec, 92 W/mm^2, dendrite size 6 μm. (b) cladding speed 40 mm/sec, 573 W/mm^2, dendrite size 2 μm.

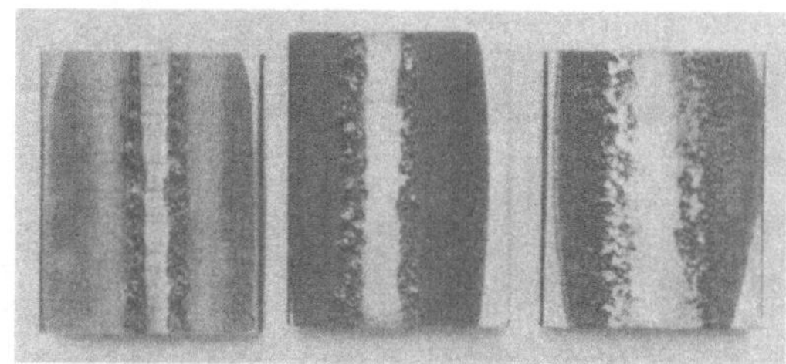

FIGURE 17. Progressive elimination of cracking by preheating the substrate. Clad-iron boron (1000 HV) substrate - mild steel.

Interdendritic cracking was observed in stainless clad layers produced at high cladding speeds (>20 mm/s) with high power densities (>366 W/mm^2). Crack-free clad layers were produced at lower power densities coupled with slower speeds.

7.7. Chemical composition/homogeneity/dilution

Figure 18(a,b) illustrates the distribution of alloying elements in a 316 stainless clad layer and in the interface region, showing no macrosegregation and negligible dilution.

One may define the dilution as the compositional difference between the injected powder and the clad layer. Very low dilution was observed near the clad surface, with an overall dilution of about 5% typical. Also, Fig. 19 shows that even with high penetration, dilution is mainly confined to the interfacial region, indicating perhaps the "calmness" of the process. However, work from Takeda (6) using copper markers to illustrate the flow within the clad track suggests that there is considerable mixing turbulence.

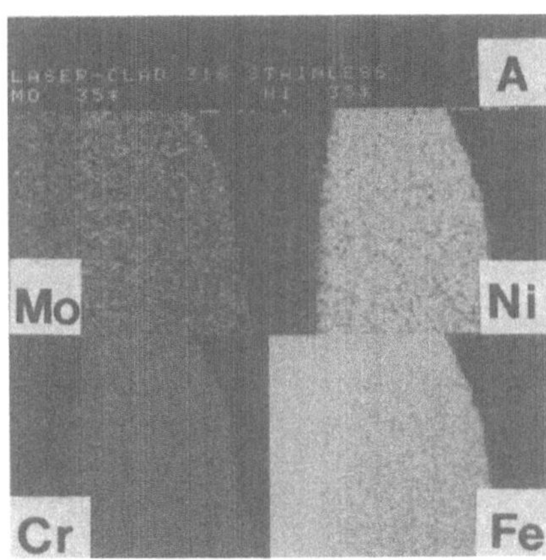

FIGURE 18. (a) X-ray digimap of alloying elements in a stainless 316 clad layer.

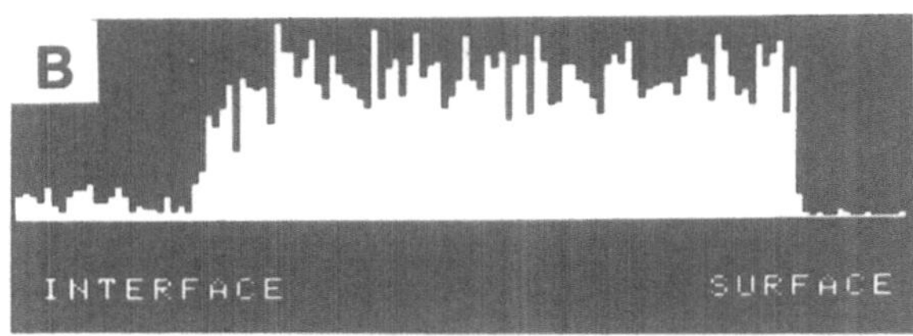

FIGURE 18. (b) line scan of chromium across the clad/substrate interface.

8. OTHER CLAD/SUBSTRATE COMBINATIONS

In addition to stainless/mild steel, the following clad/substrate combinations were produced using the laser:

Note: Stellite SF6 is a cobalt-based hardfacing alloy

(a) Nickel/mild steel
(b) Bronze/mild steel
(c) Stellite SF6/brass
(d) Chromium/titanium
(e) Stainless/aluminum
(f) Iron boron/mild steel
(g) Stellite SF6/mild steel
(h) Mild steel/stainless

Some porosity but good bond strength

Cracking plus delamination in "e"

9. CONCLUSIONS

The process may be evaluated in terms of economic, engineering and quality assurance aspects.

Engineering aspects present less of a problem since they are mostly similar to other laser-processing applications which have already found industrial acceptance; except perhaps aspects of powder injection, which have now been developed to a reliable level.

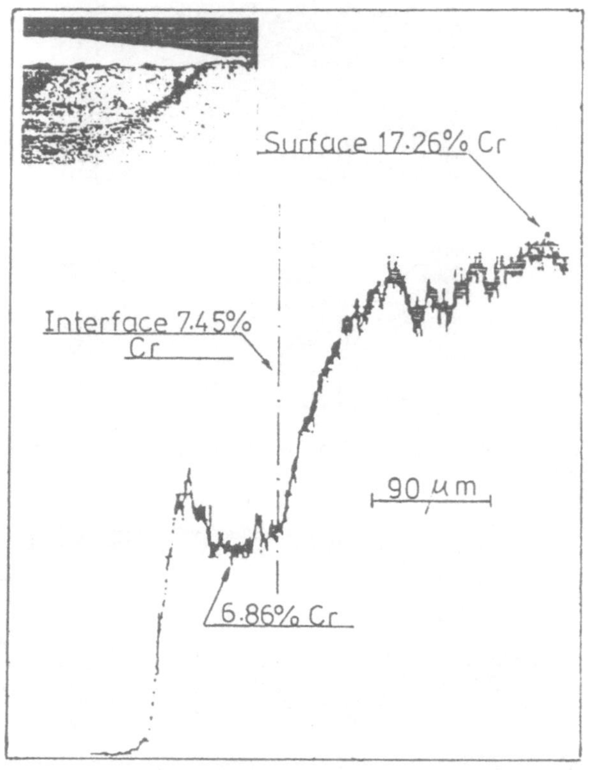

FIGURE 19. Crystal spectrometer scan of chromium across the thickness of a clad layer with high penetration.

From a metallurgical/physical evaluation of a representative clad/substrate combination of austenitic stainless steel and mild steel, there is conclusive evidence that clad layers of acceptable quality can be produced using the laser. Similar data is being found for other systems.

From the economic assessment there is no doubt that laser cladding is best suited for treatment of small confined areas, such as valve seatings, turbine blade edges, wear surfaces of tools, etc. Deposition of thin coatings of expensive materials is also a good application. Laser cladding of large areas may be cost effective if adaptive automation of the process can be achieved, whereby the process will automatically correct itself for heating effects on the substrate.

REFERENCES

1. J. Powell, Proc. Conf. on "Surface Engineering with Lasers," London, May 1985, Paper 17, publ. Metal Society, London.
2. V. M. Weerasinghe and W. M. Steen, "Laser Cladding with Pneumatic Powder Feed, Proc. 4th Int. Conf on Laser Processing, Los Angeles, Jan. 1983.
3. V. M. Weerasinghe, Ph.D. Thesis, London University, 1985.
4. S. Dallaire and P. Cielo, "Pulsed Laser Treatment of Plasma Sprayed Coatings," Met. Trans B V 13B N E Sept. 1982, pp. 479-483.
5. H. Bhat, R. A. Zatorski, H. Herman and R. J. Coyle, "Laser Treatment of Plasma Sprayed Coatings, Proc. 10th Int. Conf. on Thermal Spraying, Essen, W. Germany, pp. 2-6, May 1983, Publ. Deutscher Verlag für Schweisstechnik GmbH Dusseldorf, W. Germany, 1983.
6. T. Takeda, W. M. Steen, and D. R. F. West, "in situ Clad Alloy Formation by Laser Cladding," Proc. LIM 2, Burmingham, UK, March 1985, publ. by IFS Publications Ltd., Bedford UK.
7. J. Powell and W. M. Steen, "Vibrolaser Cladding," Laser in Metallurgy, edited by K. Mukherjee and J. Mazumder, publ. Met. Soc. of AIME, Warrandale, PA, USA, pp.93-104.
8. M. MacIntyre, "Laser Hardfacing of RB 211 Turbine Blade Shroud Interlocks," Proc. 2nd Int. Conf. on Applications of Lasers in Material Processing, Jan. 1983, Los Angeles, USA.
9. M. Eboo and A. E. Lindemanis, "Advances in Laser Cladding Technology," LIA Conf., Los Angeles, March 1985.
10. W. M. Steen, Laser Cladding," Metals and Materials Tech., to be published.
11. UK Patent No. app. 84 25716, Quantum Laser Corp., USA.
12. J. Powell, Ph.D. Thesis, Univ. of London, 1983.
13. V. M. Weerasinghe and W. M. Steen, Computer Simulation Model for Laser Cladding by Powder Injection, Conf. Proc. ASME, Boston, Nov. 1983.
14. G. C. Lim and W. M. Steen, "Measurement of Temporal and Spatial Power Distribution of a High-Powered CO_2 Laser Beam," Optical and Laser Tech., June 1982.
15. A. L. L. Brochure, Hans Gressel weg. Munchen - 8000, W. Germany, 1982.
16. J. N. Kamalu, Ph.D. Thesis, Univ. of London, 1981.
17. J. Alexander, Ph.D. Thesis, University of London, 1982.
18. R. Castro and J. J. Cadenet, Welding Metallurgy of Stainless and Heat-Resisting Steels, Cambridge Univ. Press, 1974.

LASER GAS ALLOYING

B. L. MORDIKE
Institut für Werkstoffkunde und Werkstofftechnik, Agricolastrasse 2, D-3392 Clausthal-Zellerfeld, FRG

Key Words: titanium, nitriding, carburized

1. FUNDAMENTAL ASPECTS

Traditionally, laser surface alloying has been a two-step process in which an alloying element has been deposited onto the surface and subsequently laser melted into the substrate (1). The composition of such a layer is dependent on the thickness of the substrate melted. The homogeneity of the layer is ensured by long-range convection as well as short-range diffusion. It is also possible to alloy by heating the substrate in an apropriate atmosphere (2,3,4). Unless the surface is melted, there is very little alloying, as the rate of diffusion in the solid is low. The convection effect is then absent. If melting takes place, alloying over considerable distances becomes possible. The precise mechanism of absorption/desorption in each particular case differs depending on the nature of the gas-metal system. However, the behavior in general can be described by the fundamental law of mass action.

Consider a general reaction $uA + vB \rightleftharpoons wC + xD + \Delta H$ with equilibrium constant

$$K_c = \frac{[C]^w \cdot [D]^x}{[A]^u \cdot [B]^v}$$

In dilute gaseous systems the concentrations can be replaced by the partial pressures, e.g., for $N_2 + 3\ H_2 \rightleftharpoons 2\ NH_3$

$$K_p = \frac{P^2_{NH_3}}{P_{N_2} \cdot P^3_{H_2}}$$

The laser can heat a surface extremely rapidly, and since K is a strong function of temperature, the reaction proceeds rapidly. The gas atmosphere can be chosen so the reaction proceeds either in the forward or reverse direction. Controlled processing with oxidizing, neutral or reducing atmospheres is called gas alloying. In the following some examples will illustrate the application of the law of mass action.

Draper, C.W. and Mazzoldi, P. (eds.), Laser Surface Treatment of Metals. ISBN 90-247-3405-3.

Consider the nitriding of titanium:

$$Ti + \frac{1}{2} N_2 \rightleftharpoons TiN + \Delta H$$

In order to control the process, the nitrogen gas is diluted by an inert gas, e.g., argon, which does not take part in the reaction. Starting with pure titanium, nitriding will proceed so long as the partial pressure of nitrogen in the atmosphere is equal to or greater than that prescribed by the law of mass action. For further nitriding it is necessary to increase the partial pressure of nitrogen by increasing the concentration of N_2 in argon. A change in temperature, i.e., change in laser power, changes the equilibrium vapor pressure. A particular nitrogen/argon mixture would therefore nitride pure titanium, be neutral for a particular TiN concentration in Ti, and denitride more concentrated TiN contents.

Figures 1 to 3 show titanium specimens with successive passes at constant power and constant gas conditions. The micrographs show that the TiN content approaches a plateau value, Fig. 2. Figure 3 shows the effect of increasing the nitrogen concentration at constant power. The amount of TiN increases continuously.

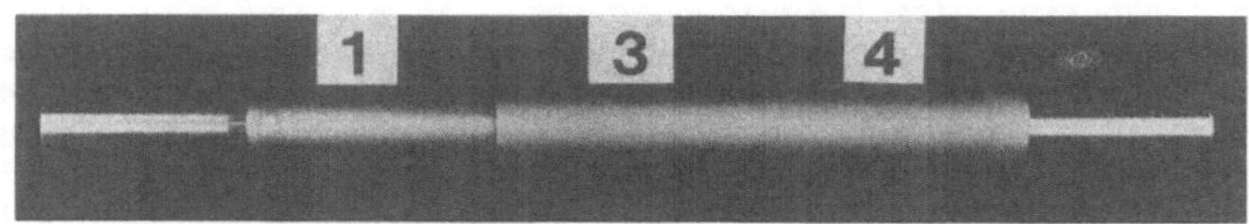

FIGURE 1. TiAl6V4 (IMI 318) test sample laser gas nitrided with constant power and gas composition, 10% N_2 in argon, 1 pass, 3 passes and 4 passes. Specimens are 15 cm long.

The micrographs show that the structure formed on gas nitriding consists of dendritically solidified TiN and interdendritic α'. In the instance of IMI 318 Ti- alloy, X-ray distribution maps show that the vanadium and aluminum has segregated. In the case of pure titanium this segregation is absent, but the behavior is otherwise completely analogous. A heat-affected zone can be observed below the melted layer in which β has transformed to α'. The quantity and size of the TiN precipitates increase with each successive pass. The depth of hardening and hardness increases with longer interaction times, see Fig. 4. The hardness as a function of TiN concentration is shown in Fig. 5.

If the surface of a nitrided specimen is melted in an inert atmosphere, denitriding takes place, as predicted by the law of mass action as shown in Fig. 6. Carburizing titanium is an analogous process: For example, in argon/methane mixtures titanium carbide is formed and similar hardness-depth profiles are obtained (Figs. 4,5). Decarburization in an inert atmosphere is also possible.

A reaction with oxygen is also possible but the surface tends to crack. There is more than one species of oxide and the oxide forms as a massive crystal throughout the whole melted layer.

With a suitable mixture of methane and nitrogen, carbonitrides are produced. These form as dendrites within a titanium matrix. All the examples discussed so far contain one hardening phase. The various

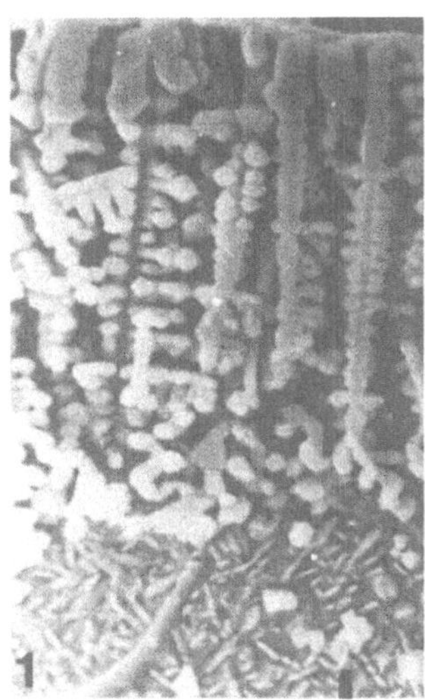

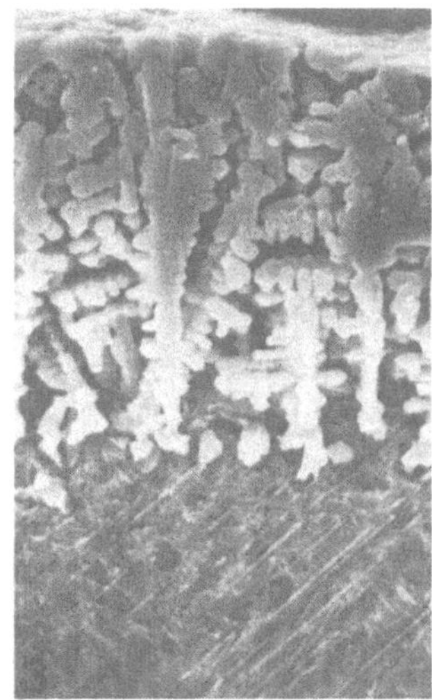

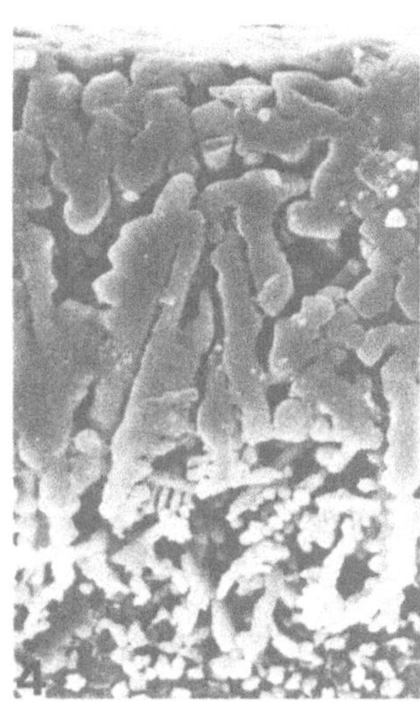

FIGURE 2. SEM micrographs of laser gas nitrided TiAl6V4 corresponding to Fig. 1. With increasing number of passes the thickness of the dendrites increases and the layer becomes denser.

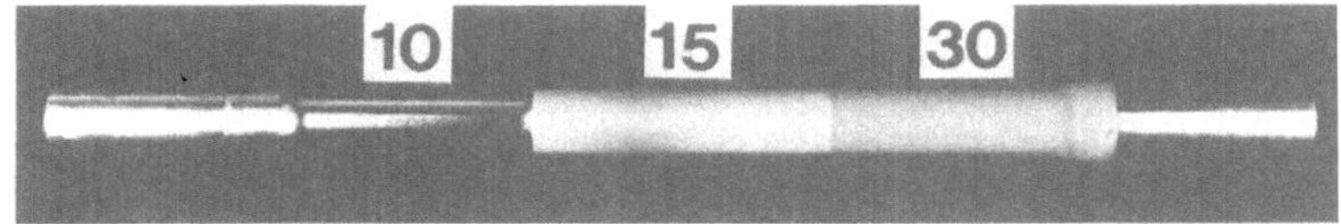

FIGURE 3. TiAl6V4 test sample laser gas nitrided with constant power, all single pass, increasing N_2 content, 10%, 15%, 30% in argon.

phases have been identified by X-ray measurement, Fig. 7. Successive passes with nitriding and carburizing atmospheres produce a layered structure of nitrides and carbides. Figure 8 shows typical micrographs for a nitride layer produced on a carbide layer and vice versa. Small amounts of oxygen mixed with the carburizing or nitriding gas do not prevent the formation of carbide or nitride, as these precipitate out at higher temperatures. On the other hand, it affects the color and surface finish.

2. EXPERIMENTAL ASPECTS

Figure 9 shows the effect of feed rate on melt depth for various atmospheres, power densities and specimen temperature. The maximum depth for a Coherent Everlase 650 W CO_2 laser is about 0.5 mm. The surface roughness as a function of the principal parameters is shown in Table 1.

The roughness depends on the initial roughness, gas flow rate and angle of impingement and composition. Surface-treated components and

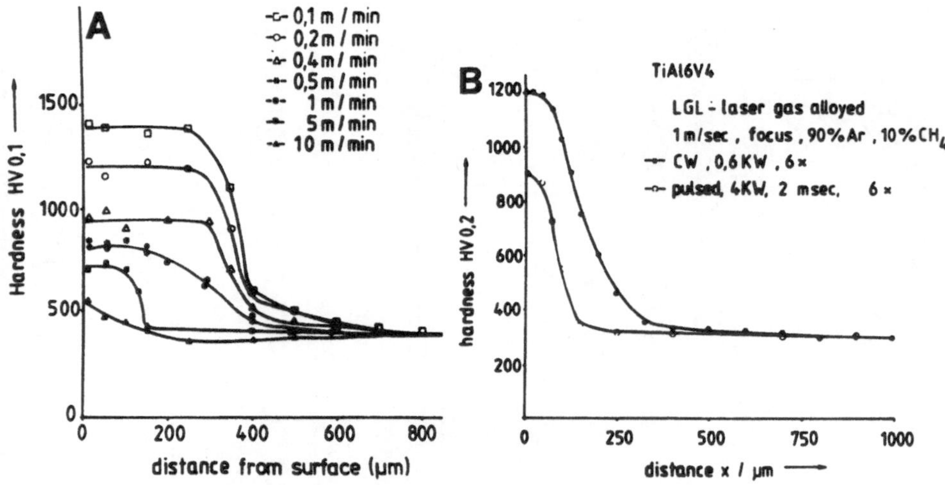

FIGURE 4. Hardness profiles of laser gas-alloyed TaAl6V4. (a) nitrided, (b) carburized.

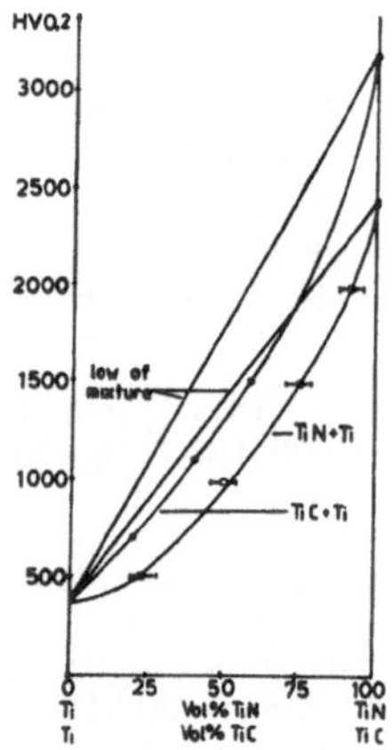

FIGURE 5. Hardness as function of TiN or TiC content.

specimens are shown in the following photographs. All slopes have been crack free and distortion free surface melted. Suitable fixing and support devices must sometimes be developed to prevent distortion, Fig. 10.

3. PROPERTIES

The effect of surface melting and gas alloying on the surface roughness is shown in Fig. 11. Surface treatment would not be expected to change the tensile, compressive properties to any extent, as the surface layer is a very small fraction of the total area. This is confirmed by

TABLE 1. Properties of laser gas-alloyed titanium, IMI 318 (TiAl6V4) after processing in various treatment gases.

No.	Treatment Conditions	Color	Rough-ness	Micro-hardness	Macro-hardness	Micro-structure	Phases	Comments
0	Starting material	Silver	7.75	336	296	equiaxed grains of α,β-Ti	α',β-Ti	
1	1 x molten	yellow	38.8	594	879	TiN-dendrites in dendrite armspacing 5-6 μm	α'-Ti + TiN	dense layer
2	8 x molten under N_2	yellow golden	12.9	956	934	TiN-dendrites in dendrite armspacing 5-6 μm	α'-Ti + TiN	uniform dense layer cracks starting at hardness impr.
3	1 x molten under CH_4 + argon (7.5% CH_4)	dark gray	12.8	527	528	TiC-precipitation in α'-matrix	α'-Ti + TiC	insufficient layer
4	8 x molten under CH_4 + argon (7.5% CH_4)	light gray	12.1	625	770	dendrite arm-spacing 1-2 μm	α'-Ti + TiC	uniform dense layer
5	1 x molten under O_2 + argon (7.5% O_2)	dark gray	15.9	387	373	(30 μm)	TiO + Ti_2O	non-uniform dense layer
6	3 x molten under CH_4 + argon then 1 x under argon	silver	18.1	469	257	above the dendritic TiC-layer is a layer with α'-Ti + TiC-precipitations (30 μm)	α'-Ti + TiC	dense layer, no brittleness
7	3 x molten with CH_4, then 3 x O_2 + Ar	gray	16.6	475	386	80 um fine TiC-dendr. TiO + Ti_2O (60 μm)	TiO + Ti_2O after grind. TiC	insufficient layer
8	6 x molten (N_2 + CH_4 + argon)	gray	31.3	497	545	Ti(N,C)dendrites	Ti(N,C)	dense layer

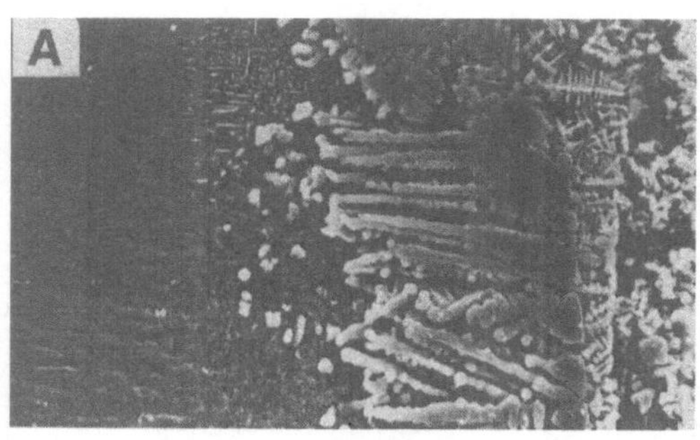

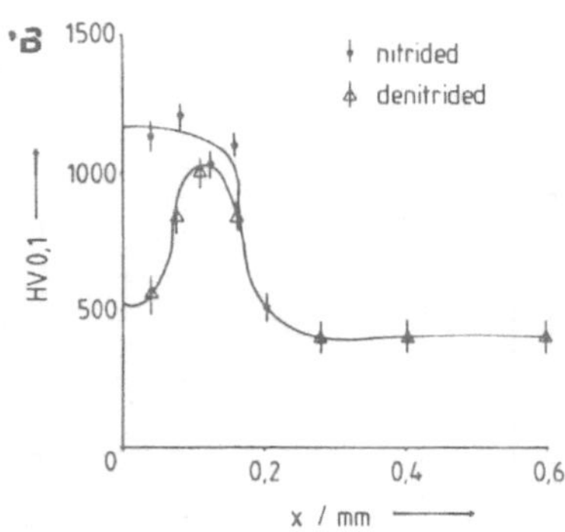

FIGURE 6. Denitriding of nitrided TiAl6V4. (a) micrograph, (b) hardness profile.

experiment; the change in yield stress and ultimate stress is within the expected scatter. The ductility, however, is markedly reduced. Cracks form along the length which penetrate the HAZ and mostly stop in the ductile material. This restricts without suppressing the necking behavior and thus reduces the elongation. Since fatigue cracks are initiated on the surface, it would be expected that laser treatment would change the fatigue behavior. If it is possible to produce compressive stresses in the surface, than an improvement in fatigue behavior would result. All surface-melted layers on titanium should show tensile residual stresses and hence power fatigue properties. The precise crack initiation conditions differ with the type of layer, e.g., carbonitrided, carburized, nitrided, etc. Figure 12 shows the fatigue curves, stress number of cycles to failure (S-N) for push-pull and rotation bending for various surfaces. In both types of loading surface treatment reduces the fatigue limit. Oxygen causes the largest reduction in fatigue limit, probably due to the nature of the oxide film. The effect of other atmospheres is less, even melting in an inert atmosphere reduces the limit. The fracture surface shows the typical fatigue fracture features (Fig. 13).

One of the weaknesses of titanium is the relatively poor surface properties. In particular, scuffing wear is a problem. This is the main reason for surface treatment. Increasing the hardness of the surface layer improves the resistance to penetration and thus the resistance against ploughing wear and erosion. Preliminary results indicate an improvement in resistance to rolling wear and adhesive wear.

The corrosion resistance of titanium is relatively good. Surface gas alloying produces in general a further improvement. TiN and TiC are both nobler than Ti, which leads to a displacement of the corrosion potential. They passivate at lower current densities (10-100 times less). Melting in an inert gas reproduces the conditions for pure titanium. These results are collated in Fig. 14.

4. GAS ALLOYING IN OTHER SYSTEMS

The principles of gas alloying are the same for all systems, from noble metal contact materials where a component is selectively oxidized to iron carbon alloys which are carburized to enjoy the benefits of martensitic hardening. The application to the latter system will be discussed in more detail. Among the most interesting applications are those of the Fe-C-system: (a) increasing the carbon content of low carbon steels (C15). These are usually shaped by pressing and can only be hardened after this operation. Gas alloying would replace a conventional method, e.g., case carburizing. (b) producing ledeburitic layers on steels to provide wear-resistant surfaces. Figure 15 shows layers of different composition which have been produced on Armco iron (10% CH_4 in Ar). Four passes are needed for ledeburite and at least six for massive cementite. The tensile behavior of Armco iron coated with ledeburite is similar to that of unmelted Armco iron (e.g., yield point, ductility) see Fig. 16. The fatigue limit - tension and rotation bending is improved. This is probably due to the creation of compressive stresses in the melted layer. Compressive streses can be produced if transformations take place in the solidified layer. The improvement in wear properties on producing fine ledeburitic layers is well known and has been discussed earlier in this chapter by H. W. Bergmann.

REFERENCES

1. C. Draper, Int. Metals Rev. (1985).
2. B. L. Mordike, H. W. Bergmann, and N. Gross, Z. Werkstofftechnik 14, 253 (1983).
3. H. W. Bergmann, Z. Werkstofftechnik, in preparation.
4. Deutsche Patentschrift Nr. P 34 40335.
5. A. Walter, I. Folker, W. M. Steen, and D. R. F. West, Surface Engineering 1, 23 (1985).

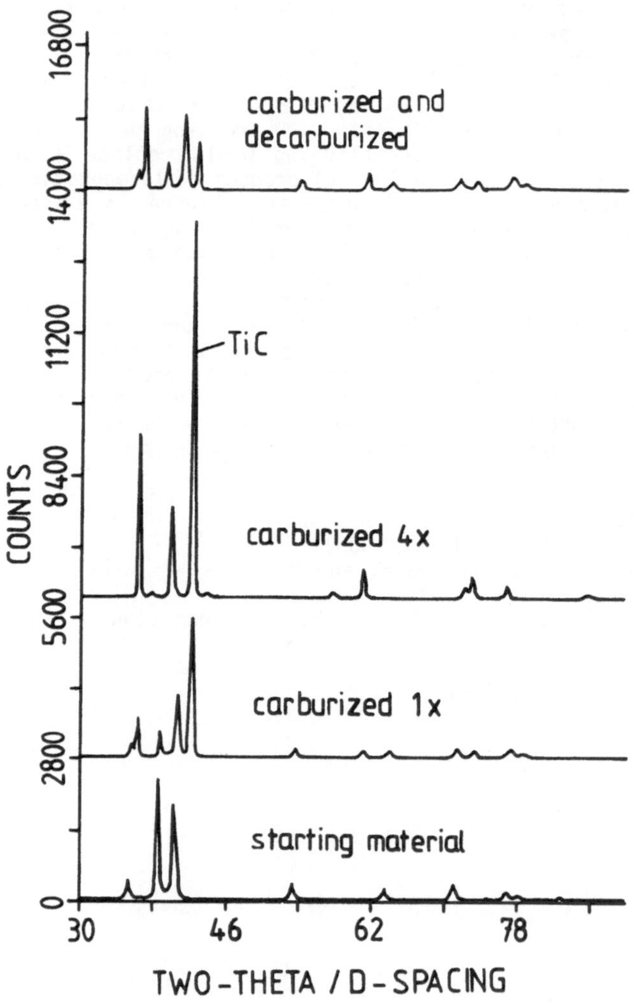

FIGURE 7. X-ray diffraction pattern for various treatments, Cu radiation.

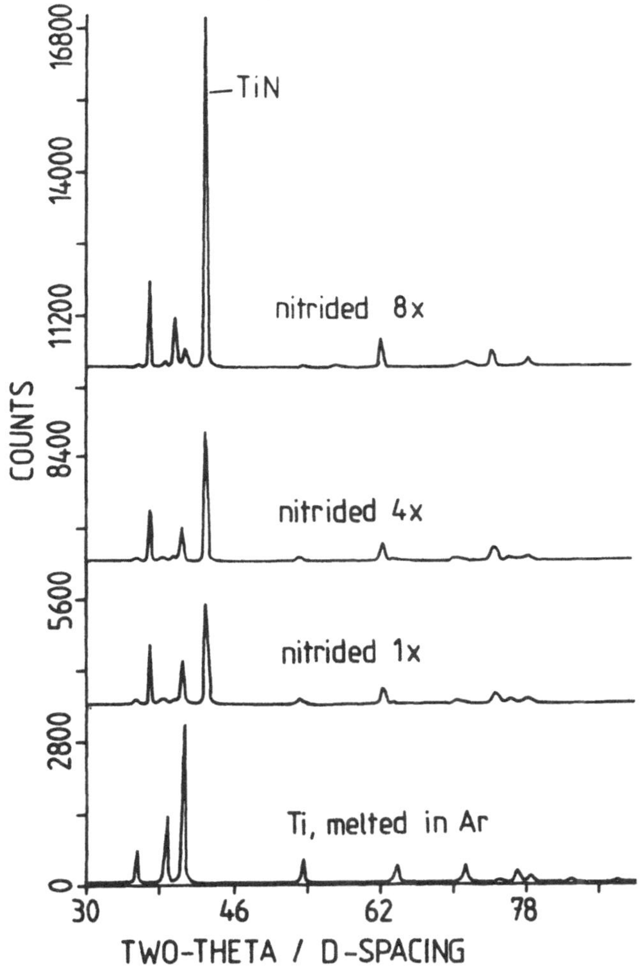

FIGURE 7. X-ray diffraction pattern for various treatments, Cu radiation.

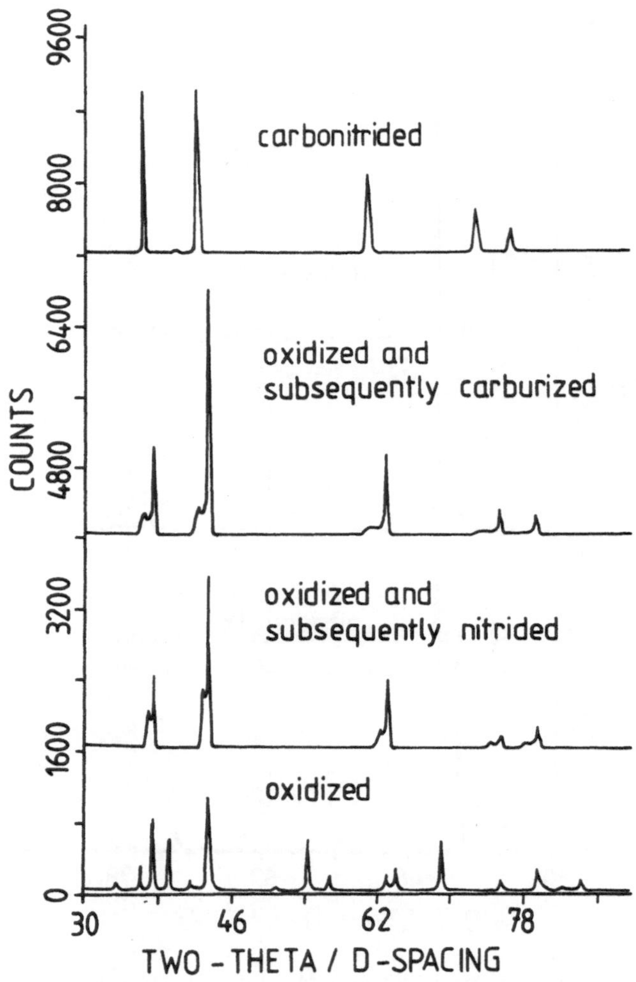

FIGURE 7. X-ray diffraction pattern for various treatments, Cu radiation.

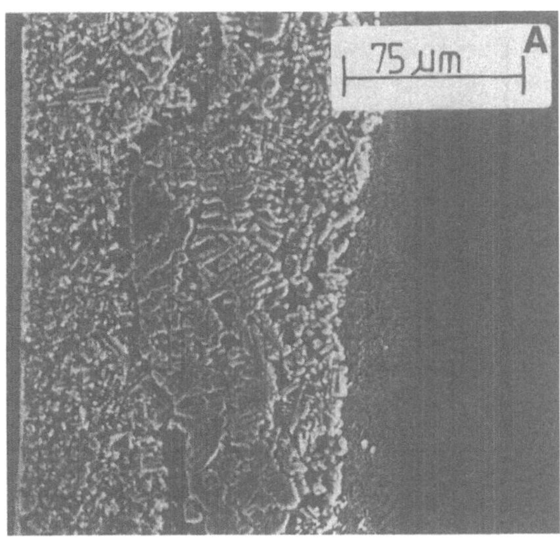

FIGURE 8. SEM-micrographs of sequentially carburized and nitrided TiAl6V4. (a) N_2, CH_4.

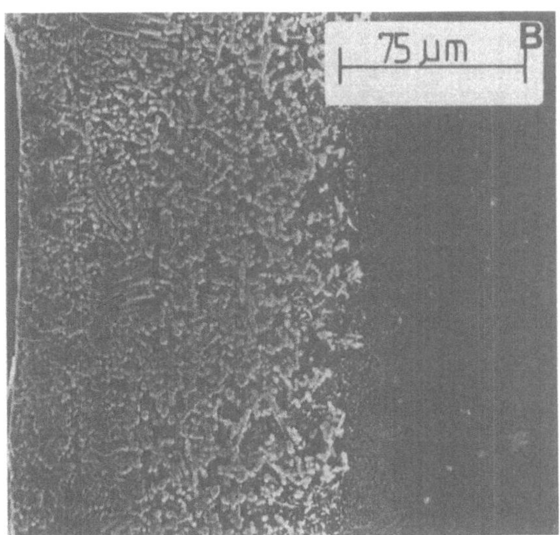

FIGURE 8. SEM-micrographs of sequentially carburized and nitrided TiAl6V4. (b) CH_4, N_2.

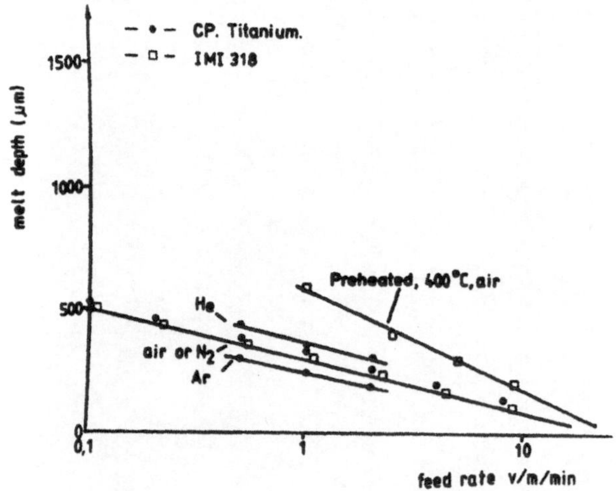

FIGURE 9. Melt depth as a function of feed rate.

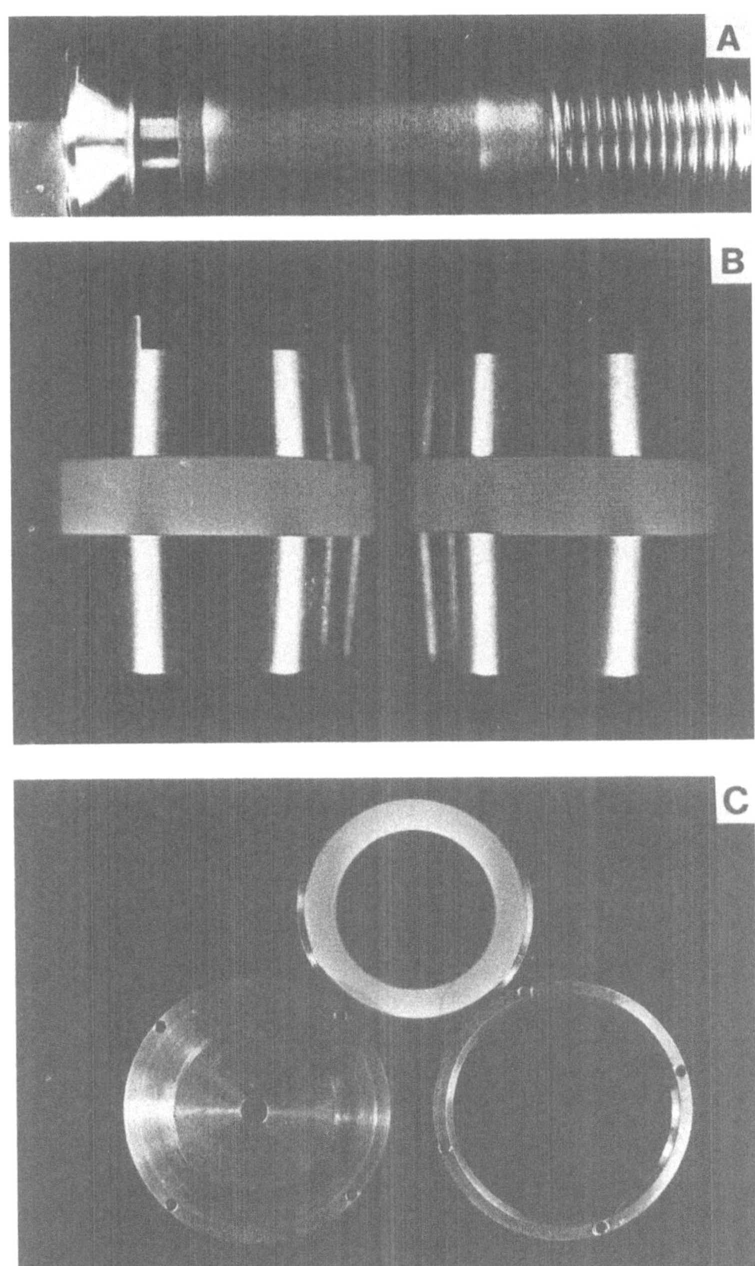

FIGURE 10. Selection of gas-alloyed TiAl6V4 components and support used for (a). (a) fastener/bolt, (b) rolls, (c) ring and support.

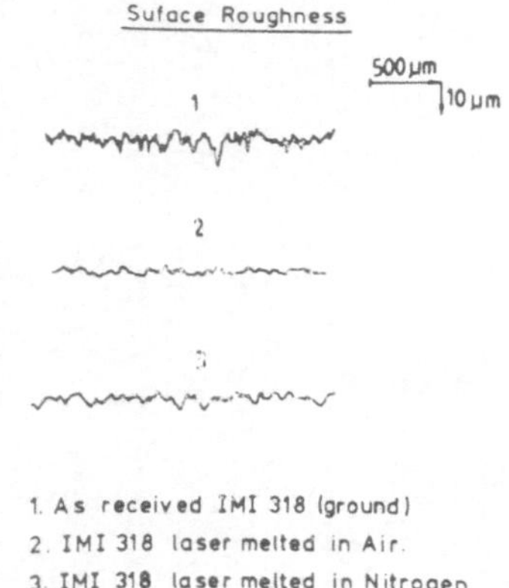

FIGURE 11. Roughness profiles for optimized process.

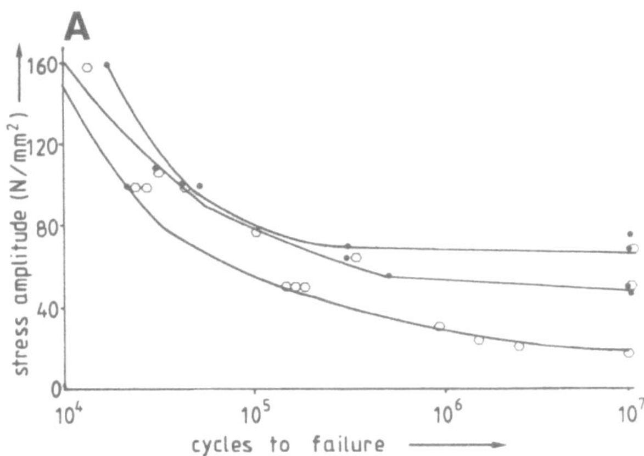

FIGURE 12. S-N curves for various laser gas-alloyed specimens.
(a) pull-pull tests.

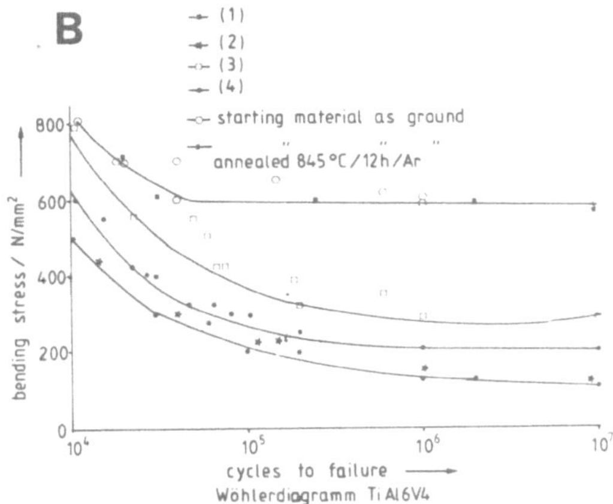

FIGURE 12. S-N curves for various laser gas-alloyed specimens.
(b) rotational bending tests.

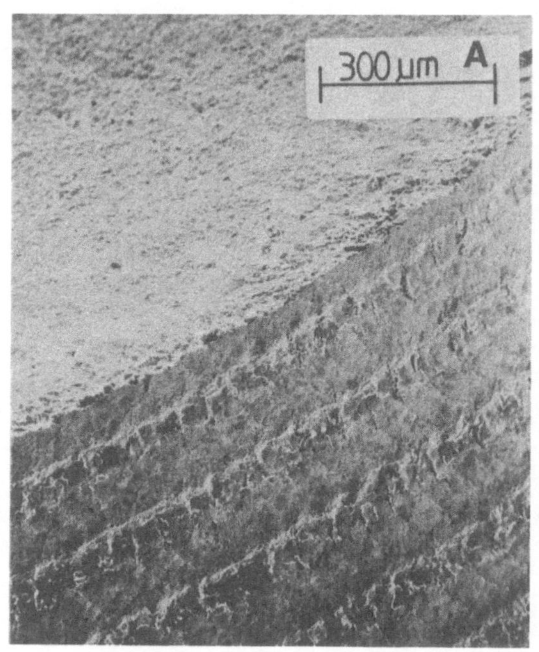

FIGURE 13. Fatigue fracture surface of gas-alloyed TiAl6V4. Push-pull mean stress 800 N/mm^2. (a) nitrided.

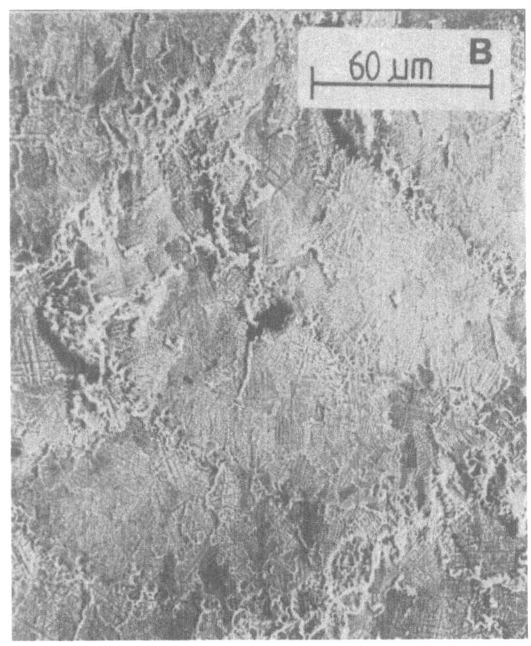

FIGURE 13. Fatigue fracture surface of gas-alloyed TiAl6V4. Push-pull mean stress 800 N/mm^2. (b) selected area of (a).

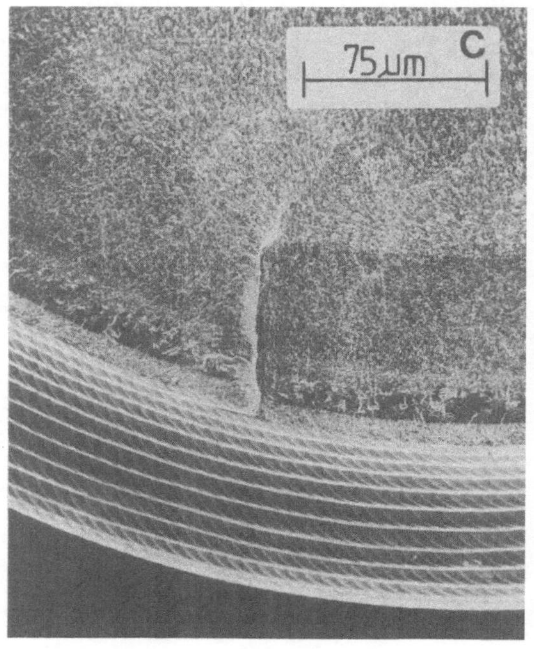

FIGURE 13. Fatigue fracture surface of gas-alloyed TiAl6V4. Push-pull mean stress 800 N/mm^2. (c) denitrided after nitriding.

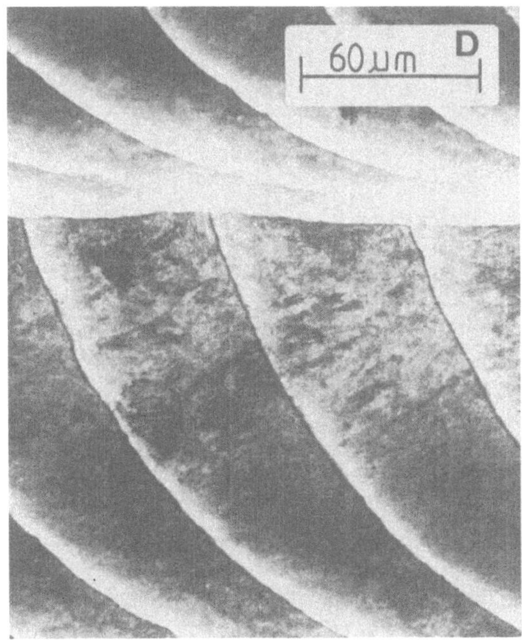

FIGURE 13. Fatigue fracture surface of gas-alloyed TiAl6V4. Push-pull mean stress 800 N/mm². (d) selected area of (c).

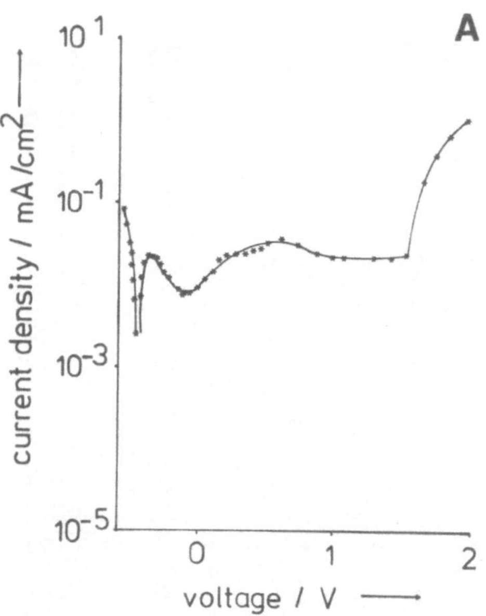

FIGURE 14. Corrosion behavior of TiAl6V4 after different treatments. (a) initial untreated material.

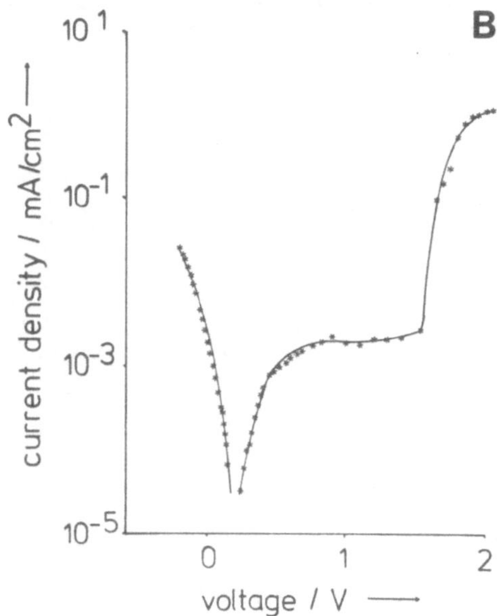

FIGURE 14. Corrosion behavior of TiAl6V4 after different treatments. (b) nitrided.

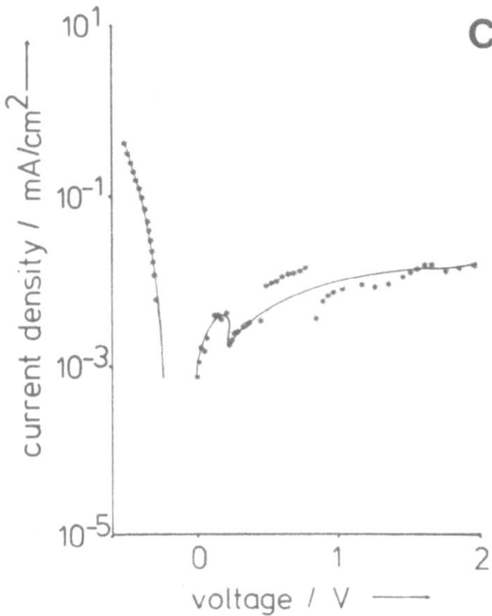

FIGURE 14. Corrosion behavior of TiAl6V4 after different treatments. (c) denitrided after nitriding.

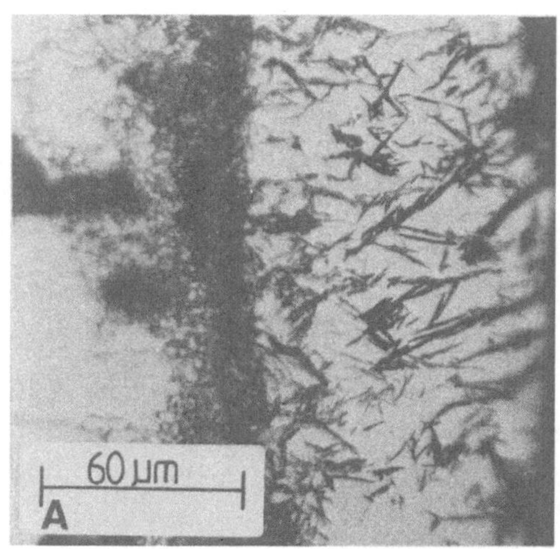

FIGURE 15. Microstructures of carburized Armco iron. (a-d) increasing carbon content.

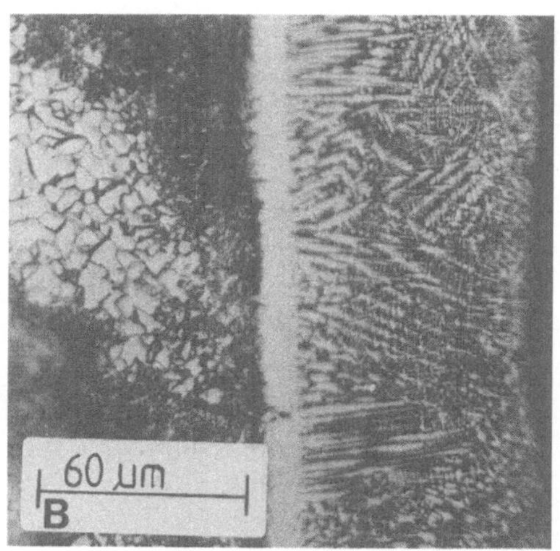

FIGURE 15. Microstructures of carburized Armco iron. (a-d) increasing carbon content.

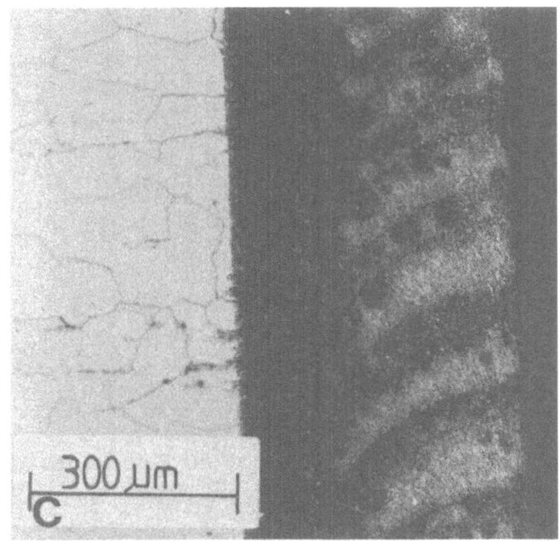

FIGURE 15. Microstructures of carburized Armco iron. (a-d) increasing carbon content.

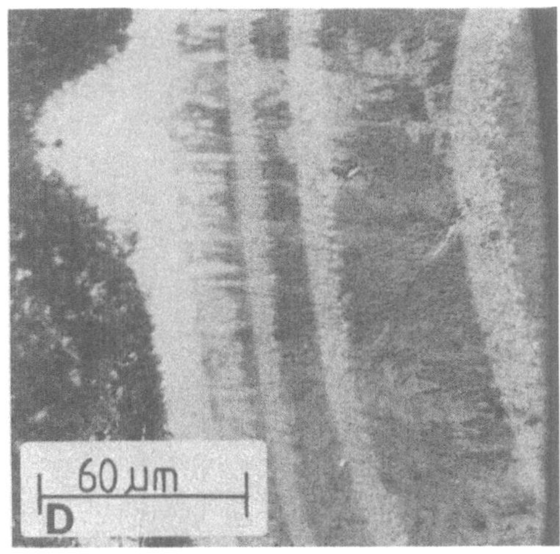

FIGURE 15. Microstructures of carburized Armco iron. (a-d) increasing carbon content.

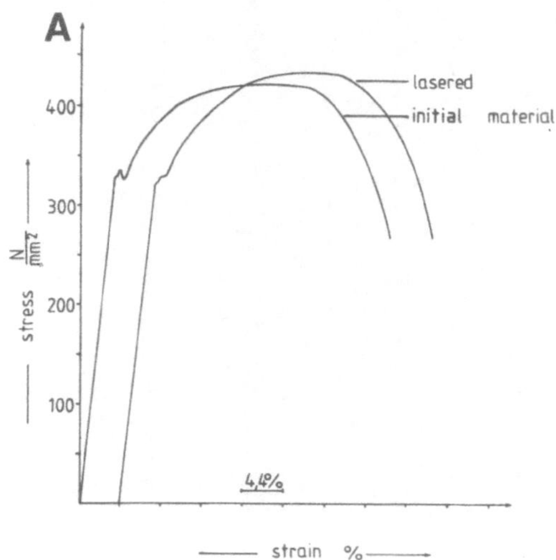

FIGURE 16. Mechanical properties of gas-carburized Armco iron.
(a) tensile test, (b) rotation bending test.

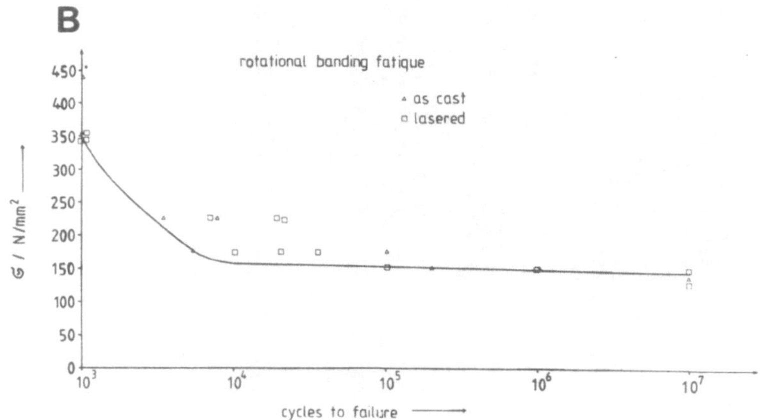

FIGURE 16. Mechanical properties of gas-carburized Armco iron.
(a) tensile test, (b) rotation bending test.

LASER HEAT TREATMENT OF IRON-BASE ALLOYS

D. S. GNANAMUTHU AND V. S. SHANKAR
Rockwell International Science Center, 1049 Camino Dos Rios, Thousand Oaks, California 91360

Key Words: mode, polarization, beam shaping

ABSTRACT

Laser heat treatment of iron-base alloys is influenced by factors such as beam intensity profile, beam absorptance, heat conduction, and core microstructure of workpiece. In this article a number of techniques designed to improve the efficiency of the laser heat-treatment process are presented. Methods to obtain a laser beam profile with uniform intensity involve the use of beam-integrating optics with Fresnel number higher than 10. Approaches to increase beam absorptance involve the use of infrared energy-absorbing coatings or the use of linearly polarized laser beams. A numerical solution to the three-dimensional, time-dependent, heat conduction equation is used to calculate and experimentally validate the heat-affected and hardened zone profiles in finite-length workpieces. The numerical solution uses an implicit time-accurate finite-difference procedure based on Newton iteration and triple approximate factorization. Core microstructure influences the hardened depth that can be obtained by laser heat treatment. This is due to the influence of carbon diffusion distance for a specific core microstructure on the rate of structural transformation for surface hardening.

1. INTRODUCTION

Laser heat treatment offers controllable surface processing methods for either hardening or tempering of iron-base alloys. Surface hardening through martensitic phase transformation is intended to increase resistance to wear and fatigue and, in addition, to obtain a surface with a high residual compressive stress (1,2). Surface tempering through precipitation of carbides from the martensitic phase is intended to lower surface hardness and thus make the surface layers less brittle. CO_2 and Nd:YAG laser beams are suitable for surface hardening and tempering. Nd:YAG lasers emit radiation at a wavelength of 1060 nm with power levels during continuous operation ranging from 200 to 500 W. CO_2 lasers emit radiation at a wavelength of 10,600 nm with power levels during continuous operation up to 15,000 W. Laser heat treatment requires power densities typically less than 10^4 W/cm^2 such that the workpiece surface is not melted. The normal spectral absorptance of a polished iron surface is reported to be nearly 5% for 10,600 nm wavelength (CO_2 laser beam) and nearly 35% for 1200 nm (near Nd:YAG laser beam's wavelength) (3). Therefore, infrared energy-absorbing coatings are used to improve laser beam absorptance. Laser heat treating is done by pulsed or continuous-wave laser beams. Due to short irradiation times with a pulsed beam, thin heat-affected zones are obtained. With a continuous-wave beam, a wide range of irradiation times can be used to obtain desired thicknesses of heat-affected zones.

Due to the precise heat deposition possible through laser processing, specifically designed differential surface-hardened patterns can be obtained. The geometry of surface-hardened patterns is based on specific applications. The hardened patterns can be stripes of parallel lines, stripes of wavy lines, or series of squares and circles. These patterns provide a surface with periodic hardness variation. Figure 1 shows the variation of hardness and ductility along a differential surface-hardened workpiece. In Figure 1 the top view illustrates patterns of untreated regions with lower hardness and higher ductility, while patterns of hardened regions have higher hardness and lower ductility. Along the interface between the untreated and hardened surface, a localized band of tempered zone can be identified, especially when the steel's core hardness is about Rc 40 (4). The side view in Figure 1 shows the cross-sectioned profile of the surface-hardened region. Along the subsurface layers in Figure 1, hardness is a maximum at the surface and gradually decreases along the hardened casing until the core hardness is reached, whereas the variation of ductility is just the opposite. An example of differential surface hardening is the enhancement of wear resistance of lubricated sliding surfaces involving two metals. In this instance, it would be preferable to have the contacting surfaces with large areas of hard and small areas of soft zones. This concept is used in the application of a spiral, surface-hardened pattern along the inner diameter of cylinder liners for locomotive diesel engines (5).

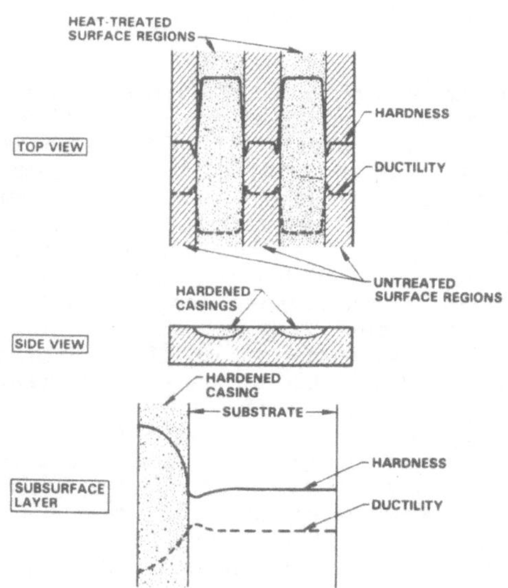

FIGURE 1. Hardness and ductility variations along a differential surface-hardened pattern.

The factors that are important for laser heat treatment are intensity profile of laser beam, laser beam absorptance, heat conduction from the surface into the substrate, and solid-state diffusion causing structural transformation of surface and subsurface layers. These are discussed in the following sections.

2. INTENSITY PROFILE OF LASER BEAM

The spatial distribution of the electromagnetic field inside the optical cavity of a laser is described by resonant electromagnetic modes. Figure 2 illustrates some of the transverse electromagnetic (TEM) modes in cylindrical and rectangular coordinates (6). Beam divergence, beam diameter, and intensity distribution along the plane of the laser beam's cross section are governed by the transverse modes. The lowest order mode is TEM 00, which has a Gaussian-like intensity profile. The beam operating from a laser in TEM 00 can be focused on a workpiece surface to the smallest spot diameter to achieve the highest power density. A beam with TEM 01* has a ring of intense energy surrounding a circle with no intensity; this mode is also commonly referred to as a "donut" mode. Selection of any one of these modes is controlled by adjustment of resonator mirrors in the laser's optical cavity. Lasers operating below 1500 W produce lower order mode beams while those operating above 1500 W produce higher order mode beams. For surface heating applications, low-order laser beams with patterns illustrated in Figure 2 are not completely suitable because of lack of uniform intensity distribution. A uniformly intense beam is needed to obtain uniform surface heating and thus avoid localized surface melting.

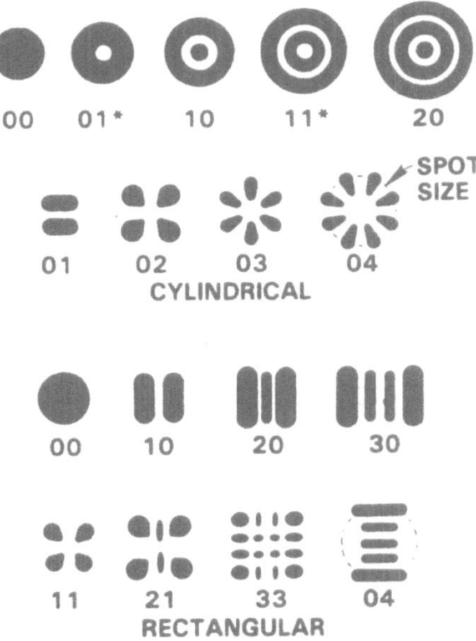

FIGURE 2. Transverse mode patterns in cylindrical and rectangular coordinates (Ref. 6).

2.1. Optical integration

Optical integration methods are used to obtain laser beams with uniform spatial intensity. This method involves dissecting the original beam into a large number of "segmented" beams and superpositioning the "segmented" beams at a common focal point through the use of a beam integrator. A beam integrator has a number of small mirror segments mounted on a base plate. Each mirror segment is positioned to be close-fitting to an adjacent segment to minimize laser beam loss between segments. As an example of the optical integration process, an ideal Gaussian beam can be dissected into four parts of equal size, as illustrated in Figure 3. These four "segmented" beams, with equal intensity distribution, are superimposed at the focal plane; two "segmented" beams with one orientation and the other two with opposite orientation, resulting in near-perfect intensity averaging. This example assumes that the original beam is symmetric. It is well known that available laser beams are rarely symmetrical as in the foregoing special example. In such cases, the laser beam is optically adjusted to illuminate as many segments as possible in a beam-integrating mirror. The uniformity of intensity for an integrated beam will be $\pm$ 1/N, where N is the number of segments that are illuminated by the beam. For example, in a 32-segment beam-integrating mirror, 25 segments will be fully or partially illuminated by the beam (7). The resulting uniformity will be $\pm$ 1/N (i.e., $\pm$ 4%). Diffraction and interference occur when beam integrators are used. The edge of each mirror segment gives rise to diffraction effects, and the multiplicity of "segmented" beams leads to interference fringes. The number of diffraction peaks in an integrated beam is given by the Fresnel number N_f:

$$N_f = \frac{W^2}{4\lambda} \frac{1}{|R_o|} + \frac{1}{|R|} \tag{1}$$

where:

W = segment width
λ = wavelength of laser beam
R_o = effective source distance from the segment
R = effective image distance from the segment

The Fresnel number should be as large as possible to obtain uniform intensity in an integrated beam. Typically, the Fresnel number ranges between 6 and 12 for infrared wavelengths.

2.2. Optics for beam shaping and focusing

The optics integrated to a laser to obtain a uniformly intense beam for surface heating applications are illustrated in Figure 4. The optics consist of a flat mirror, a spherical convex mirror, and a spherical concave beam-integrating mirror. All these mirrors are water cooled to dissipate heat arising from beam absorptance. The convex mirror enables the output laser beam (from the laser system) to be expanded in order to fully illuminate the face of the beam integrator, so that efficient beam integration can result. The beam integrator optically segments the laser beam into several small beams. Each of these "segmented" beams is superimposed at the focal point where the workpiece surface is positioned. The beam integrator has a reflectivity of better than 96% for CO_2 laser beams and is constructed of pure molybdenum. Lower reflecivity of

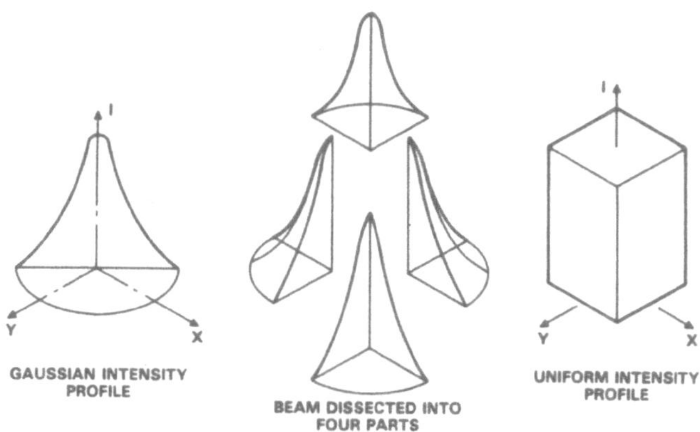

FIGURE 3. Gaussian beam dissected and integrated to a uniformly intense beam profile.

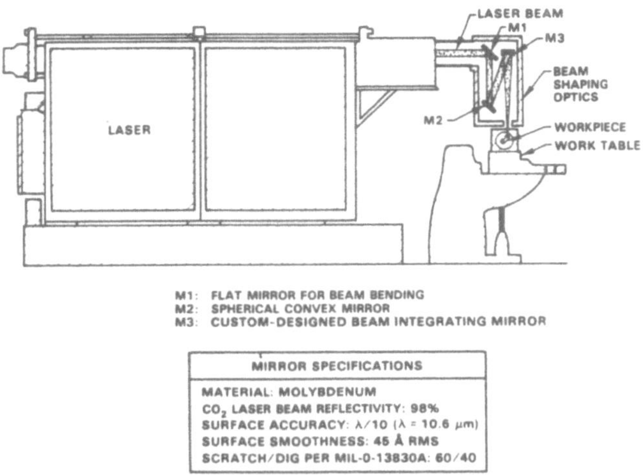

FIGURE 4. Integration of optical tooling to a 5 kW laser for surface heating.

beam-integrating mirrors is due to the beam absorption along the edges of mirror segments. From this optical concept, several modifications can be incorporated to obtain specific beam sizes and shapes such as square, rectangle, and super ellipse. As an example, by using a beam integrator with rectangular segments, a focused, rectangular, cross-sectioned laser beam can be obtained (7).

3. LASER BEAM ABSORPTANCE

To increase laser beam absorptance along metal surfaces, the following approaches are used: (1) metal surfaces painted with infrared energy-absorbing coatings and subsequently processed by a laser beam, and (2) uncoated metal surfaces processed by a linearly polarized laser beam.

3.1. Infrared energy-absorbing coatings

Coatings having high absorptance for infrared radiation must possess the following characteristics for increased efficiency during laser heat treatment (8): (1) high thermal stability, (2) good adhesion to workpiece surface, (3) chemically passive to workpiece, (4) proper coating thickness, (5) high heat transfer coefficient for heat conduction from coating to workpiece, and (6) easily applied and removed.

3.1.1. Spray coatings. Several commercially available paints, such as Krylon 1602, exhibit low normal spectral reflectance for 10,600 nm wavelength (CO_2 laser beam) (9). These paints in general contain carbon black and sodium or potassium silicates and are applied to metal surfaces by spraying. Thicknesses of paint coatings range from 10 to 20 μm.

3.2.1. Chemical conversion coatings. Chemical conversion coatings, such as manganese, zinc or iron phosphate, absorb infrared radiation. Phosphate coatings are obtained by treating iron-base alloy workpieces with a dilute solution of phosphoric acid mixed with other chemicals (10). Through this treatment, the surface of the workpiece is converted to an integrally bonded layer of crystalline phosphate. Phosphate coatings may range in thickness from 2 to 100 μm; weight of the coating may range from 0.02 to 5 mg/cm^2 of coating surface. Depending on the workpiece geometry, phosphating time can range from 5 to 30 minutes. Phosphate coatings can be prepared with a fine or coarse microstructure.

In terms of chemical passiveness and ease of coating application, silicates containing carbon black are more effective than the phosphate coatings. Figure 5 schematically illustrates the reaction of coating compounds (e.g., manganese phosphate) with workpiece surface and subsequent formation of low melting compounds which can penetrate along the grain boundaries over several grains below the surface.

3.2. Linearly polarized laser beam

Metals have lower reflectance for linearly polarized electromagnetic radiation (11). The basis of this optical phenomenon has been applied to the heat treatment of uncoated iron-base alloy workpieces by using a CO_2 laser beam (12). An unpolarized laser beam can be linearly polarized by using proper reflecting optics (13). When an unpolarized laser beam is incident on a metal miror at a specific angle of incidence, the reflected beam will be linearly polarized, as illustrated in Figure 6. This special angle of incidence is called the polarizing angle. When the beam is linearly polarized, the dominant vibration direction is perpendicular to the plane of incidence. The plane of incidence is defined as the plane that contains both the incident laser beam and the normal to the reflecting surface.

The electric vector $\bar{E}$ of the linearly polarized beam has components parallel (E_p) and perpendicular (E_s) to the plane of incidence. Figure 7 illustrates absorptance as a function of the angle of incidence for iron (13). At an angle of incidence between 70° and 80°, the absorptance is between 50 and 60% for E_p and 5 to 10% for E_s. Thus, by directing a linearly polarized laser beam at an angle of incidence

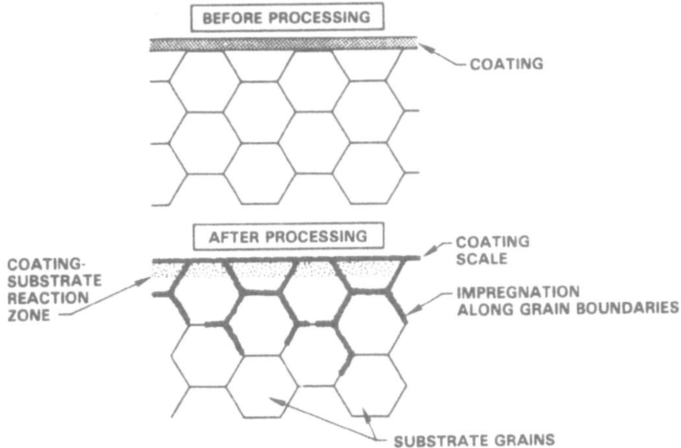

FIGURE 5. Potential reaction of infrared energy-absorbing coating with substrate during laser heat treatment. These reactions can be prevented by the use of chemically inert coatings.

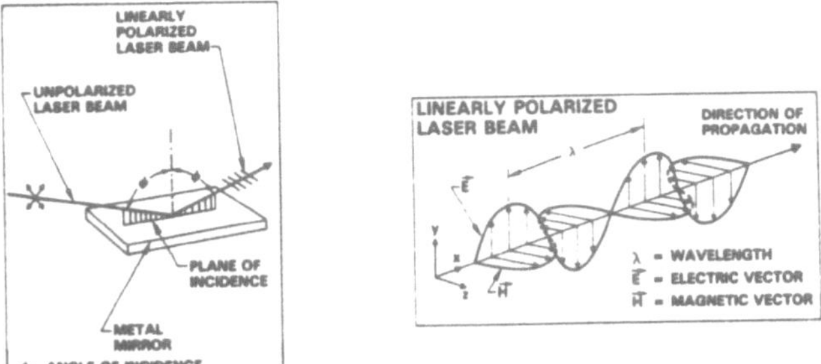

FIGURE 6. Conversion of an unpolarized laser beam to a linearly polarized beam by reflection at a specific angle of incidence (adapted from Ref. 13).

greater than 45°, substantial absorptance by iron-base alloys is possible. A potential drawback of this method is the significant laser beam power loss during conversion of an unpolarized laser beam to a linearly polarized beam.

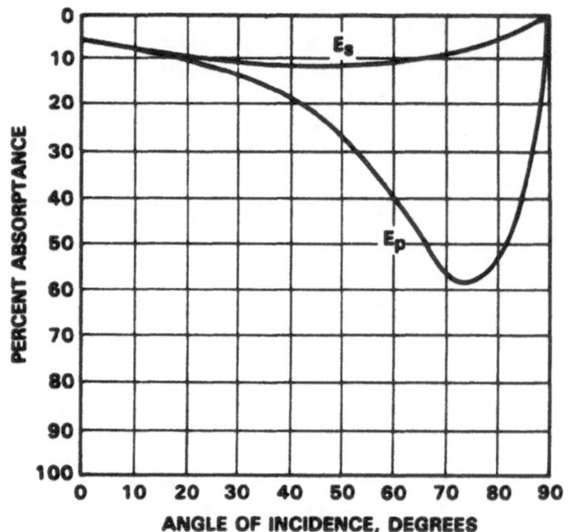

FIGURE 7. Effect of the angle of incidence of a linearly polarized laser beam on absorptance by iron-base alloys (Ref. 12).

4. THREE-DIMENSIONAL, TIME-DEPENDENT, HEAT CONDUCTION MODEL

A computational model simulating the laser heat treatment process has been developed by Shankar using the three-dimensional, time-dependent, heat conduction equation (14). This numerical approach is general in that it allows treatment of finite- or infinite-length workpieces with arbitrary cross section, laser beams with variations in power density distribution, beams with various cross-sectional shapes, arbitrary motions of a workpiece, and temperature dependence of the thermal and optical properties of a workpiece.

Figure 8 illustrates a rectangular workpiece subjected to a laser beam with a super-elliptical cross section. The coordinate system (t', x', y', z') is fixed to the workpiece that is undergoing a motion, and the coordinate system (t, x, y, z) is fixed to the laser beam that is stationary. The energy balance equation in the coordinate system (t', x', y', z') can be written as

$$q_{t}' + E_{x}' + F_{y}' + G_{z}' = 0 \tag{2}$$

where

$$q = \rho H , \quad E = \kappa \frac{\partial T}{\partial x'} , \quad F = \kappa \frac{\partial T}{\partial y'} , \quad G = \kappa \frac{\partial T}{\partial z'}$$

and ρ is the density of the workpiece, κ is the thermal conductivity, H is the enthalpy given by C_pT where C_p is the specific heat of the material, and T is the temperature. For treatment of arbitrary-shaped workpieces undergoing complex motion, a coordinate transformation of the form

$$\xi = \xi(x', y', z', t') \tag{3}$$

$$\eta = \eta(x', y', z', t')$$

$$\zeta = \zeta(x', y', z', t')$$

$$\tau = t'$$

may be necessary. After transformation, Eq.(2) can be written in the form

$$\bar{q}_r + \bar{E}_\xi + \bar{F}_\eta + \bar{G}_\zeta = 0 \tag{4}$$

where

$$\bar{q} = q/J$$

$$\bar{E} = (q_{\xi t} + E_{-x} + F_{-y} + G_{-z})/J$$

$$\bar{F} = (q_{\eta t} + E_{-x} + F_{-y} + G_{-z})/J$$

$$\bar{G} = (q_{\zeta t} + E_{-x} + F_{-y} + G_{-z})/J$$

$$J = \text{Jacobian of the transformation} = \frac{\partial(\tau, \xi, \eta, \zeta)}{\partial(t', x', y', z')}$$

4.1. Infinite-length workpiece

The stationary coordinate system fixed to the laser beam and the moving coordinate system fixed to the workpiece are related by constant velocity, U, of workpiece motion during simple translation by

$$\begin{aligned} x &= x' + Ut \\ y &= y' \\ z &= z' \\ t &= t \end{aligned} \tag{5}$$

Using Eq.(5), Eq.(4) becomes transformed to

$$\rho C_p \frac{\partial T}{\partial t} = \nabla\cdot(\kappa\nabla T) - U\rho C_p \frac{\partial T}{\partial x} \tag{6}$$

The time derivative term in Eq.(6) represents the rate of change of enthalpy per unit volume. The term $\nabla\cdot(\kappa\nabla T)$ represents conductive

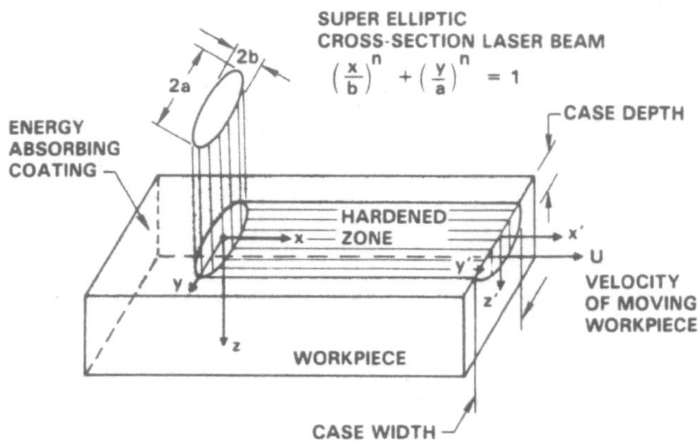

FIGURE 8. Coordinate system used for the numerical formulation of laser heat-treatment process.

heat transfer, and the last term in Eq.(6) represents the heat transfer due to motion of the workpiece. For an infinitely long workpiece, where end effects are not important, the temperature distribution with respect to the stationary cordinate system (x,y,z) can be assumed to be steady. This reduces Eq.(6) to the form

$$\nabla \cdot (\kappa \nabla T) = U \rho C_p \frac{\partial T}{\partial x} \tag{7}$$

4.2. Finite-length workpiece

For treatment of finite-length workpieces, where end effects are important, it is easier to work with a coordinate system fixed to the workpiece. Since laser heat treatment of finite-length workpieces is of practical interest, the solution procedure pertinent to the time-dependent heat flow equation of the type given by Eq.(4) is discussed here. Assuming that thermal conductivity, material density, and optical properties (beam absorptance) are weakly dependent on temperature and also that there is no surface melting, Eq.(4) can simply be written as

$$R(T) = 0 \tag{8}$$

where T is the temperature distribution in the workpiece at a given time level "n" and R is the discretized functional representation of Eq.(4). For a finite-length workpiece, the heat flow is highly time dependent because of the finite dwell time of the laser beam. To produce a meaningful simulation of the heat-affected or hardened zone profile, Eq.(8) will have to be satisfied at each time level to within a given tolerance level. The solution procedure involves a Newton iteration to solve Eq.(8) by linearizing the equation about a known neighborhood state T^*

$$R(T^*) + \frac{\partial R}{\partial T}^* (T - T^*) = 0 \tag{9}$$

To start a Newton iteration, initially T^* can be assumed to be T^n in Eq.(9). As an illustration of R and $(\partial R/\partial T)$, let us consider the heat flow equation, Eq.(2)

$$\beta \frac{\partial T}{\partial t} - \nabla^2 T = 0 \tag{10}$$

where $\beta = \rho(C_p/\kappa)$ and ∇^2 is the Laplacian. For Eq.(10), the following can be written (see Fig. 9):

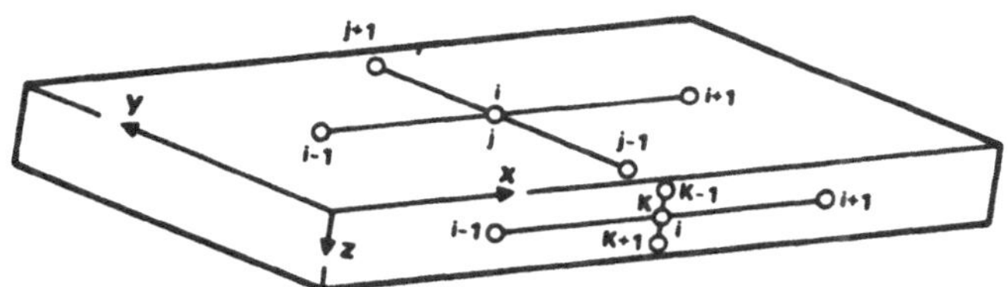

FIGURE 9. Grid indexing across workpiece.

$$R(T^*) = \beta \left\{ \frac{T^*_{i,j,k} - T^n_{i,j,k}}{\Delta t} \right\} - \left\{ (T^*_{i+1,j,k} - 2T^*_{i,j,k} + T^*_{i-1,j,k}) \big/ \Delta x^2 \right\}$$

$$- \left\{ (T^*_{i,j+1,k} - 2T^*_{i,j,k} + T^*_{i,j-1,k}) \big/ \Delta y^2 \right\} \tag{11}$$

$$- \left\{ (T^*_{i,j,k+1} - 2T^*_{i,j,k} + T^*_{i,j,k-1}) \big/ \Delta z^2 \right\}$$

and

$$\frac{\partial R}{\partial T}^* = \frac{\beta}{\Delta t} - \frac{\partial^2}{\partial x^2} - \frac{\partial^2}{\partial y^2} - \frac{\partial^2}{\partial z^2} \tag{12}$$

Equation (12) is a differential operator. Solving for $(T - T^*)$ from Eq.(9) by a direct inversion of $(\partial R/\partial T)$ is difficult because it involves computational molecules in all three directions. Thus, simplifications to the form of $(\partial R/\partial T)$ are essential for computational ease. In terms of computational speed, the approximate factorization technique is preferred because the information is more implicitly coupled. To achieve ΔT values less than 10^{-2} at a given time level, 5 to 10 internal Newton iterations may be required.

4.3. Approximate factorization

$$\frac{\partial R}{\partial T} \approx 1 - \frac{\Delta t}{\beta}\frac{\partial^2}{x^2} \quad 1 - \frac{\Delta t}{\beta}\frac{\partial^2}{y^2} \quad 1 - \frac{\Delta t}{\beta}\frac{\partial^2}{z^2} = L_x L_y L_z \tag{13}$$

In this procedure, Eq.(9) is solved in three steps.

$$L_x L_y L_z \quad T = - R(T^*), \qquad T = T - T^* \tag{14}$$

Step 1

$$L_x \bar{\Delta} T = - R(T^*)$$

Step 2

$$L_y \widehat{\Delta T} = \bar{\Delta} T$$

Step 3

$$L_z \Delta T = \widehat{\Delta T}, \qquad T = T^* + \Delta T$$

Since at convergence $\Delta T \longrightarrow 0$ at a given time level (for time accuracy), the extra terms introduced by the triple approximate factorization are of no concern because the right-hand side $R(T^*)$ in Eq.(14) is not altered.

4.4. Boundary conditions

For a finite-length workpiece, computational solution to the heat flow model, Eq.(4), requires boundary conditions along the entire surface of the workpiece. Three types of boundary conditions can be prescribed at a boundary surface, as illustrated in Figure 10.

(1) Dirichlet condition, where the temperature T is decribed.
(2) Neumann condition, where the heat flux q_n in the inward normal direction to the boundary surface is prescribed by $q_n = - \kappa \frac{\partial T}{\partial n}$.
(3) Mixed-type condition, where a combination of Neumann and Dirichlet boundary conditions is prescribed. This is usually done when the energy balance at a boundary surface is applied, and accounts for heat entering by convection and heat leaving by conduction.

At the top surface of the workpiece subjected to laser heating and boundary points directly inside the laser beam cross section, the following condition (Neumann type) is applied

$$- \kappa \frac{\partial T}{\partial z} = \frac{Q_0 \eta}{A} \tag{15}$$

where Q_0 is the laser beam power, A is the beam cross-sectional area, and η is the local absorptivity factor having a value in the range of 0.75 to 0.99.

In the computational simulation of a finite-length workpiece, at all boundary points outside of the laser beam, a mixed-type boundary condition illustrated in Figure 10 is applied. The surface heat loss during laser heat treatment is reported to be insignificant compared to the total amount of heat absorbed by the workpiece (15).

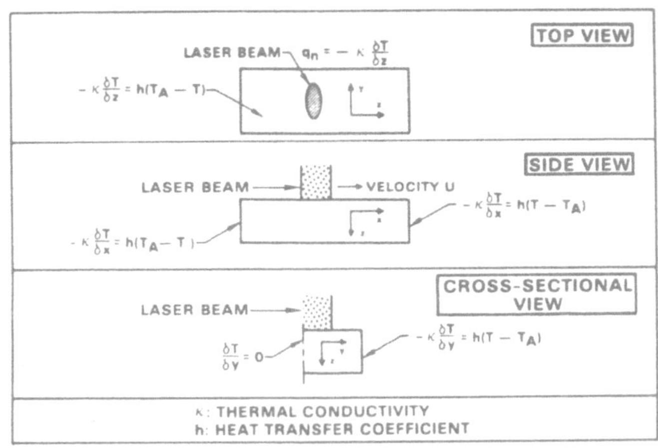

FIGURE 10. Boundary conditions used to solve the heat conduction equation.

4.5. Validation of heat-conduction model

To validate the computational heat conduction model, rectangular workpieces (AISI 4140 steel) with nominal dimensions 100 mm long (x), 50 mm wide (y), and 12 mm thick (z) were used. Length and width dimensions of steel plates varied within $\pm$ 3 mm. The steel plates had a tempered martensitic core microstructure of hardness ranging from Rc 36 to 42. The surface finish of these machined plates was typically 3 μm RMS. The surfaces were spray coated with Krylon 1602 paint to enhance absorptance of the CO_2 laser beam. Surface-hardening experiments were conducted by using a Spectra-Physics Model 975 continuous-wave CO_2 laser system. Surface-hardened stripes were obtained by scanning these plates at a specific travel speed under a focused elliptical cross-sectioned laser beam of 5000 W power.

The workpiece was modeled by using a 61 x 21 x 21 grid. The laser beam was modeled by a super-elliptical cross section with major axis 2a and minor axis 2b. A typical calculation for a finite-length workpiece was done in 50 time steps. For a 100 mm long workpiece undergoing a travel speed of 2 mm/s, the time step used in solving the heat flow equation, Eq.(4), was 1 second. The numerical method being implicit in nature, the solution is stable even for larger Δt. As Δt is increased, more internal Newton iterations will be required to converge the temperature at each time level for accuracy. By using a 61 x 21 x 21 grid, a typical calculation, with 5 to 7 internal iterations and Δt based on a total of 50 time steps, required 120 seconds on the CDC 176 machine.

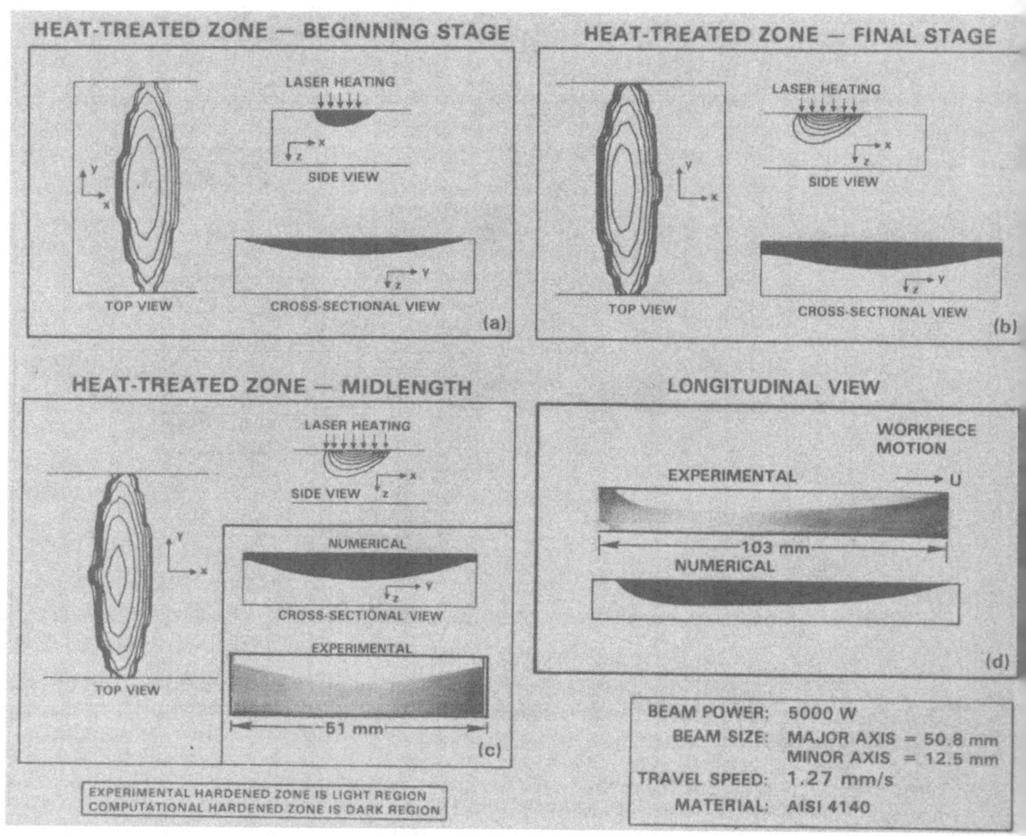

FIGURE 11. Finite workpiece simulation of hardened zone profile showing time accuracy for (a) beginning stage, (b) midlength, and (c) final stage of laser heat treatment. The longitudinal view (d) shows the increase in case depth along workpiece length.

Figure 11 shows the temperature distribution in a finite-length workpiece at various time levels for the laser beam size (a = 25.4 mm, b = 6.25 mm) and travel speed of 1.27 mm/s. Figure 11(a) shows the temperature distribution at the beginning stage of the laser heat-treatment process. Only temperature levels above the transformation temperature of 723°C are shown. Figure 11(b) shows the temperature distribution when the laser beam is at the midsection of the workpiece. The depth and width of heat penetration in the cross-sectional plane at this time level compare very well with experimental data. Figure 11(c) shows the temperature distribution at the final stage of the heat treatment process just before the beam is shut off. The laser beam's minor axis is large; hence, the depth of heat penetration continuously increases along the longitudinal direction of the workpiece, as illustrated in Figure 11(d). These results demonstrate a time-accurate calculation for laser heat treatment. Figures 12 and 13 show cross-sectional views of profiles of heat-affected and hardened zones along the midlength of steel plates for the case of b = 6.25 mm and b = 2.5 mm, respectively. All these numerical results are in good agreement with experimental data for a wide range of case depths.

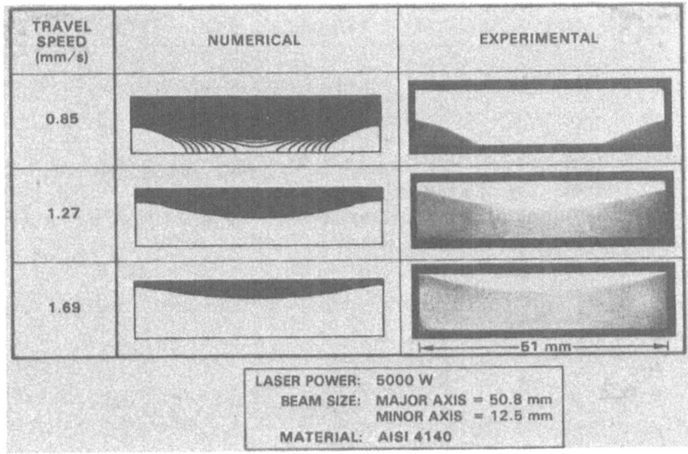

FIGURE 12. Comparison of numerical and experimental cross-sectional views of hardened zones at workpiece's midlength, showing the effect of workpiece travel speed for a laser beam of 12.5 mm minor axis and 500 W of beam power.

5. STRUCTURAL TRANSFORMATION FOR SURFACE HARDENING

Diffusion-controlled structural transformations during laser heat treatment are transformation of ferrite and pearlite to austenite, and homogenization of carbon among austenite grains during the heating cycle. Transformation of austenite having adequate carbon content to martensite occurs without diffusion during the cooling cycle, especially if the cooling rates are high enough. When iron-base alloys are processed by using high heating rates, Figure 14 shows that the eutectoid transformation temperatures Ac_1 (723°C) and Ac_3 are substantially raised (16). The increase in Ac_1 may be associated to the pearlite colonies transforming to austenite grains by a diffusional process involving "end" dissolution of Fe_3C plates (i.e., the dissolution process is the reverse of austenite transformation to pearlite) (17). Figure 15 shows the process by which Fe_3C plates dissolve during heating. The time required for the dissolution of Fe_3C plates during an isothermal treatment is dependent on the diffusion of carbon and is governed by the

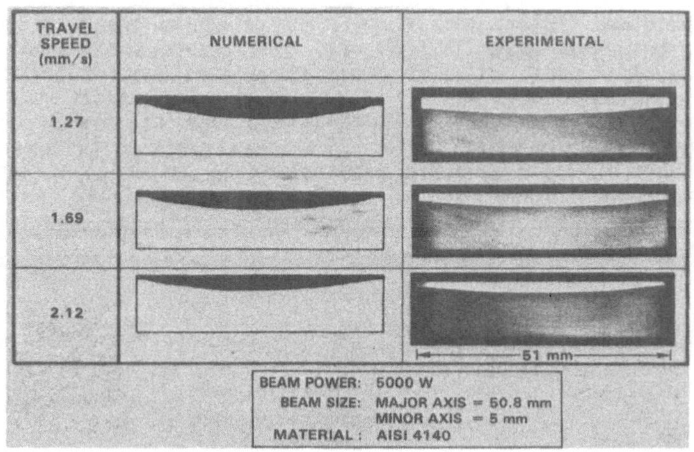

FIGURE 13. Comparison of numerical and experimental cross-sectional views of hardened zones at workpiece's midlength, showing the effect of workpiece travel speed for a laser beam at 5 mm minor axis and 5000 W of beam power.

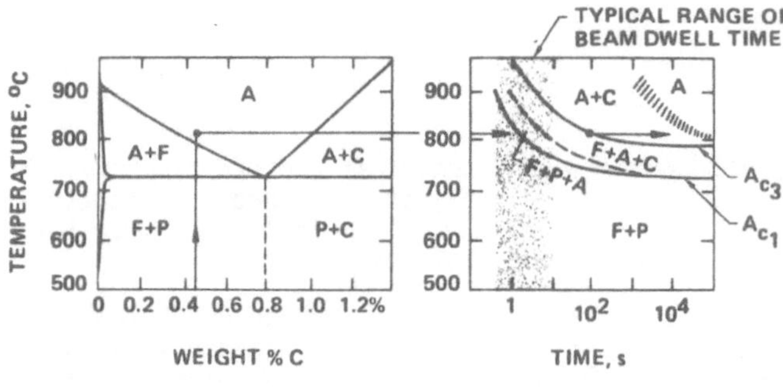

FIGURE 14. Structural transformation on heating a 0.45% carbon steel (Ref. 16).

expression $Ld = 2 Dt$, where t = time at temperature, L = radius of pearlite colony, d = spacing of Fe_3C plate, and D = diffusion coefficient of carbon in ferrite. When L and d are small, the dissolution of Fe_3C is rapid during heating. By sweeping a uniformly intense laser beam along a workpiece surface, thermal cycles are developed along the

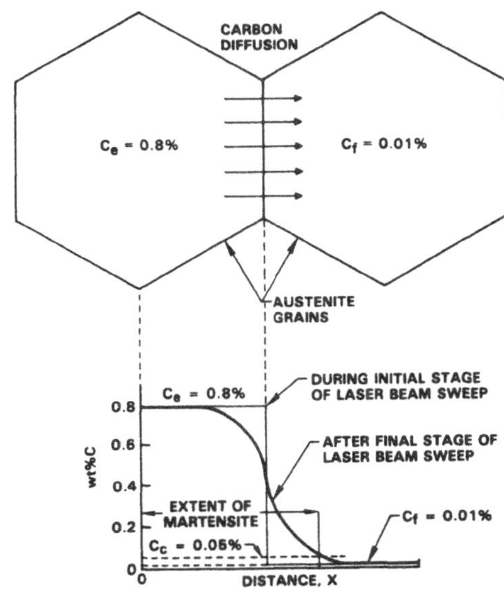

FIGURE 15. Transformation of pearlite to austenite (Ref. 17).

surface and subsurface layers, and the process conducted under these conditions is no longer isothermal. Therefore, the factor Dt should be modified to account for the temperature dependence of D and the time dependence of temperature during a thermal cycle. For diffusion during a thermal cycle, the factor Dt is represented by

$$\int_0^t D_o e^{[-Q/RT(t)]} dt \qquad (16)$$

where D_o = pre-exponential diffusion constant, Q = activation energy for diffusion, R = gas constant, and T = temperature.

During thermal cycling, when temperature is above Ac_1, austenite grains are formed from pearlite colonies. Depending on temperatures relative to Ac_3, part or all of the ferrite grains are transformed to austenite grains. Austenite grains formed from pearlite contain 0.8% carbon (c_e), and those austenite grains formed from ferrite contain a negligible amount of carbon (c_f). When austenite grains with varying concentration of carbon are adjacent to each other, carbon diffusion occurs from grains with concentration c_e to those grains with concentration c_f. When the cooling rates are high enough, regions containing carbon in excess of 0.05% will transform to martensite (18). The analytical solution to the one-dimensional diffusion equation is

$$c(x,t) = \frac{c_e + c_f}{2} - \frac{c_e - c_f}{2} \operatorname{erf} \frac{x}{2\sqrt{Dt}} \quad (17)$$

where $c(x,t)$ = carbon concentration at distance, x, and time, t.
Equation (17) can be further simplified by approximating that

$$\operatorname{erf} Z = 1 - e^{(-Z\sqrt{\pi})} \quad \text{for} \quad 0.2 < Z < 2 \quad (18)$$

and using $c(x,t) = c_c$ (i.e., $c_c = 0.05\%$), and considering $c_e << c_f$ to obtain the following equation

$$x = \frac{2}{\sqrt{\pi}} \ln\left\{\frac{c_e}{2c_c}\right\} \sqrt{Dt} \quad (19)$$

As mentioned earlier, the factor Dt for a thermal cycle is best represented in an integral form. The above equation shows that homogenization of carbon through diffusion among several austenite grains will depend on the grain size. This is because if the austenite grain size is small, then the diffusion distance, x, will also be small, as shown in Figure 16.

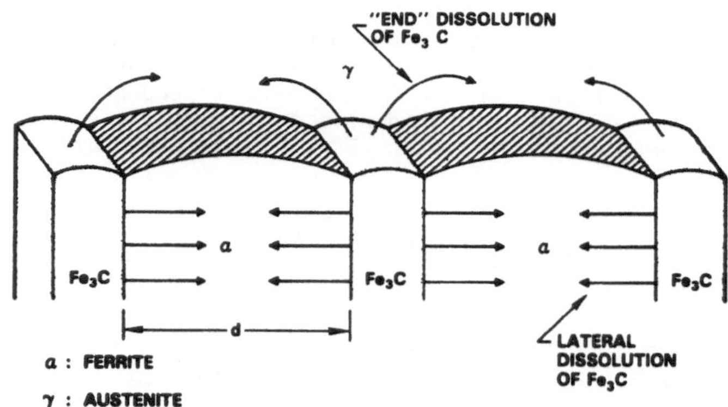

FIGURE 16. Carbon concentration profile in austenite grains during homogenization (adapted from Ref. 18).

Austenite grain size depends on the size of ferrite grains and pearlite colonies in the workpiece (prior to laser heat treatment), and the temperature-time cycle induced during laser heat treatment. Table 1 illustrates that when workpieces have a tempered martensitic or bainitic microstructure prior to laser heat treatment, the carbon diffusion distance is very small, and deep surface-hardened casings are obtained. When the workpiece microstructure contains spheres of Fe_3C and ferrite (e.g., spheroidized microstructure), carbon diffusion distance needed for homogenization of austenite is significantly long; therefore, surface-hardened casings will be negligibly thin. Thus, proper workpiece microstructure is desirable for efficient surface hardening as well as for providing the workpiece core with suitable properties (e.g., ductility, fracture toughness, and machinability) for specific applications.

6. CONCLUSIONS

(1) The factors that are important for laser heat treatment are intensity profile of laser beam, beam absorptance, heat conduction from the surface into subsurface layers, and structural transformation in workpieces along the regions subjected to a thermal cycle.

(2) A laser beam with uniform spatial intensity is desirable to obtain uniform surface heating and thus prevent localized surface melting. Beam integration methods by using optics with Fresnel number higher than 10 are used to obtain a laser beam with intensity variation of $\pm$ 1/N, where N = number of mirror segments in a beam integrator illuminated by the beam.

(3) Absorptance of CO_2 laser beam by iron-base alloy surfaces is increased by using paints such as Krylon 1602 that contain black and sodium or potassium silicates and are applied to a thickness ranging from 10 to 20 μm.

(4) A linearly polarized CO_2 laser beam is highly absorbed by uncoated iron-base alloy surfaces when the angle of beam incidence is greater than 45°. A disadvantage of this method is that during conversion of an unpolarized laser beam to a linearly polarized beam, there is significant loss of beam power.

(5) A computational model simulating the laser heat-treatment process uses the three-dimensional, time-dependent, heat conduction equation. The numerical approach is valid for finite- or infinite-length workpieces with arbitrary cross sections, laser beams with variations in power density distribution, beams with various cross-sectional shapes, arbitrary motions of a workpiece, and temperature dependence of the thermal and optical properties of the workpiece. Comparison of the calculated profiles of heat-affected and hardened zones is in good agreement with experimental data. This computational method does not assume workpiece geometry; therefore, the analysis is widely applicable to the surface heating of a desired component.

(6) Thermal cycles developed along the surface and subsurface layers induce solid-state diffusion, causing structural transformation for surface hardening. The rate of transformation of ferrite and pearlite to austenite, and homogenization of carbon among austenite grains is controlled by carbon diffusion. The depth of a heat-affected and hardened zone is governed by the response of the workpiece core microstructure to specific thermal cycles along subsurface layers.

ACKNOWLEDGMENTS

This investigation was supported by Rockwell IR&D Projects 815 and 826-5 at the Science Center. The authors thank Dr. M. R. James and Dr. P. R. Newman of the Rockwell International Science Center, and Mr. R. L. Pierce of Spawr Optical Research, Inc., for useful technical discussions.

REFERENCES

1. D.S. Gnanamuthu, C.B. Shaw, Jr., W.E. Lawrence, and M.R. Mitchell, "Laser Transformation Hardening," ISSN: 0094-243X/79/500173, American Institute of Physics (1979).
2. A. Solina, M. DeSanctis, L. Paganini, A. Blarasin, and S. Quaranta, J. Heat Treating 3, 193 (1984).
3. Thermal Radiative Properties, edited by Y. S. Touloukian and D. P. DeWitt (IFI/Plenum, New York, 1970), Vol. 7, p. 329.
4. D. S. Gnanamuthu and R. J. Moores, "Laser Heat Treatment of Track Components in Combat Vehicles Phase I," Final Report, DTIC No. AD A102761.
5. G. Eberhardt, "Survey of High Power CO_2 Industrial Laser Applications and Latest Laser Developments," Proceedings of the First International Conference on Lasers in Manufacturing, Brighton, England, edited by M. F. Kimmitt (IFS (Publications) Ltd., England, and North-Holland, New York, 1983), p. 13.
6. Solid-State Laser Engineering, edited by W. Koechner (Springer-Verlag, New York, 1976), p. 173.
7. D. D. Dourte, R. L. Pierce, and W. J. Spawr, "Optical Integration with Screw Supports," U. S. Patent No. 4,195,913 (April 1, 1980).
8. A. J. Hick, "Rapid Surface Heat Treatments - a Review of Laser and Electron Beam Hardening," Heat Treatment of Metals 1, 3 (1983).
9. Thermal Radiative Properties, edited by Y. S. Touloukian and D. P. DeWitt (IFI/Plenum, New York, 1972), p. 525.
10. Metals Handbook, Vol. 2, Heat Treating, Cleaning and Finishing (American Society for Metals, 1964), p. 531.
11. Fundamentals of Optics, Fourth Edition, edited by F. A. Jenkins and H. E. White (McGraw-Hill, New York, 1976), p. 535.
12. F. Dausinger, W. Müller, and P. Arnold, "Laser Beam Surface Treatment Process for Materials of Large Reflectivity," U. S. Patent No. 4,414,038 (November 8, 1983).
13. Polarized Light, edited by W. A. Shurcliff (Harvard University Press, 1966), p. 78.
14. V. S. Shankar and D. S. Gnanamuthu, "Computational Simulation of Laser Heat Processing of Materials," AIAA-85-0390, AIAA 23rd Aerospace Sciences Meeting, Reno, 1985.
15. S. Kou, D. K. Sun, and Y. P. Le, Metall. Trans., A 14A, 643 (1983).
16. A. Rose and B. Strassburg, Stahl und Eisen 76, 976 (1956).
17. M. F. Ashby and K. E. Easterling, "Transformation Hardening of Steel Surfaces by Laser Beams," National Technical Information Service, PB84-205533 (1984).
18. M. F. Ashby, K. E. Easterling, and W. B. Li, "Modeling the Laser Transformation Hardening of Steel," Laser Processing of Materials - Conference Proceedings, edited by K. Mukherjee and J. Mazumder, (The Metallurgical Society of AIME, 1985), p. 225.

TABLE 1. Effect of workpiece microstructure on surface-hardened depth.

MICROSTRUCTURE OF CAST IRON	MICROSTRUCTURE OF STEEL	REQUIRED DISTANCE FOR CARBON DIFFUSION	SURFACE-HARDENED DEPTH
GRAPHITE + TEMPERED MARTENSITE	TEMPERED MARTENSITE	LOW	HIGH
GRAPHITE + BAINITE	BAINITE	LOW	HIGH
GRAPHITE + PEARLITE	PEARLITE + FERRITE	MEDIUM	MEDIUM
GRAPHITE + FERRITE	SPHEROIDIZED Fe_3C + FERRITE	HIGH	LOW OR EVEN NEGLIGIBLE

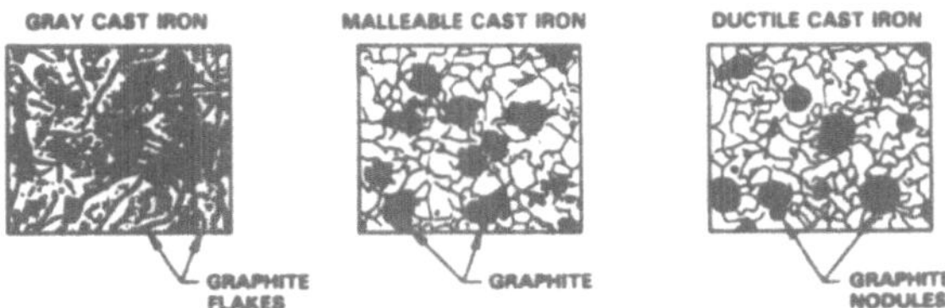

RESIDUAL STRESSES INDUCED BY LASER SURFACE TREATMENT

C. CHABROL AND A. B. VANNES
INSA, Calfetmat, France

Key Words: residual stresses, transformation hardening

1. INTRODUCTION

The laser, used as a heat source, has great potential as a tool for surface treatment. This can be solid state transformations or transformations involving the liquid state with or without changes of composition. This paper deals essentially with transformation hardening without melting for various steels. Such treatments are characterized by the microstructure, hardness and residual stresses. The overlap effect in a surface produced by multi-passes has also been studied. In addition, some residual stress results are presented for the case of cladding.

TRANSFORMATION HARDENING

2. EXPERIMENTAL PROCEDURE

2.1. Materials

The materials studied were a medium carbon steel (steel A), two alloy steels (B,C) and a micro alloy steel with vanadium (D). Their compositions are given in Table 1. They were heated (annealed, quenched and tempered at different temperatures between 400 and 600°C) so that the effect of initial microstructure on laser treatment could be studied.

2.2. Laser Treatment

Transformation hardening was carried out using two continuous CO_2 lasers, so that the influence of beam shape and energy profile could also be studied:

- A laser with maximum power 15 kW, situated in the Fiat Research Center in Torino (Italy): integrator optics gave a rectangular power distribution (Figure 1).

- The other with maximum power 5 kW, situated in Etablissement Technique Central de l'Armement (ETCA) in Arcueil (France): a cylindrical mirror enabled wider zones to be treated, but the energy profile was inhomogeneous (Figure 2).

Rectangular rod-shaped specimens, 20 and 30 mm thick, were treated by a single pass. Before treatment, they were covered with a graphite layer in order to improve the absorption coefficient at 10.6 μm wavelength.

The power density was varied between 1 and 3 kW/cm^2 and interaction times between 0.3 and 3.0 seconds.

One of the limitations of a laser is the narrowness of the beam and hence the treated zone. Some surfaces were prepared by three passes with little overlap. A defocused beam was used. The energy profile, apart from two peaks, was reasonably homogeneous (Figure 3).

TABLE 1. Composition of the studied steels

Wt% Steel	C	Cr	Ni	Mo	Mn	Si	Cu	S	P	Sn	Al	V
A	0.47	0.10	0.08	0.02	0.69	0.27	0.11	0.022	0.009	0.02	0.01	-
B	0.37	1.05	0.17	0.24	0.69	0.38	-	0.003	0.009	-	-	-
C	0.35	1.72	3.84	0.37	0.35	0.41	0.09	0.005	0.009	-	-	-
D	0.47	0.12	0.14	0.03	0.80	0.31	0.14	0.03	0.02	-	0.02	0.11

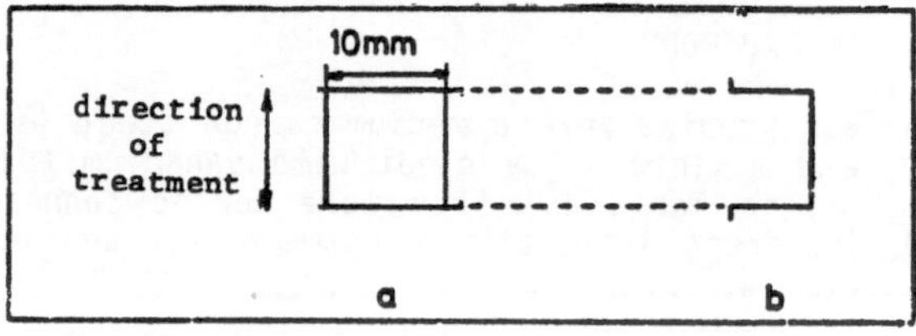

FIGURE 1. Beam impact in a plexiglas plate (a) and energy profile (b).

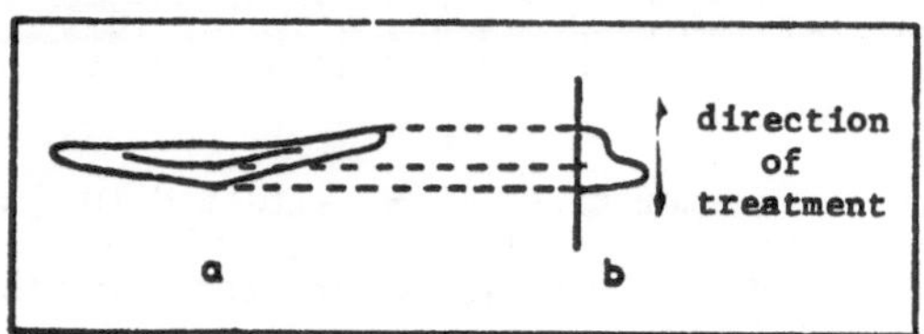

FIGURE 2. Beam impact in a plexiglas plate (a) and energy profile (b).

2.3. Determination of the residual stresses

The distribution of residual stresses was determined by the Leluan method (1). This destructive method enables the stress value in each layer of the material to be determined. It consists of removing layers of material by chemical machining which does not create any residual stresses itself and maintains the initial symmetry of the specimen.

The initial equilibrium of the residual stresses in the specimen is thus destroyed. The method consists of analyzing the equilibrium re-establishment in the specimen after machining. The return to equilibrium

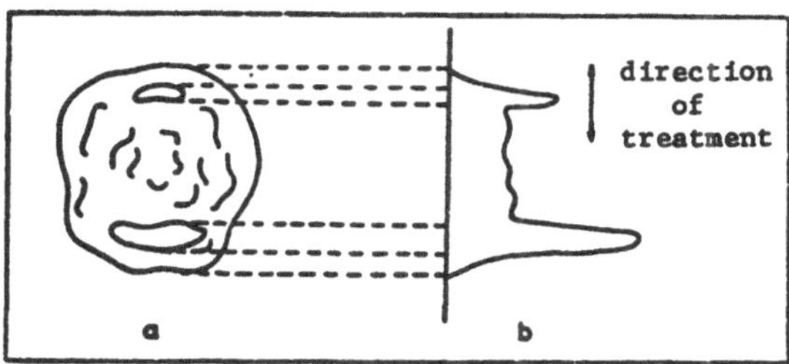

FIGURE 3. Beam impact in a plexiglas plate (a) and energy profile (b) used for multi-run treatment.

is described by elasticity theory. The initial residual stress field can be calculated assuming isotropy by measuring the strains during re-establishment of equilibrium on the side of the specimen opposite to the machined surface:

$$\sigma^{i}_{L,T} = \bar{\sigma}^{i}_{L,T} + \sum_{j=1}^{i-1} \Delta\sigma^{j}_{L,T}$$

with: $\sigma^{i}_{L,T}$ = initial stress existing in the ith layer in longitudinal and transverse directions,

$\bar{\sigma}^{i}_{L,T}$ = stress which remains in the ith layer after the ith-1 layer has been removed.

$\Delta\sigma^{j}_{L,T}$ = stress variation in the ith layer during removal of the jth layer ($j < i$).

3. RESULTS

The depths of treatment range from a few tenths of a millimeter to about 1.5 mm, depending on the initial microstructure of the steel and the laser treatment parameters.

3.1. Hardness

Figures 4 and 5 present hardness profiles as a function of case depth in steel B for a single pass for various initial microstructures and specimen speeds.

A wide scatter of hardness values in the treated zone is observed, especially for the annealed structure; also a very sharp drop at the limit of that zone, a hardness trough for quenched and tempered structures followed by the value for the substrate. The specimen speed controls essentially the depth of treatment but not the maximum hardness value.

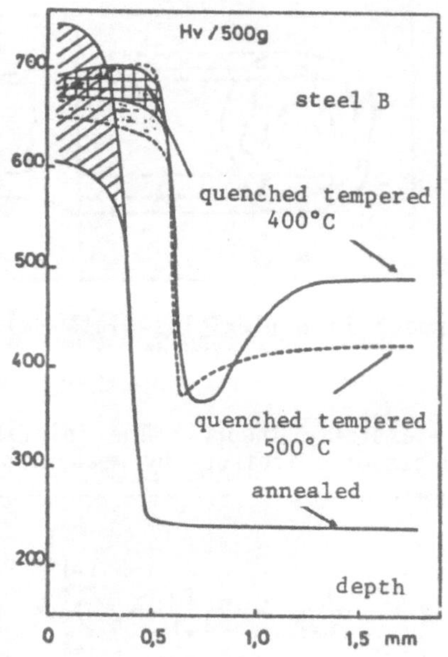

FIGURE 4. Hardness versus case depth for different initial microstructures of steel B.

3.2. Residual Stresses

Figure 6 presents the residual stress distribution in the annealed steel A. σ_L and σ_T are the longitudinal stresses - parallel to the direction of displacement - and the transversal stresses - perpendicular to the direction of displacement. Their development in the depth is quite similar.

The influence of microstructure and specimen speed on the stress profiles is investigated for the steel C (Figures 7 and 8).

The stresses are always compressive in the treated zone and tensile directly beneath it. The depth at which the stress is zero agrees with the hardened depth, as determined by the 550 HV hardness value.

Quenched and tempered structures show similar profiles with a high tensile peak, whereas the annealed structures show a broad peak with a lower maximum value. The specimen speed, as well as the power, does not have any significant influence on the value of the maximum stress. It simply decreases the depth at which the stress is zero.

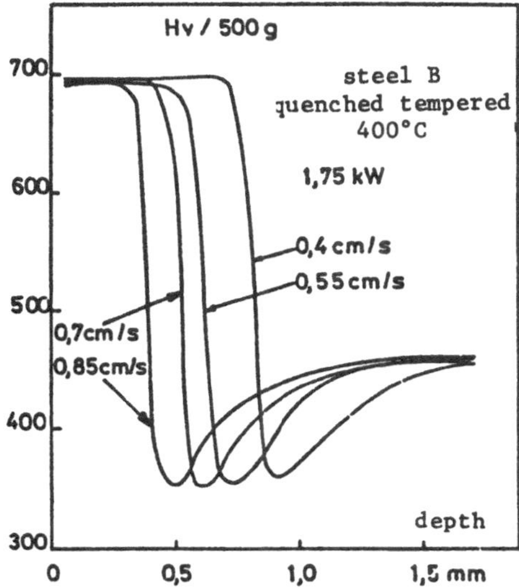

FIGURE 5. Hardness versus case depth for different scan velocities.

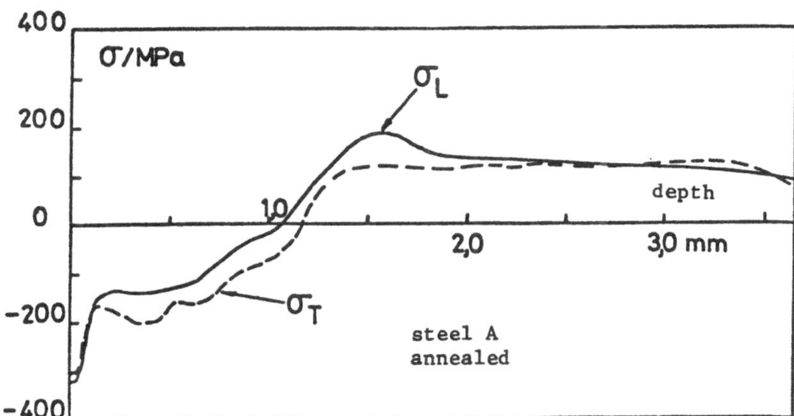

FIGURE 6. Residual stress distribution in annealed steel A treated with 2 kW at 1 cm/s.

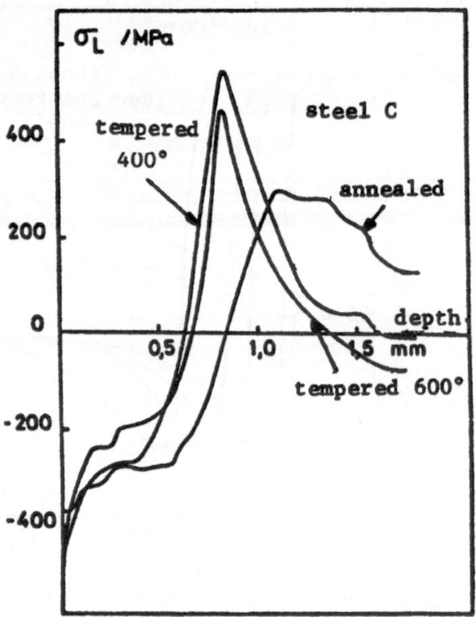

FIGURE 7. Residual stress distribution for different microstructures of steel C.

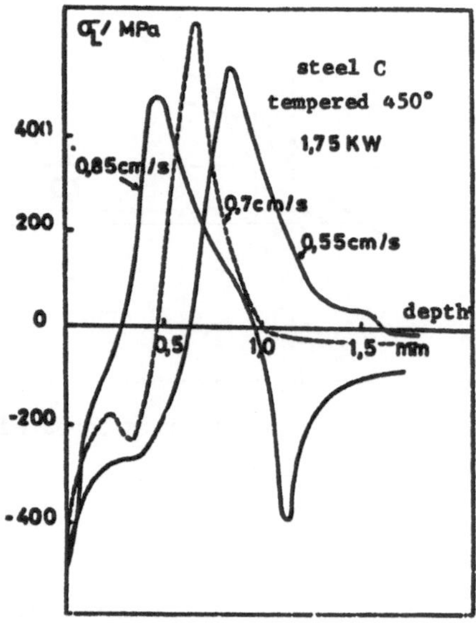

FIGURE 8. Residual stress distribution for different scan velocities.

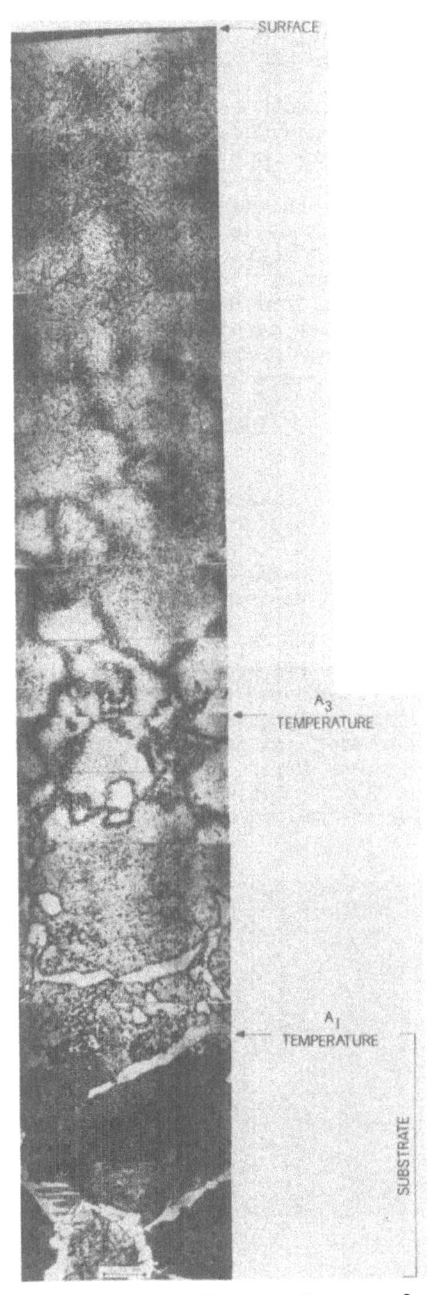

FIGURE 9. Micrograph of the treated zone in annealed steel A treated with 2 kW at 1 cm/s.

4. DISCUSSION

These results are in agreement with the microstructural observations. The optical microscopy of the treated zone in the annealed steel A (Figure 9) shows, from the substrate to surface, the following features:

- A classical annealed structure consisting of ferrite and pearlite.
- A zone of incomplete austenization: the temperature was just above A_1; martensite appeared in the pearlitic regions but individual ferrite grains remained.
- A "marbled" structure, in agreement with complete but heterogeneous austenization; dark martensite of low carbon content with a hardness of about 490 HV, which originated from ferritic regions, whereas pearlitic colonies produce light martensite of high carbon content and thus high hardness (780 HV). The time above the A_3 temperature was insufficient for much carbon to diffuse from the high carbon austenite to austenite formed from ferrite. The hardness values of these different martensites change with the depth according to the carbon diffusion. Near the surface, a greater homogeneity was achieved, the temperature being higher. Such structures have also been observed by different authors (2,3).

A similar morphology is observed in the annealed microalloy D (4,7) except for the smaller grain size and the presence of carbides remaining in the treated layer.

Quenched and tempered structures lead to more homogeneous structures. They present an additional heat-affected zone due to the laser treatment below the treated layer, where the temperature ranges from the initial tempering temperature to the A_1 temperature. This zone is characterized by a fall in hardness and high tensile residual stress values.

In the alloy steels, tempered martensite and carbides situated on the martensite boundaries are observed in the substrate (Figure 10a). In the treated zone, carbides remain. Dwell time and temperature are not large enough to dissolve them. Spheroidization occurs. This is the reason why the surface hardness is lower than that which could be expected for an alloy of this carbon content.

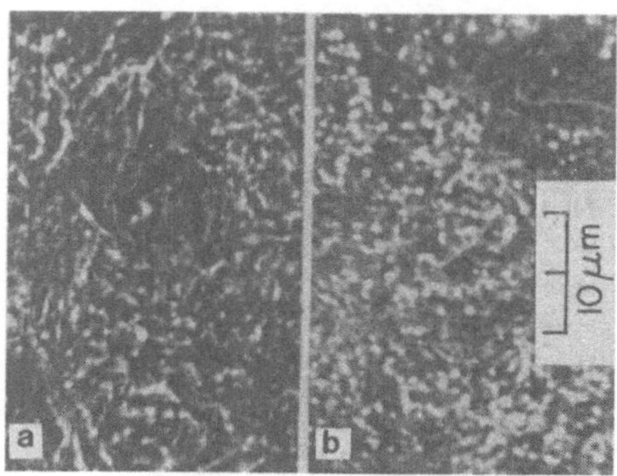

FIGURE 10. SEM micrographs of substrate and treated zone in steel C, quenched and tempered at 600°C.

All these heterogeneities are due to the high rate of heating. On one hand, the very high heating rate displaces the transformation temperatures to higher temperatures in comparison with conventional heat treatments. Time-temperature austenization curves proposed by Orlisch et al. (5) show a rise in austenizing temperature of about 100-150°C for heating rates ranging from 1000 to 2000°C/s. On the other hand, the time spent above the A_3 temperature is very short, which limits carbon diffusion and dissolution of carbides and hence leads to heterogeneous structures (Figure 11).

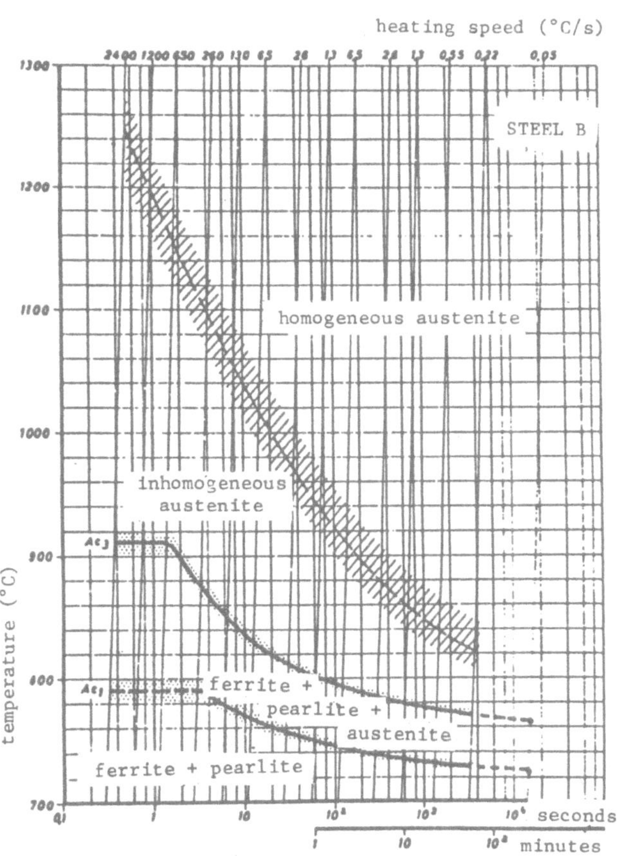

FIGURE 11. Time-temperature-austenization curve of steel B.

In this work the residual stresses depend essentially on microstructural transformations rather than thermal effects.

The stress fields show a point of inflection in the first few tenths of a millimeter depth. It indicates a discontinuity in the development of stresses. Consequently, the field can be divided into several blocks: block No. 1 the first few tenths of a millimeter, block No. 2 the remainder of the treated zone, block No. 3 the tension zone, block No. 4 the substrate. This last block can be neglected because of the very low stress value. Block No. 1 corresponds to a very acicular martensite structure, block No. 2 consists of a bainitic martensite, and block No. 3 is either a ferrite + pearlite zone or a tempered region, depending on the initial microstructure. The stresses arise in order to accommodate the strains resulting from the volume changes on transformation. They are, consequently, compressive near the surface, also compressive in the rest of the treated zone, but less pronounced and tensile in the underlying layer. This was the case in all the specimens studied.

4.1. Surface produced by a multi-pass laser treatment

The passes were made without cooling between each pass. The material becomes preheated by the previous pass and the treated zone becomes wider and thicker for the final passes.

The centerline of each pass shows hardness profiles versus case depth analogous to those for single-pass specimens (Figure 12). Nevertheless, the profile under the surface at 0.2 mm depth (Figure 13) demonstrates the pronounced heterogeneity of the treated layer in agreement with microstructural evidence, i.e.,

- In the pass: a heterogeneous structure similar to the one described for a single-pass specimen and characterized by a wide scatter in hardness.

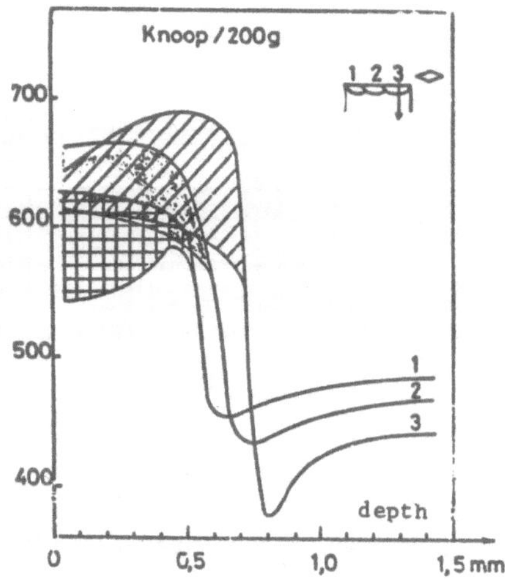

FIGURE 12. Hardness versus case depth in the 3 passes of a quenched and tempered 450°C steel C.

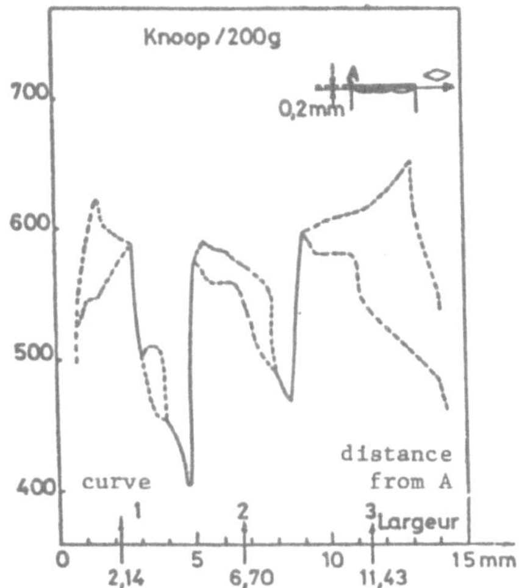

FIGURE 13. Hardness below the surface along the width of the multipass sample of Fig. 11.

- In the overlapping zone: the preheating due to the previous pass results in higher temperatures; it enables better dissolution of carbides and thus a higher degree of hardenability, and hence higher hardness values.
- The sharp drop in hardness is explained by a tempering due to a pass on a previously hardened zone.

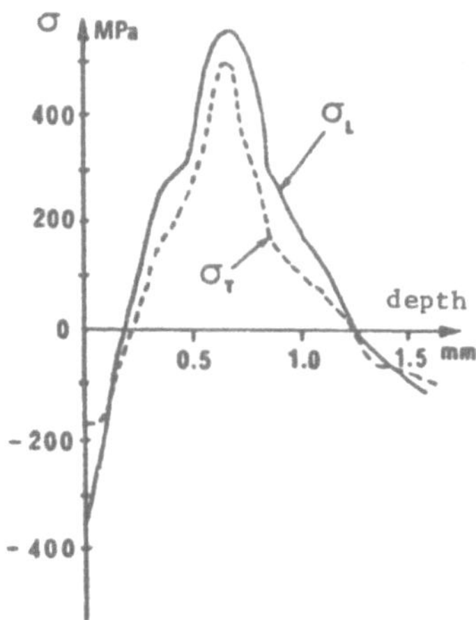

FIGURE 14. Residual stress distribution of the multipass sample of Figures 11 and 12.

The Leluan method used give profiles and maximum values of residual stress fields similar to those obtained for single-pass samples (Figure 14). This method, however, only determines the average of stress value in the machined layer. Residual stress X-ray diffraction experiments (6) carried out at ETCA confirmed the surface heterogeneities as revealed by hardness measurements. The bead is on the average in compression, but the tempered zones in tension, whereas the residual stress becomes zero in the ovelapping zone.

These results show the negative consequences of this method of treatment. Heterogeneities characterized by a softening (7) and tensile stresses due to tempering of the surface can be produced.

5. CONCLUSIONS

Based on the experimental results, it is possible to make some observations on laser transformation hardening without melting of hypoeutectoid steels:

(1) Microstructures observed in the treated zone are martensitic, characteristic of classical hardening but with some peculiarities:

(a) Martensite is heterogeneous as a result of the non-uniform austenite. This heterogeneity is related:
- directly to the initial structure
- to the transformation curves which are displaced to higher temperatures.

(b) It is impossible to dissolve all the carbides with a treatment not involving melting. Incomplete dissolution changes the carbon content in the matrix locally and, therefore, its hardenability. Nevertheless, undissolved carbides can be considered as hard inclusions which are favorable in wear applications.

(2) The analysis of residual stress fields confirms microstructural observations. Their shape changes with the material and treatment conditions, but they correlate with microstructural transformations.

Compressive stresses, always observed in the treated layer, improve the mechanical behavior. Tensile stresses which appear below the treated zone are not pronounced in annealed structures which are otherwise very heterogeneous. Quenched and tempered materials, however, are more homogeneous and the tensile stresses much more pronounced and potentially dangerous due to the fact that they facilitate crack initiation.

Based on the microstructural and residual stress observations, laser transformation hardening leads to better results in a plain medium carbon steel than in an alloy steel. Multi-pass laser treatment shows softening and tensile stresses at the surface; both should be avoided in practice.

The experimental results demonstrate the fact that the quality of treatment is determined by a number of parameters which include:

- energy profile of the beam,
- lower density arriving at the specimen,
- absorption coefficient of material and absorbing coating,
- stability of these parameters during treatment,
- thermal properties of material and their change with temperature,
- transformation temperatures during heating of the steel characterized by its composition and microstructure.

A knowledge of these parameters is useful in a study of thermal cycling and determination of the treated depth. This appears to be the most important parameter in transformation hardening from the point of view of microstructure and residual stresses. Residual sresses and, in particular, the maximum value of the tensile stresses must be taken into account because of their importance in the operational behavior of a component. Methods of prediction must be developed (8).

CLADDING

Studies* (9) were also carried out on residual stresses produced during laser cladding. The main difference, compared with the transformation hardening case, is that the material is no longer isotropic because the elastic constants of the cladding material are necessarily different from those of substrate.

A model has been developed to calculate the stresses. It takes into account specific conditions of the material, i.e., the cladding of well-defined thickness, with an elastic modulus E_c and a Poisson ratio μ_c, and for the substrate E_s and μ_s.

The residual stresses were also determined using the Leluan method with electrochemical machining adapted for the cladding material.

Cladding of Co-base powder and another of Ni-base powder was produced on a martensitic steel with a CO_2 laser with powers 4 to 5 kW. The powder was injected into the laser beam and the cladding was produced with three passes, each about 5 mm wide.

In all cases, the experimental results (Figures 15 and 17) show tensile stresses in the cladding and compressive stresses in a substrate. An intermediate zone characterized by a tensile peak is also observed. This is confirmed by hardness measurements (Figures 16 and 18) in the intermediate zone. At the present time, the interpretation of this peak is not complete.

ACKNOWLEDGMENTS

The authors thank Mr. Cantarel, Mr. Coquerelle and Mr. Gerbet of ETCA, Mr. Pizzi and Mr. Antona of Fiat, Mr. Dumas and Mr. Com-Nogue of CGE for their collaboration in this work.

---

* This study was carried out with the collaboration of Laboratoires de Marcoussis and the Fiat Research Center.

REFERENCES

1. A. Leluan, Revue du Gami, Mecanique, Juin Juillet (1969), p. 19-24.
2. A. Mulot and J. P. Badeau, Traitement Thermique, Revue de Metallurgie 136, 47-67 (1979).
3. M. F. Ashby and K. E. Easterling, Acta Metallurgica 32, 1935-1948 (1984).
4. C. Chabrol, These de Docteur Ingenieur, Lyon, Juin 1985.
5. J. Orlisch, A. Rose, and P. Weist, Atlas zur Wärme - behandlung der Stähle, (Düsseldorf, 1973), Vol. 3.
6. G. Maeder, J. L. Lebrun, and J. M. Sprauel, Materiaux et Techniques, Avril-Mai (1981), pp. 135-149.
7. E. Navara, B. Bengtsson, W. B. Li, and K. E. Easterling, Third Inernational Congress on Heat Treatment of Materials, Shanghai, China, Nov. 7-11, 1983, p. 240-244.
8. A. Solina, M. de Sanctis, L. Paganini, A. Blarasin, and S. Quaranta, J. Heat Treating 3, 193-204 (1984).
9. J. Hernandez and A. B. Vannes, to be published.

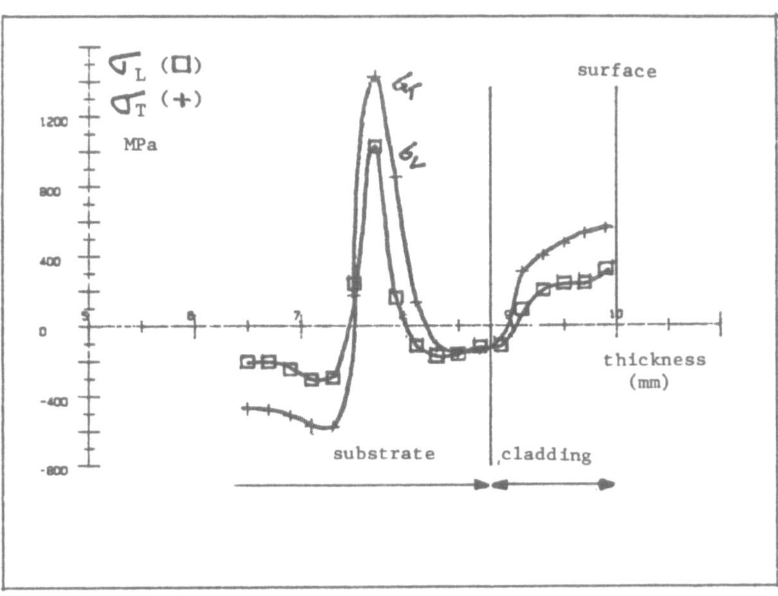

FIGURE 15. Residual stress field of Grade F stellite powder cladding.

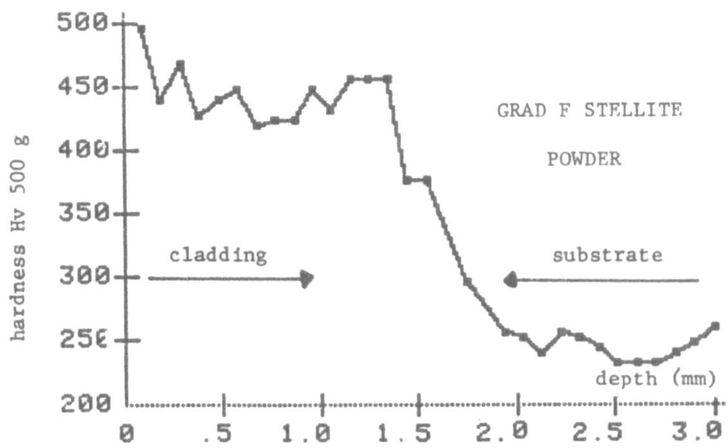

FIGURE 16. Hardness profile associated to the cladding of Figure 15.

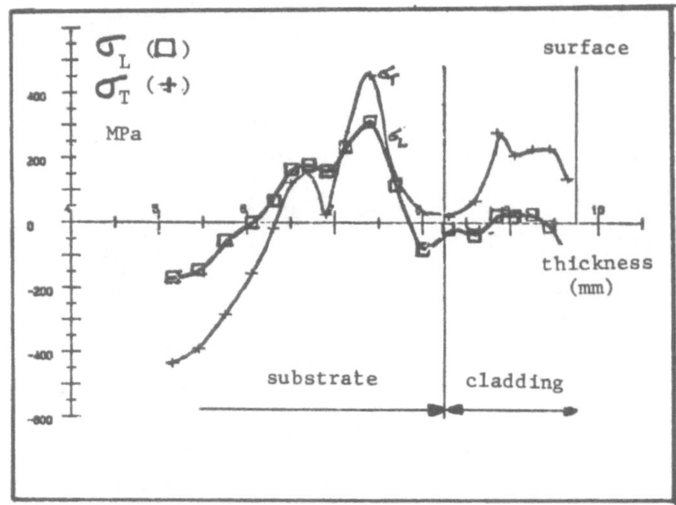

FIGURE 17. Residual stress field of nickel powder cladding.

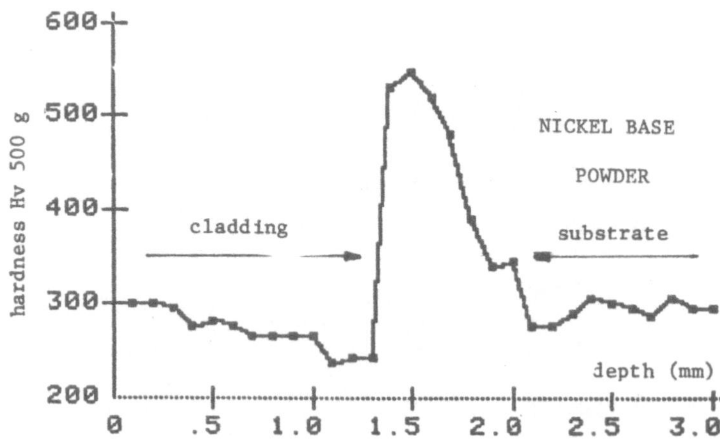

FIGURE 18. Hardness profile associated to the cladding of Figure 17.

LASER SURFACE MELTING AND ALLOYING OF TITANIUM

J. Folkes, D. R. F. West, and W. M. Steen
Imperial College, London, UK

Key Words: melting, alloying, titanium, nitriding, carburizing

1. INTRODUCTION

In recent years there has been rapid development in the use of lasers for the surface treatment of metals (1-3). Titanium is particularly susceptible to oxidation during this process, but it can be treated successfully under normal laboratory conditions providing that a good shrouding system is used. The result is that a flat, relatively smooth surface profile can be obtained. The depth of melting can be controlled by varying the laser parameters. Surface alloying may also be successfully achieved by using either preplaced powders, such as carbon, or electroplated layers, such as nickel, or by introducing an alloying gas into the shrouding system, such as nitrogen (4). A combination of these processes may also be used, as in the case of carbonitriding. The resultant alloyed zone modifies the surface characteristics of the substrate. Nickel affects the electrochemical properties, nitrogen affects the hardness and, consequently, the wear properties of the metal. Nitriding is discussed in detail here and an indication of the structure of the melt zone is given.

2. EXPERIMENTAL PROCEDURE

Surface melting and alloying were carried out using a 1 kW cw CO_2 laser (Control Laser Ltd.), operated in the range 1-1.8 kW. The alloys studied were C.P. Ti, IMI 205:Ti-15Mo, IMI 318:Ti-6Al-4V, and "10-2-3":Ti-3Al-2Fe-10V. Samples of thickness $\approx$7 mm with a machined finish were traversed relative to the laser beam at speeds (V) from 2 to 400 mm/sec and beam diameters (d) from 0.4 to 3.0 mm. The effective shrouding involved a central argon jet and an outer general flow of argon (5). Structural studies included electron microscopy (TEM) of thin foil prepared parallel to the laser-melted surface.

3. RESULTS AND DISCUSSION

3.1. Surface melting

Figure 1 shows a typical keyhole melt zone. Plasma effects improve the coupling efficiency of the beam, giving an increased penetration. This increase occurs at traverse speeds below $\approx$120 mm/sec for a focused beam (Fig. 2), where the incident power density on the surface is on the order of 1.2 mW cm^{-2}. For wider beams conduction-limited-type zones form with a flat surface profile and less pronounced surface rippling (Fig. 3). The crystal growth mechanism is best revealed in the retained β alloys (Ti-15Mo and Ti-10-2-3).

3.2. Ti-15Mo

The crystal growth is epitaxial from the β grains in the substrate, in a direction approximately normal to the zone interface (Fig. 3(b)).

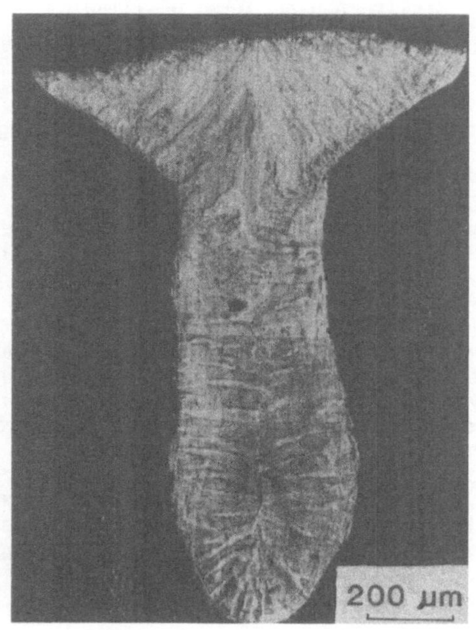

FIGURE 1. IMI 550. Keyhole melt zone showing columnar crystal growth.

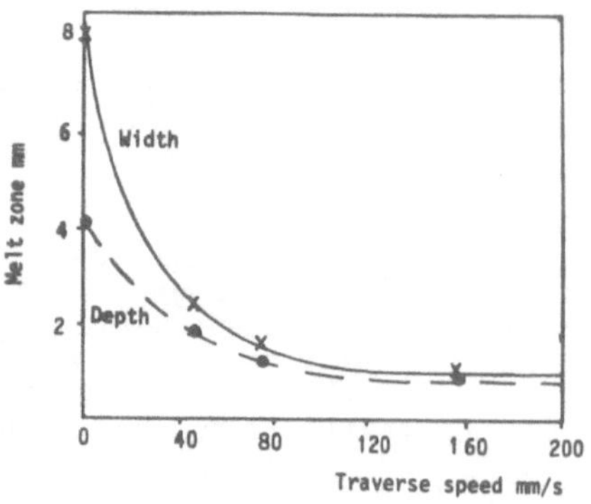

FIGURE 2. IMI 318. Depth and width of melt zone vs. traverse speed 1.6 kW, d, 0.4 mm.

A featureless region at the melt interface was interpreted as plane front growth resulting from the very high ratio of temperature gradient to solidification rate (6). The bulk of the zone showed cellular/dendritic

FIGURE 3. (a) Ti-15Mo. Transverse section of laser melt zone.

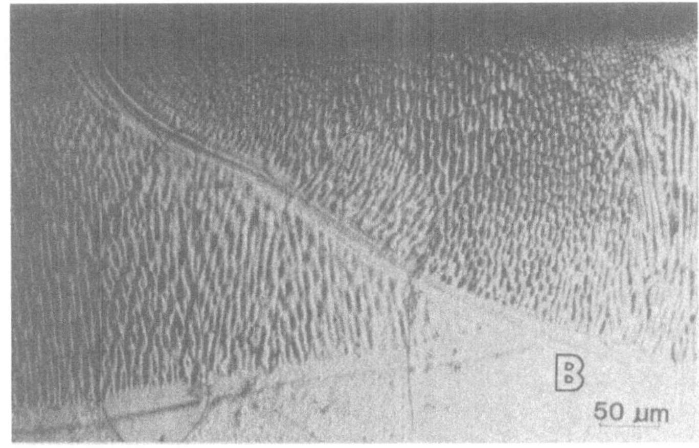

FIGURE 3. (b) Transverse section showing partially overlapping melt zones.

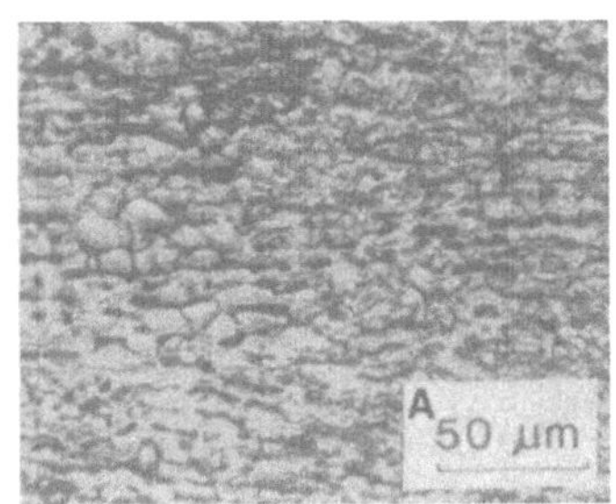

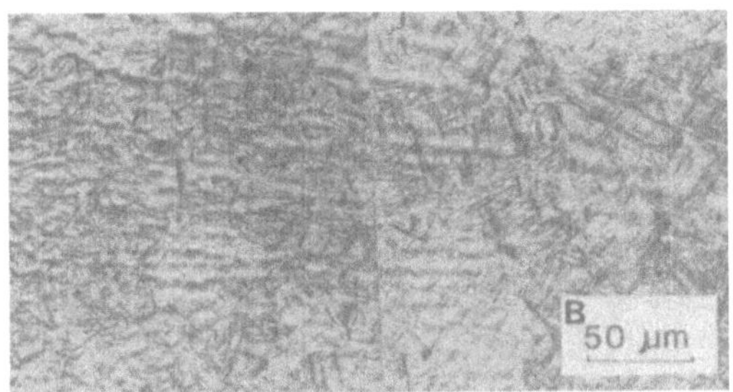

FIGURE 4. (a) IMI 318 region of HAZ adjoining substrate, (b) IMI 318 region of HAZ adjoining melt zone.

growth with no clear secondary arm spacing as shown in Fig. 4. The intercell spacing ranged from ≈0.5 to 5 μm for the conditions studied, decreasing with increasing cooling rate. Thin foil compositional analysis of a Ti-15Mo processed sample (with intercell spacing ≈0.5 μm) showed Mo values varying from 18-11.5 wt%. 18 wt% is attributed to the cell centers, in reasonable agreement with previous work on more slowly solidified materials (7).

3.3 Ti-6Al-4V

In C.P. titanium and in the near α and α+β alloys, the β martensite transformation, on cooling rapidly in the solid state, obscures the IMI cellular structure, except in IMI 550 where it may be revealed by deep etching. TEM of the melt zone showed a martensitic structure as shown in Fig. 5. Plates of a twinned substructure were common, suggesting the presence of some orthorhombic α". The plates were finer than in conventionally quenched material. Selected area diffraction evidence was consistent with the martensite, having formed with the normal Burgers relationship to β. In the substrate adjacent to the melt zones, there is a region in which a rapid heating rate ($\approx 10^4$K/s) occurs. The temperature is raised between α+β/β transus and the solidus. In Ti-6Al-4V the original α regions appeared to become martensitic as the distance from the unaffected substrate increased (Fig. 4(a,b)). This change is interpreted as involving rapid transformation of α to β followed by martensite formation on cooling. In this region the calculated time of heating in the β range is too short to allow significant diffusion to occur between the "reverted" α regions (solute-poor) and the original β regions (solute-rich). As the melt zone temperature is approached, the temperature reaches values where diffusion produces β of relatively uniform composition and the martensite then forms on cooling. Thin foils taken from this area confirmed the presence of β grains with α' plates extending into them (Fig. 6(a)). In some foils taken higher up in the HAZ, this region is nearly completely martensitic. The area adjacent to the β grain was also martensitic and highly twinned (Fig. 6(b)).

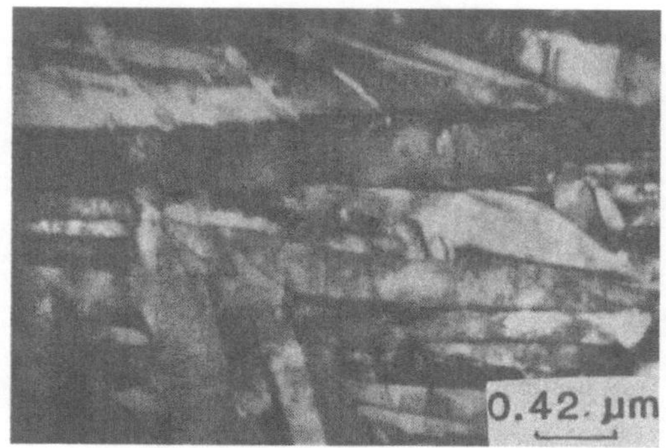

FIGURE 5. IMI 318 martensitic structures of melt zones TEM

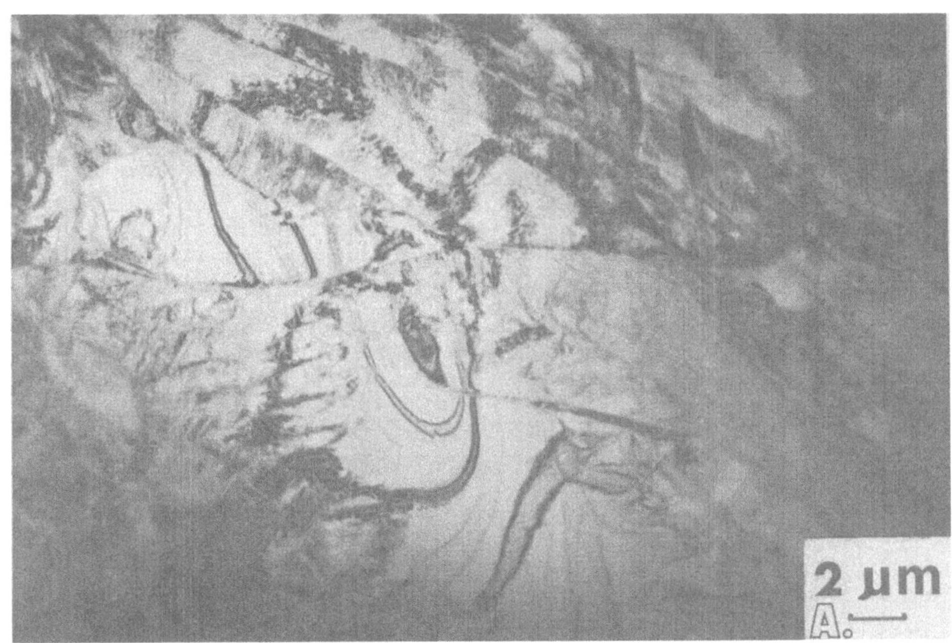

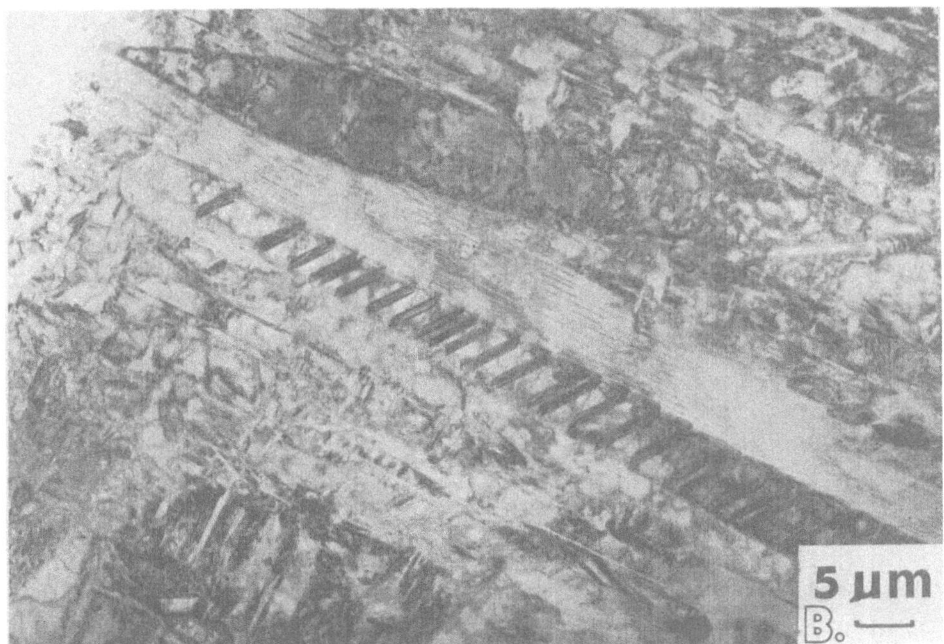

FIGURE 6. (a) IMI 318 original β regions (solute-rich) and "reverted" α' regions (solute-poor) of HAZ (b).

3.4. 10-2-3

Ti-10V-2Fe-3Al is a high-strength near β forging alloy which, when surface melted, forms a martensitic melt zone in high-speed runs (100 mm/sec), with some α particles remaining stable within the melt zone itself (Fig. 7). For slower tracks partitioning within the melt is observed, becoming coarser towards the top of the melt zone. It also becomes coarser at slower speeds. Less α particles are seen within the melt zones. The presence of these particles is accounted for by their small size and high content of α stabilizers. The treating time is too rapid for all the particles to melt, and so on cooling they remain "stable" within the melt zone. At faster speeds the interaction time is shortened so more particles are present. The α particles have, however, transformed to martensite (Fig. 8(b)), compared to the initial α+β base structure (Fig. 8(a)), as a result of the rapid cooling from above the β transus.

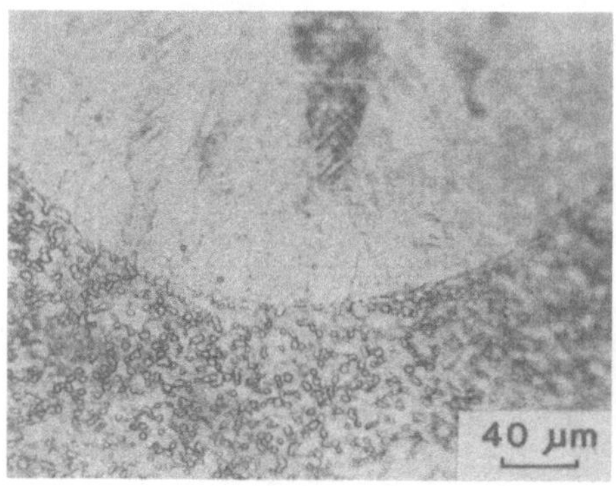

FIGURE 7. Ti-10-2-3. Transverse section of laser melt zone.

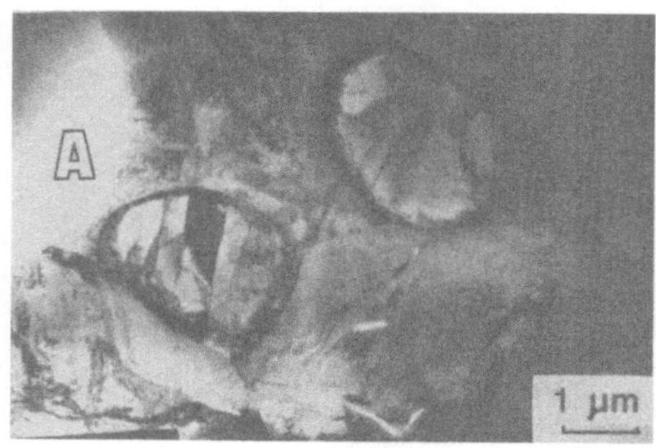

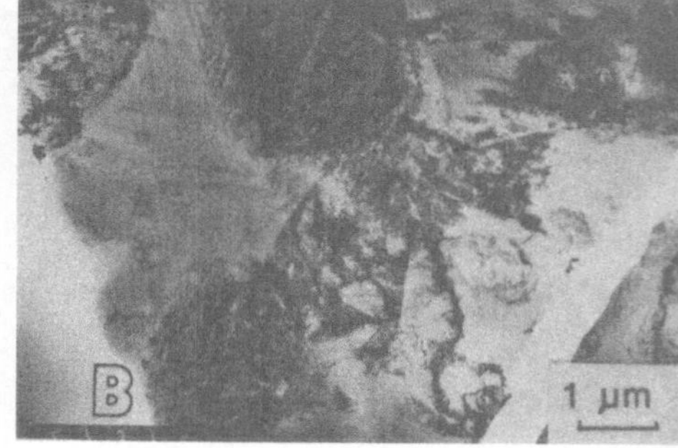

FIGURE 8. (a) Ti-10-2-3 α+β structure of substrate TEM,
(b) Ti-10-2-3 α'+β structure of melt zone.

4. SURFACE ALLOYING

Surface hardening techniques include laser alloying and cladding. An important approach to improve the wear resistance of titanium alloys has been to laser surface melt in nitrogen or air to form a layer of TiN. (Katamaya et al. (8,9)). Improvement in corrosion resistance to some acids was also obtained. Here the effects were studied of laser melting in gaseous nitrogen using the double-cone gas shroud.

4.1. Titanium Nitride

Nitriding was done on C.P. Ti and Ti-15Mo alloy using various flow rates of nitrogen (110-250 cm^3/sec), a power of 1.7 kW, d = 1.5 mm and V = 25 or 50 mm/sec. Single-track regions resulted in a zone as shown in Fig. 9(a,b,c). The light etching dendritic zone ($\approx$580 HV), extending from the surface downwards, were deduced to be dendrites of TiN formed as a result of the decreasing nitrogen content with increasing distance below the surface. For nitrogen contents of $\approx$15 at% in the liquid, TiN can nucleate at the surface and this decreases the liquidus leading to constitutional supercooling and dendritic growth. The nitrogen distribution is influenced by the mixing effects derived from surface tension forces and from the impingement of the nitrogen jet on the surface. The liquid remaining between the TiN dendrites will solidify by the advancement of the main solidification front from the base of the melt zone. The presence of TiN dendrites in the lower regions of some melt zones is attributed to high nitrogen levels attained from convective effects. The remainder of the zone is either α or α' in C.P. Ti ($\approx$420 HV) or cellular/dendritic β in Ti-15Mo ($\approx$420 HV). Repeated nitriding of such zones results in a fully dendritic structure after three passes at V = 25 mm/sec and five at V = 50 mm/sec. Some cracking was observed. At focused beam similar effects are observed. With partially overlapping tracks a progressive increase in nitrogen was observed, with overlap, by increased amounts of TiN. These zones were analyzed by X-ray diffraction. A lattice parameter of 0.4223 nm was obtained for the nitride with both C.P. Ti and Ti-15Mo substrates. The X-ray spectra of the alloyed C.P. substrate showed the presence of some "split" peaks deduced to be from the C.P. titanium in the form of an orthorhombic martensite. The martensite would have formed by nitrogen enrichment of the C.P. Ti which on rapid cooling reverts to martensite. The Ti-15Mo lattice parameter remained unchanged on nitriding. High microhardness values were measured on the top surfaces of the tracks $\approx$1000 HV and wear tests (10) indicated encouraging wear properties.

4.2. Carbonitriding

The laser has the potential to alloy carbon in the form of graphite dag and nitrogen, by the gas shroud at the same time. The zones obtained are similar to those of the nitride and have high hardness. The use of such zones is for wear resistance and again its potential is being evaluated.

5. SUMMARY AND CONCLUSIONS

Laser surface melting of titanium alloys can produce conduction limited crack-free melt zones of smooth surface profile and depths of up to $\approx$0.3 mm. The mechanism of solidification was predominately cellular dendritic and in the near α and α+β alloys, the melt zones were martensitic with a fine plate size. In the HAZ reversion of α or α' to β occurred followed by α' formation on cooling. Laser melting in nitrogen

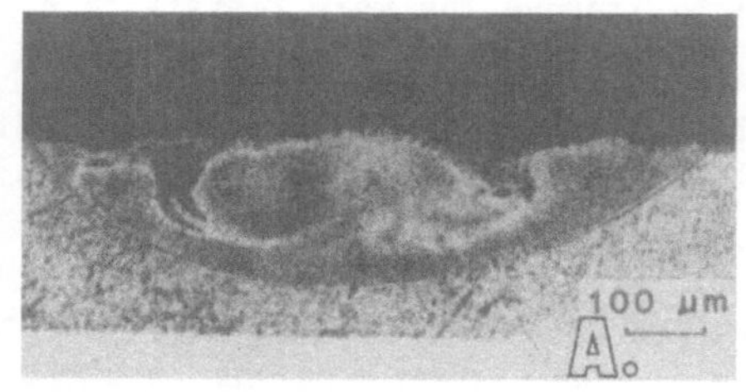

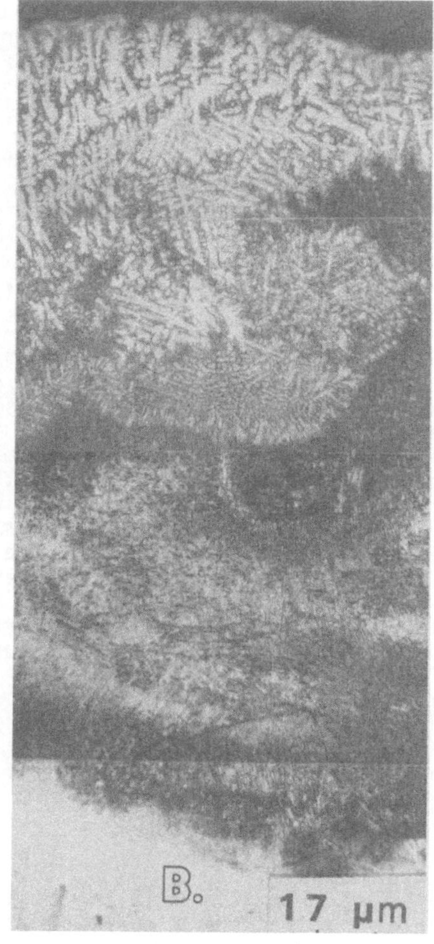

FIGURE 9. N_2 alloyed material; single pass, (a) Ti-15-Mo substrate, (b) C.P. Ti substrate, TiN dendrites at top surface.

forms TiN in the surface layers with hardness levels of ≈1000 HV. Laser melting in nitrogen with a carbon surface layer produces predominately dendritic melt tracks with surface layer hardness ≈1500 HV.

ACKNOWLEDGMENTS

Acknowledgments are made to the S.E.R.C. and Rolls Royce, Barnoldswich, for support and to Dr. H. M. Flower.

REFERENCES

1. R. A. Bayles et al., "Applications of Lasers in Materials Processing," ASM, 127 (1979).
2. P. Moore et al., "Application of Lasers in Materials Processing," ASM, 259 (1979).
3. C. W. Draper, "Lasers in Metallurgy," Conf. Proc. Met. Soc. AIME, 67 (1981).
4. Walker et al., Surface Engineering, 1, 23 (1985).
5. H. C. Man, Ph.D. Thesis, University of London (1985).
6. B. H. Kear, E. M. Breinan, and L. E. Greenwald, Met. Tech. 6, 121 (1979).
7. J. I. Nurminem and H. D. Brody, "Ti Science and Technology," 1893 (1973).
8. S. Katayama et al., Proc. 3rd Int. Conf. on "Welding and Melting by Electron and Laser Beams," Lyons (1983).
9. S. Katayama et al., ICALEO 1983, LIA, Los Angeles, (Nov. 1983).
10. Rolls Royce Aerospace, private communication.

LASER SURFACE ALLOYING OF STAINLESS STEEL WITH CARBON

C. MARSDEN, D. R. F. WEST, AND W. M. STEEN
Imperial College, London, UK

Key Words: alloying, stainless steel, carburizing

1. INTRODUCTION

In recent years considerable interest has developed in the surface alloying of materials using lasers to modify and improve their surface properties. The recent review by Draper (1985) (1) includes reference to work with pulsed solid-state lasers and with multi-kilowatt, continuous-wave (cw) lasers. Using the latter, much work is reported on alloying ferrous-based materials with Cr, Ni and Mo, often to high concentrations.

The reason for the intense interest in this area of research is because transition metal additions account for roughly one third of the cost of highly alloyed steels, and surface alloying could reduce that consumption by 90-99%, leading to considerable savings.

Relatively little work has been carried out in the area of introducing carbon into the surface layers of ferrous substrates to increase their hardness.

Walker (2,3) has reported surface-alloyed regions containing up to 6 wt% C on pure iron substrates using dag graphite coatings. Mordike et al. (1983) (4) alloyed C10 (0.010 wt%) and ST22 (low carbon steel with U.T.S. 220 N/mm^2) steels with carbon by melting in atmospheres of CO_2 or acetylene. All compositions up to the formation of Fe_3C were achieved.

The study reported here forms part of a detailed program on carbon alloying of a steel using graphite coatings and powder injection. The substrate was a 420 stainless steel (~ 13 wt% Cr - 0.2 wt% C).

This type of steel finds applications in the power-generating industry, e.g., in turbine applications. This investigation aimed to obtain basic information on structural changes and surface hardening with a view to the improvement of erosion resistance.

2. EXPERIMENTAL PROCEDURE

Specimens of 420 stainless steel were in the form of flat discs 10 mm thick and 30 mm in diameter, the surfaces of which were grit-blasted to give a uniform surface finish.

Laser treatments were carried out using a Control Laser 2 kW CO_2 machine typically operated between 1.0 and 1.6 kW.

The first set of specimens were treated in an inert atmosphere to produce laser-melted tracks. These were produced at speeds between 10 and 20 mms^{-1} under a beam of 2.0 mm diameter and powers between 1.0 and 1.6 kW.

The second set of specimens were alloyed by injection of a fine carbon powder (50-75 μm particles) through a 3.2 mm tube directly into the melt pool. A beam diameter of 3.0 mm was employed and specimens were processed at speeds and powers between 10 and 80 mms^{-1} and 1.0 and 1.6 kW, respectively.

The third set of specimens were alloyed by means of a carbon coating to observe three effects:

(1) Effect of varying traverse speed with constant beam diameter and power,
(2) Effect of varying coating thickness for a constant beam diameter and power at varying speeds,
(3) Effect of re-laser alloying the same track at a constant beam power and diameter and traverse speed up to a maximum of 16 times.

For (1) a series of runs were carried out using a 1.6 kW, 2.0 mm beam with traverse rates varying from 10 mms^{-1} to 400 mms^{-1}.

For (2) a series of specimens were prepared whereby the thickness of coatings varied in the ratio 1:2:3:4. These specimens were then processed at the same time under a 1.6 kW, 2.0 mm beam at traverse rates from 10 mms^{-1} to 100 mms^{-1}.

For (3) a series of runs were carried out under a 1.6 kW, 2.0 mm beam at 10 mms^{-1}. Alloyed tracks were produced; the carbon was then re-applied and the area re-treated. In this way, a series of tracks was produced that had been treated between 1 and 16 times.

Microstructural observations and microhardness measurements (100 g load) were made on traverse sections of the laser-treated zones. Cryogenic treatments were given to some of the laser-treated specimens.

3. RESULTS

3.1. Melted tracks

Figure 1 shows one of a number of unalloyed laser-melted tracks. The etched structure consisted of light cells separated by a thin film of dark material. Typical cell spacings were of the order of 3-4 μm for traverse speeds 10-20 mms^{-1}, indicating cooling rates of between $0.7\text{-}1.5 \times 10^3$ Ks^{-1} from the liquid state, after Brower et al. (1970) (5).

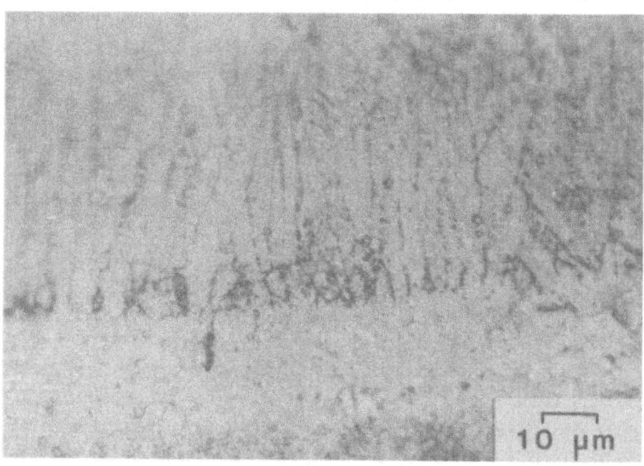

FIGURE 1. Transverse section of unalloyed melt track. Power 1.4 kW, speed 20 mms^{-1}, diameter 2.0 mm.

The laser-melted tracks have a typical hardness of ≈600 HV. Light microscope observations of etched specimens did not reveal a martensitic structure although this is expected from previous work by Lamb (1985) (6). Further work, e.g., transmission electron microscopy, will be carried out. There is a heat-affected zone below the melted region. Between this HAZ and the melted region exists a zone ≈25-50 μm thick from which epitaxial growth of cells occurs.

3.2. Alloyed tracks by injection of carbon powder

Figure 2 shows a typical structure of a laser melt track alloyed by carbon powder injection.

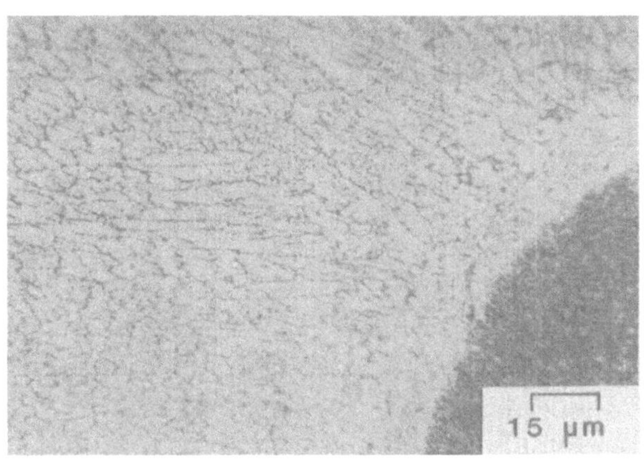

FIGURE 2. Transverse Section of melt track alloyed by carbon powder injection. Power 1.6 kW, speed 15 mms^{-1}, beam diameter 3.0 mm.

Cell spacings of ≈3-5 μm were observed for tracks produced under beams of 1.0 to 1.6 kW at traverse speeds between 10 and 80 mms^{-1}, indicating cooling rates ranging from $0.4\text{-}1.5 \times 10^3$ Ks^{-1}.

The structures of the laser-alloyed tracks and their hardnesses were very similar to those produced by laser melting.

The zone between the melted zone and HAZ was similar to that produced in laser melting and varied in thickness from ≈20 to 160 μm.

Figure 3 shows the variation of depth of the melted zone with speed and laser power. It can be seen that the depth of melted zone varies proportionally with laser power and inversely with speed.

3.3. Alloyed tracks by single-cycle treatments

Figure 4 shows the depth of melt zone against traverse speed for single-cycle treatments using an identical beam of 1.6 kW power and 2.0 mm diameter, with a uniform thickness of carbon coating. Traverse speeds varied from between 10 and 400 mms^{-1}, but virtually no melting occurred at speeds in excess of 200 mms^{-1}.

The structures produced at the different speeds were very similar and hardness values for all tracks were ≈600 HV. The structures contained ≈80% of dendrites, interpreted as austenite, and the remaining

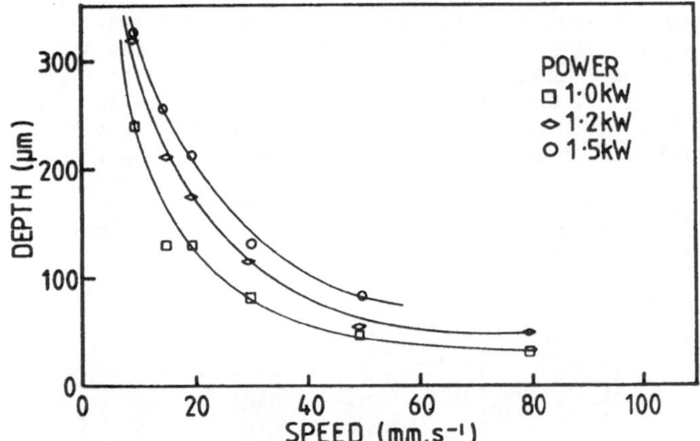

FIGURE 3. Depth v. speed for different beam powers during alloying by carbon powder injection. Beam diameter 3.0 mm.

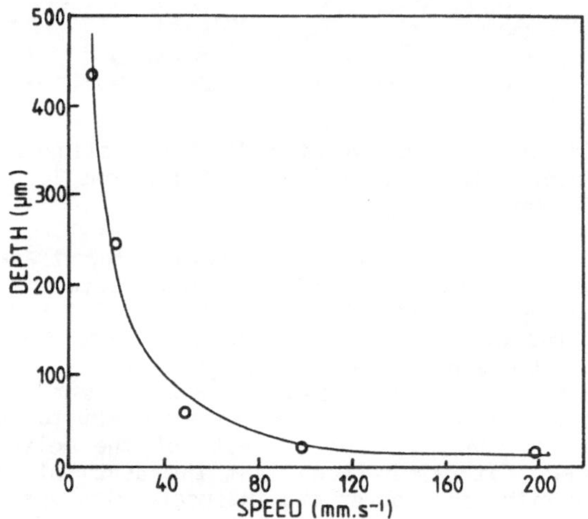

FIGURE 4. Depth v. speed for single alloying cycle treatments by carbon coating. Power 1.6 kW, beam diameter 2.0 mm.

interdendritic area was interpreted as carbide-containing. No lamellar eutectic structure was identified with either light or scanning electron microscopy, but the difficulties of etching the 13% Cr material should be borne in mind. The hardness values of approximately 600 HV were similar for all traverse speeds.

The secondary dendrite arm spacings (λ) were found to vary from $\approx 1.8\ \mu m$ (for the tracks produced at 10 mms^{-1}, indicating cooling rates of the order $5 \times 10^3\ Ks^{-1}$) to $\approx 0.6\ \mu m$ (for the 200 mms^{-1} tracks, indicating a cooling rate of $\approx 6 \times 10^4\ Ks^{-1}$).

The microstructures were not uniform throughout the melted zones. Light etching areas were observed, indicative of convective flow effects in the liquid state; Draper (1985) (1) has recently reviewed work on such flow effects. It is not yet known whether compositional as well as structural variations are present. Figure 5 shows a secondary electron image of such a region from a transverse section, and Figure 6 shows an optical image of such a region from a longitudinal section at 90° to the surface.

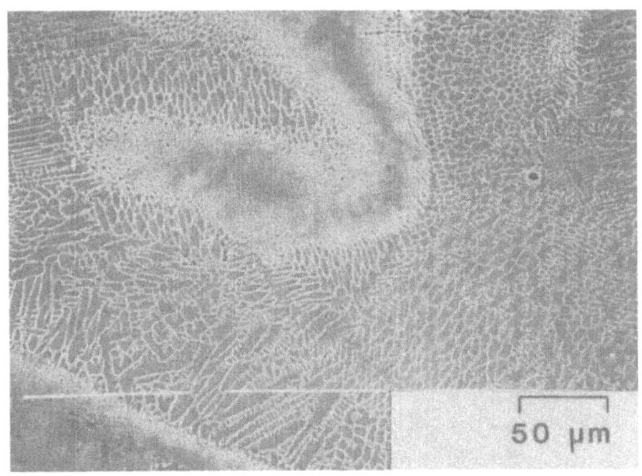

FIGURE 5. Secondary electron image of a transverse section of a melt track alloyed by carbon coating showing a light etching region, indicative of convective flow in the liquid state. Power 1.6 kW, speed 20 mms^{-1}, beam diameter 2.0 mm.

Two different areas between the HAZ and melted zone were observed, the first being similar to that already mentioned, indicating epitaxial growth from the substrate. The second feature involved a distinct region, interpreted as austenitic, suggestive of planar solidification, from which cells or dendrites developed epitaxially. Typical thicknesses of this austenitic "ring" were 3-8 μm. There was no obvious relationship between speed of traverse and the formation of this region, but its formation tended to be favored at the base of the melt tracks.

Figure 7 shows the depth vs. traverse speed for specimens treated under identical laser conditions, but with different carbon coating thicknesses. The mass per unit area of carbon varied from $1.6\text{-}10.2 \times 10^{-5}\ g\ mm^{-2}$ and the laser conditions were a beam of 2.0 mm diameter and 1.6 kW power. Traversing speeds varied between 10 and

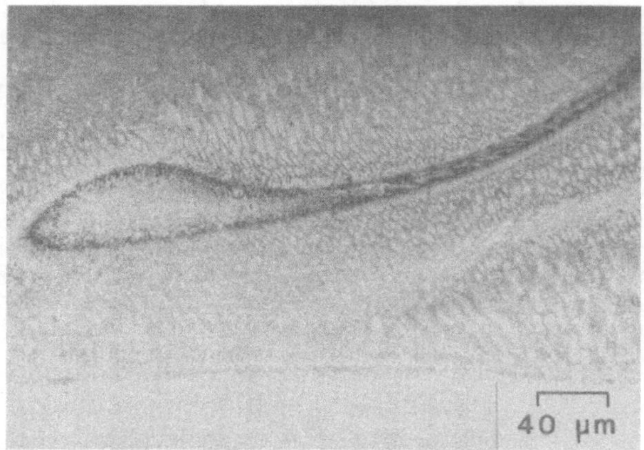

FIGURE 6. Longitudinal section of a track alloyed by carbon coating showing evidence of convective flow in the liquid state. Power 1.6 kW, speed 10 mms^{-1}, beam diameter 2.0 mm.

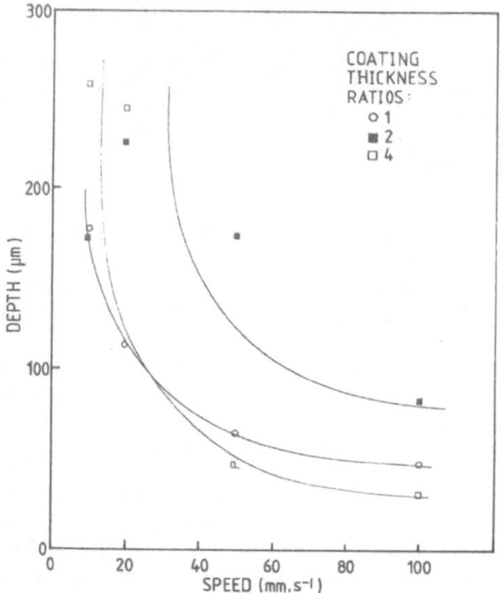

FIGURE 7. Depth v. speed for different coating thicknesses. Power 1.6 kW, beam diameter 2.0 mm.

100 mms^{-1}. Though there is considerable scatter, the graph follows the expected hyperbolic relationship. All the alloyed tracks displayed hypoeutectic structures, consisting of dendrites (austenitic) and interdendritic regions (assumed to contain carbides), Figure 8.

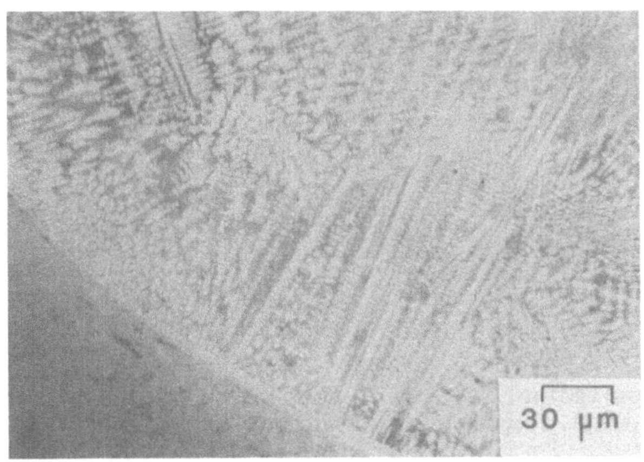

FIGURE 8. Transverse section of track alloyed by carbon coating, showing dendrites (austenite) and interdendritic regions (assumed to be carbides). Power 1.6 kW, speed 20 mms^{-1}, beam diameter 2.0 mm.

In the shallow edge regions of some tracks, a hypereutectic structure containing primary carbide particles was noted. The secondary dendrite arm spacings in the hypoeutectic samples varied from 1.6 to 0.85 μm, indicating cooling rates of about 7-30 x 10^3 Ks^{-1}, respectively. The secondary dendrite arm spacing did not vary detectably with depth in any of the tracks, though in some tracks there was more eutectic at the top than at the bottom, Figure 9. HAZs with planar and epitaxial features were observed. Figure 8 displays the former. Figure 10 is a longitudinal section at 90° to the surface, showing dendritic alignment and an HAZ with planar features.

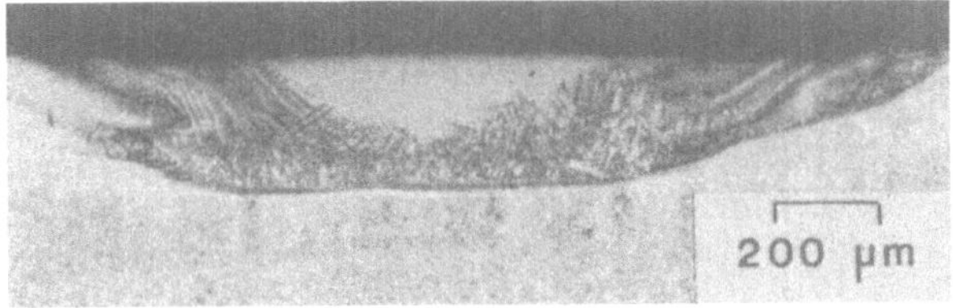

FIGURE 9. Transverse section of melt track alloyed by carbon coating, showing a greater proportion of eutectic at the top of the section than at the bottom. Power 1.6 kW, speed 10 mms^{-1}, beam diameter 2.0 mm.

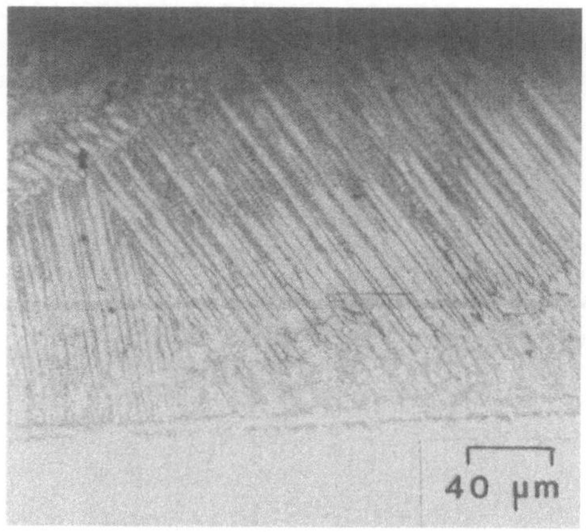

FIGURE 10. Longitudinal section of melt track alloyed by carbon coating, showing alignment of dendrites and an HAZ with planar features. Power 1.6 kW, speed 10 mms^{-1}, beam diameter 2.0 mm.

3.4. Alloyed tracks by multicycle treatments

The multicycle laser treatments produced structures ranging from hypoeutectic to hypereutectic. In the specimens treated between 1 and 2 cycles, the structures were similar to those reported above. As the number of cycles increased, the quantity of carbon alloyed increases, leading to the formation of a smaller proportion of austenite dendrites and a corresponding increase in the proportion of interdendritic material assumed to be eutectic. The structure produced after four cycles was predominantly eutectic. After seven or more cycles the structures were hypereutectic, Figure 11, and suffered from cracking and porosity, with the extent of porosity increasing with successive laser treatments above seven cycles.

Figure 12 shows average hardness of the melt zone against number of treatment cycles. The hardness increased as the carbon content of the treated zones increased.

Figure 13 shows the hardness as a function of depth below the melt surface for a selection of different numbers of cycles. The microhardness values show considerable scatter in the melt zone and no clear trend or variation with depth is detected.

HAZs with both the epitaxial and planar features are observed; the planar tended to be observed in those specimens treated with more than one cycle. The scatter of hardness values through the depth of a treated zone suggests a degree of heterogeneity. This can also be seen in the structures, due mainly to the melt pools created by successive laser cycles penetrating to different depths.

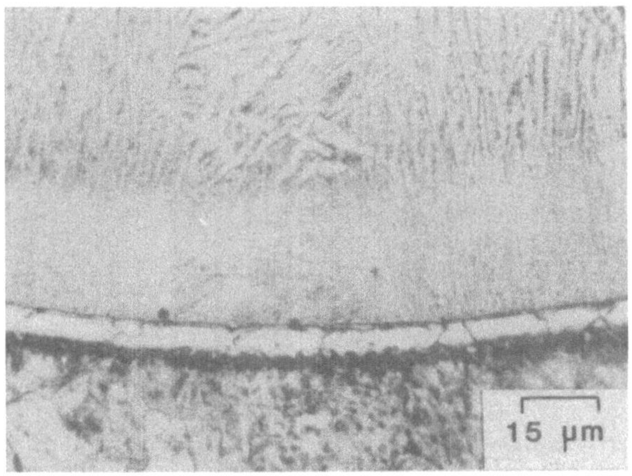

FIGURE 11. Transverse section of multi-cycle treatment melt track alloyed by carbon coating, showing a hypereutectic structure and an HAZ with planar features. Power 1.6 kW, speed 10 mms^{-1}, beam diameter 2.0 mm.

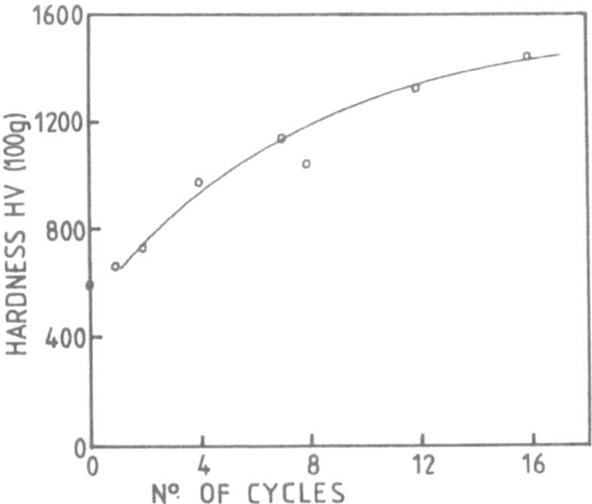

FIGURE 12. Average hardness v. number of treatment cycles. Power 1.6 kW, speed 10 mms^{-1}, beam diameter 2.0 mm.

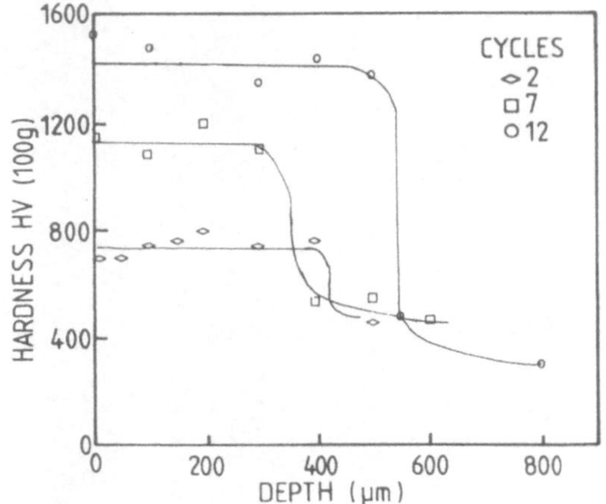

FIGURE 13. Hardness v. depth for different numbers of treatment cycles. Power 1.6 kW, speed 10 mms^{-1}, beam diameter 2.0 mm.

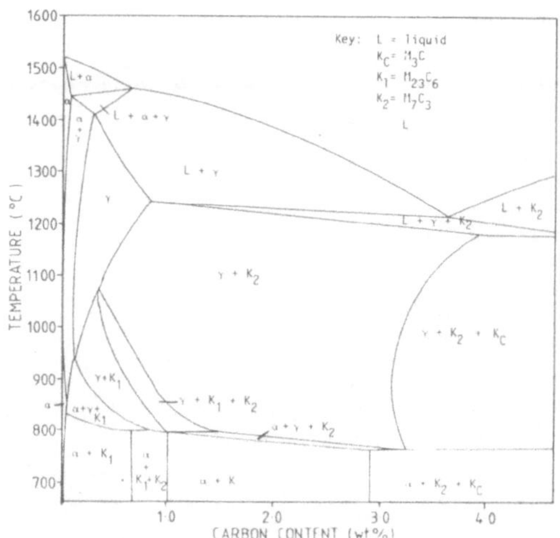

FIGURE 14. Section of the Fe-Cr-C phase diagram at 13.0 wt% Cr.

4. DISCUSSION

4.1. Solidification

Figure 14 shows a section of the Fe-Cr-C phase diagram at 13.0 wt% Cr after Bungardt (1958) (7). 420 stainless steel has a carbon content of ≈ 0.2 wt%. On solidification, the primary phase is α(b.c.c.); on cooling under equilibrium conditions in the solid state α transforms to γ (F.C.C.), and the final structure at room temperature would consist of $\alpha + M_{23}C_6$. When the solid-state cooling rate increases sufficiently, γ will transform to martensite.

Theoretically, if the cooling rate from the liquid state is sufficiently high, the possibility exists of preventing the solid-state formation of γ, and of the α being retained down to room temperature. As indicated in the results, the phase constituting the cells in the laser-melted alloys has not been firmly identified but is expected to be martensite (M. Lamb) (6). The observed dark regions between the cells indicate the occurrence of C and Cr segregation during cooling, leading to a small amount of eutectic formation; the eutectic may be in divorced form.

As the carbon content of the alloy is increased, a variety of phases form on solidification. The maximum solid solubility of carbon in γ is ≈ 0.8 wt% in equilibrium. For a carbon content of 1.0 wt% the phases expected to be present at the completion of solidification would be austenite dendrites and eutectic ($\gamma + M_7C_3$). Transformations subsequently occurring in the solid state would depend on the cooling rate, and retention of austenite can result at sufficiently high cooling rates due to the low Ms temperature. As the carbon content of the alloy progressively increases, the proportion of eutectic present on solidification would increase, until at ≈ 3.7 wt% C the solidification structure would be fully eutectic, which has so far remained unresolved by light microscopy and scanning electron microscopy. Beyond the eutectic composition primary carbides (M_7C_3) and eutectic would solidify, the carbide width being ≈ 3 μm.

The structures were similar to those produced by Walker et al. (1984) (3) in Fe-C alloys.

4.2. Solid-state transformation

The alloying additions to any steel have a profound effect in lowering of the martensite start (Ms) temperature. According to Pickering (1976) (8) the Ms temperature of a Fe-0.1 wt% C - 12 wt% Cr alloy is about 300°C and is depressed below this value for the base material according to the equation:

$$- [47.4(\text{wt\% C} - 0.1) + 17(\text{wt\% Cr} - 12)] = \Delta Ms$$

The above gives a Ms temperature of ≈ 240°C for the 420 base material (2 wt% C, 13 wt% Cr), a Ms of ≈ 0°C for a carbon content of 0.7 wt% and a Ms of ≈ -190°C for a carbon content of 1.1 wt%. Thus martensite formation will not occur when a hypoeutectic structure solidifies and cools rapidly to room temperature; austenite retention will occur.

Lamb (1985) (6) reported martensitic structures without alloying 420 base material on laser melting under certain conditions. Previous work by Bee and Wood (1982) (9) on rapid solidification of 12 wt% Cr steels by pendant drop melt extraction and melt spinning, producing cooling rates of between 10^5 and 10^6 Ks^{-1}, concluded that the as-quenched structures were similar to those produced by similar means. With increasing carbon content the constituent phases were martensite (0.14 wt% C), martensite and austenite (0.45 wt% C) and austenite and M_7C_3 (0.87 and 1.25 wt% C). The above results show that no martensite would be expected to form in 13% Cr alloys containing more than ≈0.8 wt% C on cooling to room temperature, agreeing with the results by Pickering (8) stated earlier.

Molian (1985) (10) has laser-alloyed a 0.2 wt% C steel with quantities of chromium up to ≈10 wt% Cr; he concluded, on the basis of TEM observations, that the microstructures were essentially dislocated lath martensite irrespective of composition (up to 10 wt% Cr) and cooling rate. Molian (1985) (11) has also estimated cooling rates in laser surface alloying processes as a function of depth of melt zone. The results of the present work do not correlate closely with those published by Molian (11), due most probably to different power densities being employed. Figures 3, 4 and 7 show the relationship between depth and speed for different power densities. The large degree of scatter shown in Figure 7 is thought to be due to a complicated plasma formation caused by a breakdown in shrouding.

4.3. Hardness

Walker et al. (1984) (2), on alloying pure iron with carbon, reported hardnesses of ≈470 HV on hypoeutectic structures cooled to room temperature or hardnesses of 650 HV on cooling to -196°C. This is attributed to the formation of martensite in the primary austenite, associated with an Ms temperature close to room temperature. Similar results have been reported by Christodoulou et al. (1983) (12) on alloying 1 C - 1.4 Cr steel with carbon. No significant increase in hardness from ≈600 HV was noted in the present work when hypoeutectic structures were cooled to -196°C from room temperature, suggesting no transformation of the austenite had occurred. This is consistent with the carbon content being greater than about 1.1 wt% when the Ms temperature is ≈-190°C. These hardnesses are possible due to fine cells and the presence of fine intercellular carbides.

Considering the hypereutectic compositions produced in the present work, the hardness increased with increasing carbon content from ≈800 HV to 1500 HV. Walker et al. (1984) (2) reported hardnesses of ≈900 HV for hypereutectic structures containing ≈50% primary carbides; this correlates approximately with hardnesses found in the present work in hypereutectic structures containing ≈50% primary carbides.

5. CONCLUSIONS

(1) The Laser Surface Alloying of 420 steel (13 wt% Cr, 0.2 wt% C) by means of carbon coatings enables high concentrations of carbon to be introduced into the substrate. Carbon levels ranging from hypoeutectic to hypereutectic and up to ≈4 wt% C can be readily achieved. However, significant porosity and cracking occurs in the hypereutectic structures.

(2) The rapid solidification rates associated with laser processing, produce very fine structures, whose features depend on carbon content, mixing conditions in the melt and cooling rate, e.g., secondary arm spacing of austenite ranges from 2 to 0.6 μm, indicative of cooling rates of 5-60 x 10^3 Ks^{-1}. These were produced under processing conditions between 1.0 and 1.6 kW and species of 10 to 700 mms^{-1}.

(3) The martensitic transformation does not take place in the hypoeutectic structures even on cooling to -196°C.

(4) Hardness values of ≈600 HV can be achieved at hypoeutectic levels and up to ≈1500 HV in hypereutectic structures.

ACKNOWLEDGMENTS

The authors thank the Scientific Engineering Research Council and C.E.G.B. (Central Generating Electricity Board) Scientific Services, Gravesend, for supporting the work.

REFERENCES

1. C. W. Draper and J. M. Poate, International Metals Reviews 30, 85 (1985).
2. A. Walker, H. M. Flower, and D. R. F. West, J. Mater. Sci. 20, 989 (1985).
3. A. Walker, D. R. F. West, W. M. Steen, Metals Technology 11, 399 (1984).
4. B. L. Mordike, H. W. Bergmann and N. Grob, Z. Workstofftech 14, 253 (1983).
5. W. E. Brower, R. Starhan, M. C. Fleming, A. C. F. Cask, Met. Res. J. 12, 176 (1970).
6. M. Lamp, Ph.D. Thesis, Imperial College, London (1985).
7. K. Bungardt, E. Kunze, and E. Horn, Archiv. f. das Eisenhuttenwessen 3, 193 (1958).
8. F. B. Pickering, International Metals Reviews 21, 229 (1976).
9. J. V. Bee and J. V. Wood, Met. Sci. 16, 268 (1982).
10. P. A. Molian, J. Mater. Sci. 20, 2903 (1985).
11. P. A. Molian, J. Mater. Sci. Lett. 4, 265 (1985).
12. G. Christodoulou, A. Walker, W. M. Steen, and D. R. F. West, Metals Technology 10, 215 (1983).

CARBURIZATION OF STEEL SURFACES BY LASER TREATMENT

E. RAMOUS
Istituto di Chimica Industriale, Universita di Padova, Italy

Key Words: absorptive coatings, modeling, microstructures

1. INTRODUCTION

Interest in the application of laser beams for surface treatment of steels is rapidly increasing. Generally, high-power, continuous-wave CO_2 lasers are used, with beam integrators or other optical devices such as oscillating mirrors, to obtain a uniform distribution of the energy of the beam on square or rectangular areas, typically 10 x 10 mm.

However, the machined or finished surface of steels to be treated does not present a sufficient absorptivity for the wavelengths used. Therefore, the surface must be coated by a suitable material to improve its absorptivity. The properties and the behavior of such coatings under the irradiation by laser are very important for the practical feasibility of the treatment. Actually, the coating properties determine the effective absorption of the surface to be treated and, consequently, the ratio of the incident energy exploited for the surface treatment.

Moreover, knowledge of the absorption coefficient is necessary to the application of any thermal model, and to test the correspondence between calculated and experimental data. Other interesting problems about the absorption coefficient are its dependence upon surface temperature and other treatment parameters, e.g., power density, interaction time, etc.

2. ABSORPTION MEASUREMENTS

Measurement of the surface temperature under laser irradiation is quite difficult. But the absorption of irradiated surfaces can be deduced by examining the thermal transient of thin slabs of steel, 0.8 mm thick, as an example.

It is well known from thermal models (1), derived from the traditional Carslaw and Jaeger equation (2), that this thickness cannot be considered as semi-infinite, but "finite," i.e., the temperature on the rear surface of the irradiated sample changes within the interaction time. It can be demonstrated (1), see Fig. 1, that in a fraction of the interaction time, the temperature difference between irradiated and rear surface becomes constant, and this difference can be easily calculated. Therefore, the temperature of the irradiated surface can be deduced from the measurement of the rear surface temperature by a thermocouple. Finally, from the temperature variation, the absorption coefficient can be calculated by a simple calorimetric balance.

Some results are summarized in Fig. 2, where absorption coefficients of different coatings relative to graphite are indicated. The most interesting coatings appear to be graphite and silica. In Fig. 3 the absorption coefficient of a steel surface, coated by graphite, is shown vs. interaction time and corresponding calculated temperature of the irradiated surface. It is evident that α is not a constant: increasing

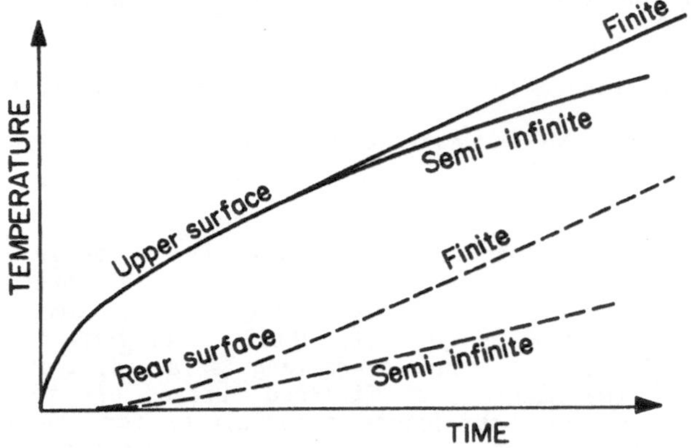

FIGURE 1. Calculated surface temperatures vs. time for samples of "semi-infinite" and "finite" thickness, under laser irradiation.

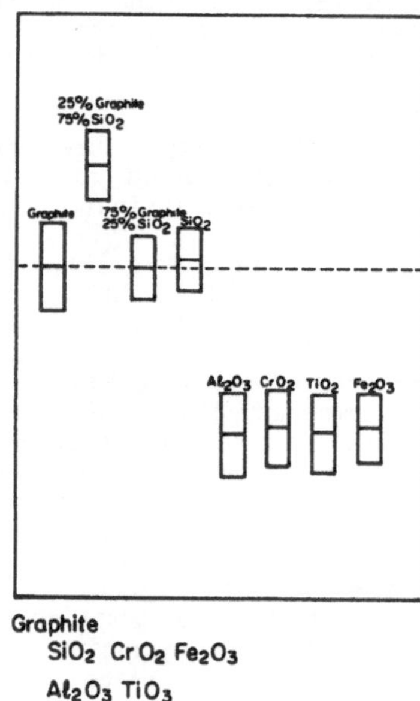

FIGURE 2. Comparison of absorption properties of different coating materials (graphite as reference).

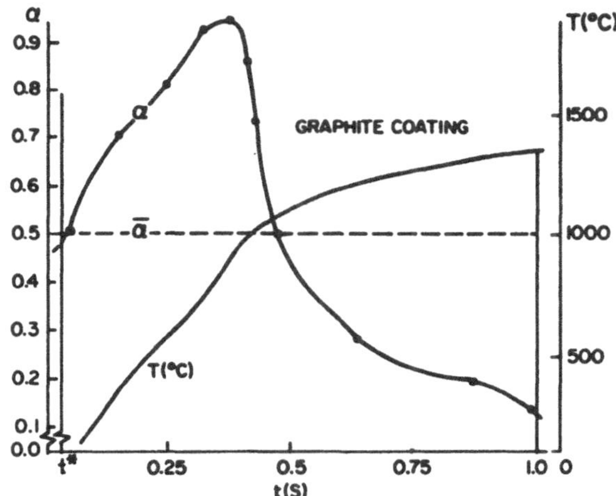

FIGURE 3. Absorption coefficient and thermal history of a steel surface coated by graphite.

both with temperature (interaction time) up to a maximum, at about 1000°C on the irradiated surface, then it decreases to lower values, corresponding to that of an uncoated metallic surface.

This behavior can be related to exothermic oxidation reactions occurring between graphite and surrounding air's oxygen. At lower temperatures α maintains high values, but over 1000°C the coating is destroyed and α decreases.

In Fig. 4 the absorption behavior of a composite coating of graphite and silica dag is shown. This type of coating gives better absorption results in a wide range of surface temperatures. The good performance of this composite coating may be explained as follows: Presumably graphite offers a beneficial effect at low temperatures, and silica, which possibly melts but remains on the surface, is unaffected by oxidation reactions, and continues to work as an absorptive coating at high temperature.

These results give indications of the best practical application of the examined coatings. The graphite appears more useful in surface treatments for transformation hardening, where the maximum temperature on the surface does not exceed 1000-1100°C. Silica graphite coatings work better in treatments where higher surface temperatures are required. Figure 5 presents results on transformation hardening of a 0.4% C steel coated with graphite and graphite-silica mixtures.

3. SURFACE CARBURIZATION

Graphite dag, as already discussed, is extensively used as coating material for metallic surfaces to improve absorption of laser radiation during surface treatments. However, the presence of the graphite can induce a carbon enrichment by diffusion in the surface layers. In transformation hardening of steels this can induce damage such as a higher

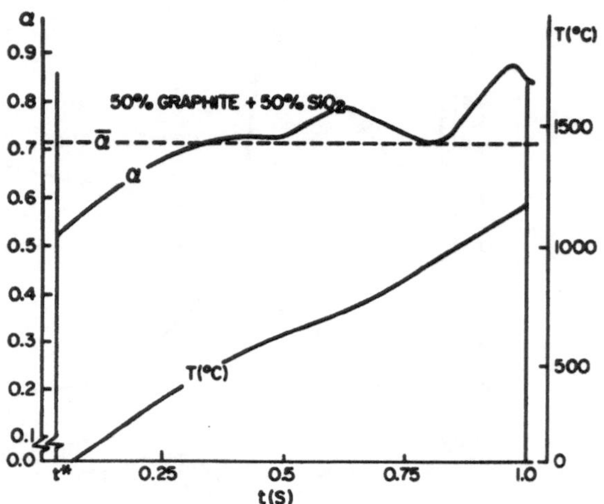

FIGURE 4. Absorption coefficient and thermal history of a steel surface coated by mixed graphite-silica dag.

content of retained austenite and some little localized melting (3,4) as a consequence of the lowering of the melting temperature, increasing the carbon content.

Therefore, two questions arise for investigation:

(a) What is the effective thickness of the carbon-enriched layers in the surface treatment of steels by power lasers, using graphite dag coatings?

(b) Is there a possibility of obtaining surface carburization, only by solid-state diffusion, using the laser heating?

3.1. Mathematical Model

The carbon diffusion in the surface layers during laser heating can be decribed by Fick's second law, x being the direction normal to the surface:

$$\frac{\partial c}{\partial t} = D \frac{\partial^2 c}{\partial x^2} \tag{1}$$

The value of the diffusion coefficient D is temperature dependent, according to an "Arrhenius equation" like:

$$D = D_o e^{-E/RT} \tag{2}$$

D_o being not dependent on temperature variation. Our calculations were performed with these simplified assumptions:

(a) Means values for the physical properties of the base material (ARMCO iron) in the considered temperature range.

(b) Surface temperatures were evaluated by the thermal model of heat diffusion in a slab, of semi-infinite thickness, heated from the surface by an external source of heat (4).

(c) 0.6 was taken as the absorption coefficient of the laser radiation.

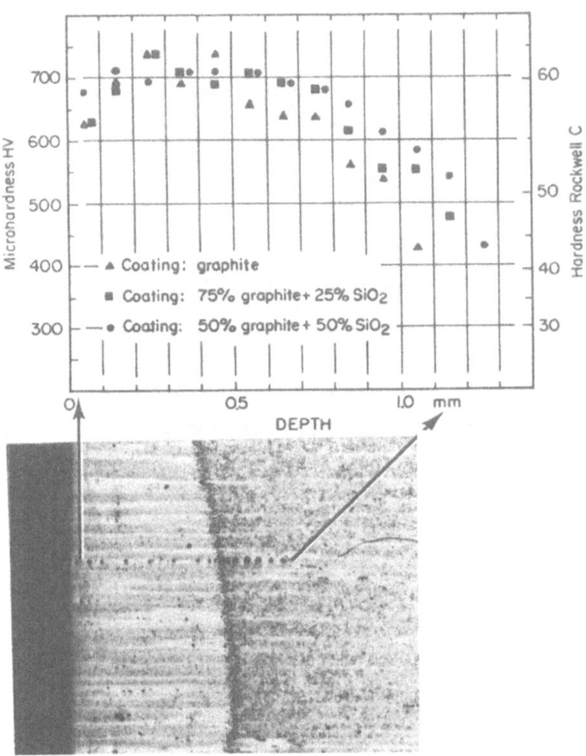

FIGURE 5. Microstructure and hardness profile of 0.4% carbon steel, laser treated by transformation hardening, with different coating materials. Maximum transformed case depth is about 1 mm.

3.2. Results and discussion

Results obtained by calculations and experimental tests are summarized in Table 1. The values of the diffusion path were calculated by the aforementioned mathematical model. The indicated values correspond to the depth where the carbon content is reduced to 10% of the values reached on the surface.

Comparison between the experimental results (see, for example, microstructures in Fig. 6) and calculated data confirm the validity of the mathematical model used. Indeed, the maximum disagreement between experimental and calculated diffusion paths does not exceed 10%.

TABLE 1.

Sample	F_o(W/mm^2) Intensity of Absorbed Radiation	Inter-action Time (sec)	T_{max} °C	Carbon Diffusion Path (mm)	
				Calculated	Experimental
1	20.00	1	1548	0.037	0.04
2	3.0	20	1051	0.049	0.055
3	3.4	20	1174	0.068	0.07
4	3.8	20	1330	0.08	0.09
5	4.1	20	1422	0.12	0.13
6	4.5	20	1546	0.17	0.17

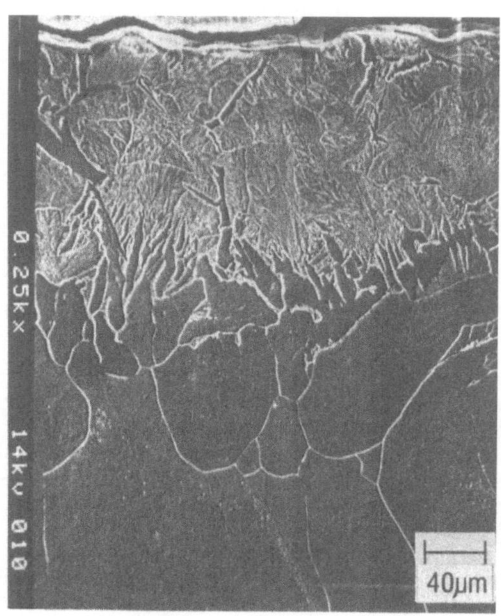

FIGURE 6. Microstructures of ARMCO iron samples surface carburized by laser treatment (solid-state diffusion).

Moreover, by the second series of tests, the possibility of obtaining, by laser heating with the highest interaction time, a noticeable carbon enrichment on iron and steel surfaces by solid state diffusion, without melting, is shown. Technological implications of this possibility are obvious.

On the contrary, the results of the first tests show that the harmful effects derived from the graphite dag are almost irrelevant in steel surface transformation hardening. Indeed, in this second case the carbon diffusion path is very small because in this type of surface treatment by laser, the used interaction time must be very short.

Deeper carburized layers can be obtained by heating the surface above the melting point. Structures of these carbon-alloyed layers are very similar to the "white cast iron": iron carbides in a matrix of austenite and martensite (Fig. 7). Surface hardness and wear resistance are significantly increased; however, melting and resolidification processes damage the smoothness of the surface.

REFERENCES

1. S. Kou, D. K. Sun, and Y. P. Le, Metall. Trans 14A, 643 (1983).
2. H. Carslaw and J. Jaeger, Conduction of Heat in Solids (Oxford Press, London, 1978), pp. 50,112.
3. R. Menin, E. Ramous, and M. Magrini, Proc. 4th Int. Conf. Rapidly Quenched Metals, Sendai, August 1981, edited by T. Masumoto and K. Suzuki (Japan Institute of Metals, Sendai, 1982) p. 193.
4. A. V. LaRocca, in Proceedings of the 5th Int. Symposium on Gas Flow and Chemical Lasers, Oxford, August 1984, edited by A. S. Kaye and A. C. Walker (Adam Hilger Ltd., Bristol, 1985), p. 83.

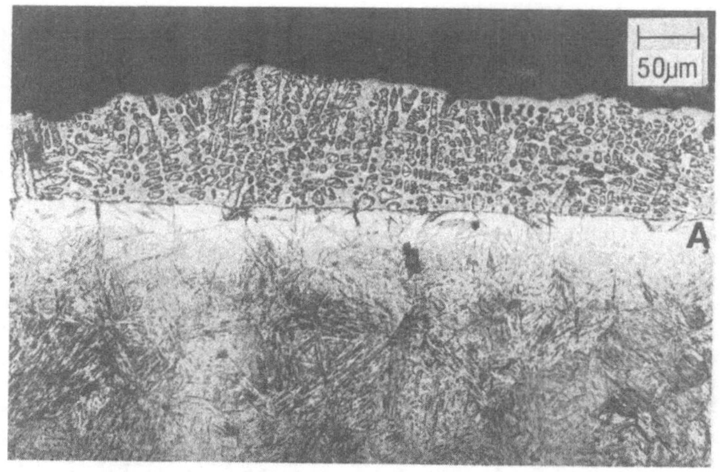

FIGURE 7. Microstructure (A) and hardness profile (B) of 0.4% carbon steel surface layer, laser melted and carbon alloyed.

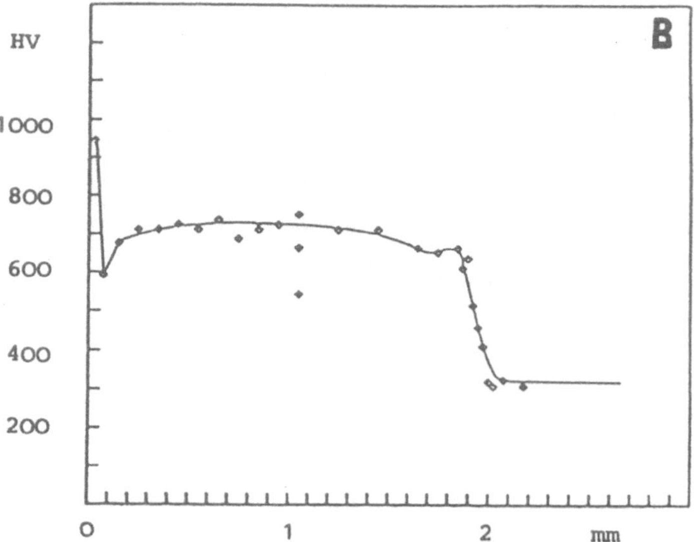

RAPID SOLIDIFICATION OF SURFACE LAYERS MELTED BY CW LASER

L. GIORDANO AND E. RAMOUS
Istituto di Chimica Industriale, Universita di Padova, Italy

Key Words: rapid solidification, stellite coating, carbon steels

1. INTRODUCTION

Rapid solidification processing (RSP) commonly results in departures from conventional microstructures, giving an improvement of grain refinement and chemical homogeneity (1). Fine-grained structures generally have improved strength and reduced anisotropy. Chemical homogeneity deriving from non-equilibrium-extended solutions offers opportunities for subsequent heat treatments to produce the final microstructures of desired properties.

High-density heating devices, such as laser beams, allow rapid melting and subsequent solidification to be obtained in surface layers, producing typical effects of RSP in a surface treatment. The range of attainable surface modifications is enlarged by the possibility to introduce other elements by surface alloying during melting (2).

However, the microstructure resulting from the RSP by laser surface melting is strongly dependent on the thermal transient induced into the surface layers. Therefore, the application of this surface treatment requires a suitable knowledge of the relationships between the laser treatment parameters, the induced thermal transient and the influence of thermal conditions during solidification on resulting microstructure.

In the following, laser surface melting of cast-iron, high-carbon steels and stellite coatings is described.

2. EXPERIMENTAL

An AVCO CO_2 15 kW cw laser was used. The beam was focused by a "beam integrator" that supplies a rectangular spot of adjustable dimensions (typically 10 x 10 mm). A movable table allows the sample to be moved at a constant velocity beneath the fixed laser spot.

The tests were carried out using a power density between 5 and 15 kW/cm^2, and different interaction times, in the range between 0.2 and 10.0 s, defined as the time necessary for the spot to cover a distance corresponding to its dimension in the direction of displacement. The effective power arriving on the sample surface was measured, before each treatment, with a cone calorimeter. To improve the radiation absorption, the surface of the sample was covered by a graphite dag.

The thermal transients induced into the samples during the laser surface treatment were registered by thermocouples inserted into the bulk of the samples. After treatment the samples were examined by optical and SEM microscopy, X-ray diffraction, and in some cases, by Mössbauer spectroscopy (using the X-ray backscattered radiation).

3. CAST-IRON TREATMENT

3.1. Materials

The tests have been carried out on samples of gray iron with flake graphite, the composition of which is given in Table 1.

TABLE 1.

C	Si	Mn	Cr	Ni	S	P	Sn
3.10	2.16	0.50	0.19	0.08	0.041	0.028	0.11

The structure turns out to be type A graphite and of dimensions contained between 3 and 5 of the ASTM scale in a pearlitic matrix.

3.2. Treatment conditions

The laser parameters, power densities and interaction time have been chosen on the basis of data derived from a mathematical model of the thermal transient induced by a laser beam on the surface layers. Obviously, more than one pair of values (power density/interaction time) could give the same molten depth concerned (1-2 mm).

After some preliminary tests we chose to work with a power density of about 4.5 kW/cm^2 and consequent interaction time between 1 and 8 s to obtain suitable surface-melted layers.

3.3. Results and discussion

In Fig. 1 the microhardness profiles along a transverse section are reported (3). In the samples of lesser thickness, the hardness improvement of the surface-melted layer is greatly reduced. Only in the samples

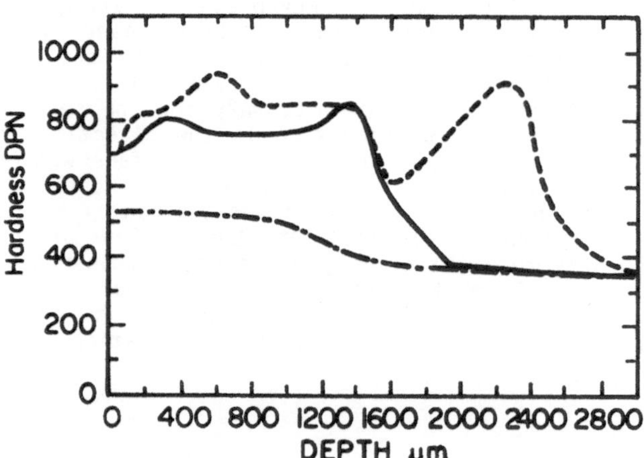

FIGURE 1. Microhardness profiles of laser-melted, cast-iron samples. Power density = 4.5 kW/cm^2, dwell time = 2.8 s, a = slab thickness. ------ a = 27 mm, ______ a = 11 mm, _ . _ . _ . a = 5.4 mm.

of sufficient thickness, over about 10 mm, did the laser melting and subsequent self-quenching induce a noticeable surface hardening. With the greatest sample thickness over 20 mm, the maximum hardness decreased and the hardness profile appeared more discontinuous.

These different patterns correspond to very different microstructures in samples of various thickness. In effect, the laser surface melting parameters (power density and interaction time) determine the depth of the melted layer, but the final microstructure (and hardness profile) is determined by the self-quenching rate, which depends on the workpiece thickness. In the thinner samples the quenching rate is not sufficient to reach the critical rate for martensite transformation. Then the structure of the melted layer is only slightly modified and contains small quantities of cementite and fine pearlite. Indeed, the structure obtained in larger workpieces is typical of white cast iron, with primary cementite and dendrites of transformed austenite in the melted zone, as shown in Fig. 2(c). But in these samples also the unmelted transition layer between the melted zone and the base material appears transformed into martensite with variable quantities of retained austenite (Fig. 2(d)). This latter zone was found to favor initiation of microcracks going towards the surface of the workpiece. The martensite structure appears in the transition zone, under the melted layer, only where the critical quenching rate for hardening was exceeded. The formation of these macroscopic faults can be avoided by choosing the treatment conditions to control the cooling rate. This is confirmed by the results we obtained on workpieces with intermediate thickness between 10 and 20 mm. In these workpieces the martensitic transformation was confined to the melted layer. The transition zone presented a transformation structure, but it was bainite, refined pearlite and a little martensite. In these samples, with intermediate thickness, both the structure and the hardness profile of the superficial layers were satisfying, and microcracks have not been found. In pieces of high thickness, the formation of microcracks can be avoided by reducing adequately the cooling velocity by pre-heating of the workpiece.

In our experiments cast-iron workpieces with thickness ranging between 10 and 20 mm were directly surface-hardened by laser melting. From these experiments the values of penetration depth vs. interaction time are given in Fig. 3. Short interaction times led to the formation of microcracks while with long interaction times a decrease of hardness in the melted zone was noted. The structures obtained for short and long interaction times are analogous to those met with in the preceding case respective to sample thickness. In the samples where the quantity of retained austenite is negligible, it was noted that in the melted zone, increasing the interaction time also increases lamellar spacing of the pearlite, derived from the transformation of austenite.

After the removal of 0.1 mm of surface material by means of grinding, the latter were subjected to wear tests in order to verify the tribological behavior of the melted layer subject to low specific load values but a high number of alternate cycles of stress typical of the slide-bed couple. As a material for comparison, cast iron G32 was chosen. The behavior of laser-melted cast iron has been compared with that of samples of induction-hardened steel and sulfurized steel. In our test condition wear of laser remelted cast iron was reduced from 2 to 4 times in comparison with other material examined.

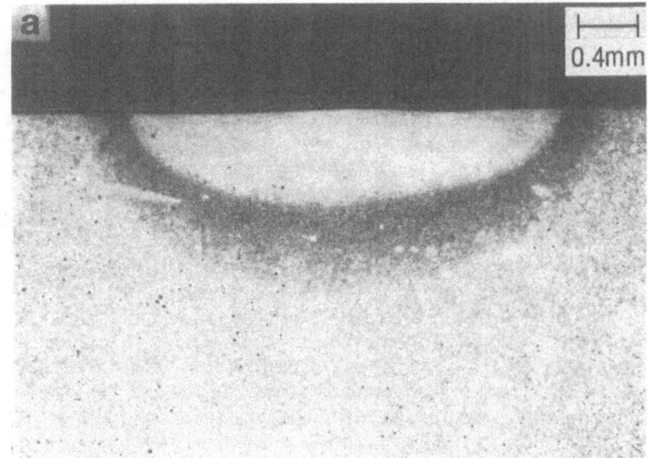

FIGURE 2. Structures of laser-melted surface layers of cast irons: (a) cross-sectioned view.

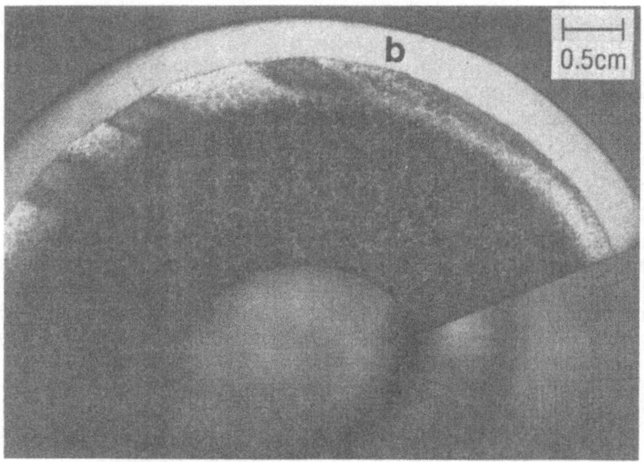

FIGURE 2. (b) surface normal view.

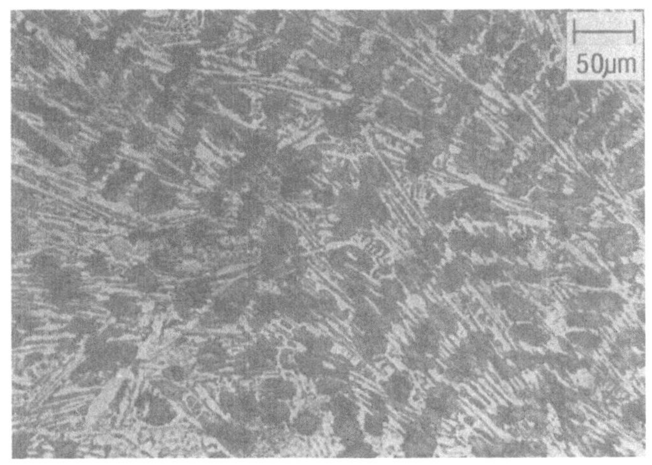

FIGURE 2. (c) melted zone.

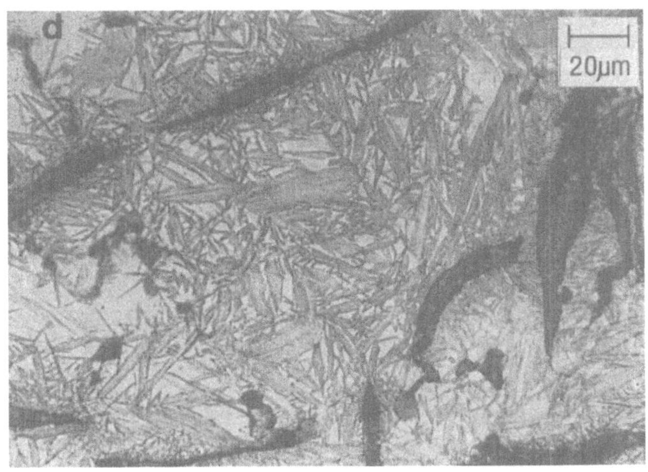

FIGURE 2. (d) HAZ.

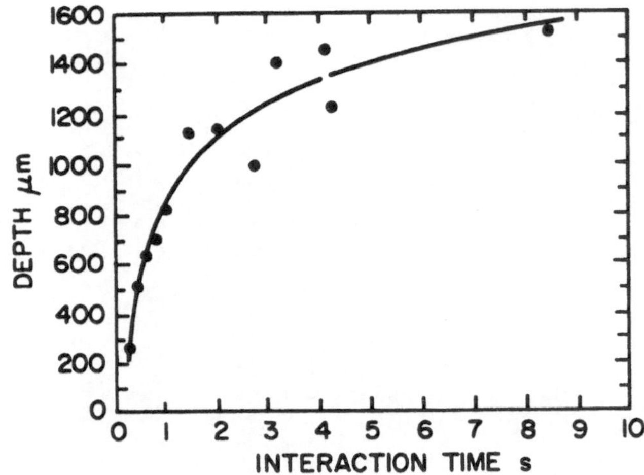

FIGURE 3. Laser melting of cast iron: interaction time vs. melt depth.

4. HIGH CARBON ALLOY STEEL TREATMENT

The surface melting by laser was examined in the same way on high carbon alloy steels: 52100, AISI A2 and D3. The aim of the work was to study the possibility of obtaining metastable surface layers with mainly austenitic structure. This, being metastable and supersaturated with carbon, would be transformed with subsequent heat treatment to structures of improved hardness and toughness. Reported here are the results concerning the AISI A2 steel, as a typical example, the composition of which is shown in Table 2.

TABLE 2. Average composition of AISI A2 steel.

C	Cr	Mn	Si	Mo	V
1.0	5.0	0.7	0.3	1.0	0.2

4.1. Treatment conditions

The treatment conditions investigated were a specific power of 15 kW/mm^2 and interaction time between 0.1 and 0.8 s, the spot area was 8 x 10 mm. Layers that were laser melted only and laser melted followed by subsequent heat treatment have been examined by light microscope and SEM. Metastable, oversaturated austenite was also examined by X-ray diffraction and Mössbauer spectroscopy.

4.2. Results

4.2.1. Surface melting. Micrographic observations of all the samples show a molten surface layer characterized by a remarkable variety of structures: needle-shaped, dendritic, cellular. The outer part of the molten layer of sample treated with interaction time of 0.2 s, for instance, was observed to have present ferrite needles oriented more or less perpendicularly to the surface, and a zone directly below and adjacent formed by a network of δ-ferrite and carbides surrounded by austenitic islands.

Analyzing the melted region of specimens treated at 0.3 and 0.2 s, respectively, we can identify three zones: the first one composed of austenitic dendrites and austenite plus carbides, the second one formed only by austenite, and the third one consisting of the heat-treated zone.

The prevalent structure of specimens treated at interaction times of 0.6 and 0.3 s is undoubtedly the dendritic one. On the other hand, the specimen at 0.6 s, besides presenting a more considerable melted region, shows a very homogeneous cellular structure formed by austenitic grains surrounded by δ-ferrite and carbides (Fig. 4(a)). Only the specimen at 0.6 s, with a very homogeneous structure, displays a regular microhardness profile. The X-ray diffraction analysis of specimens at 0.3 and 0.2 s established that the dendritic structure is composed of carbides and little ferrite, however, in the needle-shaped zones. The predominance of austenite was confirmed, and the Mössbauer spectroscopic analysis confirmed as well the carbon supersaturation of that phase.

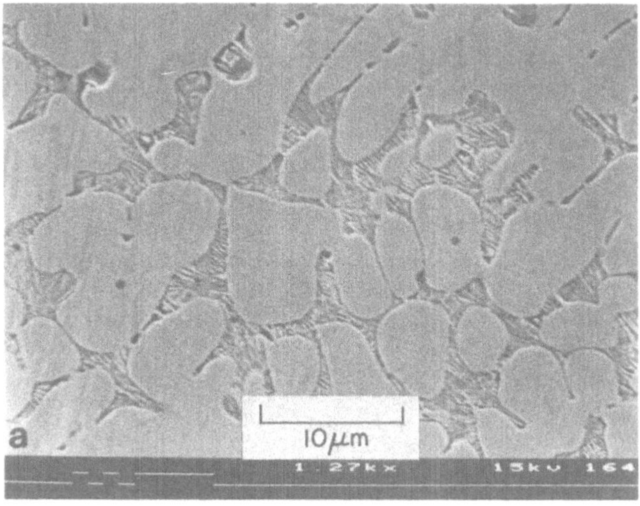

FIGURE 4. Microstructures of high-carbon steel melted layer: (a) laser-melted.

4.2.2. 550° Treatment. The destabilizing treatment at this temperature gave rise to different results on various specimens.

In fact, the microhardness profile (Fig. 5) of specimens 2 and 3 shows a decreasing trend moving from the outside to the inside of the melted structure, with surface-microhardness values that are higher than 900 HV.

On the other hand, for specimen 1 the transformation of the cellular austenite confirms its higher homogeneity, with microhardness values higher than 700 HV affirmed. The micrographic observation (Fig. 4(b)) shows how there is a further carbide precipitation at the same time as austenite is transformed into ferrite.

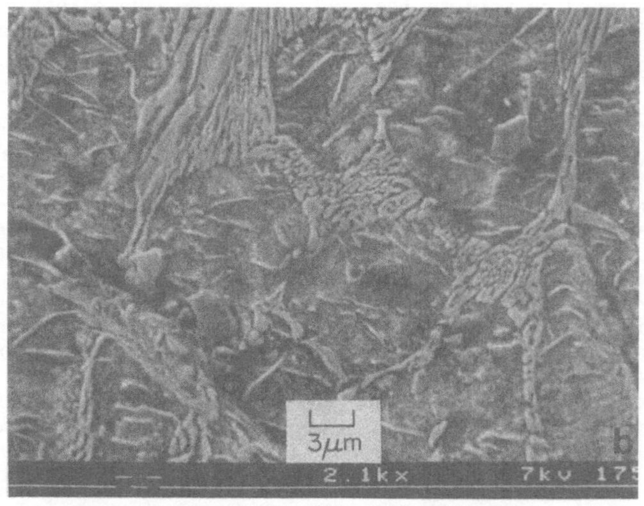

FIGURE 4. Microstructures of high-carbon steel melted layer: (b) laser-melted and heat-treated.

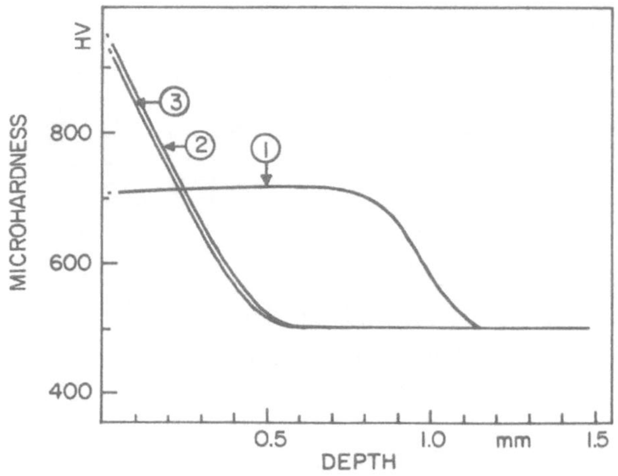

FIGURE 5. Microhardness profiles of samples after laser melting and post laser heat treatment at 550°C. Laser treatment parameters 15 kW/cm^2 and interaction time: sample 1, 0.2 s; sample 2, 0.4 s; sample 3, 0.8 s.

Tentative treatment below 500°C proved insufficient to obtain significant transformation of the metastable austenite. Treatments of many hours produced only partial transformation of the cellular austenite to bainite.

From our tests we can observe that it is possible to obtain, by laser melting and subsequent heat treatment, surface layers with increased hardness on high carbon alloy steels, maintaining a high toughness in the bulk of the workpiece.

The best structure for the laser-melted layer to seek for a useful application of such a process is the cellular one. The reasons for such a choice can be summarized in a few comments: the possibility of removing a surface layer during the finishing process, the homogeneity of the structure of the hardness, and the absence of cracks. In order to obtain such results, one needs to operate with longer interaction times and slower cooling speeds. These latter parameters obviously depend also on the thickness of the pieces, and it is obvious that the cellular structure is the more difficult treatment.

5. STELLITE COATINGS ON AUSTENITIC STEELS

Coatings of F and SF 6 stellites on samples of AISI 304 stainless steel were examined. The nominal compositions of alloys used are shown in Table 3.

TABLE 3. Compositions of materials studied (weight %)

Material	Co	Cr	W	C	Ni	Fe	Si	B
AISI 304 steel	-	18	-	<0.06	9	Bal	<1	-
Stellite F	Bal	25	12	2.0	22	1	1	-
Stellite SF6	Bal	19	8	0.7	13	-	3	1.7

5.1. Laser coating parameters

The effect of laser-operating parameters on the deposition of stellite by surface melting has been investigated (5). In hardfacing by laser, the minimum power density of the laser should not only melt the coating powder completely, but also enable the liquid coating to wet the substrate. When low-power lasers with beam diameters of a few millimeters are used, the coating can be obtained by multiple adjacent tracks. Using higher power lasers (at least 3-5 kW), it is possible to cover zones as wide as 10 mm or more in a single track. In each case, the optimum operating conditions have to be assessed so that the coating powder is melted and a uniformly distributed and even coating layer is produced. It is very important to obtain a smooth and regular coated surface to reduce subsequent finishing operations.

The optimum laser parameters to satisfy these requirements clearly depend on the thickness of the deposit to be obtained. For stellite hardfacing by high-power lasers on extended surfaces by a single pass, the operating conditions are given by a relatively limited range of power density and coverage values, as already discussed (5). The 2-3 mm thick deposits investigated in this work were obtained with a laser having a power density of 0.12 kW/mm^2, a coverage of 8.3 mm^2/s and a 10 x 10 mm spot.

Figure 6 shows a cross-sectional view of the stellite deposits obtained by laser after electrolytic etching. The solidification microstructure consists mostly of primary dendrites with some secondary branching. The dendrites are grouped in clusters with a common growth direction, the preferred direction generally lying in a plane approximately perpendicular to the surface, but not always in a direction normal to the surface.

The main microstructural differences between the stellite coatings applied by laser and more traditional techniques can be deduced from Figures 6(a) and (b). The laser deposits have:

. a much smaller and more uniform dendrite spacing,
. much smaller interdendritic carbide particles,
. a much reduced volume fraction of interdendritic carbides.

These microstructural differences are a direct consequence of the higher cooling rate obtained by laser hardfacing.

The high-power density of the laser beam can produce surface melting with very short interaction times, 0.1-1 s under our conditions. Consequently, the cooling rates, by transmission to the almost heat-unaffected base material, can be very high.

Over the range of laser-processing parameters examined, the primary and secondary dendrite arm spacings averaged 70 and 8 μm, respectively (Fig. 6(a)). The dendrite spacing can be related to the cooling rate during solidification. Comparison of our results with the dendrite spacing of rapidly solidified stellite alloys by melt spinning indicates cooling rates between 500 and 5000 K/s in our laser-melted coatings. By comparison, the cooling rate of the TIG coating can be similarly estimated as 10 K/s; the cooling rate of the coating applied by oxyacetylene torch must be lower still, resulting in the observed coarser microstructure and larger primary carbides (Fig. 6(b)).

5.2. Microhardness measurements

The dendrite size of the laser-applied coatings generally increases with increasing energy supplied during melting, as already observed elsewhere (5). These different microstructures present different surface hardnesses. The influence of the laser-melting parameters on surface hardness is shown in Figure 7. The higher values correspond to lower interaction times, i.e., to higher cooling rates during solidification and finer dendrites.

5.3. Transition zone between coating and base material

The very small interaction time and the well-defined power density of laser heating enables the melted depth of the base material to be finely controlled. Therefore, correct choice of the laser hardfacing parameters allows a very narrow transition zone between coating and base material to be obtained. This suggests that limited mixing occurs between the two alloys during laser melting. This is confirmed by the concentration profiles of the alloying elements cobalt, chromium, iron, nickel and tungsten obtained from microprobe analysis of the transition zone. The thickness of the interdiffusion zone of iron, for instance, is in the range 14-20 m. This confirms that laser surface melting does not allow the dilution of coating material by iron coming from the steel substrate.

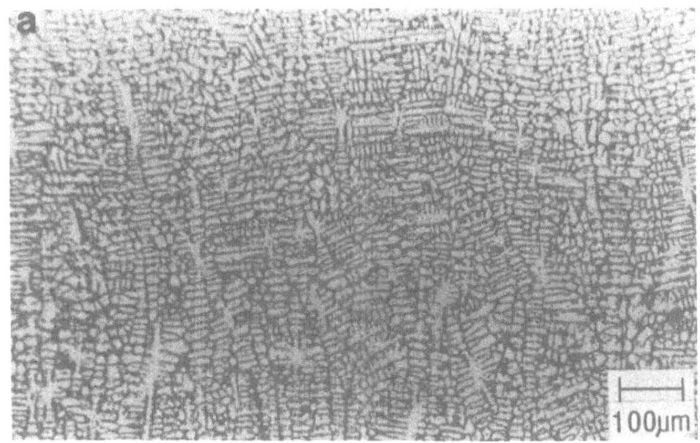

FIGURE 6. Microstructures of stellite coatings: (a) laser.

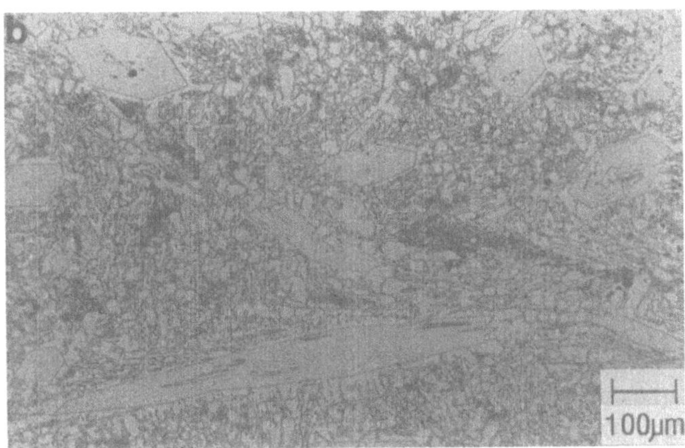

FIGURE 6. Microstructures of stellite coatings: (b) oxyacetylene.

Therefore, the specific properties of wear and corrosion resistance of the stellite alloy coating can be maintained.

REFERENCES

1. J. F. Wallace, J. Metals 15, 372 (1963).
2. B. H. Kear, E. M. Breinan, and L. E. Greenwald, Metals Techn. 6, 121 (1979).
3. A. Tiziani, P. Meneghello, V. Tagliaferri, P. Munarei, and M. Magrini, Proc. 2nd Int. Cong. Heat Treatment of Materials, Florence (1982) Ed. AIM - Milano, p. 847.
4. A. Tiziani, L. Giordano, and E. Ramous, Proc. ASM Conference on Laser in Materials Processing, Los Angeles (1983), p. 108.
5. L. Giordano, E. Ramous, A. Tiziani, M. Cantello, and F. Pasquini, Proc. 3rd Int. Conf. Heat Treatment of Materials, Shanghai (1983), 9.22.
6. F. Duflos, J. F. Stohr, in Rapidly Solidified Amorphous and Crystalline Alloys, edited by B. J. Kear, B. C. Giessen, and M. Cohen (North Holland, NY, 1982), p. 167.

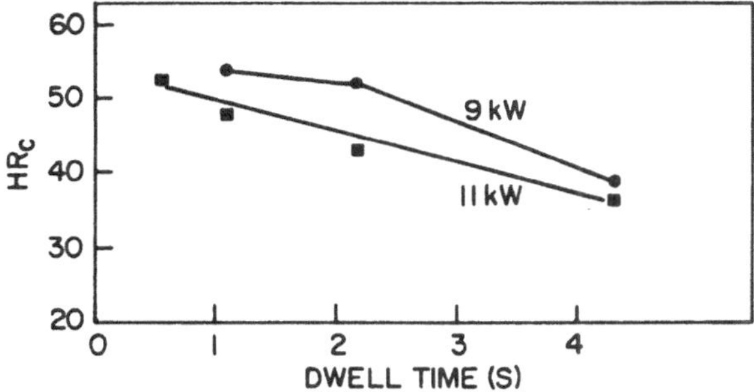

FIGURE 7. Surface hardness of stellite coatings.

LASER SURFACE TREATMENT FOR ELECTROMECHANICAL APPLICATIONS

J. COM-NOUGUE AND E. KERRAND

Laboratoires de Marcoussis, Centre de Recherches de la C.G.E.,
91460 Marcoussis, France

Key Words: chromium steel, residual stress, absorptive coatings

1. INTRODUCTION

Materials such as chromium steels and low-alloy steels are used for electromechanical applications, particularly in turbines where they may be subjected to several types of surface degradation during operation: erosion, fatigue and wear, for example. As a consequence, the surface properties of these materials must be improved.

This paper describes three laser processes - transformation hardening, surface melting, and cladding - which can offer an answer to the above-mentioned problems. For each laser technique, we have investigated the influence of the processing parameters on the metallurgical properties of two chromium steels and a low-alloy steel used in steam turbines. Results are discussed primarily in terms of the geometry, structure and hardness of the treated zones. Besides the parametric study, we have also investigated a numerical solution of the heat-conduction equation in order to predict the parameters relevant to transformation hardening and monitor the process.

2. LASER SYSTEMS

2.1. Lasers and workstations

The lasers used in these investigations were located in two different laboratories.

One series of laser tests was performed at Etablissement Technique Central de l'Armement of Direction des Recherches et Techniques (DRET) with a transverse flow system delivering 5 kW of maximum output power. The beam has a nominal diameter of about 50 mm and a slightly oval shape with a heterogeneous energy profile characterized by two peaks in diametrically opposite positions.

The other experiments were made with a 3 kW CO_2 source at the laser laboratory of the CGE Research Center where two CO_2 lasers (1 and 3 kW) connected to a (3+1)D workstation with CNC are already used (Figure 1). This 3 kW system is based on a fast axial flow system with a "stable resonator" optical cavity. The beam is characterized by a divergence close to 1 mr, and its profile has an approximately truncated Gaussian shape with a nominal diameter of about 25 mm. Eventually this laboratory will have a third CO_2 source with a maximum output power of at least 7 kW, which is presently under development at the Research Center. The source uses the same fast axial flow technique as the 3 kW laser but with a U -type "unstable resonator" optical cavity. The monomode annular output beam will have an external diameter of approximately 72 mm.

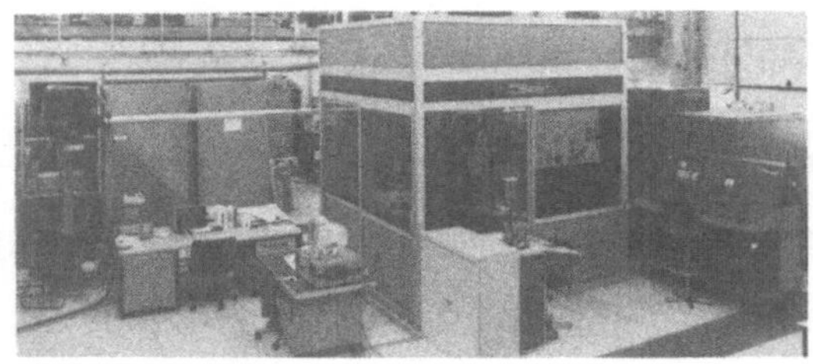

FIGURE 1. Laser laboratory of the CGE Research Center.

During the tests, the workpieces were traversed under the stationary laser beam on an x-y movement table capable of controlled constant traverse speeds up to 30 cm/sec. Accessory apparatus, such as laser optics or powder feed mechanism, can be added as required by the application.

2.2. Beam shaping optics

In addition to the use of a defocused beam in all the laser processes, two other beam shapes were tested in the case of transformation hardening: (i) a semielliptic one (27 mm x 4 mm) obtained by means of a cylindrical mirror and used with the 5 kW laser, and (ii) a system incorporating a kaleidoscope beam integrator which could produce a uniform laser power density over a rectangular (6 mm x 3 mm) or square (6 mm x 6 mm) area on the workpiece.

This integrator, which gives a sharp beam profile (65% of energy in a 5.5 x 5 mm area with a constant power density), has been used with the 3 kW laser up to now.

2.3. Power feeding device

The workstation is fitted out with a system similar to those used in plasma coating. It consists of a vibratory module linked to the powder holder by means of a feed screw which sends the powder at a uniform rate into a small chamber. An inert gas flow then injects the powder into a flexible tube towards the nozzle where the laser beam is partially focused with a ZnSe lens. The powder particles are melted in the laser beam before reaching the surface to be coated.

3. MATERIALS

The two chromium steels (S1,S2) which were investigated exhibit a tempered martensitic structure characterized by a microhardness of 350 and 315 HV, respectively. Table 1 gives the chemical composition of each one as well as the composition of a low-alloy steel (S3) which was also investigated and which presents a quenched-tempered structure with a microhardness of 280 HV.

Two commercially available coating powders were also chosen for the study (Table 2): (i) a cobalt-base alloy (P1) with a nodular shape and particle size between 25 and 125 μm, and (ii) a nickel-base alloy (P2) composed of irregular grains, the size of which ranges from 25 to 100 μm.

TABLE 1. Chemical composition of steels used (% concentration by weight)

	C	Cr	Mn	Mo	Ni	P	S	Si	V	W
S1	0.1	1.75	0.72	1.6	2.7	0.025	0.003	0.23	0.3	
S2	0.21	11.73	0.48	0.98	0.51	0.019	0.007	0.34	0.3	0.02
S3	0.1	0.8	0.4	0.8	0.5	0.03	0.03	0.4	0.15	

TABLE 2. Chemical composition of coating alloy materials (% concentration by weight)

	C	Si	Cr	Co	Fe	W	Ni	Mo
P1	1.2	1.2	29.00	63.0	1.0	4.5		
P2	0.02	0.8	17.0		5.0	5.0	56.0	17.0

4. CHARACTERIZATION

After the laser treatment, the morphology and metallurgical characteristics of the treated zones were determined by optical microscopy supplemented by Vickers microhardness profiles on polished and etched metallographic samples.

On selected specimens treated by laser hardening, the residual stresses were measured in the hardened zones by means of an X-ray diffraction method (1). Further, the variations in chemical composition of tracks produced by laser powder cladding and the level of the dilution in the base material were examined by electron microprobe analysis.

5. TRANSFORMATION HARDENING

5.1. Experimental procedure

Series of trials were carried out over a wide range of laser power, beam diameters and traverse speeds and with various absorbing coatings. The laser power ranged from 1.7 to 3.5 kW for travel speeds between 4 and 20 mm/s. All three steels were treated by using a semi-elliptic beam as well as a beam defocused at a 16 mm diameter in the case of the 5 kW laser. The S2 chromium steel was also investigated by using the 3 kW laser with a defocused or homogenized beam at power levels between 1.8 and 3 kW and traverse speeds ranging from 5 to 30 mm/s.

In addition, several surface preparations were selected to enhance the optical absorption of the 10.6 μm infrared radiation. Before the laser trials, the top surface of the workpieces was sprayed with graphite or black paint. Absorption measurements at 10.6 μm gave 55 to 60% absorptivity for black paint compared with 40-50% in the case of graphite.

TABLE 3. Defocused beam frp, tramsverse laser. Case depths and surface widths for the hardened zones.

Material	P (kW)	V (mm/s)	Hardened Zone (mm)	
			Depth	Width
S1	2.5	5	0.96 (1)	8
	2.5	7.5	0.6	5.8
S2	2.5	5	0.8 (1)	7
	2.5	7.5	0.45	4
S3	2.5	5	1 (1)	7.5
	3	15	0.2	2.4
S1 (2)	3	10	1.36	9.2
S2 (2)	3	10	1.06	9.3
S3 (2)	3	10	1.2	8.2

(1) Slight surface melting
(2) Tests performed with a black paint coating

5.2. Results

5.2.1. Defocused beam. The defocused beam, which is characterized by a very heterogeneous distribution of the energy, produces hardened zones with a lenticular shape. Table 3 gives some results for the maximum depth and surface width of the treated zones obtained on the three steels investigated. In some cases, the treatment brought about a slight surface melting. Furthermore, it has also been noted that better performances were achieved with the paint coating than with the graphite spray. For example, case depths greater than 1 mm were achieved in all materials at 3 kW and 10 mm/s without any surface melting. The microstructure produced in the hardened zones appears to be a fine-grained martensite. An X-ray diffraction analysis has also shown that: (i) some austenite was present in these zones just below the workpiece surface, and (ii) in cases where a melting had occurred (graphite coating) cementite was also produced. Microhardness profiles were determined on the various hardened zones and are shown in Figures 2 and 3 for the two chromium steels. Values of 500-560 HV for S1 and 560-700 HV for S2 were achieved just below the surface or under the thin molten zone where it is present. The profiles generally show a step near the surface followed by a continuous decrease down to the base metal. After laser treatment the low-alloy steel exhibits maximum hardnesses ranging from 450 to 500 HV.

In the tests performed with the fast axial flow laser, the beam of which has a nearly Gaussian energy profile, the hardened zones are characterized by a constant depth over nearly their whole width. Such a beam will be suitable to treat homogeneously large surfaces for which it is necessary to make successive tracks. Table 4 gives data measured on the S2 chromium steel precoated with a black paint. It shows that a coverage rate up to 80% (hardened zone width/laser spot diameter) can be achieved with this beam profile whereas this rate was only 50% with the heterogeneous beam profile. The greatest case depth was 1.2 mm, obtained with a laser power of 2.1 kW and a speed of 5 mm/s.

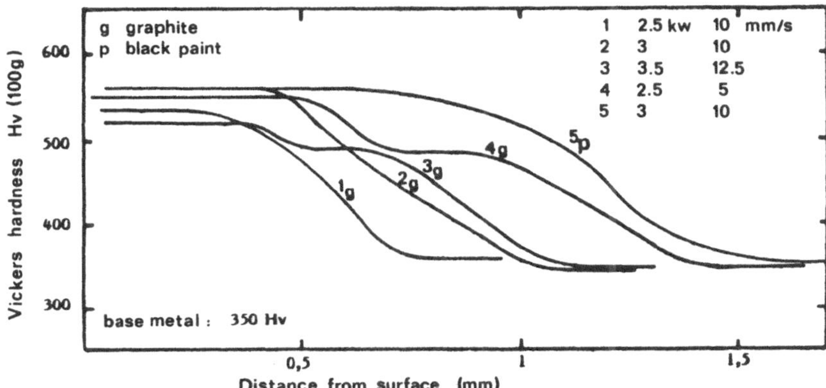

FIGURE 2. Hardness profiles on cross sections of hardened zones and base metal of S1 after various laser treatments performed with a defocused beam.

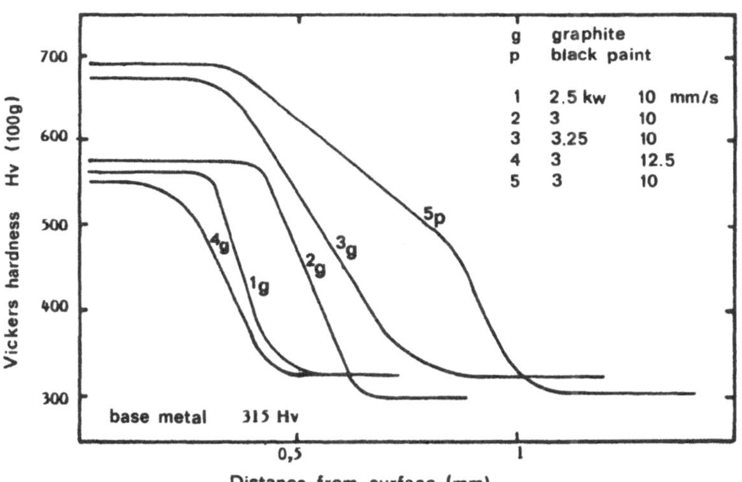

FIGURE 3. Hardness profiles on cross sections of hardened zones and base metal of S2 after various laser treatments performed with a defocused beam.

TABLE 4. Nearly Gaussian beam from axial laser. S2 chromium steel.

Beam ϕ(mm)	P (kW)	V (mm/s)	Hardened Zone (mm)	
			Depth	Width
8	1.8	5	1.06	6.2
	2.1	11.6	0.58	4.4
	2.4	18.3	0.52	4.5
	2.8	25	0.39	6.4
10	2.1	5	0.96	8.4
	2.4	11.6	0.76	7.2
	2.8	18.3	0.54	7.5
12	2.1	5	1.2	9.2

TABLE 5. Semi-elliptic beam. Case depths and surface widths for the hardened zones.

Material	P (kW)	V (mm/s)	Hardened Zone (mm)	
			Depth	Width
S1	2.4	7	0.7 (1)	16.1
	2	7	0.54	15.7
S2	2.4	7	0.57 (1)	15.7
	2	7	0.57	10.8
S3	2.5	4	0.8 (1)	17.7
	2	8.5	0.2	8.9

(1) Slight surface melting

5.2.2. Semi-elliptic beam. In the case of the tests performed with the transverse flow laser, a semi-elliptic beam gives hardened zones with a constant depth over nearly the whole treated width. Table 5 gives the geometrical characteristics of these zones as a function of the operating conditions. These results show that hardened depths up to 0.8 mm could be achieved with widths of less than 16 mm, compared to the width of 27 mm of the laser spot. The microhardness profiles show the hardness just below the surface to be 475-500 HV on the S1 steel and 525-725 HV for the S2 steel.

Figure 4 compares the behavior of the steels investigated, and it must be pointed out that the same energy threshold for hardening is observed for all of them. It must also be noted that this threshold depends on the intensity distribution in the laser beam.

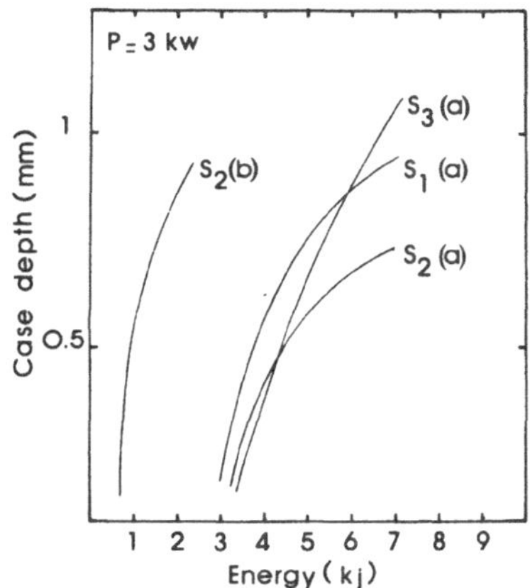

FIGURE 4. Evolution of the case depth in different steels (chromium steels: S1-S2, low-alloy steel: S3) as a function of the laser energy: (a) defocused beam, P = 3 kW, graphite; (b) semi-elliptic beam, P = 2 kW graphite.

5.2.3. Uniform beam integrator. The tests performed up to now with the kaleidoscope beam integrator in association with the axial flow laser showed no improvement compared to the results achieved with a focusing lens. This probably results from the particular energy profile of this source, and the value of this integrator would be more obvious if used with a more heterogeneous laser beam.

With regard to the efficiency of each type of beam shape, the corresponding results show the importance of, and the need to have, a good energy distribution in the beam to achieve better performances in the field of surface treatments.

5.2.4. Determination of the residual stresses in the hardened zones. The stresses resulting from hardening treatments performed with a semi-elliptic beam have been measured on S2 steel (i) on the treated sample surface perpendicular to the travel direction, and (ii) as a function of the depth.

It has been observed that the martensite formation and the volume increase induce compressive stresses on the surface that can be as high as 600 MPa, about 3 mm to each side of the hardened line axis, followed by a continuous decrease towards the edges of the hardened zone which is 14 mm wide. As a function of the depth, the treated zone exhibits compressive stresses with a peak value of 600 MPa just below the surface, followed by a continuous decrease towards a zero value at the interface between the hardened zone and the bulk material. It must be noted that as the compressive stresses decrease, the hardness decreases to reach the hardness of the base material where tensile stresses are observed at a depth three times larger than the case depth. These tensile stresses exhibit a peak value of 600 MPa at 1 mm below the surface. Figure 5 shows a typical evolution of the residual stresses with the corresponding hardness profile in a S2 steel treated at 2 kW and 7 mm/s.

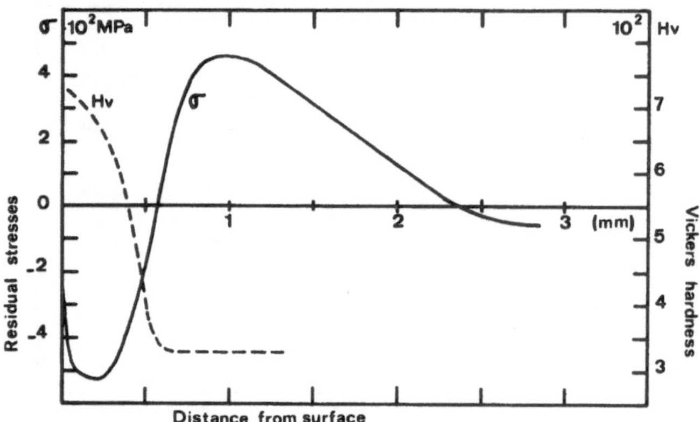

FIGURE 5. Evolution of the residual stresses and hardness in the hardened zone as a function of depth (semi-elliptic beam, S2 steel, 2 kW, 7 mm/s).

5.3. Heat flow

In the theoretical part of this study, an extension of the numerical solution of the steady-state heat conduction equation for constant thermal properties is given (3).

The objective of this investigation was to provide a numerical analysis for the three-dimensional heat conduction equation for a moving beam with a random energy distribution. In order to account for the random energy profile, the beam is considered as composed of $N_1 \times N_2$ zones in which the power density of each zone is supposed to be constant and independent of that in the surrounding zones.

If X_i and Y_i are the centerpoint coordinates of an elementary zone and B_i, L_j, respectively, its half-length and width, the temperature increase at an (x,y) point due to all surface elements (4) is:

$$T = T_0 + \frac{1}{k\sqrt{\pi}} \sum_{i,j} Q_{i,j} \int_0^{\infty} \left[\exp - \frac{z^2}{16\varepsilon^2}\right] \left\{ \mathrm{erf}\left(\frac{y - y_j + L_j}{4\varepsilon}\right) - \mathrm{erf}\left(\frac{y - y_j - L_j}{4\varepsilon}\right) \right\}$$

$$\left\{ \mathrm{erf}\left(\frac{x - x_i + B_i}{4\varepsilon} + \frac{V\varepsilon}{\alpha}\right) - \mathrm{erf}\left(\frac{x - x_i - B_i}{4\varepsilon} + \frac{V\varepsilon}{\alpha}\right) \right\} d\varepsilon$$

where:

i,j : subscripts denoting two principal directions
$Q_{i,j}$: heat actually absorbed in (i,j) area: $P_{i,j}/4\ B_iL_j$
η : absorption coefficient
α : $k/\rho\, C_p$ (α thermal diffusivity, k thermal conductivity, ρ density, C_p specific heat)
V : speed of the workpiece along the x direction

T_0 is the base temperature prior to heating and (i,j), respectively, vary from 1 to N_1 and 1 to N_2. The different terms of the equation were evaluated by numerical integration to determine the temperature distribution.

The random energy distribution was determined by an accurate molding of a burn pattern on plexiglass obtained by irradiation with the CO_2 laser beam, and in each zone the power density was evaluated from the incident power using the relative depths of the pattern.

The computer model predicts the workpiece maximum temperature reached during the treatment and its correlation with the case depth. In order to allow a comparison with the experimental data, the temperature increase was calculated for the defocused beam of the transverse laser with B = 8.25 mm and L = 6 mm at selected processing power/speed values. The chosen grid mesh includes nine zones (beam with two energy peaks in the travel direction) and the theoretical analysis was performed for a chromium steel (S2) with the following thermal properties (300 K):

Thermal conductivity: $k = 29$ W/m/°C
Thermal diffusivity: $\alpha = 0.06$ cm^2/s

Figure 6 gives the relation between experimental and theoretical case depths for the defocused beam. A very good agreement is obtained between the experimental results and the mathematic model, in spite of an approximation in the determination of the workpiece initial temperature before each trial and of the beam profile. Figure 7 shows the temperature increases as a function of time at the top and the bottom of the heat-affected zone. The experiment was conducted with 3000 W and 10 mm/s on a surface coated with a black paint (56% absorptivity). The temperature curve exhibits two peaks corresponding to the energy peaks in the beam spot. The influence of such an energy distribution shows that it can be used to increase the time duration above the A_3 temperature (formation of uniform austenite) with an appropriate shaping of the beam.

Further, the calculation developed with the computer model indicates that the maximum temperature reached on the workpiece surface never exceeds the melting point of the material when the hardening treatment is performed at 3 kW and 10 mm/s on a surface coated with graphite or a black paint. Consequently, the slight melting actually observed for these conditions on graphite-coated surfaces probably results from a reaction of the graphite spray itself under the laser beam.

6. SURFACE MELTING

6.1. Experimental

The surface melting technique can locally produce microstructural modification impossible to achieve by conventional heat treatment and which can improve the mechanical properties of workpiece surfaces for applications where fatigue, wear and localized corrosion are concerned. This process is presently under evaluation in the case of a chromium

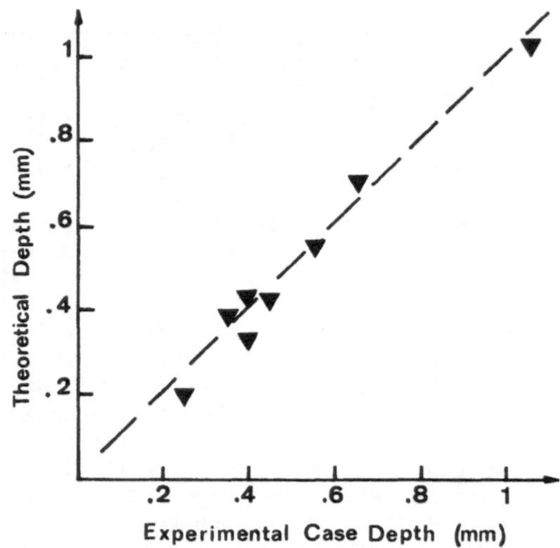

FIGURE 6. Relation between experimental and theoretical hardened depths (defocused beam).

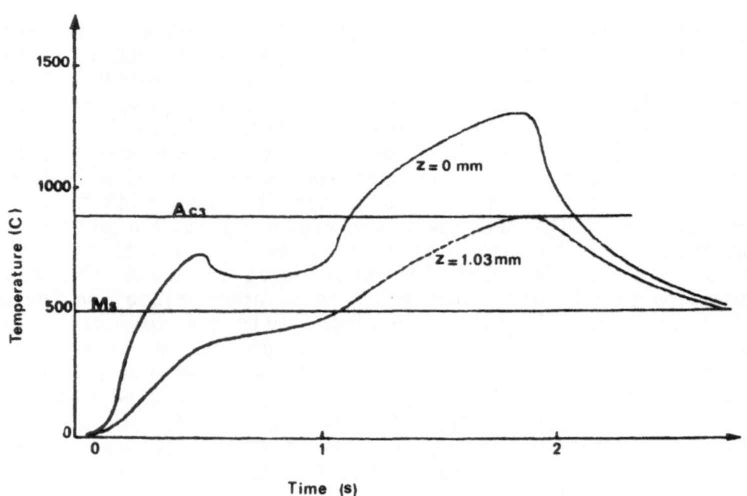

FIGURE 7. Calculated thermal cycles at the top of the bottom of the heat-affected zone (defocused beam, P = 3 kW, V = 10 mm/s, T_0 = 20°C, black paint coating, steel S2.

steel (S2) and a low-alloy steel (S3). Tests have been carried out in order to investigate the influence of the following parameters: laser powers ranging from 2.5 to 4.5 kW and travel speeds between 5 and 100 mm/s. For these experiments, the beam diameter was varied between 2.5 mm and 5 mm. Before the treatment the sample surface was shot-blasted to produce a constant absorptivity. A helium shield gas was used to avoid surface oxidation of the molten zone during the rapid solidification. Further, no sample preheat was performed before the laser surface melting.

6.2. Results

No cracking of the sample's surface has been observed after the laser treatment. The various tests resulted in two different geometries of the molten zone: (i) a thin, lenticular shape obtained with processing conditions close to the hardening treatments, and (ii) a more complex morphology, similar to that for welding, by using higher power densities.

Laser surface melting of the two steels produced a fine cellular structure. In particular, an oriented basaltic growth can be observed in the center of the molten zone due to limited overmelting with a significant temperature gradient. The edges of this zone exhibit a fine-grained equiaxial structure resulting from significant overmelting with a high temperature gradient. Such structures are seen in Figures 8 and 9 for the S2 steel treated with 3 kW in 10 mm/s.

FIGURE 8. Structure in the center of the molten zone (S2 steel, P = 3 kW, V = 10 mm/s).

The microhardness profiles have been determined in the various treated zones for both steels and are shown (i) as a function of the depth for S2 steel (Figure 10), and (ii) parallel to the width of the track for S3 steel (Figure 11). Values up to 725 HV for S2 and 520 HV for S3 were achieved in the molten zones. These microhardnesses are similar to those measured in the steel hardened by a solid-state transformation. However, the hardness profiles from the two steels generally exhibit a decrease

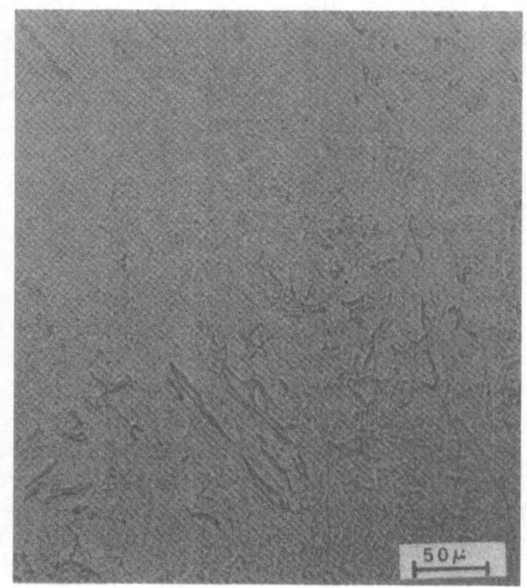

FIGURE 9. Structure at the transition zone between the molten zone and the heat-affected zone (S2 steel, P = 3 kW, V = 10 mm/s).

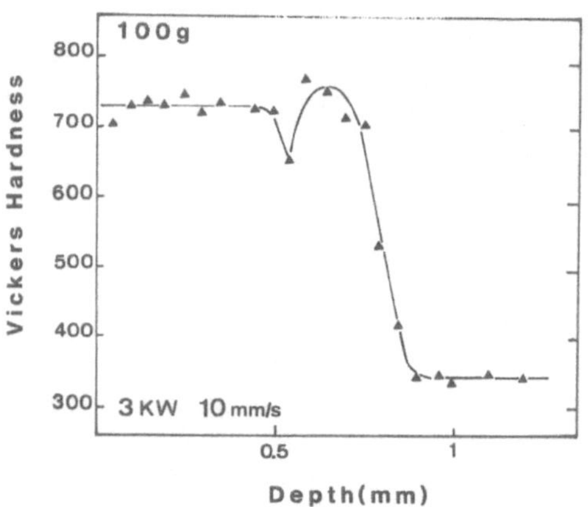

FIGURE 10. Hardness profile of S2 steel after laser surface melting (P = 3 kW, V = 10 mm/s).

in a transition zone between the molten zone and the heat-affected zone (see Figures 10 and 11). This evolution confirms the metallographic observations which show a modification of the structure in the transition zone.

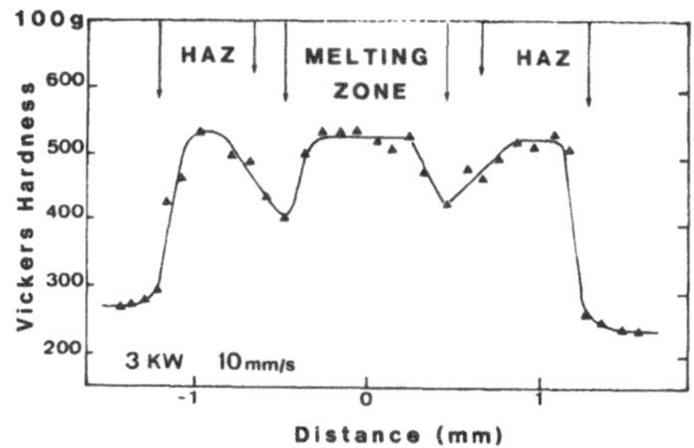

FIGURE 11. Hardness perpendicular to the treated surface of S3 steel (P = 3 kW, V = 10 mm/s).

7. CLADDING

7.1. Experimental procedure

Tracks were produced in which the clad was laid down over a chromium steel substrate (S2) by a technique based on powder injection into the laser beam. A set of processing conditions has been tested with two powders and, in particular, a cobalt base (see Table 2). The tests were performed with laser powers ranging from 3 to 4.5 kW for traverse speeds between 5 to 10 mm/s. The spot diameter of the defocused beam was about 3 mm on the workpiece. The powder feed rate was between 5 g/mm and 20 g/mm. Samples were not preheated before the laser cladding.

7.2. Results

The coatings are characterized by a regular, slightly rough surface free from cracks. An important effect of the traverse speed on the deposit shape was observed. Coatings were produced with thicknesses between 200 and 700 microns. Furthermore, it was found that in the case of the 5 kW laser, the heterogeneous beam profile results in relatively small cladding widths compared with the beam spot size (50-60%).

The cobalt-base cladding is characterized by a very fine dendritic structure which locally has micropores of about 1 µm in diameter.

In some cases, significant melting of the substrate occurred during the laser cladding, producing a dilution of the deposit in the base metal. However, if the steel was only superficially molten during the deposition, a good metallurgical bonding between the cladding and the substrate was achieved. Surface analyses show a rapid variation of the cobalt, chromium and iron concentrations at the interface between the coating and the metal, confirming this good metallurgical bonding.

Vickers microhardness profiles were determined as a function of depth. Values of 600-780 HV, approximately constant over the whole thickness of the deposit, were achieved in the cobalt-base cladding. An example is given in Figure 12 for S2 steel treated at 4.5 kW and 7 mm/s.

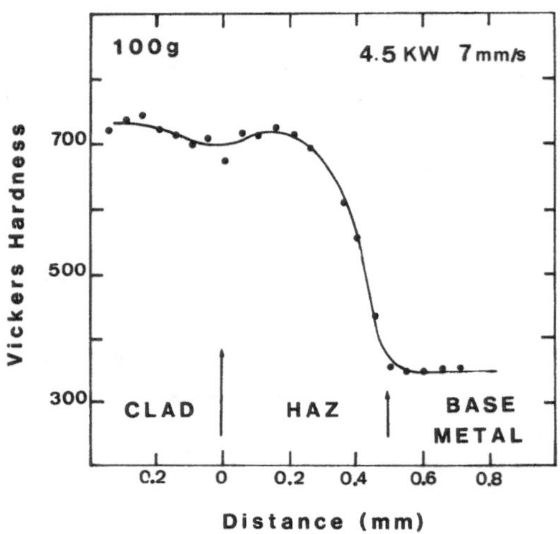

FIGURE 12. Microhardness in the clad layer and the metal near the interface (P = 4.5 kW, V = 7 mm/s).

8. CONCLUSION

An investigation of laser treatments such as hardening, surface melting and cladding of two chromium steels and a low-alloy steel has been performed using various beam shapes with two CO_2 lasers (5 kW and 3 kW).

The laser-hardening treatments have shown the importance of, and the need to have, a suitable energy distribution in the beam to achieve good performances.

It has also been observed that better results were achieved when black paint was used as an absorbing coating. Further, the energy threshold below which no hardening effect is produced was found to depend on the intensity distribution in the beam.

Examination of the residual stresses induced by laser hardening has shown that compressive stresses were produced in the case depth and tensile stresses in the bulk material.

A numerical solution of the three-dimensional heat-conduction equation has been determined for a laser beam with a random intensity distribution. Very good agreement was obtained between the experimental results and the theoretical values.

Results obtained on laser cladding have shown, in particular, the possibility of producing layers which have good metallurgical bonding to the substrate without significant dilution. Further, it was found that the traverse speed has an important influence on the shape of the deposited layer.

REFERENCES

1. G. Maeder, J. L. Lebrun, and J. M. Spranel, "Present Possibilities for the X-ray Diffraction Methods of Stress Measurements, NDT International, 235,247 (1981).
2. L. Barral, J. L. Lebrun, J. Com-Nougué, and E. Kerrand, "Détermination des contraintes résiduelles sur un acier a 12% de chrome traité par laser, SMF Journées d'Automne, 465 (1984).
3. J. Com-Nougué and E. Kerrand, "Laser Transformation Hardening of Chromium Steels: Correlation between Experimental Results and Heat Flow Modeling," ICALEO, Boston (1984), pp. 112,119.
4. H. S. Carslaw and J. C. Jaeger, Conduction of Heat in Solids, Second Edition (Oxford University Press, London, 1978), p. 270.

EDITED QUESTIONS - CHAPTER 5

H. BERGMANN - Monday, 9/9/85

Q. What are some of the processing parameters used on the rocker arm example?
A. Scan speed 1 m/min cold
5 m/min hot
A zig-zag scanning pattern with 60-70% overlap between passes
Total time 20 sec/rocker arm

Q. Why the pile-up of material at edges? Is it a material property or scanning problem?
A. Scan problem. You cannot extend beyond edge of a piece because gravity would induce a flow of material down the side. The laser dwells longer at the end of a scan where it turns around.

Q. Is the roughness at the surface due to incomplete solution of graphite?
A. Yes, you must specify the size of the starting graphite particles in order to control the final surface roughness after laser melting.

Q. Does the fatigue correlate with the residual stress?
A. Yes.

Q. Does the grinding change the fatigue?
A. Yes, you change the stresses.

Q. How does the deviation from symmetry depend on the scanning velocity?
A. The velocity determines the magnitude and direction of the thermal gradients in the piece. Scanning in one direction or both directions changes the symmetry.

Q. Have you studied passivation in the amorphous Fe-Cr-C alloy?
A. Yes, we observed similar properties to melt spun alloys, except that melt spun had a greater amount of pitting.

Q. Did you investigate the influence of an increase in processing speed on the levels of residual stress?
A. Yes, but it's not well understood. Work is continuing in this area.

W. STEEN, Monday, 9/9/85

Q. Does ablation deposition always travel away from the laser toward the surface?
A. Yes, the laser flux is unidirectional and it only ablates the face of the particles the laser hits.

Q. Are you implying that if the substrate doesn't melt, the cladding won't stick?
A. It will stick, but very poorly.

Q. How does one know the absorption coefficient of a particle?
A. The "guessed" absorption coefficient does not affect the overall thermal calculation significantly.

Q. Is it important to control the carrier gas flow in the vicinity near the surface?
A. Yes, the direction of the flow is critical, as shown by the catchment efficiency curve.

Q. Have you attempted cladding with amorphous metal powders?
A. No, (comment - Mordike - yes, they have deposited the powders during pulsed laser melting of surfaces).

Q. Have you measured the thermal shock resistance?
A. Only in a few special cases. None of the samples showed chipping or flaking of the clad.

Q. How does working closely with industry affect graduate student work, especially in regard to (1) deadlines, (2) patents etc., and (3) proprietary material?
A. (1) The students enjoy it but don't enjoy the deadlines imposed. Sometimes the extra money makes it worthwhile.
(2) This is settled prior to the work being done.
(3) If the work is very sensitive, the university is not the place for it. It should go to a contract lab. Without open communication, nothing is gained or learned, which is bad for the student. Also, the security of a university lab cannot be as tight as a contract lab.

Q. Have you tried cladding with oxides such as Al_2O_3?
A. Yes, presently Al_2O_3, in the past SiO_2. The results are mixed depending on the substrate. Cracking can result.

B. MORDIKE, Thursday, 9/12/85

Q. What type of laser was used?
A. A Coherent Everlase model 525, rated at 500 W.

Q. Were the samples exhibited (Fig. 1) used for bending tests?
A. Special tensile rotation-bend and push-pull specimens were used.

Q. When $\beta \rightarrow \alpha$ transformation occurs on cooling. Does it have any effect on the mechanical properties of the layer?
A. Will be explained/discussed later.

Q. In the SEM slide of the nitride (Fig. 2), were the dark regions pores or etching effects?
A. Etching effects.

Q. C.V.D. TiN coatings - are their properties comparable to the laser-formed TiN?
A. We have not directly compared them.

Q. Was nitrogen or ammonia used to form nitrides, and did you have a problem with hydride formation?
A. "Pure" nitrogen in argon was used. To form carbides, methane was used. No hydrides were detected.

Q. Were the oxide samples formed by melting in air or oxygen?
A. Oxygen diluted to 10% in inert gas.

Q. How much overlap on the tracks was used?
A. 70% overlap.

Q. What microhardness load was used? (see graph in Figs. 4, 5 and 6)
A. 0.2 gram.

Q. Were the threads (Fig. 10a) on the samples shown treated?
A. No.

Q. How long does it take to laser process the sample (Fig. 10b)?
A. At 600 W takes 1 min to cover 1 mm^2.

Q. Define ground surface as a starting finish.
A. As received from the factory.

Q. Was acetylene a problem when used for gas alloying? What about oxidation reactions in the path of the laser?
A. "Safe" enough.

Q. Did you find that the Everlase laser was a "good" laser? You appear to get smooth surface finishes - could this laser be used as a general workhorse laser?
A. We had problems in that the laser was designed in America, made in England and serviced in Germany. We had long downtimes.

Q. Titanium oxides are white, nitrides are gold. Why are your samples black?
A. Good question! Only happens in air processed samples.

Q. How do you look for hydrides and what effect do they have on the structure?
A. X-ray techniques detect the hydrides and they have a catastrophic effect on the structure. (Platelets and prismatic planes mentioned!)

Q. Could you comment on surface roughness?
A. We try to obtain surfaces that need no further machining - an example would be car valve seats we have worked on with a German manufacturer.

D. GNANAMUTHU, Wednesday, 9/4/85

Q. Are you aware of silicate coatings used by other investigators?
A. As these are highly absorbing coatings at 10.6 um, they certainly are of interest in other labs. They happen also to be water soluble and hence are easy to apply provided the substrate is clean.

Q. Could you comment on how fatigue properties are measured?
A. We have measured fatigue properties of the specimens using a cantilever bending technique. The specimens were surface hardened using overlapping tracks. Manganese phosphate was used as the energy-absorbing coating.

J. FOLKES, Monday, 9/9/85

Q. What does CLA stand for?
A. Center Line Average

Q. Do you observe cracks in the TiN system?
A. Yes, some cracking was observed.

C. MARSDEN, Monday, 9/9/85

Q. What are the interdendritic phases?
A. They are believed to be a eutectic, M_7C_3.

Q. Have you looked at microprobe analysis of the swirl area?
A. No. However, we may be able to detect changes in chromium concentration.

Q. How does the melt depth compare between the powder injections and coatings?
A. The best coupling was to the coatings, then the powders, and finally the grit-blasted. The melt depths correlate with coupling.

Q. When was liquid nitrogen quenching done (Section 4.3)?
A. At the end of each set of scans, not after each scan.

Q. Do you see any evidence for the formation of amorphous phases?
A. No.

Q. Have you investigated the corrosion properties of the samples?
A. No, but Cr_7C_3 may form which may increase the corrosion susceptibility.

Q. Why not use nitrogen as a cover gas?
A. It is hypothesized that nitrides may form.

E. RAMOUS (First Talk), Monday, 9/7/85

Q. Did the sodium in the water glass coating produce a plasma?
A. Yes.

Q. How did you measure the carbon diffusion length?
A. By the structure. The length was defined as when the carbon concentration goes to 10% of the surface concentration.

Q. Have you seen δ-ferrite in the carburizing of your surface?
A. Yes.

Q. One could think of carbon diffusion driven by a temperature gradient. What do you think your model would say for short interaction times?
A. The model overestimates steady state but we feel that this could be a driving force.

Q. Does the thickness of the carburized coating depend more or less critically on final composition?
A. Yes, along with many other things.

Q. From a practical point of view, for thin coatings, the heat flows into the substrate, not radially. Therefore, the coating will not make up for inhomogeneous beams. Is this correct?
A. Yes.

E. RAMOUS (Second Talk), Monday, 9/9/85

Q. Did you observe similar effects mentioned previously, such as increased hardness in PLM vs. Ti6 etc.?
A. The samples could not be compared because the compositions used were not the same, especially the carbon.

Q. Did you heat the samples after PLM?
A. No, the main goal was to obtain a metastable bainite structure using the laser.

Q. How does the melt size and processing time of the layer obtained compare to TIG etc.?
A. The sizes were 1-1.7 mm for a single pass (depth)
10 mm wide
Did not compare to TIG.

Q. How do you know you don't form bubbles?
A. By the use of shielding gas, since the bubbles come from impurities.

E. KERRAND, Monday, 9/9/85

Q. What is the power loss in the kaleidoscope?
A. Approximately 20-30%.

Q. How were the abs. losses measured?
A. Thermocouple calorimetry.

Q. How do you explain the oscillations in the temperature vs. time plot?
A. The beam is inhomogeneous and is scanned in a direction aligned with the two intensity maxima.

Q. Is it important as to the entry point of the powder relative to the laser/melt puddle?
A. Yes, for our experiments the powder injection follows the beam.

CHAPTER 6 - APPLICATION TO INDUSTRY

CHAPTER INTRODUCTION - C. W. DRAPER

Representatives from three corporations known to be leaders in the application of lasers were invited to this NATO Institute. Their lectures provided great insight, particularly to the non-industry students in attendance, into the many difficulties faced by proponents of laser processing, especially when one tries to actually place that technology on the factory floor.

Dr. La Rocca, from FIAT's Central R&D staff, describes several applications related to increased wear behavior and performance in FIAT automotive engines. He describes a thermal modeling method employed by FIAT engineers to better understand the laser-part-heat flow geometry. In addition, Dr. La Rocca describes the use of the hemispherical reflector in improving the energy utilization of stellite powder cladding to exhaust valves.

Mr. Macintyre of Rolls-Royce has considerable experience with TIG welding, the electron beam and the laser in the field of aircraft engine production. His lecture provided valuable insight into the added difficulties of this industry in overcoming the expense associated with the extensive testing required by governmental aviation authorities. This applies not just to material changes, but also manufacturing changes.

Dr. Roessler of General Motors Research Laboratories presented a broad brush look at the types of applications that have proven to be practical in the automotive industry. Although this text does not contain a paper by Dr. Roessler, we appreciate the time and effort that goes into the preparation of lectures.

All the speakers from industry deserve a special thanks. Permission to speak on areas bordering on the proprietary is often difficult to obtain in the industrial sector. We apreciate that extra effort.

DEVELOPMENTS IN LASER MATERIAL PROCESSING FOR THE AUTOMOTIVE INDUSTRIES

A. V. LA ROCCA
FIAT AUTO, Central Staff, Turin Italy

Key Words: thermal modeling, spherical mirror concentrator, automotive welding

1. NOMENCLATURE

c	=	Specific heat	(joule g^{-1} $°C^{-1}$)
D	=	Thermal diffusion length	(mm)
F	=	Intensity of impinging radiation	(W mm^{-2})
F_o	=	Intensity of absorbed radiation	(W mm^{-2})
K	=	Thermal conductivity	(W mm^{-1} $°C^{-1}$)
ℓ	=	Slab thickness	(mm)
R	=	Reflectivity	(o)
t	=	Time	(sec)
T	=	Temperature	(°C)
z	=	Abscissa in the direction of slab thickness	(mm)
α	=	Thermal diffusivity = $K/\rho c$	(mm^2 sec^{-1})
ρ	=	Mass density	(g mm^{-3})
τ	=	Duration of irradiation	(sec)

2. INTRODUCTION

Of the discoveries of this century the laser stands as one of the most important for the variety and economical impact of its applications. In those related to manufacturing, the object of this talk, the laser is used as a source of electromagnetic radiation possessing an extremely high power density. Therefore, the other characteristics of laser radiation, such as monochromaticity and coherence, are only used indirectly by giving better collimation and focusability to the laser beam, thus making more effective its manipulation by optics (especially of the refracting type, i.e., lenses) and its concentration in very small focusing spots where the awesome power density of the beam can reach extremely high values 10^7-10^9 watt/cm^2.

The very high power density of the beam is translated into a "surface heat source" of similar density when the beam interacts with a material, because it gets absorbed by the material in an extremely thin layer which for metals is of the order of 10^{-6} cm.

This fact is used in all the working processes performed with the laser, which involving heat energies can be called, at least for metals, of the metallurgical kind. The most important work processes are:

- Surface heat treating
  . by phase transition (metallurgical and/or physical)
  . cladding
  . alloying
- Welding
- Cutting
- Drilling
- Deburring
- Assist conventional metal working

By looking first at surface heat treatments, the advantages brought by the laser will become clear. The very high intensities of the heat source, established on the surface by laser beam impingement, translate into high heat fluxes which cause very fast temperature rises and sharp thermal gradients, by which the heat deposition is localized in a region very close to the irradiated surface.

Very fast processing times and unique process properties are obtained because of two effects:

(1) The heat energy is localized where this work has to be performed. Therefore, it is no longer necessary to heat the entire piece to the high temperature required for phase transition. Only a very small percentage of the material (1/1000 to 1/100) needs to be heated. Therefore, the rather low efficiency of the laser (about 10%) becomes irrelevant, and productivity gains by a factor of 10 to 100 become possible.

    Furthermore, and sometimes even more important, when one deals with costly pieces in the semifinished state, by avoiding heat flow into the bulk of the piece, no heat-induced damage occurs. Distortions, cracks or stresses, which otherwise could result in costly reworking or scrapping of the piece, are avoided.

(2) Very high temperature gradients are reached in the treated layer, resulting in greater driving forces. This induces rapid transformation and greatly enhanced material properties. Because the process has been freed of the influence of many outside variables, high quality can be maintained within very strict limits.

In colloquial terms, the laser introduces in the thermal processes the impulsuve phenomena which have proved so useful in all aspects of life involving mechanical forces.

The advantages that the laser brings from an energetic standpoint, which finally translate also in higher productivity, can be seen to apply also to the other processes, even though in a manner less obvious than for the surface treatments.

In welding, the process efficiency, defined as the ratio of the energy needed to make the weld (i.e., heat and melt the metal forming the weld) to the heat lost into the metal by conduction (losses by convection and radiation to the ambient being much smaller), ranges from 5-15% for the conventional processes, the higher values corresponding to those with higher power densities.

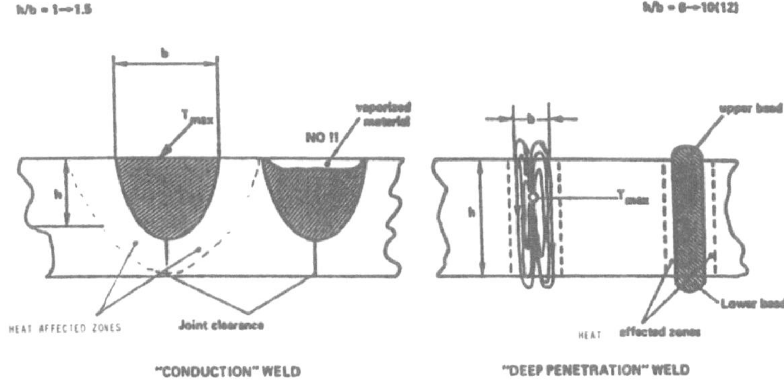

FIGURE 1. The two types of laser welding.

The laser can perform two types of welds (see Fig. 1). The conduction weld is obtained by keeping the heat source on the surface, that is, by avoiding vaporization of the material. In this case, low power densities are used ($< 10^4$ W/cm^2), the weld profile is controlled by heat conduction from the surface into the material, resulting in welds which show an aspect ratio (ratio of depth to width) of order 1 to 1.5. In this case, the heat-affected zone on the sides of the weld might be as thick as half the weld or more.

By increasing the power density (10^5-10^6 W/cm^2), a drastic change in the type of weld achievable with the laser occurs. The aspect ratio becomes much higher (5-12), the thickness of the heat-affected region decreases to a fraction of the weld width (1/4-1/6). This indicates a large increase in process efficiency in spite of the fact that by increasing the power density, part of the material has been vaporized and some of this vapor has been excited and ionized (processes energywise much more expensive than melting, respectively, ten and a hundred times more).

The answer for the increased efficiency, which now may range as high as 85 to 90%, has to be sought in some other intervening phenomena which drastically changed the mechanism of heat conduction to the metal surrounding the weld. These phenomena are made possible by the very high power density and the ensuing extremely fast heat fluxes in the material. The extremely high temperature gradient established between the central core of ionized material, through the surrounding excited, overheated vapor and overheated melted material, causes fast impulsive motions.

A pattern of mass flow in a circulatory, antisymmetrical motion (with respect to the axis of the weld cross section) is forced in the weld cavity (the so-called keyhole), causing heat to be transferred within it in the manner of a heat pipe, that is, by mass and latent heats of phase transformations. In this case, besides melting and vaporization, excitation and ionization processes are by far much larger. Thus those phenomena which were thought to be a source of loss prove to be essential to the high efficiency of the process. Also, it becomes clear that most of the ionized, excited and overheated vapor must be recovered in the weld cavity and only a very small part (less than 1%) lost into the ambient.

The resulting effect of the extremely high "equivalent conductivity" established in the weld cavity is to make the surrounding metal appear as having a very low conductivity and thus to perform as an insulator, thereby reducing the heat flow to the bulk of the material (see Fig. 2).

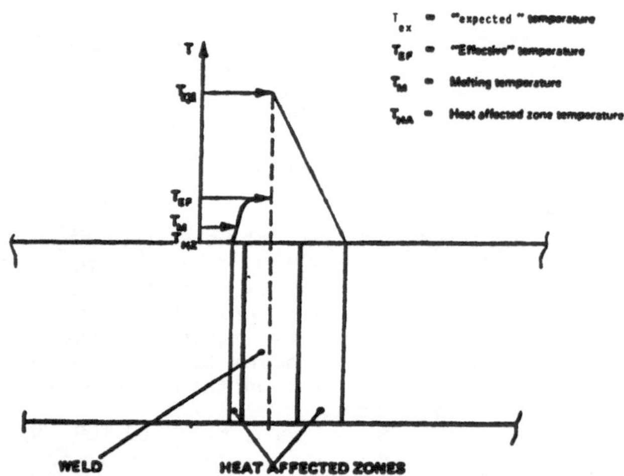

FIGURE 2. The postulated reasons for the improved efficiency of the deep penetration welding.

The postulated effects arising from and increased heat absorbance with heat sinks represented by the change of phase latent heats:

- The sensible heat, that is the one measurable in terms of an "expected temperature" T_E for a given power intensity F is depressed significantly to the "effective" temperature T_{EF}.
- A large "effective" conductivity is obtained in cavity by transport of mass and latent heats of phase changes.
- The higher capability of absorbing and conducting heat established, at a sustained sufficiently high T_{EF}, in the molten region cause reflections of the temperature front from the solid region. Less heat is transmitted compared to that of a material with uniform material properties under the same slope of the temperature profile.

This is the mechanism by which much higher (5 to 8 times) energy efficiency is achieved in the deep penetration laser welding in comparison to conventional welding. But the energy efficiency refers to the unit mass of the weld. Thus for making a proper comparison, the energy efficiencies must be multiplied by the aspect ratio of the welds obtainable by the different methods. Therefore, it becomes easy to justify the claims in greater productivity ranging up to 30 times that of conventional methods, as stated by authoritative users such as the U.S. Naval Research Laboratory and the U.S. Navy F.M.C. facility, among others.

Because increased productivity by a factor less than two already fosters equipment replacement in conventional production facilities, the incredibly high productivity increases made possible by laser processing lead to the expectation that they will have a revolutionary effect on all aspects of production on which they might impact. These expectations are reinforced by the fact that the increases in productivity come along with a host of very significant advantages, the most important of which are the following:

Advantages of laser processing

- Improvements in product quality.
- Reduction in material and processing costs.
- High productivity.
- Improved environmental conditions (by reducing or eliminating noise, fumes, lubricating and refrigerating fluids, chips, etc.).
- Flexibility, controllability and easy automation of the processing tool (laser beam) and of the production system (eventually multistation) incorporating the laser.
- Capability of performing the metallurgical processing at the very stations of the mechanical working line (with great implications on logistics, work and space savings).
- Capability of easily being incorporated in the first flexible manufacturing complexes.

The reasons for these advantages follow from the characteristics of the laser beam as a working tool hereafter described.

Characteristics of the laser beam as a working tool

1. Transfers energy fluxes of extremely high intensity.
2. Acts at a distance and in the ambient atmosphere; conversely, it can be applied, through an appropriate window, to a workpiece in vacuum.
3. Applies its energy to any surface which is optically reachable.
4. Saves processing energy.
5. Eliminates or reduces the damage caused by dispersion of thermal energy in the workpiece.
6. Reduces or eliminates post processing finishing operations (also because it does not cause vibrations).
7. Performs as an unwearable or self-restoring tool.
8. Performs in a "clean" manner (no noise, fumes, dust, chips, lubricating/refrigerating fluids, vibration, etc.).
9. Possesses no inertial mass, thus a quick response to command (intensity, position, shape of the beam).

10. Does not require, in order to apply its energy, the motion of mechanical means of sufficient mass and rigidity to ensure precision and efficiency to the process.
11. Is ideally suited for automation.
12. Renders the metallurgical processes, often today the most troublesome and "off line," compatible with mechanical work stations and lines.

These advantages explain why the laser is sometimes used advantageously even at the level of power obtainable from conventional sources (e.g., arc torch, plasma torch, etc.).

In conclusion, the advantages that the laser brings to material processing are many and significant. Furthermore, they interact synergistically, making it unnecessary to strive for the maximization of a single advantage (say: the productivity increase).

Instead, it must be emphasized that in studying the introduction of each application, use must be made of "system engineering criteria" to properly evaluate the total impact of the many and often not obvious implications. They might prove elusive, inasmuch as they require the acquisition of a new perspective on the ways of producing and also designing the product, as well as reorganizing the layout and the procedures of the production plant. This perspective is quite often different from the current ones and becomes possible only after the introduction of the new tool.

Thus a significant revolution also at the level of the entire production system (comprising the product and the production facilities) could be a consequence of laser technology having really "stepped into" the mass production industries, and foremost among them the automotive industries.

Some very successful applications have already opened the way. As an illustration of one of them, Fig. 3 taken from LaRocca (1) shows the fully automated multi-station laser systems used by FIAT AUTO at the Mirafiori plant for the welding of several types of syncro gears. A number of these systems take care of almost the total production of such parts. In several years of industrial use, significant improvements in part quality, performance, cost savings, and the practical elimination of scraps have resulted.

3. THE ACTIVITIES IN FIAT AUTO

The FIAT AUTO S.p.A. has been one of the first European corporations to foresee the importance of laser technology since the early seventies.

After a period of intensive collaboration with laboratories abroad, foremost among them the AVCO Everett Laboratory in the USA, FIAT proceeded in establishing its own Laser Laboratory Center at C.R.F. (Centro Ricerche Fiat) in Orbassano, a Turin suburb, equipping it with an AVCO HPL - 15 kW CO_2 laser source, around which was constructed a multistation processing facility. Fiat was also very active in promoting the starting of a National High Power Laser Program under the sponsorship of the C.N.R. (Centro Nazionale delle Ricerche), participating in the activities of the program since its onset in 1978. For this purpose another laser application center was established at the R.T.M. Institute (Istituto Ricerche Tecnologiche Meccaniche) in Vico Canavese, at that time jointly held in equal parts by FIAT, Olivetti and Finmeccanica. Also, this center was equipped with an AVCO HPL - laser source of 15 kW, and complemented with a multi-station processing setup and several other

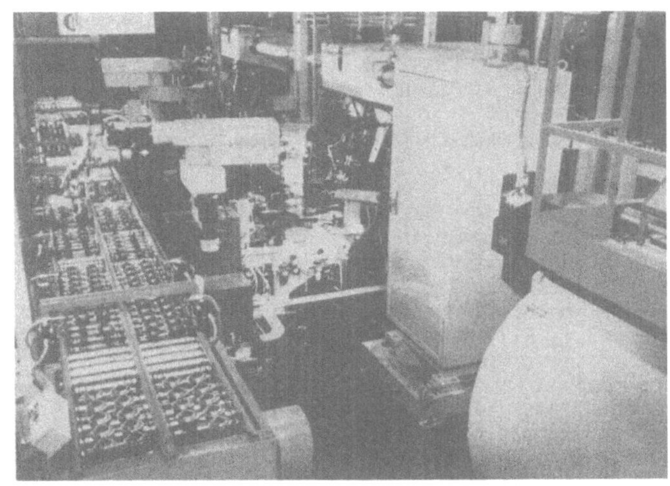

FIGURE 3. The two-station, fully automated, robot-served laser system built by Comau, for the welding of Synchro-gears for FIAT AUTO, S.p.A., shown in operation at FIAT Mirafiori Plant, Turin, Italy.

laser sources. This facility became the High Power Laser Application Center of the National C.N.R. Laser Program.

The development activities in the technology were conducted by FIAT with its own funds, with applied research funds of the I.M.I. (Italian Mobiliary Institute) and with C.N.R. funds. Both the C.R.F. and R.T.M. facilities were used, while active collaboration was established with the other governmental, university and industrial research institutes.

Foremost among them are the CISE of Segrate - Milano, the Universities of Turin, Padova, Naples, Bologna, the C.S.M. (Centro Studi Metallurgici) etc.

The activities conducted by FIAT have been wide ranging to cover all the significant aspects of this new and very complex technology.

Among them one can list:

- Physico-mathematical models of the time-dependent, unsteady thermal fields established in the material by interaction with the laser beam.
- Theoretical and experimental studies of laser material interaction of the mechanism of plume generation and of the ensuing energy partition of laser beam power among the intervening processes.
- The effects and the methods of gaseous shielding of the parts to be treated; methods and devices for mass additions for some laser processes.
- Methods and devices for real time "on line" diagnostics of beam characteristics while processing at full power.

- Methods and devices for utilization of beam reflection and scattering for process enhancement and diagnostic.
- The development of the various laser processes for several parts and components brought to the point of giving specifications for industrial applications.
- The definition of complete laser processing system specifications.
- The construction, installation and operation of laser processing systems in the production lines.

We will deal briefly with only some of them.

4. THERMAL FIELD MODELING

A normalized solution has been formulated for the one-dimensional heat equation for the case of no internal sources nor skins, and with only a flux of intensity F_0 entering at $z = 0$. The form of this solution becomes quite effective because of the reference made to the unique and unequivocal process parameter which is the duration τ of the heating phase; soon it will become evident that this parameter also sets the conditions for the subsequent cooling phase.

To it correspond particularly meaningful values of the field variables (temperature and its derivates, depth, etc.) to which it is appropriate to refer. For example, a physical parameter of particular importance is the maximum temperature obtained at the surface at time τ. Also, particularly important is the diffusion length at time D_τ.

$$D_\tau = 2\sqrt{\alpha\tau} \tag{1}$$

and consequentially also the ratios:

$$z_n = \frac{z}{D_\tau} \tag{2}$$

$$t_n = \frac{t}{\tau} \tag{3}$$

Thus using a most simple normalization criteria, that is, by making the ratio of homogeneous physical quantities, starting from the most meaningful, i.e.:

$$T_n = \frac{T(z,t)}{T(o,\tau)} = \frac{\text{current temperature}}{\text{maximum temperature}} \tag{4}$$

and using the pertinent normalized variables of Eqs.(1-4), one can write a complete normalized field solution over the entire duration of the process as:

$$T_n = \sqrt{\pi}\sqrt{t_n}\left\{\text{ierfc}\left\{\frac{z_n}{\sqrt{t_n}}\right\} - \sqrt{t_n - 1}\;\text{ierfc}\left\{\frac{z_n}{\sqrt{t_n - 1}}\right\}\right\} \tag{5}$$

of which the graphical representation in the (T_n, t_n) plane is given in Fig. 4.

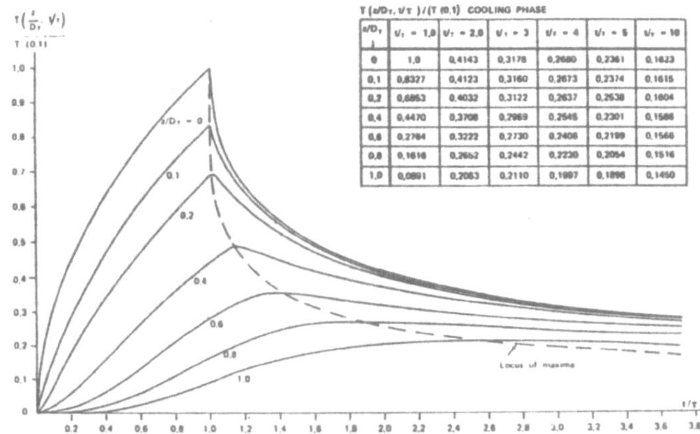

T (z/Dτ, t/τ)/(T (0,1) COOLING PHASE

z/Dτ	t/τ = 1,0	t/τ = 2,0	t/τ = 3	t/τ = 4	t/τ = 5	t/τ = 10
0	1,0	0,4143	0,3178	0,2680	0,2361	0,1623
0,1	0,8327	0,4123	0,3160	0,2673	0,2374	0,1615
0,2	0,6853	0,4032	0,3122	0,2637	0,2538	0,1604
0,4	0,4470	0,3708	0,2969	0,2545	0,2301	0,1586
0,6	0,2784	0,3222	0,2730	0,2406	0,2199	0,1566
0,8	0,1616	0,2662	0,2442	0,2230	0,2054	0,1516
1,0	0,0891	0,2063	0,2110	0,1997	0,1896	0,1450

FIGURE 4. The semi-infinite thickness slab normalized solution: heating and cooling phases.

Because of the normalization criteria employed, this diagram acquires universal significance in describing the one-dimensional thermal flow field for any homogeneous, isotropic material, of which the physical properties are maintained constant over the entire process duration and for whatever value of the incoming flux F_0, constant over the heating duration.

Looking at the cooling phase, one can see that it is conditioned by the heating duration τ, which sets all the initial values.

All the cooling curves for various z_n tend asymptotically to zero for t_n tending to infinity. Thus they show a tendency to converge; this is already quite noticeable for $t_n = 10$. Quantitatively, this is reported in the table within Fig. 4.

Starting from the singular point ($z_n = 0$, $t_n = 1$) which corresponds to the absolute maximum value of the temperature, a dashed curve originates which is the locus of the relative maxima for the z_n = const curves and is given by the equation:

$$z_n = \sqrt{\frac{1}{2} t_n(t_n - 1) \ln \left\{\frac{t_n}{t_n - 1}\right\}} \tag{6}$$

This curve, which tends to ∞ for $t_n \rightarrow 1$, exists only for times subsequent to the end of the irradiation. It shows that at the right side of the vertical line $t_n = 1$, exists a region, which is that below the curve, where the material continues to be heated. Only the region above the curve undergoes cooling.

The curve marks a boundary between two regions which are experiencing contrasting thermal stresses. The pertaining amount of mass involved and energy released, the tensional and elastoplastic properties, the average temperature of the two regions evolve differently with time, causing in the immediate neighborhood of the curve a dangerous situation, in which contrasting stresses of thermal and metallurgic nature can cause microcracks and singular morphologies of the microstructure.

The zone deserves to be studied with attention, using for example computer programs capable to analyze thermal and metallurgical stresses, and using as first input data, those of the thermal field.

5. THE NOMOGRAM

In performing heat treatments by laser, some of the conditions imposed for performing the process are often not explicit. As a consequence, their implications in forcing unique solutions in the ensuing thermal field are not clearly perceived. As a matter of course in obtaining desired characteristics at the surface ($z = 0$) and of the treated layer up to a depth z_l of the piece, specific values of the temperature are prescribed at these two values of z. The imposition of two conditions to be simultaneously reached at the time of the irradiation, makes the system (considering all equations, including those of the imposed conditions) become determined with the duration τ of the irradiation serving as the independent variable. The connection which is binding together the system of equations lends itself to be represented in the form of a nomogram quite useful to clarify their interaction by putting in evidence the logical path by them implied.

The nomogram is illustrated in Fig. 5. The path to be followed is that of the line marked with arrows, which starts from the first quadrant. From it, for each value of the ratio between the temperature

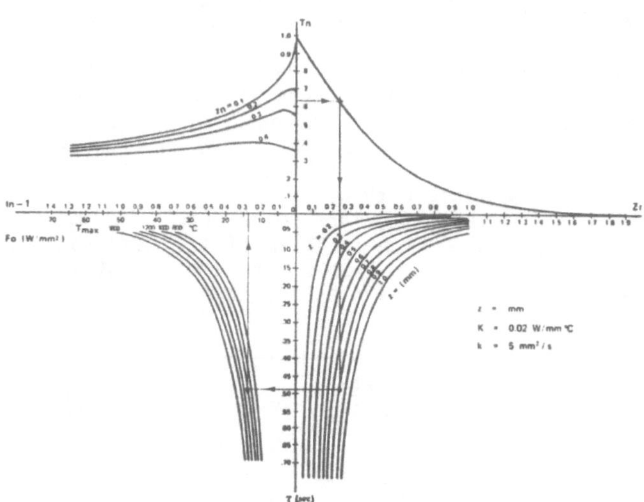

FIGURE 5. The nomogram for the semi-infinite thick slab.

reached at the end of the irradiation at the surface $T(0,\tau)$ and that $T(z_1,\tau)$ reached at a prescribed depth z_1, can be obtained a single value of the depth number (z_1/D_τ). In turn, in the second quadrant this parameter allows determination of a single value of the irradiation time τ, by reading the thickness z_1 in mm on a family of curves in which the proper physical constant properties of the prescribed material have been introduced. In the third quadrant the value of τ determines the incoming flux F_0(W cm^{-2}), which is obtained by reading the prescribed maximum surface temperature $T(0,\tau)$ in °C on the family of curves which has been evaluated using the given physical properties of the material. The fourth quadrant reproduces in the plane (T_n, t_n) the part relative to the cooling phase of the diagram of Eq.(5) previously discussed and illustrated in Fig. 4. It binds together the temperature and the normalized times $t/\tau > 1$ to the conditions reached at the end of the irradiation.

Because of the fact that for a given material this path is unique, the results depend on the initial point, that is, on the selection of the temperatures which have to be simultaneously reached for two values of z ($z = 0$, $z = z_1$) at the time τ.

Passing now to consider the cooling phase, one can say, first of all, that it has to take place in times short enough to obtain, in the entire region to be treated, the desired phase transitions. For example, in the case of iron alloys, the material has to be brought above the temperature T_{AC} for austenite transformation, and then cooled quickly enough to reach the appropriate temperature (M_F, M_S) for martensite transformation, without intersecting in the T.T.T. (Temperature, Time, Transformation) diagram the C.C.T. (Continuous Cooling Transformation) curves, or the Bain curves, obtained by an instantaneous temperature drop followed by an isotherm transformation.

Thus in the fourth quadrant can be placed metallurgical curves such as in Fig. 6, where the nomogram is presented with non-normalized temperatures in the first and fourth quadrant, the latter having also the τ time given in sec. In this manner it is easier to place the Bain or C.C.T. curves pertinent to the material, the properties of which had been used to evaluate the curves of the second and third quadrants. Also to be noticed is that in Fig. 6 the cooling curves are given only for the surface, each one for the corresponding maximum temperature, while in Fig. 5 they are given for various normalized depths z/D_τ.

One can see how for times of irradiation $\tau > 1.5$ sec. the C.C.T. curves, which are given in terms of τ, start to be intersected by the surface cooling curves, showing that in these cases it is impossible to obtain self hardening of the material.

The usefulness of the nomogram comes first in giving insight into the interrelations existing between operational parameters and process results, with a first link to the metallurgical phenomena which are conditioning those results. As such, it is also useful in giving, with satisfactory approximation, quantitative information on the self-hardening depth obtainable for the various materials and corresponding windows of the operational parameters.

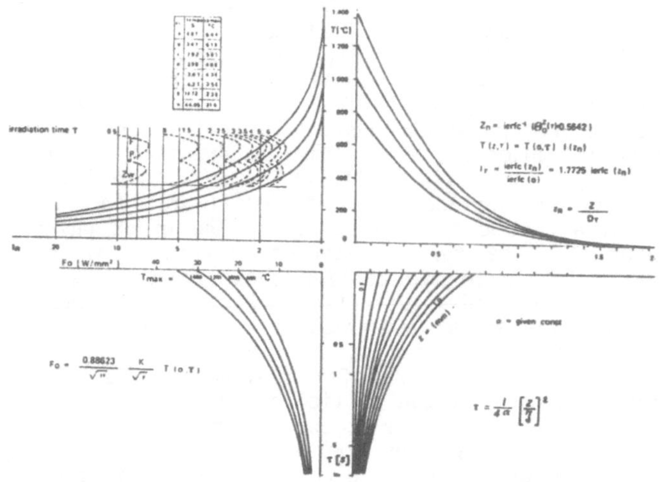

FIGURE 6. The nomogram for the semi-infinite thickness slab.

6. THE FINITE THICKNESS SLAB

When the thickness becomes finite, i.e., smaller or comparable to the value of thermal diffusion length $D = 2\sqrt{\alpha t}$, the flow conditions are changed. In the finite slab the flow is stopped by the back surface and reflected back. Thus while the field equation remains unchanged, the boundary conditions need to be modified, changing the second in z, now written for $z = \ell$

$$\begin{aligned} F_o(t) &= -K \frac{\partial T}{\partial z} \qquad \text{for } z = 0 \\ 0 &= -K \frac{\partial T}{\partial z} \qquad \text{for } z = \ell \end{aligned} \tag{7}$$

the change in boundary conditions is sufficient to alter the solution given in Eq.(5) into (2)

$$T(z,t) = T(z,t)\Big|_{\ell=\infty} + \frac{F_o D}{K} \sum_{n=1}^{\infty} \left\{ \text{ierfc}\left(\frac{2n\ell - z}{D}\right) + \text{ierfc}\left(\frac{2n\ell + z}{D}\right) \right\} \tag{8}$$

Thus the new solution is given by two terms: The first can be recognized as that for the semiinfinite thickness case; the second performs as a corrective term $B(z,t)$ given as an infinite series. The physics of the situation will clarify that there is no problem in dealing with it, being naturally truncated by implicit conditions.

It is easy to understand that the basic physical difference occurring in the finite thickness case is that the temperature front, blocked by the adiabatic back face, is made to bounce back and forth between the two faces. The corrective terms describe these reflections, $\beta(o,t)$ from the front face, $\beta(\ell,t)$ from the back face.

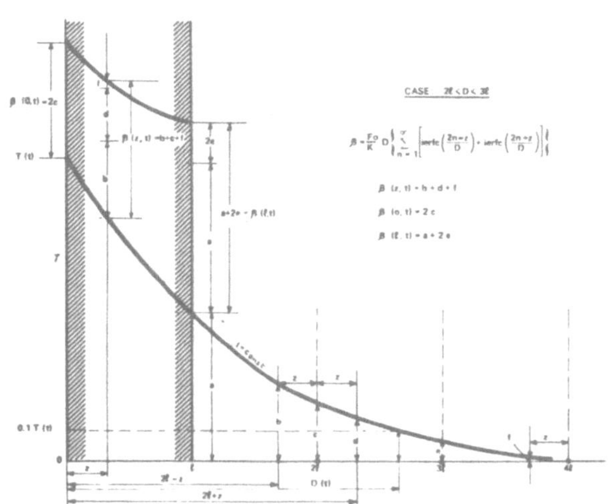

FIGURE 7. The corrective term ß for the finite thickness solution.

A graphical construction which brings back within the slab the area under that portion of the infinite solution curve which extends beyond ℓ is given in Fig. 7. From it, it is easy to see how the boundary conditions are automatically respected at the faces. The equations for the normalization vs. $T(0,\tau)_\infty$ and z/D_τ can be written, extended also for the cooling phase, following the procedure used in treating the semi-infinite thickness case. In this manner one gets:

$$T_n = \sqrt{\pi}\ \sqrt{t_n}\left\{\text{ierfc}\left(\frac{z_n}{\sqrt{t_n}}\right) + \sum_{n=1}^{\infty}\left[\text{ierfc}\left(\frac{2n\ell_n - z_n}{\sqrt{t_n}}\right) + \text{ierfc}\left(\frac{2n\ell_n + z_n}{\sqrt{t_n}}\right)\right]\right\} \tag{9}$$

$$- \sqrt{\pi}\ \sqrt{t_n - 1}\left\{\text{ierfc}\left(\frac{z_n}{\sqrt{t_n - 1}}\right) + \sum_{n=1}^{\infty}\left[\text{ierfc}\left(\frac{2n\ell_n - z_n}{\sqrt{t_n - 1}}\right) + \text{ierfc}\left(\frac{2n\ell_n + z_n}{\sqrt{t_n - 1}}\right)\right]\right\}$$

where the following short notations for the normalized parameters have been used:

$$\ell_n = \frac{\ell}{D_\tau}\ ; \qquad t_n = \frac{t}{\tau}\ ; \qquad z_n = \frac{z}{D_\tau}\ ; \qquad T_n = \frac{T(z,t)}{T(0,\tau)_\infty}$$

The equation gives in the plane T_n, t_n, a family of normalized curves parametric in ℓ_n. Some are illustrated in Fig. 8.

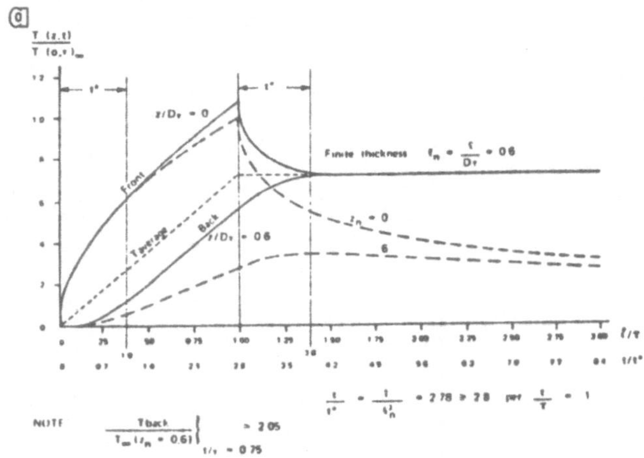

FIGURE 8a. The normalized $(T/T_{max})_\infty$ vs. (t/τ) diagrams for semi-infinite E thin plates.

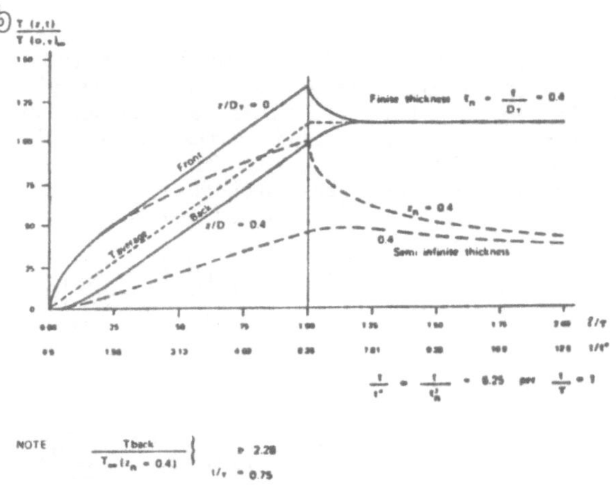

FIGURE 8b. The normalized $(T/T_{max})_\infty$ vs. (t/τ) diagrams for semi-infinite E thin plates.

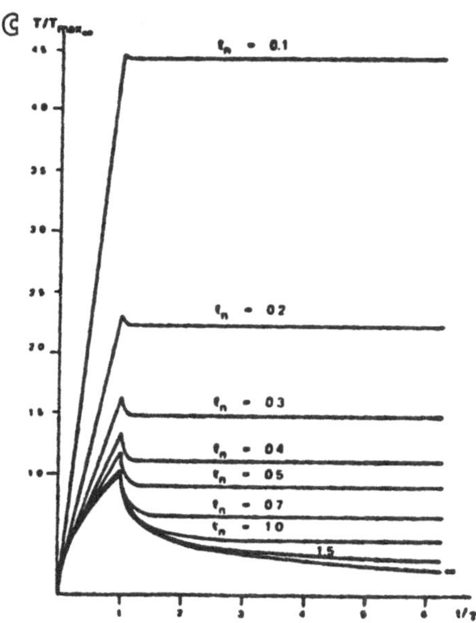

FIGURE 8c. The normalized $(T/T_{max})_{\infty}$ vs. (t/τ) diagrams for semi-infinite E thin plates.

From considerations ensuing from the energy conservation imposed by the adiabatic back face, these statements can be made:

(1) There exists for the workpiece, an average temperature $\bar{T}(t)$ at time t, and a corresponding average heating rate $\dot{\bar{T}}$, independent of t, given as:

$$T = \frac{F_o t}{\rho c \ell} ; \qquad \dot{T} = \frac{F_o}{\rho c \ell} \tag{10}$$

(2) The solution will become quasi steady, i.e., the temperature profile will no longer change with z but only with time. While the character of the equation indicates that this condition will be reached exactly for $t \rightarrow \infty$, it also can be shown that approximations quite acceptable for engineering purposes are obtained for times which correspond to ratios $\ell/D = 1$.

(3) Because energy in the form of sensible heat is absorbed by the piece, the temperature profile must be curved. The divergence constant in the z curve will be a parabola.

(4) Hence a parabolic profile will be established within the slab and it will translate in the T direction without changing in shape. This means that each of its points will move with the same heating time rate, which must be the previously defined $\dot{T}$ mean average heating time rate.

(5) The parabolic profile implies also a constant temperature difference between front and back faces; that is, proportional to F_0/K while the $\dot{T}$ is proportional to $F_0/\rho c$. Hence the possibility of separating the physical constants and corresponding effects.

Hence the properties of the temperature profile constructed in Fig. 7 are now understood. It can be argued that it is advantageous to select for the time t^* at which a constant temperature time rate is obtained (and correspondingly a parabolic temperature profile get established within the slabs) the time at which $D^* = \ell$ or $t^* = \ell^2/4\alpha$.

In this case the expression for the parabolic profile becomes:

$$T_n^*\left\{\frac{z}{\lambda}, \frac{t}{t^*}\right\} = \frac{\sqrt{\pi}}{2}\left\{\left\{\frac{z}{\ell}\right\}^2 - 2\frac{z}{\ell}\right\} + \frac{T(o,t)}{T(o,\tau)_\infty} \tag{11}$$

and the difference between front and back face temperatures is found to be:

$$\Delta T\Big]_{z/\ell=1}^{z/\ell=0} = \frac{\sqrt{\pi}}{2} = 0.8862 \tag{12}$$

of which two thirds are given by the difference between front face temperature and mean temperature

$$\Delta T\Big]_{z/\ell=0.4226}^{z/\ell=0} = \frac{2}{3}\frac{\sqrt{\pi}}{2} = \frac{\sqrt{\pi}}{3} \tag{13}$$

and one third between average and back face temperature

$$\Delta T\Big]_{z/\ell=1}^{z/\ell=0.4226} = \frac{1}{3}\frac{\sqrt{\pi}}{2} = \frac{\sqrt{\pi}}{6} \tag{14}$$

where the properties of the parabola allow to write the value of z/ℓ corresponding to $\bar{T}$ as $\bar{z}/\ell = 0.4226$.

Thus the temperature vs. time is given for $t > t^*$ by three parallel lines with angular coefficient $\sqrt{\pi}/4$, that is the one of the $\bar{T}$ line. The Fig. 9 shows the behavior of the finite slab in the (T_n^*, t_n^*) plane and the nomenclature used.

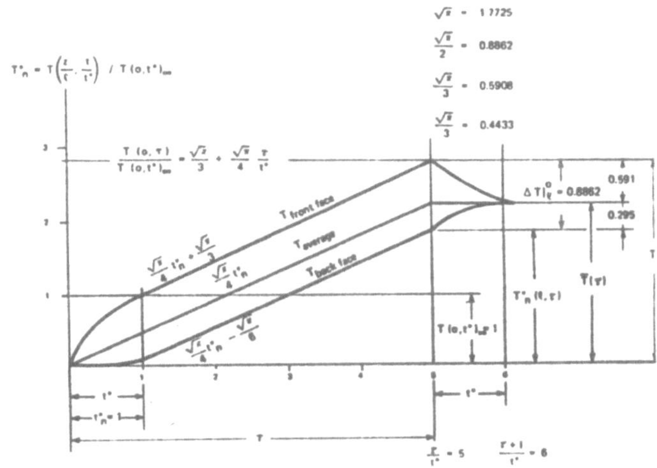

FIGURE 9. The nomenclature of the finite thickness slab solution in the (T_n^*, t_n^*) plane.

It is illustrated also the cooling phase when $t/\tau > 1$, τ being the duration of the heating phase. It can be observed how the front and back face tend to the average temperature $\bar{T}(\tau)$ reached and time τ, which will stay constant from there on, if the adiabatic and one dimensionality will apply to the case at hand. In such a case, the average temperature will be reached with good approximation in an additional time t^* following the end of the irradiation τ. The approximation will become extremely good (within the thickness of the line) at a time $\tau + 1.5\ t^*$.

7. HARDENING OF SMALL THICKNESS PARTS

The model has been useful in giving a better insight into the problems encountered in the hardening of contoured parts of small thickness such as gear and rack teeth. First of all, the reflections of the heat transient at the back face cause more than a doubling of the temperature with respect to that experienced at the same depth in a part of semi-infinite thickness. Because of this, the material would undergo annealing in case of non-simultaneous treatment of the two sides. Meanwhile at the front face a higher temperature is reached which can cause local melting. More critical yet is the fact that a much slower rate of cooling is experienced by the part. Because in judging the selection of the operating parameters much more attention is given to what happens at the front face of the piece, one may be easily led to a wrong path by being made to think of going to lower power density, which unavoidably forces longer interaction times. The result is to push the part in a metallurgical situation where no self-hardening is possible. This unpleasant situation may persist even by changing to more easily hardened materials (for example, with a higher carbon content), because the self-cooling rates have gone quite out of range.

To escape the difficulties arising from this situation one has to pay great attention to the irradiation time which has to be quite short. It becomes the true controlling parameter, determining, for a given material, if self-hardening can occur and over what depth, and for heat symmetry reasons, the necessity of simultaneously treating the front and back surface of the pieces.

As an illustrative example, one could go back and look at the case of Fig. 8a for $\ell_n = 0.4$, $\tau/t^* = 6.25$. The normalized temperature vs. t^* time diagram shows that at the end of the irradiation the front temperature is about 1.35 times that of the semi-infinite case (thus very likely causing surface melting), while the back surface has reached a temperature about 2.3 times that experienced at an equivalent depth $z/D_\tau = 0.4$ in a semi-infinite thick plate. Furthermore, in the cooling phase both faces tend to the average temperature which is reached in a time $\sim t^*$ following the end of irradiation. Because of its value in the case of the example, if the adiabatic conditions are really enforced and the one-dinensional hypothesis for the heat flow is valid, no self hardening is possible.

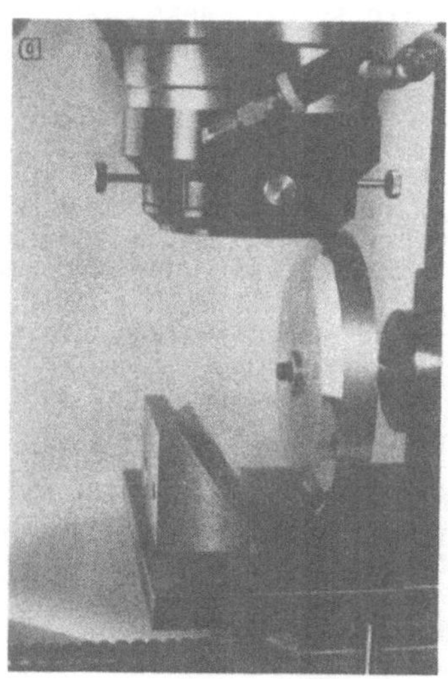

FIGURE 10. The apparatus to treat simultaneously the two sides of a rack tooth (work conducted at T.R.M. Institute, Vico Canavese, Italy, with the collaboration of Cantello M., Monico A., Manino A. and als). (a) The focusing head, the 45° beam bending mirror, and the rotating multifaced mirror giving the oscillating sweeping motion to the beam.

The tooth face must be swept along its width by a laser spot of appropriate power intensity distribution and size, to solve the problem of obtaining short irradiation times and eventual pre-heating. To do this, special optical devices, such as the one shown in Fig. 10, must be

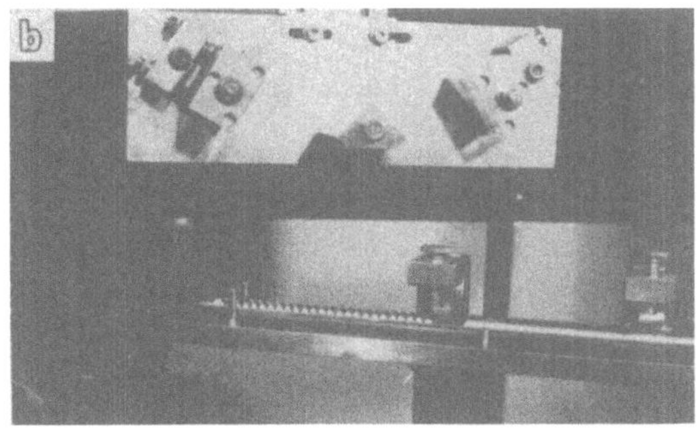

FIGURE 10. (b) The beam splitting mirrors directing the oscillating sweeping beam spots on the tooth faces.

used. It employs a multifaceted rotating mirror which produces an alternating motion of the beam. Two such mirrors symmetrically placed with respect to beam splitting and reflecting mirrors, can treat simultaneously the two faces of the rack teeth while the rack is actuated by a simple uniform translational motion. Such a device is depicted in Fig. 10. The hardness profile and the macro showing the treated region of such a tooth is given in Fig. 11. Hardened cases of 50-55 Rc for 0.5 mm thickness have been obtained with auto steering racks of C-45 steel. The implications of these developments on the hardening of small module gears are significant and relate to material substitution (less costly, more workable) and processing cost reductions, stemming from simplified logistics, elimination of large, costly and energy-wasteful installations, damaged parts reprocessing and scrap elimination.

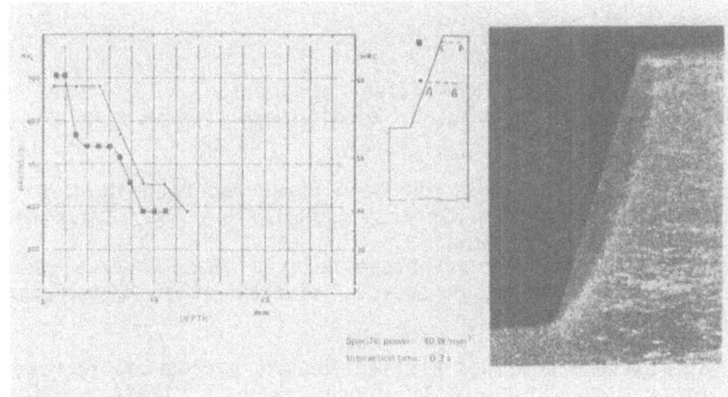

FIGURE 11. The hardness profile at two heights of a treated tooth and the macro snowing the treated region (work conducted at R.T.M. Institute, Vico Canavese, Italy, with the collaboration of Cantello M., Monico A., Manino A. and als).

8. MEANS FOR RECOVERING THE BEAM POWER REFLECTED AND SCATTERED BY THE WORKPIECE

Several advantages can be obtained by such means. Basically, they consist of a mirror-surfaced cavity which encloses the laser beam material interaction region. This cavity in the most general case must be a hemisphere, possessing a small hole through which the beam enters.

Classical optics can be used for describing the property of such a device which greatly increases the absorption of the workpiece surface by performing as a sort of a black body. The curves of Fig. 12, taken from work of C. Ferrari, of FIAT CRF, Orbassano, Italy, show that the effective absorption depends on the value of the mirror reflectivity, workpiece absorption coefficient, and typical ratio of the hole to the hemisphere areas.

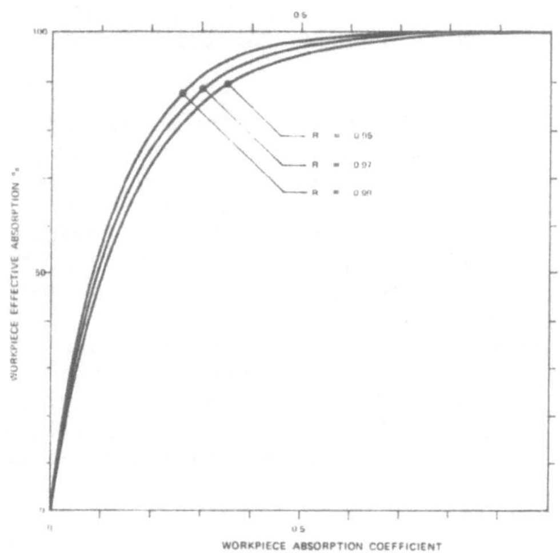

FIGURE 12. Workpiece effective absorption coefficient for various reflectivities "R" of the power recovery cavity surface.

By using such devices, the beam power has been shown to increase by a factor larger than three in treating aluminum and larger than two in the cladding of powdered stellite.

Besides the obvious advantage derived from a large reduction in the power needs of the laser source, several other significant advantages result:

(1) The surface coatings applied for the purpose of increasing the workpiece absorption are no longer needed. Their application constitutes additional steps with associated times and costs; moreover, they have been found to be responsible for some undesirable effects on the metallurgical and ensuing mechanical and fatigue handling properties of the treated parts.

(2) The processing of otherwise difficult to treat materials such as aluminum, brass, copper, etc. is made possible.

(3) Laser beam retroreflection in the laser cavity can be avoided by using non-orthogonal impingement of the beam. Degraded laser performance during processing may be induced by such reflections.

(4) Of particular relevance for surface treatment is the fact that more uniform power density distribution can be obtained in the working area; the device performs an integrating function.

(5) By spreading the working area on which redirected beam power is recovered, pre- and post-heating can be performed, significantly improving the processing quality (elimination of micro cracks, porosities; and achievement of smoother surface conditions, which in the limit may be mirror like, if formed from a liquid phase).

(6) Means of material addition can be easily incorporated in the device enhancing their performance. Of these means, those using the material in the form of powders have proved to be most effective, because of the unique combination of transparency and very high equivalent absorption of the material in that form.

(7) Means for monitoring the workpiece surface conditions can be easily incorporated in the device.

(8) Means for better use and control of the gas employed for workpiece and mirror protection can be advantageously incorporated in the device.

The beam energy recovery has been employed in the stellite cladding of exhaust valves of FIAT AUTO engines using the apparatus schematically illustrated in Fig. 13. It includes the feeding of the stellite powder carried by a bed of appropriate gases, used also to fill the cavity of the energy recovery apparatus. The feeding of the material in powder form has proven to be the most promising approach, by solving most of the problems which had been encountered in all of the previously tried approaches. They employed various types of alloys (S. F-6, F., G., 12 etc.) procured from more than one source, and various feeding means, according to the form of the material, such as: rods, wires, synthesized disks and rings, scurries and pastes.

The better absorptivity and transparency of the powder, the absence of a binder, the presence of a protective gas, eliminate the formation of porosity, reduce the power requirement, and by allowing pre-heating of the valve surface, reduce the amount of material used in the process. These effects are enhanced by the energy recovery apparatus, which has permitted reduction of the energy requirements by over 50%.

The laser cladding with the energy recovery scheme has been performed at 1.8 kW with a Spectra Physics 973 laser, using powdered stellite F and 13 sec. processing time. Previously, the valves were laser treated using an AVCO HPL laser at 6.5 kW and 8 sec. processing time. The laser-treated valves have undergone metallurgical, X-ray and ultrasonic inspections, element distribution mapping and to check the adhesion of the cladded material, thermal shock testing. Similar testing has been conducted on the T.I.G. cladded valves.

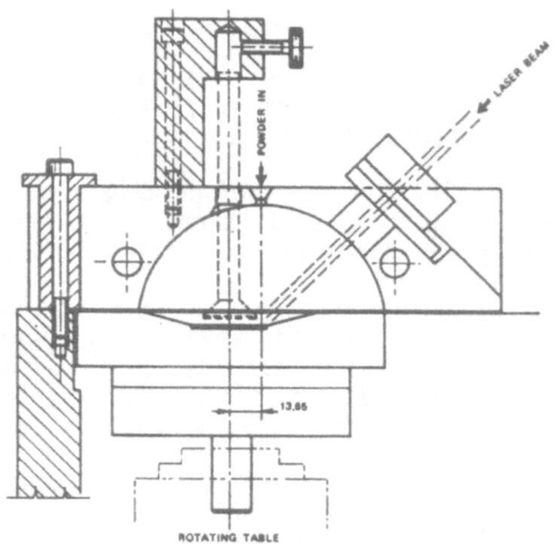

FIGURE 13. Schematic of energy recovery apparatus for laser cladding of valves (work conducted at R.T.M. in collaboration with Cantello M., Ferraro F., Manino A., and als).

The comparative tests have proven that, while the T.I.G. processing valves were satisfactory, those processed with laser showed improvements in every respect: better thickness uniformity of the cladding, improved metallurgical properties such as microstructure in the bulk and at the interface, hardness and element distributions, with particular attention given to Co, Cr and Fe concentrations.

The laser-treated valves have consistently shown much less Fe dilution of the stellite and a much better structure at the interface, which is responsible for the better adhesion of the cladding. The test results show further improvement for the laser treated with the energy recovery scheme and the stellite fed directly in power form. A typical hardness profile for a treated valve is shown in Fig. 14. All the results of the previous tests are maintained or improved, while the amount of material is further reduced (to about 30% of that used by the T.I.G.), the over-metal to be removed is estimated to be about 10-15% of that of the T.I.G. processed valves. Further improvements in material and over-metal amounts can be obtained by reshaping the groove receiving the cladding. It can be said that the process is quite attractive and ready for full industrial application.

9. CONCLUSIONS

Significant developments in methods and processing techniques have taken place, bringing closer the time in which other laser systems for material processing will make a significant inroad on the shop floor of mass production industries, to join those already proven by years of successful use in production.

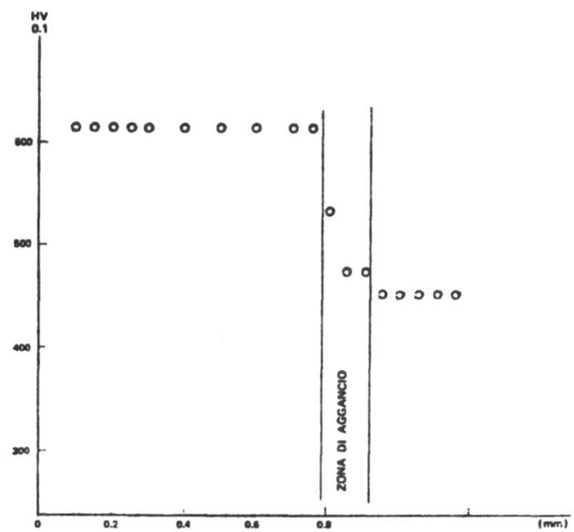

FIGURE 14. Hardness profile of a laser cladded valve.

ACKNOWLEDGMENTS

The author is grateful for the many valuable discussions and contributions of Cantello M. and his associates: Benettin, M., F., Rudilosso, S., Pasquini, of the R.T.M. Institute of Vico Canavese, Turin, Italy. The author thanks the J. Wallenberg Foundation of the Royal Swedish Academy of Engineering Sciences for the sponsorship of parts of this work.

REFERENCES

1. La Rocca, A. V., 1985, "Some Considerations on the Definition of Laser-Robotics Systems," Laser Robotics I Conference, Ann Arbor, MI, USA, April 23-24, 1985.

2. La Rocca, A. V., 1978, (ECOSA I Conference, Brighton UK) Laser Application in Machining and Material Processing, Vol. II, Appendix A: Heat Propagation in Matter.

THE USE OF LASERS IN ROLLS-ROYCE

R. M. MACINTYRE
Rolls-Royce Ltd., UK

Key Words: jet engine turbine blades, electron beam, TIG welding

ABSTRACT

This paper describes the application of a cobalt-based hardsurfacing alloy to a nickel-based gas turbine blade for aero-engine use. The prior technique, manual argon arc welding, was time consuming, critically dependent upon operator skill and suffered from a lack of reproducibility, particularly in the level of nickel dilution produced. The use of a laser and a blown-powder technique to introduce the hardsurfacing alloy enables clad deposits of optimum wear characteristics, free from heat-affected zone cracking and of a consistent quality to be produced. The process is able to be automated and run under microprocessor control.

1. BACKGROUND

The RB.211 high-pressure turbine blade is a shrouded blade manufactured from a cast nickel-based superalloy optimized for creep strength. It operates in the engine at a flame temperature of approximately 1600 K.

The tip shrouds on the blade are designed with interlocking edges to combat the wear that takes place on these edges due to blade vibration. The geometry of the interlock design is intended to place the wear face at the optimum angle and allow its area to be maximized. The wear pad size is nevertheless limited to approximately 4.5 mm by 3 mm.

Excessive wear of the interlock would lead to blade rejection on overhaul or, if allowed to go undetected, precipitate resonance leading to blade fracture. The wear pad is therefore faced with a cobalt-based hardsurfacing alloy with the objective of extending the wear resistance to at least match the designed creep life of the blade, which is targeted at 10,000 hours of service operation.

2. PRIOR TECHNIQUE

Blades were previously hardsurfaced using a manual tungsten inert gas (T.I.G.) welding process using the alloy in the form of a small-diameter wire. The cobalt-based alloy is very sensitive to dilution with nickel, as this affects the microstructure of the hardsurfaced deposit. This has a deleterious effect on the high-temperature wear resistance of the alloy. The optimum level of nickel dilution could not be achieved without a "double-pass" welding technique which involved grinding a weld preparation on the blade shroud, weld depositing the hardsurfacing alloy, partially grinding back this first deposit, applying a second layer of alloy and then finish grinding the two-layer deposit. The need to control the thickness of each layer to avoid nickel dilution from the blade material required great dexterity and control by the welder in the manipulation of the hardsurfacing wire and welding torch and great concentration for the several minutes required to produce the welded deposit. Operator fatigue and variations in individual skill led to inconsistency in the finished deposit in terms of both nickel content and deposit hardness. There were variations in the amount of material applied; the deposit sometimes extended beyond the edge of the weld preparation into the inside radius of the shroud interlock. The blade material, being very highly alloyed, is susceptible to cracking in the heat-affected zone of any weld. The T.I.G. welding technique with its relatively high total heat input tended to produce such heat-affected zone cracking in the blade material. It was felt that the laser offered the potential of a higher power density heat source able to fuse hardsurfacing alloy in powder form onto a substrate with a much lower total heat input. Initial work was carried out using pre-placed powder on a flat substrate with some success. It was, however, soon realized that the small size and shape of the interlock would prevent this application technique being used.

3. LASER HARDSURFACING

3.1. The Laser

The laser used for this work is a fast axial flow carbon dioxide laser with an output power up to a nominal rated 2 kW. It produces a parallel beam approximately 20 mm in diameter. This is delivered via a 45° mirror to a potassium chloride lens by which means it can be focused to a diameter as small as 0.3 mm, giving a power density of the order of 10^4 W/mm^2, considerably in excess of that available from a T.I.G. welding torch.

3.2. Hardsurfacing Technique

As the hardsurfacing powder could not be preplaced on the small pad area, it was decided to adopt a blown powder technique. A defocused beam is used to produce a melt pool between 1 mm and 2 mm wide, typically 1.3 mm for RB.211 blades. The hardsurfacing material, in powder form, is blown into the melt pool by a stream of inert gas from a nozzle at one side of the beam. As the powder enters the melt pool, it is fused to the base material by the laser beam. The workpiece is traversed under the beam and powder delivery nozzle as shown in the diagram to produce a bead of hardsurfacing alloy. If a rectangular or other shape pad is required, then adjacent, overlapping tracks are laid down to cover the area required. A pad of any required thickness can be built up by applying successive layers.

Powder feeds from this, by gravity, to a delivery tube where it is carried by a stream of argon gas to the nozzle. The hopper is fitted with a vibrator to ensure an even powder flow. The powder flow rate is controlled primarily by changing the metering orifice and also by varying the gas flow rate through the nozzle. The various movements required to hardsurface a turbine blade are performed using a five-axis manipulator (X, Y, Z plus two rotational axes), all axes being fitted with stepper motor drives and controlled via a microprocessor. One of the rotational axes serves to turn the blade over so that both interlocks on one blade can be hardsurfaced in a single setup. Although the control system is open-loop, it has an inherent accuracy of $\pm$ 0.02 mm.

3.3. Process Optimization

The main process parameters, which were varied during the investigatory work, were beam power, spot size, traverse speed and powder delivery rate. The influence of each of these on the quality of the hardsurfaced deposit was checked. The spot size was kept deliberately small to give a narrow bead width, enabling the required shape of wear pad to be built up very precisely. The beam power and spot size together determine the beam power density on the workpiece and this was kept between the quite close limits required to maintain good fusion of the hardsurfacing alloy to the blade material. Typical power densities used are in the range 10^2 to 10^3 W/mm^2. The power was therefore limited to less than one kilowatt for the size of pad on this blade. Once the optimum power density range had been determined, the total heat input for a given deposit using specific parameters was calculated and those parameters selected which gave a minimum heat input without too great a penalty in total processing time. The tolerance band for each of the main parameters was investigated and those parameters selected which enabled the greatest tolerances to be used commensurate with acceptable results.

The finalized technique built up each interlock in four layers, applied alternately to each side by turning the blade over, thus allowing a few seconds for each layer to cool down while a layer was being applied to the opposite interlock. All the blade movements required to complete both interlocks were contained in a programme in the microprocessor and carried out as a complete sequence in a single hardsurfacing operation, with a cycle time of approximately seventy-five seconds. The operations sequence was simplified compared to the prior technique, consisting of the grinding of a weld preparation, hardsurfacing and a finish grind.

3.4. Evaluation and Testing

Test pieces in the form of simulations of the interlock geometry or actual blades were subject to extensive laboratory examination. Hardsurfaced deposits were sectioned and examined for excessive porosity, lack of fusion to the base materials and for the appropriate metallurgical structure indicating an undiluted deposit. Test pieces and blades were checked for nickel content using energy dispersive analysis on a scanning electron microscope. Deposits were obtained which were free from porosity, fully fused to the blade material and had a nickel content only 1-2% higher than the original cobalt-based hardsurfacing alloy, a result only matched by the most rigorous execution of the conventional technique.

Hammer wear tests were carried out simulating as closely as possible the type of wear which occurred in the engine to produce wear figures for comparison with similar tests utilizing the existing technique. Finally, engine blades were hardsurfaced using the developed technique and subjected to modification approval testing and cyclic endurance testing and directly compared to conventionally hardsurfaced blades in the same engine build. These tests denonstrated wear rates at the high blade operating temperature equal to the optimum for this material composition.

4. PRODUCTION LASER HARDSURFACING

A special purpose workstation was designed solely for the hardsurfacing of turbine blades. The main factors considered in the design were as follows.

A work-handling and blade-fixturing system of low inertia to give a long operating life over tens of thousands of similar or identical operations per year. To this end aluminum was used extensively in the design. This did not involve a compromise with strength, as laser hard-surfacing, being a non-contact process, imposes no loads on the work-piece or fixture.

Maximum utilization of the laser beam, achieved by fully automating the operation of the process. With a total processing time of approximately seventy-five seconds, single-button initiation of the cycle was incorporated, freeing the operator to load a second workstation. With a simple single-clamp fixture, unloading a finished blade and loading a new one can be accomplished comfortably within a seventy-five-second cycle. Maximum utilization could therefore be achieved with a double workstation installation. Simple operation was ensured by designing the microprocessor control systems to monitor and perform the maximum possible number of functions. Separate units control each workstation, but they are interlinked so that each may monitor the position of the changeover mirror which switches the beam from one station to the other and whether a programme is being run at the other workstation. When the operator loads a blade, closes the safety guard and initiates a cycle, the microprocessor will monitor the other station and, if a programme is running, will wait until that cycle is completed before switching the beam to its own workstation and commencing the hardsurfacing operation. The operator can thus leave a workstation having initiated the cycle. Once the cycle is complete, the safety guard is opened automatically by the microprocessor, thereby indicating to the operator that the blade is ready for unloading.

In-process monitoring is carried out via the microprocessor. In addition to the changeover mirror, it monitors laser operation, the hardsurfacing powder supply, carrier gas supply and also overchecks the interlocks on the safety guard and beam path. If any aspect is unsatisfactory, the start of the hardsurfacing operation will be inhibited and the problem area indicated to the operator diagrammatically on the V.D.U. incorporated into the microprocessor control. The microprocessor programme is recorded on a magnetic tape cartridge.

5. COMPARISON WITH CONVENTIONAL PROCESS

Laser hardsurfacing produces a higher quality hardsurfaced deposit. The accurate control of the power input possible with the laser enables melting of the substrate to be controlled more closely, and minimum dilution of the hardsurfacing alloy to be achieved using a single-stage preparation. When using the manual T.I.G. welding process, deposits with minimum dilution and optimum wear performance can only be produced using a double-pass technique with an intermediate grinding operation.

Total heat input into the blade is greatly reduced. The heat-affected zone in the blade material is limited to less than 0.1 mm and problems with heat-affected zone cracking are removed. The reproducibility of the power settings, the control of the powder delivery and the precise repeatability of the processing speed and programme movements give a consistency in the finished product which cannot be matched by a manual technique.

5.1 Savings

A direct cost saving arises from the greatly reduced processing time. Compared with the previous "double-pass" T.I.G. welding technique, the laser hardsurfacing operation reduces processing time from fourteen minutes to seventy-five seconds. Despite the higher operating costs of the laser, this gives a substantial cost reduction.

Due to the greater precision of the process and the elimination of the intermediate grinding operation, material savings are considerable. It has been estimated that consumption of the expensive cobalt-based hardsurfacing material is cut by more than 50%.

Gains also accrue from the reduced number of separate operations which simplifies and shortens the manufacturing cycle, reducing inventory costs. The combination of precise control giving an optimized result and the repeatability of programme and settings giving consistency enables the process to be automated. This in turn further assures process reproducibility and enables a high throughput capability to be achieved leading to the cost savings already outlined.

EDITED QUESTIONS - CHAPTER 6

LA ROCCA, MCINTYRE

ALDO LA ROCCA

Q. What beam shape was used in the model?
A. Elliptical.

Q. How do you apply the heat transfer equation to small parts, and what about melting?
A. We use an adapted model for small parts and another for those in which melting occurs.

Q. Does the coupling of the energy recovery device change with time?
A. Yes, the inside of the dome gets dirty during processing, especially at high power densities. It is important, therefore, not to use too high a power density.

Q. Is there variation in the values of the material thermodynamic constants with T?
A. No, they are assumed to be constant.

Q. Do you use an iteration of the general solution of the heat transfer model as you go along?
A. We use it as a guide.

Q. Do you carry out experiments to confirm your parameters?
A. Yes.

Q. Do you have problems with cleaning and oxidation?
A. Yes.

Q. Is the system used to weld parts of the FIAT cars?
A. Yes. (Ed. note) Then Prof. LaRocca discussed applications of high penetration welding.

Q. Does worker resistance to introduction of lasers into industry pose a problem?
A. Yes, but also the reluctance of management to accept it.

Q. How many multikilowatt CO_2 lasers is FIAT using?
A. Several. (Ed. note - huge amount of laughing from assembly.)

MALCOLM MCINTYRE

Q. How deep is the part being treated (gear tooth)?
A. For this example 1.0 mm.

Q. Is laser hardening of the gears used?
A. No, due to expensive testing that would be required by C.A.A. for authorizing manufacturing change.

Q. Hardness value of gear?
A. 700 hv. Important to get compressive residual stresses.

Q. Is any copper detected?
A. No. The copper is chemically stripped (refers to Cu film, to stop diffusion of C into unwanted areas, being removed).

Q. How long has Rolls-Royce been using electron beam techniques?
A. About 20 years.

Q. What laser and powers are used to drill cooling holes?
A. Nd:YAG, 600 W average power.

Q. How big are the blades being treated?
A. Five to six inches long - from RB 211 engine.

CHAPTER 7. LASER SURFACE CHEMISTRY

CHAPTER INTRODUCTION - J. TARDIEU de MALEISSYE

The presence of a gaseous or liquid phase creates new conditions for laser-substrate interactions which can add a new dimension to the surface treatment of metals. The laser can be used in different ways in such systems:

- As a chemical activation source for the gas-phase decomposition, preceding the surface deposit.
- At the solid-gas interface in order to thermally produce a well-localized metallic layer on the substrate.
- With direct irradiation of surface in order to modify its chemical or electrochemical reactivity.

The three following papers are concerned with these different aspects of the laser-driven heterogeneous reactions.

The first paper deals with general physicochemical kinetic features related to gas-phase decomposition prior to its condensation as a deposit. The next paper is concerned with surface matallic films generated from laser dielectric breakdown. The last work treats of a solid phase activated by laser, coupled with an electrochemical process.

These three examples are for the most part controlled by diffusion or thermodiffusion.

Among the laser-assisted processes, gas-metal interactions represent an applied research field in rapid expansion because of the potential for applications in the microelectronic field.

Draper, C.W. and Mazzoldi, P. (eds.), Laser Surface Treatment of Metals. ISBN 90-247-3405-3.

LASER-INDUCED DECOMPOSITION OF MOLECULES RELATED TO PHOTOCHEMICAL DEPOSITION

J. TARDIEU de MALEISSYE
Laboratoire de Chimie Générale - Tour 55 et U.A.CNRS 870,
Université Pierre et Marie Curie, 4 Place Jussieu, 75005-Paris

Key Words: Energy distribution, energy transfers, gas decomposition, thermodiffusion, vapor deposition

ABSTRACT

Complex laser-gas interactions generally precede the deposition of solids on a substrate, especially in laser chemical vapor deposition. The most important interactions are presented in this paper both in their physical and chemical aspects.

The former includes the laser thermodiffusion depending strictly on the partial pressures of absorber and reactant species. The transient depletion in absorber concentration which appears during irradiation into the laser beam is discussed. The chemical aspect is considered from a kinetic viewpoint and concerns mainly the binary gaseous systems frequently involved in LCVD.

The laser-induced binary processes include photosensitized activation and decomposition of non-absorbent molecules through an infrared active but chemically inert photosensitizer.

The maximum decomposition yield dependence on the relative pressure is a common feature to laser-induced binary chemical processes. The related distribution of energy between the reactive or inert gaseous partners is finally presented and discussed in connection with this maximum.

1. INTRODUCTION

The decomposition technique and the deposition of metal films on surfaces as the result of gas-phase decomposition have developed rapidly in the past few years (1,2). The use of the laser as an activation source today competes successfully with both electron and ion beams, and its specific properties are well appreciated for many industrial processes. The laser beam can propagate through many reactive media and its spatio-temporal resolution may be adjusted exactly to the reacting system. The laser power may be directed toward the substrate in order to heat the surface, or into the homogeneous phase prior to any interaction with the substrate.

The gas-substrate techniques of interaction initiated by a laser source may be generally classified into one of three groups:

- Laser chemical etching
- Laser photochemical deposition
- Laser photothermal deposition

In fact, these techniques frequently have many features in common. After a brief description of these methods, we shall focus our attention on the gas-phase decomposition which leads to the photodeposition process and appears frequently as the rate-limiting step.

2. LASER-ASSISTED CHEMICAL ETCHING

This technique was developed recently and allows a good preparation of surfaces of ceramics, glasses and insulators used for advanced semiconductor device processing technology.

The chemical etching process involves three partners: the etching, the substrate and the laser source.

The etchant, being in contact with the solid, reacts with it under laser activation, and superficially modifies the surface. In this way, simple gases such as Cl_2, HCl or SF_6 are dissociated by laser to form Cl or F radicals (3) which will attack a silicon surface. Vibrational energy may be brought by the laser also to activate a gas which can react later with the substrate.

For example, excited SF_6 reacts with Si and produces SiF_4 (4). After its chemical modification, the surface may be treated and the etched zones removed by classical chemistry in solution.

The more common etchants are halogens (Br_2, Cl_2 and HCl), freons which can treat simple Si or Ge surfaces, or more complex substrates such as Ga-As, ZnP or CdS (5-7) after activation by an argon ion laser or a CO_2 laser.

The choice of etchant defines both the bond energy which is required for its decomposition and the corresponding laser photon energy. The process also differs, depending on whether an atomic species is released in gaseous form, which will diffuse from the surface to the inside of a substrate, or if the etchant decomposes directly at the surface.

A subsidiary role can be played by the laser which promotes dissociative chemisorption of the etchant on the surface. For example, SF_6 may be resonantly excited on the Si surface up to a high vibrational energy level, producing an etching effect (8). Few studies to better understand the etchant role and to optimize the etching process exist so far. However, important differences in the treatment result as the laser wavelength, its power, the etchant species or its pressure are varied.

3. PHOTOCHEMICAL LASER DEPOSITION (PLD)

In contrast with chemical etching, the surface is less important in PLD with respect to gas-phase decomposition.

Classical examples for PLD are given by the gas-phase photodecomposition or organometallic vapors in order to produce a high local concentration in metallic atoms. This low-pressure phase is next condensed, forming a well-localized elemental deposit on the substrate surface.

During the initial photoabsorption step, complex energy transfer, thermodiffusional and heterogeneous nucleation processes take place. The partial pressure of buffer gas which may be present can modify strongly the decomposition rate. Among the various examples of organometallic vapor photodecompositions, we can mention the decomposition of germane at 248 nm, which gives GeH_2, GeH and Ge. Also, the InI decomposition at 193 nm on nickel substrates (8) which produces In^+ and I^-.

By using excimer lasers under 200 nm of wavelength, it is possible to produce ion pairs from metal halides belonging to Group III of the periodic table. Also, photochemistry on the surface can take place at the same time as gas-phase processes and the overall kinetics become similar to the kinetics depending on the adsorption isotherms. Light energy incident on the substrate is deposited in the molecules adsorbed on the surface, a process which frequently competes with the gas-phase process. Surface photochemistry predominates at lower pressure with a long molecular free path, while the gas-phase photochemistry prevails at medium and high pressure.

4. LASER THERMAL DEPOSITION (LTD)

The laser beam is used in the LTD technique only for local heating of the substrate. The decomposition reaction can take place in the hot spot produced by the laser, and the deposit of a condensed phase, which is in general a metallic layer, is obtained in this way. LTD is carried out on non-metallic substrates such as semiconductors or insulators, by using a pulsed or cw infrared or visible laser.

Ni, Cr, Mo, Si and Au atoms at pressures ranging from 10 to 760 torr have been deposited by LTD processes (9-13). Metallic deposits from metal carbonyls and metal halides have attracted special attention for the future design of ultra large-scale integrated circuits.

$$Me(CO)_n \longrightarrow n\,CO + Me\,(s)$$

$$WF_6 + 3\,H_2 \longrightarrow W\,(s) + 6\,HF$$

$$WF_6 + 3/2\,Si \xrightarrow{\text{surface}} W\,(s) + 3/2\,SiF_4$$

It is planned that in the future, LTD can constitute a direct write process applied to the fast interconnection of device structures in integrated circuits.

The overall process can be described by a series of physicochemical steps coupled through heat and mass transport. Five essential steps may be enumerated:

1. Transport of reactant gas to the laser-heated surface area
2. Adsorption on the surface
3. Decomposition on the adsorbed surface
4. Desorption of gaseous products from the laser-heated area
5. Diffusion of gaseous products outside the decomposition zone

5. GAS-PHASE DECOMPOSITION

In PLD processes, the adsorption and desorption steps are superseded by the gas-phase decomposition, and the first step 1 becomes the final step of deposition. But whatever process is concerned, the partial or total pressure of reactants and buffer gases plays a major role in the course of reaction. Some examples and general results will illustrate its place in the gas-phase decomposition kinetics.

5.1. The role of pressure in gas-phase decomposition induced by laser

The overall pressure of reactants directly affects the collisional energy transfer which occurs between the absorber molecule and its reacting partner.

The laser beam geometry determines an intense energy gradient between the irradiated volume and its neighborhood. The pumped molecules inside the irradiated volume possess a high level of vibrational and rotational energy and lose it very rapidly by collision when they leave the irradiated zone. So, gas phase decomposition takes place in the laser beam where the first reaction steps are fast in comparison to the diffusion of excited species out of the irradiated zone. This purely physical effect constitutes in fact the rate-determining step of the reaction.

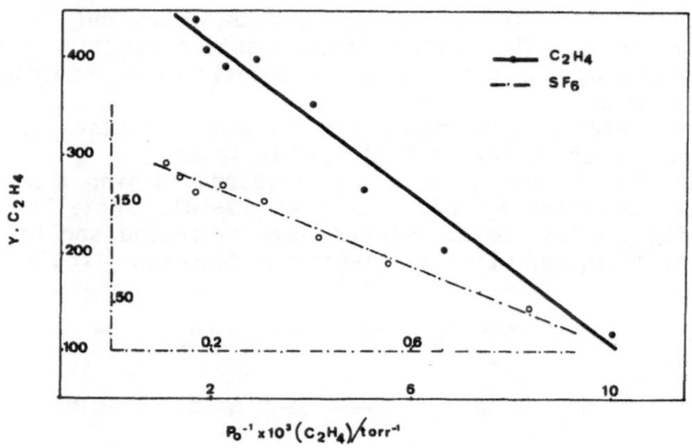

FIGURE 1. Ethylene and ethane decomposition rate versus, respectively, $[P_o(C_2H_4)]^{-1}$ and $[P_o(SF_6)]^{-1}$ (dashed line).

Ethylene decomposition can illustrate such an effect. This molecule strongly absorbs CO_2 laser radiation at 10.6 µm and decomposes, giving light molecules (CH_4, C_3H_6, C_2H_2...), condensed aromatic species and soot deposition. Its decomposition rate Y (Fig. 1) may be expressed as a function of different initial ethylene pressures by

$$Y = A - B/P_{o\ (C_2H_4)} \tag{1}$$

The quantum yield of decomposition for a given initial pressure and incident intensity I_o is defined as the following ratio:

$$(\Phi)_{P_o\ C_2H_4,\ I_o} = Y/I_{absorbed}$$

As the pressure increases, Φ tends to a limit. Then Φ_{lim}^{-1} corresponds to the average minimum photon number required for the decomposition of one molecule of C_2H_4 (Fig. 2). The relationship (1) may be understood by

$$Y_{(C_4H_4)} = [\Phi_{lim}/V_{cell}](I_{absorbed} - \zeta/[C_2H_4]_o) \tag{2}$$

V_{cell} is the cell volume corresponding to the experiment, $I_{absorbed}$ is the total laser intensity absorbed by C_2H_4, $\zeta/[C_2H_4]_o$ is the thermal diffusivity with

$$\zeta = (X/r)^2(\lambda_T/C_pT)$$

X is the smallest root of Bessel function of zero order (16), r is the cell radius, λ_T and C_{pT} are the conductivity and heat capacity coefficients dependent on T.

Thus the first term in the relation (1) is seen as the generation of decomposed molecules and the second term represents the loss by thermal diffusion of reactant molecules from the active volume.

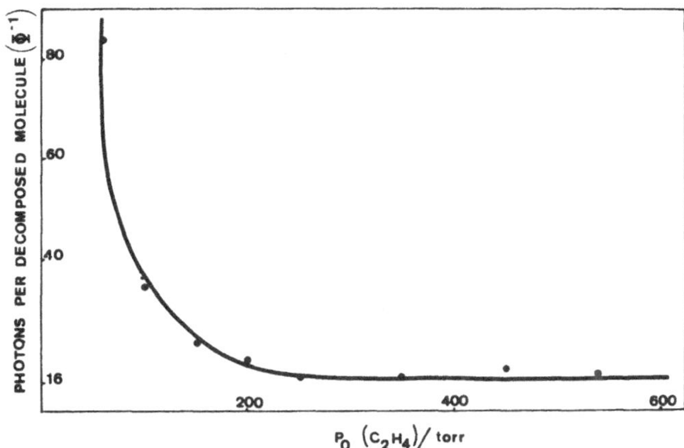

FIGURE 2. Average number of absorbed photons per decomposed molecule Φ^{-1}, versus initial ethylene pressure.

5.2. Photosensitized gas-phase decomposition

Because they don't absorb at the corresponding wavelength, various molecular species cannot be decomposed directly by laser radiation. But mixed with another molecule which can be laser pumped, these molecules decompose after collisional energy transfer. SF_6, SiF_4, BCl_3 are photosensitizers currently used, which may react sometimes as SiF_4 with their non-absorbing partner.

In the following alkane decomposition experiments, SF_6 was chosen as photosensitizer because of its strong absorption coefficient at 10.6 μm and its high thermal stability.

Ethane, propane and butane isomers in these conditions give methane, olefins and condensed deposits as decomposition products. Acetylene, photosensitized by SF_6, gives a highly powdery deposit of carbon black.

By keeping the initial pressure of ethane constant (260 torr) while the p_{SF_6} varied between 1-10 torr, a linear reaction rate dependence with $p_{o(SF_6)}^{-1}$ is obtained. This behavior is quite similar to the ethylene rate variation represented previously (Fig. 1).

These two observations may be extended to propane also and they indicate that the pumped molecule transfers its energy within a heat bath composed essentially (at 99%) by the reacting partner. The proportion of excited pumped molecules diffusing out of the beam controls the yield of decomposition at constant pressure of hydrocarbon. The more they diffuse - lower pressures - the smaller is the reaction yield.

At fixed photosensitizer pressure of 3.3 torr, the initial pressure of hydrocarbon being changed from 60 to 500 torr, the decomposition rate first increases with the pressure, goes through a maximum, then decreases (Fig. 3). For a given pressure of hydrocarbon, the reaction may be completely inhibited. This behavior is well illustrated by the butane isomers (Fig. 4). The isobutane composition is completely inhibited when the pressure increases by only 30% after its maximum. This pressure effect seems a common feature in all binary systems activated by IR lasers. The reaction rate modification brought by the variation of incident laser intensity is also illustrated in Fig. 3. The maximum yield is shifted towards higher pressures of hydrocarbon when the laser power is increased. Its quadratic dependence on the laser output power (Fig. 5) will be discussed further.

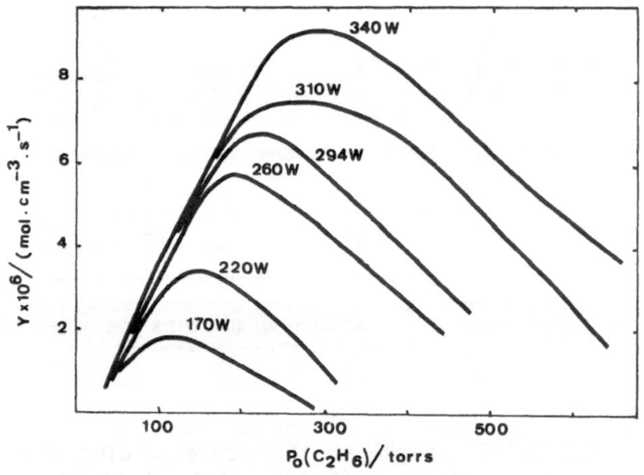

FIGURE 3. Ethane decomposition rate vs. its initial pressure at different laser power.

5.3. The role of pressure in the laser gas-phase absorption

Under cw laser irradiation of several hundred watts, pressures of ten to hundred torr and strong absorption coefficient, the Beer-Lambert law is not respected. This is the case for C_2H_4 and SF_6. By adding increasing pressures of transparent hydrocarbon from 60 to 400 torr and keeping a constant pressure of SF_6 of 3.3 torr, the overall laser absorption is profoundly modified. The absorption is found to increase much more quickly between 200 and 400 torr (Fig. 6). The energy deposited into the gaseous mixture is thermalized and rapid heat and

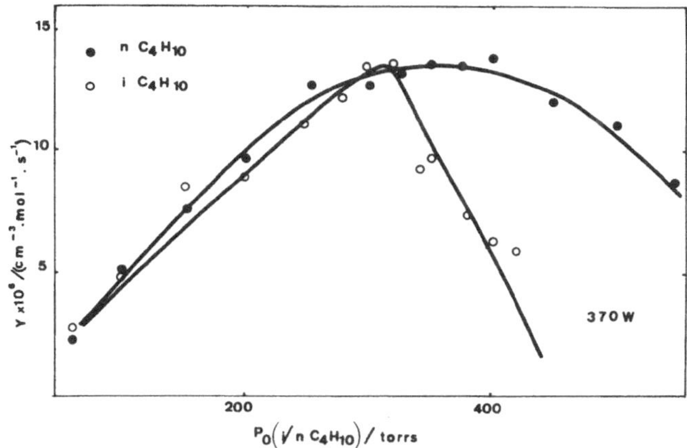

FIGURE 4. Butane isomers decomposition rates vs. their respective initial pressures.

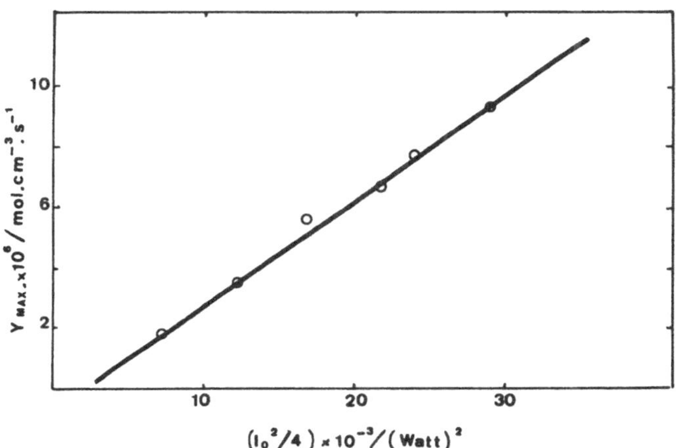

FIGURE 5. Quadratic power dependence of maximum ethane decomposition yields - ($P.SF_6$) = 3.3 torr).

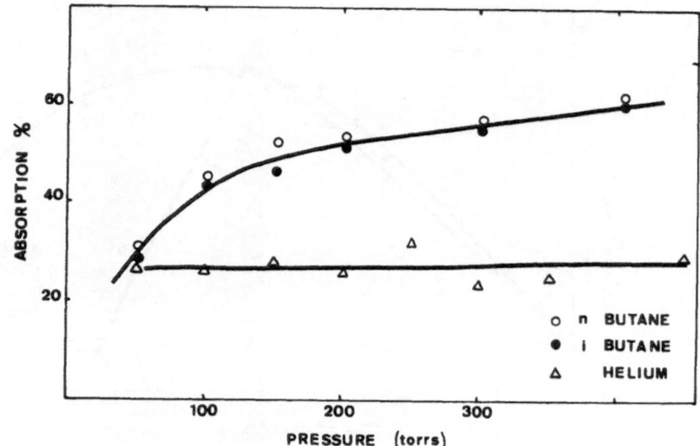

FIGURE 6. SF_6-Ar (3.3-51.7) torr adsorption as a function of transparent gas at 10.6 μm.

mass transport takes place from the irradiated volume towards the peripheral zone. The difference between the mean molecular velocities of two components in a non-uniform gas may be calculated by using the Chapman relationship:

$$\bar{c}_1 - \bar{c}_2 = -(N_1N_2)^{-1}\left\{D_{12}\nabla N_1 + N_1N_2\frac{m_2 - m_1}{m}\nabla \ln P - \frac{1}{P}\frac{n_1n_2}{n}\cdot\frac{m_1m_2}{m}(F_1 - F_2) + k_T\nabla \ln T\right\}$$

where C_j, N_j, n_j, m_j and F_j are, respectively, the mean molecular velocities, the mole fraction, the number of molecules, the molecular weight and the force acting on the j-th species. P, D_{12} and k_T are, respectively, the total pressure, the ordinary coefficient of diffusion and the thermal diffusion ratio. This expression may be simplified under cw laser irradiation and becomes:

$$N_1 = -N_1N_2\alpha_{12}\nabla \ln T \tag{4}$$

where $\alpha_{12} = k_t(N_1N_2)^{-1}$ is a complicated function of temperature. By taking an average value $\bar{\alpha}_{12}$, the transient ratio of absorbing species 1' to the buffer gas 2' in the beam may be expressed by

$$N_1'/N_2' = (N_1/N_2)(T/T')^{\alpha_{12}} \tag{5}$$

The laser intensity captured by a given concentration of absorber $(X)_0$ is a function of the buffer gas concentration $(M)_0$ and may be expressed as a combination of $\beta/(M)_0$ and $\gamma(M)_0$ terms, related, respectively, to the thermal diffusion and collisional relaxation of X:

$$(I_{absorbed})_{(M)_o} = \beta/(M)_o + \gamma(M)_o + \delta \qquad (6)$$

The coefficients β, γ and δ are determined by multiple linear regression, and the negative value obtained for β indicates unambiguously that the concentration of SF_6 inside the beam is transiently depleted during the laser irradiation (17).

The last term δ represents the laser intensity in the absence of any buffer gas effect. The absorbed intensity may be reexpressed in terms of molar fraction of absorbing species removed by diffusion or released by collision

$$(I_{abs})_{(M)_o} = (I_{abs})_{(X)_o}[1 - N(X)_{diff} + N(X)_{coll}] \qquad (7)$$

The difference between the ratio of absorber SF_6 and buffer gas, before and during the laser irradiation (Fig. 7), explains why increasing the pressure of transparent species hinders the diffusion of absorber out of the laser absorption volume and enhances the absorption.

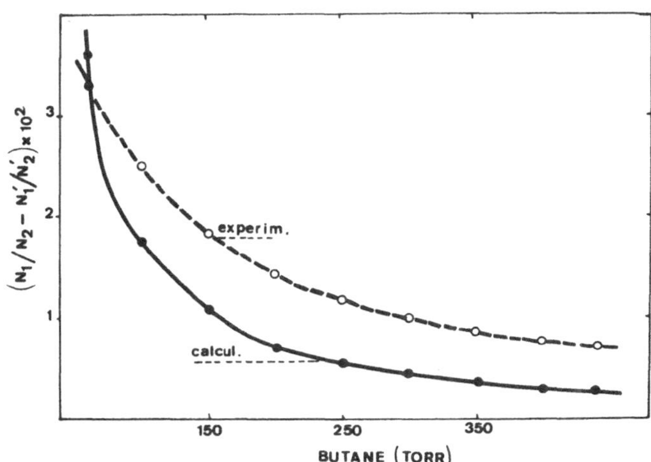

FIGURE 7. Difference between the concentration ratio $(SF_6)/(C_4H_{10})$ into the beam volume before irradiation and during irradiation vs. the initial pressure of butane.

• Calculated by using expression 5.
∘ From absorption measurements and expression 7.

5.4. Laser-absorbed energy distribution inside a binary gas mixture

It is tempting to attribute the decrease in the reaction rate after the maximum to a simple heat dilution effect due to the increase of the heat capacity of the mixture. In fact, the heat dilution is only a minor effect because heat capacity and thermal conductivity both increase with temperature and, consequently, their ratio is not very sensitive to variation of temperature. In addition, the adiabaticity of laser heating increases as the thermal diffusivity decreases, so it seems more suitable to consider the distribution of laser energy among all of the species present. When the photo steady state is established, the energy flowing continuously through the system may be divided in three parts.

The first is stored into the internal degrees of freedom of the pumped molecule; the second part is also stored via V-V collisional energy transfer into the internal degrees of freedom of B; the last part results from the V-T transfer and corresponds to the total translational energy present in the heat bath.

The laser energy Σnq deposited into the heat bath is balanced among the three previous fractions represented, respectively, by $(n_Aq)_A$, $(n_Bq)_B$ and $(nq)_T$:

$$\sum nq = (n_Aq)_A + (n_Bq)_B + (nq)_T \tag{8}$$

The reaction must occur by a bimolecular process involving the coupling of internal energies ϵ_A and ϵ_B between the two partners. The condition $\epsilon_A + \epsilon_B \geq$ activation energy, must be respected; then the reaction yield may be expressed by:

$$Y = \lambda(n_Aq)_A \cdot (n_Bq)_B \tag{9}$$

with λ as a coupling constant.

In the first approximation let us assume $\Sigma nq - (nq)_T$ constant when the concentration of B changes.

$$(n_Aq)_A = [\Sigma nq - (nq)_T] - (n_Bq)_B \tag{10}$$

The reaction yield (9) expressed as a function of (10) becomes:

$$Y = \lambda'(n_Bq)_B - \lambda(n_Bq)_B^2 \tag{11}$$

with $\lambda' = \lambda[\Sigma nq - (nq)_T]$.

The parabolic equation (11) goes through a maximum (Fig. 8) when

$$(n_Bq)_B = \lambda'/2$$

$$= (n_Aq)_A$$

and

$$Y_{max} = \lambda(n_Aq)^2{}_A \tag{12}$$

According to (10), $(n_Aq)_A = [\Sigma nq - (nq)_T]/2$

Then

$$Y_{max} \simeq \lambda[\Sigma nq - (nq)_T]^2/4 \tag{13}$$

which points out the laser intensity quadratic dependence shown in Fig. 5.

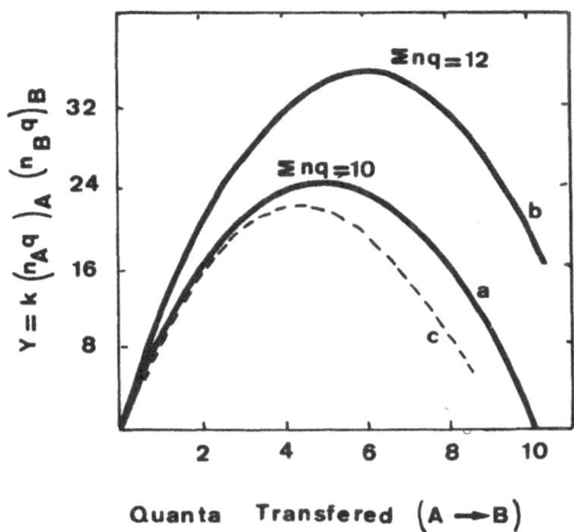

FIGURE 8. Reaction rate evolution = $\lambda(n_A q)_A(n_B q)_B$ vs. the number of quanta transferred to $B,(n_B q)_B$.

a : Σ nq = 10 quanta
b : Σ nq = 12 quanta
c : Σ nq = 10 quanta and energy loss (10%) during A⟶B internal energy transfer

An exact distribution of energy between the collisional partners is, in fact, more complex because some noteworthy effects have not been taken into account here. Among them, the intermolecular V-V energy transfer function which depends on the molecular structure of each species. Also, the overall laser energy absorption as a function of the absorbing species discussed previously (17).

The parabolic evolution of reaction yield is well illustrated by the n-butane decomposition in Fig. 4, the CO_2 formation from the SO_2-CO bireacting system, not presented here, and by other binary systems including irradiations with pulsed TEA CO_2 lasers (18,19).

The energy distribution between the two partners A and B may be restricted to a given maximum energy fraction present in B. After the maximum concentration is reached, V-T energy transfers prevail over V-V transfers and the rection yields decrease linearly with the reactant pressure as schematized in Fig. 9. This behavior is rather similar to that which is observed in the previous experimental decompositions.

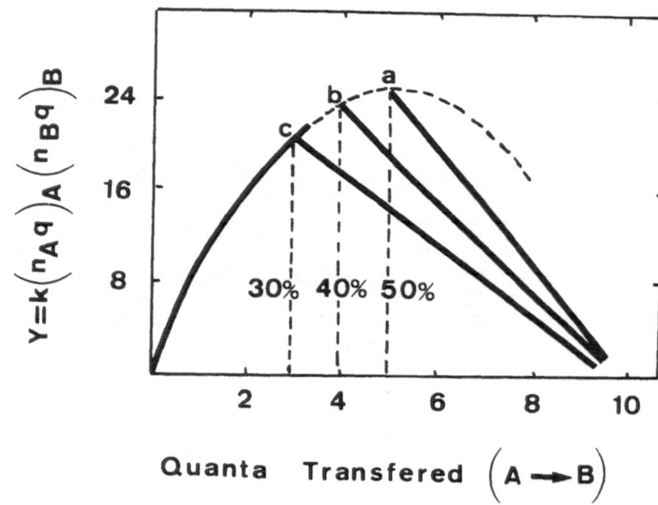

FIGURE 9. Parabolic reaction rate evolution limited by Maximum Internal Energy Transfer (MIET).

a - MIET = 50% Σ nq
b - MIET = 40% Σ nq
c - MIET = 30% Σ nq

REFERENCES

1. D. J. Ehrlich and J. T. Tsao, J. Vac. Sci. Technol. 81, 969 (1983).
2. D. J. Ehrlich, R. M. Osgood, Jr., and T. F. Deutsch, J. Vac. Sci. Technol. 21, 23 (1982).
3. T. J. Chuang, Mat. Res. Soc. Symp. Proc. 17, 45 (1983).
4. T. J Chuang, J. Chem. Phys. 74, 1453 (1981).
5. A. W. Tucker and M. Birnbaum, SPIE Proceed. 385, 131 (1983).
6. D. J. Ehrlich, R. M. Osgood, J. Deutsch, and T. F. Deutsch, Appl. Phys. Lett. 36, 698 (1980).
7. R. M. Osgood, Jr., A. Sanchez, D. J. Ehrlich, and V. Daneu, Appl. Phys. Lett. 40, 391 (1982).
8. T. J. Chuang, Vibrations at Surfaces (Plenum Press, 1983).
9. S. D. Allen, J. Appl. Phys. 52, 6501 (1981).
10. S. D. Allen and A. B. Trigubo, J. Appl. Phys. 54, 1614 (1983).
11. R. J. Von Gutfeld, R. E. Acosta, and L. T. Romankiw, IBM J. of Res. and Dev. 26, 136 (1982).
12. J. C. Puippe, R. E. Acosta, and R. J. Von Gutfeld, J. Electrochem. Soc. 128, 2539 (1981).
13. R. J. Von Gutfeld, E. E. Tynan, R. L. Melchner, and S. E. Blum, Appl. Phys. Lett. 35, 651 (1979).
14. R. Bauerle, Mat. Res. Soc. Symp. Proc. 17, 19 (1983).
15. J. P. Herman, R. A. Hyde, B. M. McWilliams, A. M. Weisberg, and L. L. Wood, Mat. Res. Soc. Symp. Proc. 17, 9 (1983).
16. R. C. L. Yuan and G. W. Flynn, J. Chem. Phys. 57, 1316 (1972).
17. J. Tardieu de Maleissye and F. Lempereur, Appl. Opt. 81, 334 (1982).
18. J. Blazejowski and F. W. Lampe, J. Phys. Chem. 88, 1666 (1984).
19. S. Kuwabara, K. Kuwata, I. Nishiyama, and I. Hamszaki, Chem. Phys. Lett. 106, 540 (1984).

METAL FILM DEPOSITION BY LASER BREAKDOWN CHEMICAL VAPOR DEPOSITION

THOMAS R. JERVIS
Materials Chemistry Group, Materials Science and Technology Division, Los Alamos National Laboratory, Los Alamos, NM 87545

Key Words: chemical vapor deposition, dielectric breakdown, film deposit, metal carbonyl decomposition

ABSTRACT

Dielectric breakdown of gas mixtures can be used to deposit homogeneous thin films by chemical vapor deposition with appropriate control of flow and pressure conditions to suppress gas-phase nucleation and particle formation. Using a pulsed CO_2 laser operating at 10.6 μm where there is no significant resonant absorption in any of the source gases, we have succeeded in depositing homogeneous films from several gas-phase precursors by gas-phase laser pyrolysis. Nickel and molybdenum from the respective carbonyls and tungsten from the hexafluoride have been examined to date. In each case the gas precursor is buffered to reduce the partial pressure of the reactants and to induce breakdown. The films are spectrally reflective and uniform over a large area. Films have been characterized by Auger electron spectroscopy, X-ray diffraction, pull tests, and resistivity measurements. The highest quality films have resulted from the nickel depositions. Detailed X-ray diffraction analysis of these films yields a very small domain size (< 5.0 nm) consistent with rapid quenching from the gas-phase reaction zone. This analysis also shows nickel carbide formation consistent with the temperature of the reaction zone and the Auger electron spectroscopy results which show some carbon and oxygen incorporation (9% and 1%, respectively). Gas-phase transport and condensation of the molybdenum carbonyl results in substantial carbon and oxygen contamination of the molybdenum films requiring heated substrates, a requirement not consistent with the goals of the program to maximize the quench rate of the deposition. Results from tungsten deposition experiments, representing a reduction chemistry instead of the decomposition chemistry involved in the carbonyl experiments, are also reported.

1. INTRODUCTION

Chemical Vapor Deposition, in which vapor phase chemical reactants deposit a coating on a substrate, has a long history of applications in metal and other coatings. Inasmuch as these processes are thermally driven, the commercial availability of high-power carbon dioxide lasers in the early 1970s made some fusion of these technologies inevitable.

In 1973 a method for local substrate heating for patterned chemical vapor deposition devised by Lydtin & Wilden was reported (1). A helical carbon resistor was fabricated on a ceramic substrate, but details of the process were not fully reported. A diagram of their apparatus is shown in Figure 1. Further development of this local heating technique was done by Christensen (2) and later by Allen and her collaborators (3) at the University of Southern California starting in about 1978. This

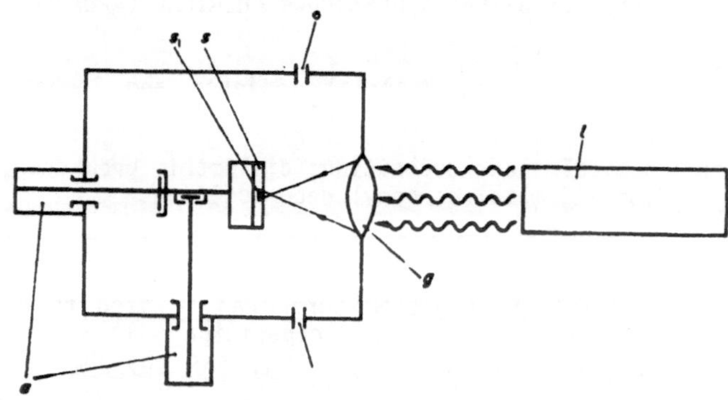

FIGURE 1. Diagram of apparatus used by Lydtin and Wilden for CVD of carbon film resistors.

group investigated a number of metal systems using both pulsed and cw carbon dioxide lasers operating in the infrared (IR) through a transparent reactant gas mixture. Writing of small-scale patterns was one goal of this work although actual patterned circuits were not produced. This is a thermal surface process with no gas-phase reaction intended.

At about the same time, a concerted effort at laser chemical vapor deposition for microelectronic applications was initiated at Lincoln Laboratories by Ehrlich, Deutsch, Osgood, Tsao, and their co-workers (4). Using visible and ultraviolet (UV) wavelengths, they narrowed the spot size to submicrometer dimensions on the substrate, and directly photolyzed reactants in the gas phase or on the substrate surface or both. This technique is illustrated in Figure 2. This work has been quite highly developed for selective doping and metallization, resulting in complete circuits having been fabricated using the laser direct writing technique.

Bauerle and his collaborators (5) at Linz have also used local illumination at visible and ultraviolet wavelengths to deposit patterns as well as single-crystal needles of metals and semiconductors.

In another application to microelectronics, Collins, Solanki, and their co-workers (6) at the Colorado State University have developed a technique for large-area depositions of metals and insulators by gas-phase photolysis of reactants by a UV excimer laser as illustrated in Figure 3. The work is also well advanced with a number of metal and insulator coatings having been produced. A principal advantage of this technique over conventional vacuum deposition methods is excellent coverage of stepped features on the substrate. The use of an excimer laser also limits the number of dissociation channels available. Higher energy processes can thus be tuned out in some cases.

Haggerty and collaborators (7) at the Massachusetts Institute of Technology and Bilenchi, Musci, and their collaborators (8) at CISE S.p.A. have used a geometry similar to that of Collins but with a carbon dioxide laser as a heat source for gas-phase pyrolysis of silane to deposit films of amorphous silicon for solar cells. In this case the

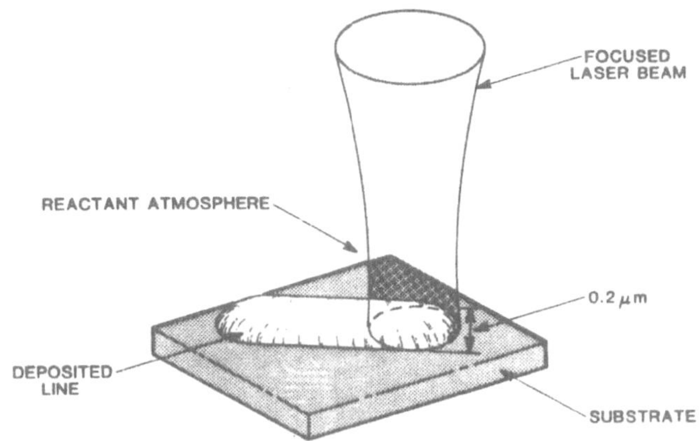

FIGURE 2. Schematic diagram of process for direct writing of very fine lines using surface activation as described by Ehrlich.

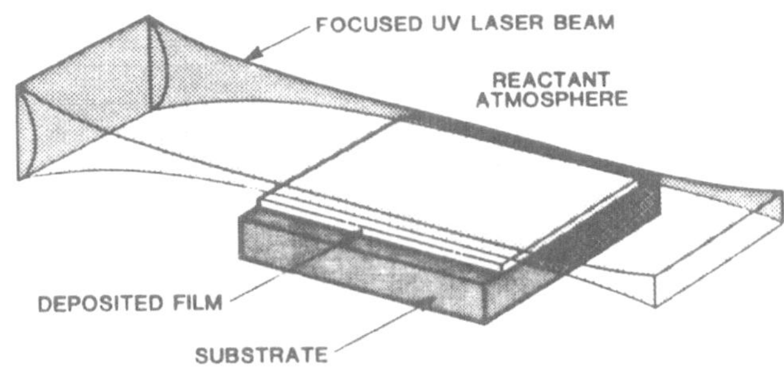

FIGURE 3. Schematic diagram of process for excimer laser CVD of large-area films as described by Collins.

10.6 micrometer radiation is at resonance with the silane, resulting in heating of the gas by multiphoton absorption.

There have thus been four basic techniques demonstrated for the use of lasers in chemical vapor deposition: gas-phase pyrolysis by resonant absorption of IR radiation, gas-phase photolysis by UV radiation, substrate heating with subsequent surface pyrolysis by IR and visible radiation, and a combination of surface and gas-phase photolysis by UV radiation. In general, the gas-phase techniques are useful for large-area depositions and the surface-focused techniques for selective area deposition.

A number of other laboratories (9-23) have also reported results on various laser chemical vapor deposition activities using one or more of these methods as well as various photoelectrochemical methods for etching or depositing films. A more complete discussion is beyond the scope of this brief introduction, but the most significant efforts in the field of laser chemical vapor deposition have been described above.

Finally, there is a substantial literature, including work on metals and alloys (24,25), on the products of chemical reactions induced by laser-initiated dielectric breakdown. The products of these reactions are generally powders. The relatively high partial pressures of the reactants in these experiments cause homogeneous nucleation and powder formation. Laser methods have also been investigated extensively for powder production (26).

2. RESULTS

We have used dielectric breakdown of gas mixtures to drive chemical vapor deposition reactions (27) in a geometry similar to that of Collins, as shown in Figure 4, resulting in the formation of metal films. The focused beam of a pulsed carbon dioxide laser operating on the 10.6 micrometer line creates a region of high electric field sufficient to break down the gas. This in turn creates a high-temperature reaction zone at a distance of 2 to 3 mm from the substrate which is at room temperature. The deposition on the cold substrate results in rapid quenching of the deposit from the gas phase and very fine grain structures. In fact, the principal goal of this work is the deposition of amorphous alloy films, and the reason for choosing this method of deposition is the promise it holds for creation of very fine grain or amorphous materials. We have chosen gas-phase processing for the advantages of relatively large area depositions, low substrate temperatures for rapid quenching of the deposited material, and spatially defined reaction volume to eliminate wall effects. Because high vacuum is not required, the chamber can be recycled with a clean substrate in a few minutes, resulting in a high throughput of films.

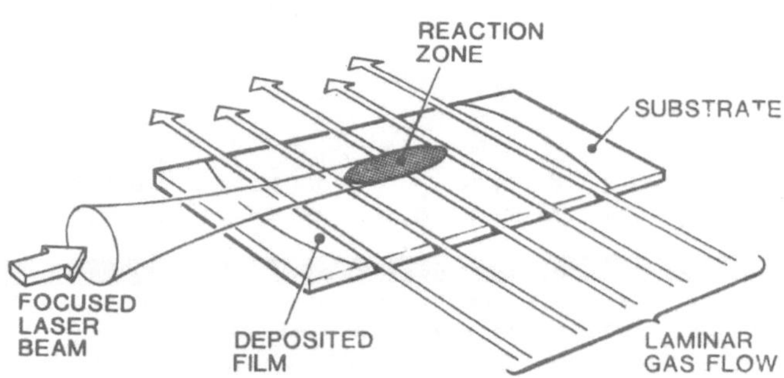

FIGURE 4. Schematic diagram of process for laser breakdown CVD.

Consideration of available source gases and the existence of known amorphous phases of Ni-Mo alloys (28-29) led to the choice of this system for initial investigation. Because $Ni(CO)_4$ is a well-understood, if highly toxic, chemical vapor deposition source, we began our investigations in this material.

We first attempted to heat the gas by resonant absorption in $Ni(CO)_4$ at 10.93 micrometers using tuned cw and pulsed CO_2 lasers in the hope that the Ni-CO bond could be broken by multiphoton absorption without dissociating the C-O bond. These experiments were not successful. We were, however, able to create dielectric breakdown conditions using the pulsed laser, and these conditions could be created without the need for tuning to a difficult line.

We have therefore pursued the use of laser breakdown for the chemical vapor deposition of metal films and have had success in this new technique for laser deposition. Using the dielectric breakdown technique, we have been able to produce films of Ni and Mo from the respective carbonyls, and W from WF_6 and H_2 by adding argon to the gas mixture. Concentrations in the case of the carbonyls were 2-3% carbonyl in argon at a total pressure of 10-20 torr. In the WF_6 experiments breakdown could only be achieved at higher pressures (15-35 torr) at concentrations of about 1% WF_6 in varying mixtures of H_2 and Ar. In all cases, total flow rates through the chamber were 30-3000 standard cm^3 per minute. Any turbulence in the chamber increases the residence time of the gas over the substrate and increases the chance of powder deposition on the substrate, hence efforts were made to insure that the flow across the substrate was laminar. The addition of argon to the gas mixture promotes the breakdown of the gas and serves to buffer the reactant species so that homogeneous nucleation does not occur in the gas phase. At high (greater than about 1 torr) partial pressures of reactant gas, powder formation occurs.

The table below shows the results of Auger electron spectroscopy depth profiles on representative samples of the films produced. The high rate of incorporation of carbon and oxygen in the Mo films is due to the condensation of $Mo(CO)_6$ on the substrate between laser pulses. Because of our interest in low substrate temperatures, we do not wish to heat the substrate to prevent this condensation. Thus, although we have been able to obtain Mo films exhibiting metallic characteristics, we have abandoned $Mo(CO)_6$ as a source and will not report detailed results on these Mo depositions. Future efforts will concentrate on the MoF_6 reduction process.

Precursor Gases	Film Composition, Atomic %
$Ni(CO)_4$, Ar	Ni 90%, C 9%, O 1%
$Mo(CO)_6$, Ar	Mo 40%, C 30%, O 30%
WF_6, H_2, Ar	W 55%, O 45%

Our work in the WF_6 system is in preparation for work in the MoF_6 system, as the two materials are similar in their thermal chemical vapor deposition behavior. Tungsten deposition rates of 0.5-1.5 nm/shot depend on WF_6 partial pressure and in part on flow rate, with greater deposition rates at lower flows. Adhesion of these films has been poor ($\sim 10^7$ dynes/cm^2), but scanning electron microscopy reveals clearly homogeneous films. The high rate of oxygen contamination in these films is uniform through the thickness of the film, indicating that the contamination is occurring during the growth process, perhaps from trace amounts in the H_2 and Ar sources. Work is continuing on this system.

Although carbon incorporation is a remaining problem in the Ni depositions, we present complete characterizations of these films, as they demonstrate the small grain size which is a principal feature of the technique and goal of the work.

Nickel deposition rates, like those for tungsten, vary from 0.5 to 1.5 nm per shot. Films as thick as 1.0 micrometer were produced although typical thicknesses were more of the order of a few hundred nm. Although a point focus is used in contrast with the line focus used by Collins, rather large area films (1 x 2 cm) were obtained. The films were fairly uniform in thickness over the deposited area with variation of about 15% over a centimeter.

Powder films, a common occurrence, can usually be identified by the appearance of the surface, but powder depositions with particle sizes of several nanometers are not obvious. Rapid determination of overall film quality and integrity was therefore done by adhesion tests. Film/substrate yield strengths of from 1.0 to 2.5×10^8 dynes/cm^2 ($1.5\text{-}3.5 \times 10^3$ psi) were obtained regularly from the Ni films. These figures demonstrate the homogeneous character of the films.

Composition results have already been mentioned. Figure 5 shows an Auger depth profile of a typical Ni film demonstrating uniform deposition. Incorporation of oxygen at the 1% level may be significant or may be the result of contamination in the Auger spectrometer.

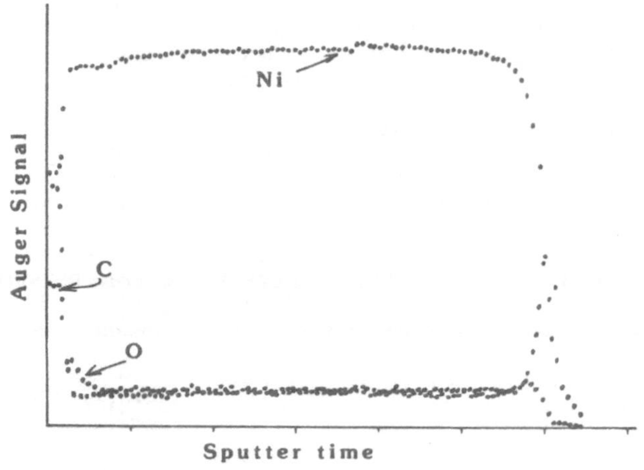

FIGURE 5. Auger depth profile of 1500 Å Ni film.

Structural analysis of the Ni films was done by digital diffractometer analysis of several films. Films of the order of a few hundred nm thickness yielded widths for the (111) Ni peak indicating a diffracting domain size of about 2.5 nm. More detailed analysis of data on a 1.0 micrometer film is shown in Figure 6. The raw data for this 42-hour scan at 0.1 degree steps is shown at the top of the figure. The strong amorphous signal is from the substrate, a glass microscope slide. A fit to the (111) and (200) Ni peaks with the amorphous background subtracted out was obtained but showed distinct fitting errors as can be seen in the figure. Figure 7 shows a three-peak fit to the same data with the addition of the Ni_3C (101) peak to the two Ni peaks. The peak height of the Ni_3C (101) is consistent with the Auger results of about 9% carbon

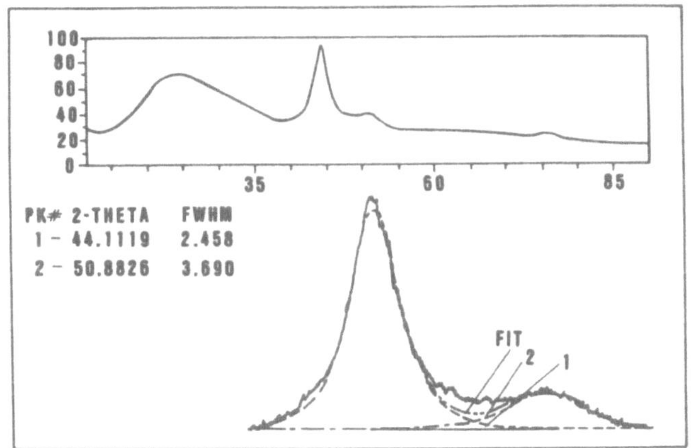

FIGURE 6. X-ray diffraction results for 1.0 μm Ni film with fit to Ni (111) and (200) peaks.

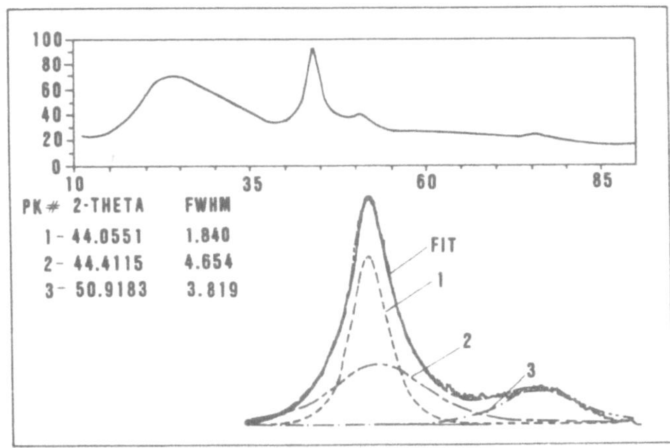

FIGURE 7. X-ray diffraction results for 1.0 μm Ni film with fit to Ni (111) and (200) and Ni_3C (101) peaks.

incorporation, leading us to believe that the impurity in the film is entirely in the carbide. Analysis of the width of the Ni peaks indicates some preferential orientation to the (111) direction and a maximum diffracting domain size of 4.7 nm. The Ni_3C peak is very broad, indicating a grain size of less than 2.0 nm. Stretching of the Ni lattice spacing due to the carbon incorporation is of the order of 1%. The diffracting domain size, which is about an order of magnitude smaller than that of comparable vacuum-deposited films, indicates that rapid quenching from the gas phase is occurring as anticipated.

Resistivity mesurements were made on Ni lines formed by lift off on glass substrates. Linewidths of from 0.6 mm to 3.5 mm and thicknesses from 40 nm to 90 nm were measured. Contact was made to the lines with silver-loaded epoxy and resistance measurements were made at line lengths from 1.2 cm to 0.4 cm. Contact resistance was measured at about 10^{-3} of line resistance. The data were reduced by linear regression of the resistance against the ratio of line length to cross-sectional area with a final figure of 5×10^{-3} ohm-cm. Variance was about 40%, reflecting what seems to be large-scale nonuniformity in the deposits. The high value of the resistivity (pure Ni has a resistivity of 6.8×10^{-6} ohm-cm) may be indicative of the presence of Ni_3C.

3. CONCLUSIONS

We have demonstrated that laser dielectric breakdown can be used to drive chemical vapor deposition reactions in both decomposition and reduction chemistries. We have also shown that the properties of the Ni films which have been most fully characterized are consistent with rapid quenching from the gas phase to the deposited film. The flexibility of the method leads us to believe that amorphous alloy films can be produced using this technique.

ACKNOWLEDGMENTS

I would like to thank R. Cordi for the Auger analysis and electron microscopy, L. Newkirk for the X-ray analysis, and J. Cost, R. Springer and J. Haggerty for useful discussions.

REFERENCES

1. H. Lydtin and R. Wilden, Microelectronics and Reliability 12, 177-178 (1973).
2. C. P. Christensen and K. M. Lakin, Appl. Phys. Lett. 32, 254-256 (1978).
3. S. D. Allen, J. Appl. Phys. 52, 6501-6505 (1981).
4. D. J. Ehrlich and J. Y. Tsao, J. Vac. Sci. Technol., B 1, 969-984 (1983).
5. D. Bauerle, Surface Studies with Lasers (Springer-Verlag, 1983), pp. 178-188.
6. K. Emery, P. K. Boyer, L. R. Thompson, R. Solanki, R. Zarnani, and G. J. Collins, Proc.-SPIE Int. Soc. Opt. Eng. 459, 9-17 (1984).
7. M. Meunier, T. R. Gattuso, D. Adler, and J. S. Haggerty, Appl. Phys. Lett. 43, 273-275 (1983).
8. R. Bilenchi, I. Gianinoni, M. Musci, and R. Murri, "Laser Induced Chemical Vapor Deposition of Amorphous Silicon," Proc. of the 4th European Conference on Chemical Vapor Deposition, Eindhoven (1983), pp.194-196.
9. M. Hanabusa, A. Namiki, and K. Yoshihara, Appl. Phys. Lett. 35, 626-627 (1979).

10. V. Baranauskas, C. I. Z. Mammana, R. E. Klinger, and J. E. Greene, Appl. Phys. Lett. 36, 930-932 (1980).
11. R. D. Coombe and F. J. Wodarczyk, Appl. Phys. Lett. 37, 846-848 (1980).
12. Y. Rytz-Froidevaux, R. P. Salathe, and H. H. Gilgen, Phys. Lett. A 84A, 216-218 (1981).
13. R. F. Karlicek, V. M. Donnelly, and G. J. Collins, J. Appl. Phys. 53, 1084-1090 (1982).
14. R. W. Andreatta, D. Lubben, J. G. Eden, and J. E. Greene, J. Vac. Sci. Technol. 20, 740-741 (1982).
15. J. T. Cheung, Appl. Phys. Lett. 43, 255-257 (1983).
16. I. P. Herman, R. A. Hyde, B. M. McWilliams, A. H. Weisberg, and L. L. Wood, Mat. Res. Soc. Symp. Proc. 17, 9 (1983).
17. W. E. Johnson and L. A. Schlie, Appl. Phys. Lett. 40, 798-801 (1982).
18. Y. Mishima, M. Hirose, Y. Osaka, and Y. Ashida, J. Appl. Phys. 55, 1234-1236 (1984).
19. C. Wanxing, W. Rugeng, X. Chungen, and W. Yugi, Chin. J. Lasers 10, 858-859 (1983).
20. R. M. Osgood, H. H. Gilgen, and P. Brewer, J. Vac. Sci. Technol., A 2, 504-505 (1984).
21. Q. Mingxin, R. Monot, and H. Van den Bergh, Sci. Sin. 27, 531-539 (1984).
22. P. J. Love, R. T. Loda, R. A. Rosenberg, A. K. Green, and V. Rehn, Proc.-SPIE Int. Soc. Opt. Eng. 459, 25-32 (1984).
23. F. A. Houle, C. R. Jones, T. Baum, C. Pico, and C. A. Kovac, Appl. Phys. Lett. 46, 204-206 (1985).
24. A. M. Ronn, Sci. Am. 240, 114-128 (1979).
25. S. M. Shin, C. W. Draper, M. E. Mochel, and J. M. Rigsbee, Materials Lett. 3, 265-269 (1985).
26. J. H. Flint and J. S. Haggerty, Proc.-SPIE Int. Soc. Opt. Eng. 458, 108-113 (1984).
27. T. R. Jervis, J. Appl. Phys. 58, 1400-1401 (1985).
28. J. L. Brimhall, L. A. Charlot, and R. Wang, Scripta Met. 13, 217-220 (1979).
29. R. P. W. Lawson, W. A. Grant, and P. J. Grundy, Nucl. Inst. & Meth. 209/210, 243-247 (1983).

COMBINED USE OF LASER IRRADIATION AND ELECTROPLATING

J. R. ROOS, J. P. CELIS, W. VAN VOOREN
Department of Metallurgy and Materials Engineering,
Katholieke Universiteit Leuven, B-3030 Heverlee, Belgium

Key Words: electrodeposition, epoxy substrate, gold plating, laser plating enhancement

ABSTRACT

The irradiation by a laser beam of a substrate used as a cathode during electrolysis causes a drastic modification of the electrodeposition conditions in the irradiated region. Interesting aspects of this technique are:

- The possibility of rapid maskless patterning,
- The possibility to enhance the plating rate in selected areas,
- The possibility to obtain electrodeposited coatings having unique structural properties.

In the present paper experiments done with a Nd:YAG laser irradiating an epoxy-Cu substrate during a gold-cobalt electrolysis will be presented. In order to use the laser energy efficiently, laser parameters (e.g., pulse frequency, power density, wavelength) and the optical and thermal properties of the material to be irradiated must be carefully selected. An optimal pulse frequency was observed which depends on the thickness of the copper substrate. Structural characteristics of the gold spots deposited will be discussed.

Based on a literature survey of laser-enhanced plating and on the present results, the mechanism of laser plating enhancement will be reviewed.

1. INTRODUCTION

Laser processing is a growing field with many applications in different areas of technology. This processing is based to a large extent on the energy available in the laser beam and on the possibility to focus and guide this beam easily. The resulting interaction is then determined by the energy housekeeping in which the following parameters play an important role: the characteristics of the laser beam, the characteristics of the irradiated material and its surrounding, the heat loss to that surrounding. The resulting energy transfer can induce a number of modifications in the surface conditions and characteristics of the irradiated material (1-3), namely:

- Mechanical modifications such as cutting, drilling and welding (4),
- Metallurgical and structural modifications:
  Thermal effects, e.g., hardening, diffusion and annealing,
  Surface melting, grain refining, production of amorphous top layers (5), alloying (6), oxidation, creation of internal stresses and modification of the surface roughness,
  The deposition of a coating.

Considering this last modification, laser applications for the deposition of a coating can be classified based on the phase condition from which the coating originates. Such a classification is summarized in Fig. 1. Wear-resistant coatings can be obtained by using a high-power CO_2 laser beam as a heat source to melt a suitable mixture of powdery metallic elements and compounds and to bind this mixture onto the substrate (7). With an injection of ceramic powders with specific characteristics (e.g., SiC or WC) into the melted zone, composite surface layers with improved wear resistance can be produced (8). Laser treatment of plasma-sprayed Ni-base alloy coatings (e.g., NiCr, NiCrAlY) can be applied to obtain denser coatings and also to induce a redistribution of elements over the coating section (9). Laser glazing of Fe-Ni-Cr-P-B powders sprayed onto a nickel substrate has also been reported (5) as well as a laser-induced formation of $CdTe_xSe_{1-x}$ semiconducting compounds (10).

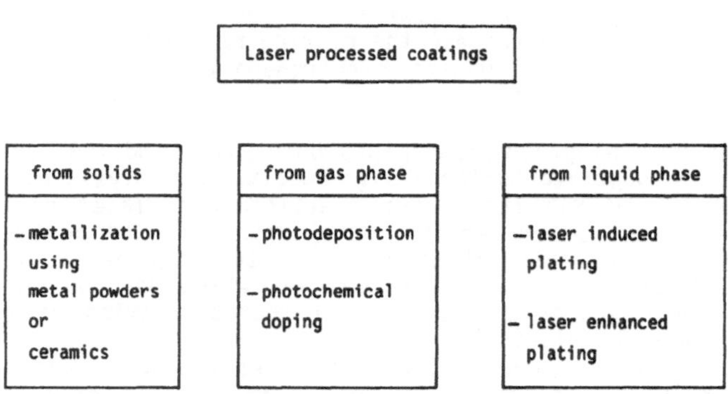

FIGURE 1. Classification of laser-processed coatings.

Besides the interaction of a laser beam with a solid surface, coatings can also be obtained based on a laser-induced photodissociation of a molecular gas in the vicinity of a gas-solid interface. In particular, low-power UV lasers of a few mW can be used for such applications in conjunction with a good focusing system. Most of the photodepositon work is related to metal production by photolysis of metal-alkyds. Since the process has a heterogeneous character, both the properties of the solid and the gas-phase kinetics have to be taken in consideration. Typical applications are in the field of semiconductors, e.g., direct doping (11), deposition of Si from SiH_4, deposition of Cr, Mo, W on Si wafers. In a different field of the coating technology, namely, chemical vapor deposition, laser-induced decomposition of $Ni(CO)_4$ into Ni has been reported and an enhanced deposition rate by a factor of 10^3 to 10^4 is claimed. UV laser photodeomposition of metal carbonyls also provides a means for maskless direct writing of refractory metals (12).

Finally, material deposition from the liquid phase can result from a laser beam irradiation. In this respect, the present paper will give a state of the art and a survey of some experiments we did to check the feasibility and potentialities of this technique for the selective plating of gold on electronic components.

2. LASERPLATING: STATE OF THE ART

The integration of lasers into the electrodeposition technology is presently occurring. The main difference between laser plating and the photodecomposition process is that it is not a gas presenting attenuation of the laser radiation, but liquids! The first attempt to use laser irradiation in combination with metal electrodeposition probably took place in December 1978 at the IBM-Thomas J. Watson Research Center (13). From these experiments it was demonstrated that the rate of plating is larger in the region of laser absorption than in the non-irradiated areas so that a pattern can be traced by a beam movement along the cathode. It was claimed that the deposition rate could be enhanced by a factor of 1000!

Going through the present literature, it seems, however, that only a very limited number of researchers are active in this area. Nevertheless, a number of potential applications of this technique can be distilled from the published work. Considering the net result of laser irradition, one can distinguish between laser-enhanced plating resulting in an increase of the plating rate, and laser-induced plating resulting in the initiation of metal decomposition. Both processes can in certain circumstances take place simultaneously. Considering the plating conditions, one can further distinguish two types of deposition techniques for which laser-induced/enhanced deposition has been experimentally verified, namely

- Enhanced electrolytic deposition,
- Induced electroless deposition or immersion plating.

Laser-enhanced electrolytic deposition of Ni, Cu and Au has been reported by von Gutfeld et al. (14-17). In general, power densities of 10^2 to 10^6 W/cm^2, depending on the optical reflectivity of the irradiated cathode used, are applied. The selection of the optical wavelength results generally from a compromise ensuring a large absorption by the cathode material and a minimum absorption by the electrolyte (Fig. 2). Ar^+ lasers (λ = 514.5 nm) should be selected in combination with green Ni and blue Cu electrolytes, while Kr^+ lasers (λ = 647.1 nm) or Nd:YAG lasers (λ = 1060 nm) should be used with light yellow-gold electrolytes. Two types of experimental setups can be distinguished: one where a thick metallic cathode is irradiated directly at the place where a coating has to be deposited (Fig. 3a), another where a transparent substrate coated with a metallic film is irradiated at the back side (Fig. 3b). The most recent development is the "Laser Jet Stream" proposed by IBM (18). This setup consists of a pressurized stream of electrolyte squeezed through a nozzle. A laser passes through the center of the stream and acts as an optical guide, keeping the laser light trapped along its length. The result of this laser irradiation, which is independent of the cell design, is a dome-shaped deposit (typical thickness 1 to 4 μm, width 0.5 mm) together with a background deposition. Potential applications are maskless laser patterning of microelectronic materials, repair of broken electrical circuits and localized plating of noble metals, resulting in appreciable cost savings.

Laser-induced electroless deposition has been reported by Al-Sufi et al. (19) for copper from copper sulfate/hydrochloric acid mixtures, by Karlicel et al. (20) for platinum and gold from an aqueous solution of chloroplatinic or chloroauric acid, and by Auerback (21) for silver from a silver nitrate/N-methyl pyrrolidone mixture. Recently, Zahavi et al. (22,23) reported the laser-induced gold deposition on silicon

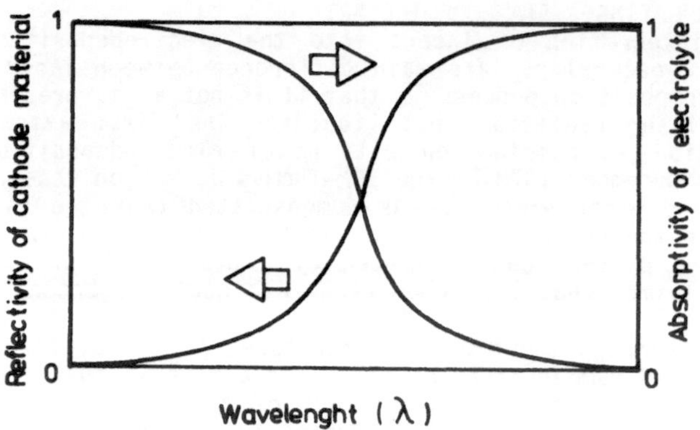

FIGURE 2. Reflectivity and absorptivity of a laser beam for cathode and electrolyte, respectively.

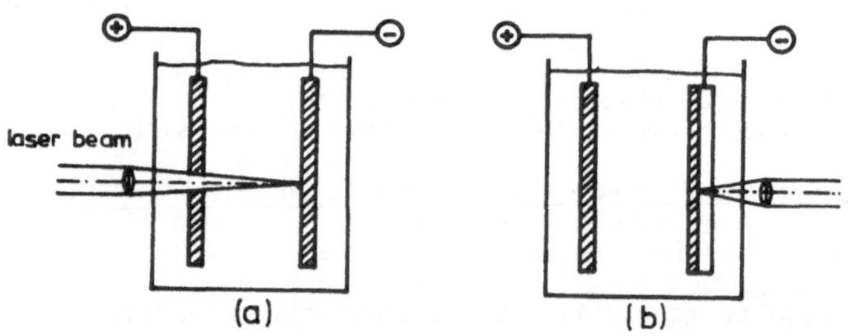

FIGURE 3. Schematic representation of (a) directly irradiated cathode, and (b) irradiated at the back.

and GaAs polyimide. The amount of gold deposited could be controlled effectively by varying the laser energy density either by inserting absorbing filters or by defocusing the laser beam. Potential applications are in the field of direct writing of electrical circuits on ceramics and nonconducting materials.

3. LASER-ENHANCED GOLD PLATING: EXPERIMENTAL PROCEDURE AND RESULTS

The effect of laser irradiation during gold plating was studied. As electrolyte, an industrial cobalt-containing gold cyanide plating solution was selected (15 g/l Au as $KAu(CN)_2$, 500 ppm Co, organic additives, pH 4.5, room temperature). Due to the addition of cobalt salts, a discoloration of the gold cyanide electrolyte from light yellow to light red takes place. At 25°C the current efficiency, determined by a gravimetric method, was found to be 22% under DC conditions. An increase in bath temperature up to 55°C results in a current efficiency increase

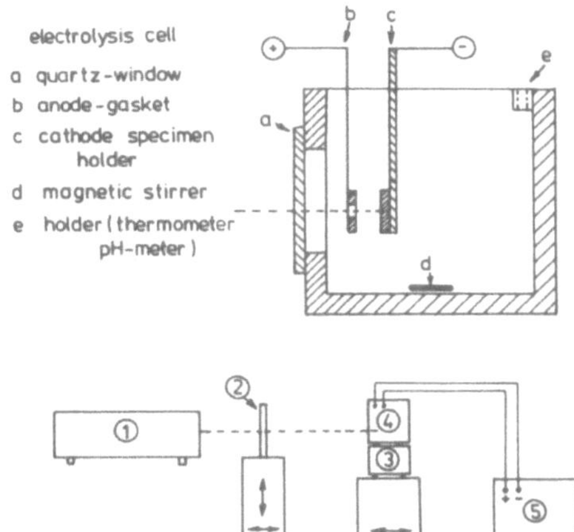

FIGURE 4. Schematic representation of the experimental laser plating setup used.

up to 50%. Most tests were performed in the galvanostatic mode at a current density of 1 A/dm^2. The experimental setup used is shown schematically in Fig. 4. The anode consists of a platinized titanium gasket. The electrolysis cell made from plexiglas contains a quartz window through which the laser beam directly irradiates the cathode surface. The current was applied by an Amel type 555B potentiostat. A Nd:YAG laser (λ = 1064 nm) was used at 32.5 or 35 A. Some typical laser beam output characteristics measured in air using photodiodes are summarized in Table 1. A constant spot size of 150 μm is taken into consideration for our calculations. The irradiation time varies between 1 and 10 min. As cathode, three different materials were selected, namely,

- A Cu-Zn sheet coated with an electroless 4 to 12 μm thick electroless Ni-P layer (24),
- An epoxy sheet coated with a 35 μm thick copper layer,
- An epoxy sheet coated with a 5 μm thick copper layer (19).

Special attention was given to the pretreatment of the cathode material in order to obtain good reproducibility. The pretreatment applied is summarized in Table 2.

A current density of 1 A/dm^2 was selected because, related to the low bath temperature selected, a large hydrogen evolution takes place at higher current densities. Laser irradiation seemed to promote this hydrogen evolution too.

TABLE 1. Characteristics of the laser irradiation applied.

Pulse Frequency (kHz)	Average Power (W)	Pulse Duration (ns)	Peak Power Density (MW/cm^2)
0.5	0.5	60	94.3
1	1.0	60	94.3
2	1.8	65	78.4
5	3.1	75	46.8
10	3.8	120	18.2
20	4.1	175	6.6
50	4.3	230	2.1
cw	4.5	-	0.025

Based on an estimated Sankey diagram showing energy losses due to undesired absorption and reflection processes, it is possible to evaluate the energy that can be transferred effectively to the cathode material. As can be seen from Fig. 5, only ~25% of the initial laser output energy can be utilized at the cathode surface. The evidence of this large

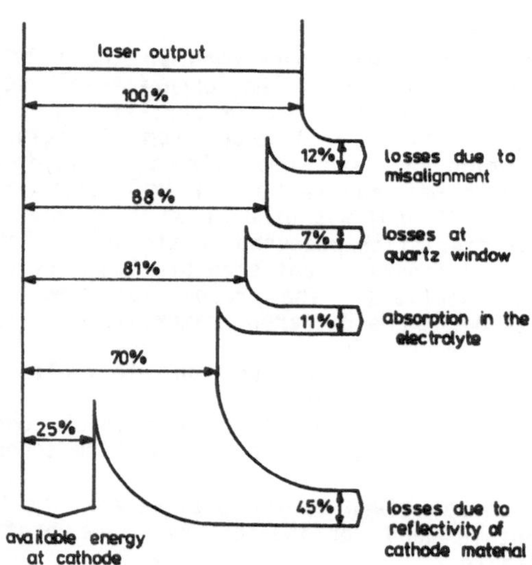

FIGURE 5. Sankey diagram for intermediate and surface-reflection losses.

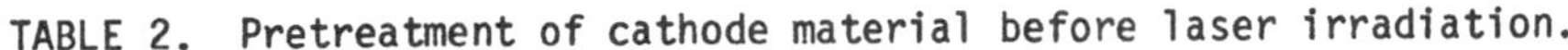
TABLE 2. Pretreatment of cathode material before laser irradiation.

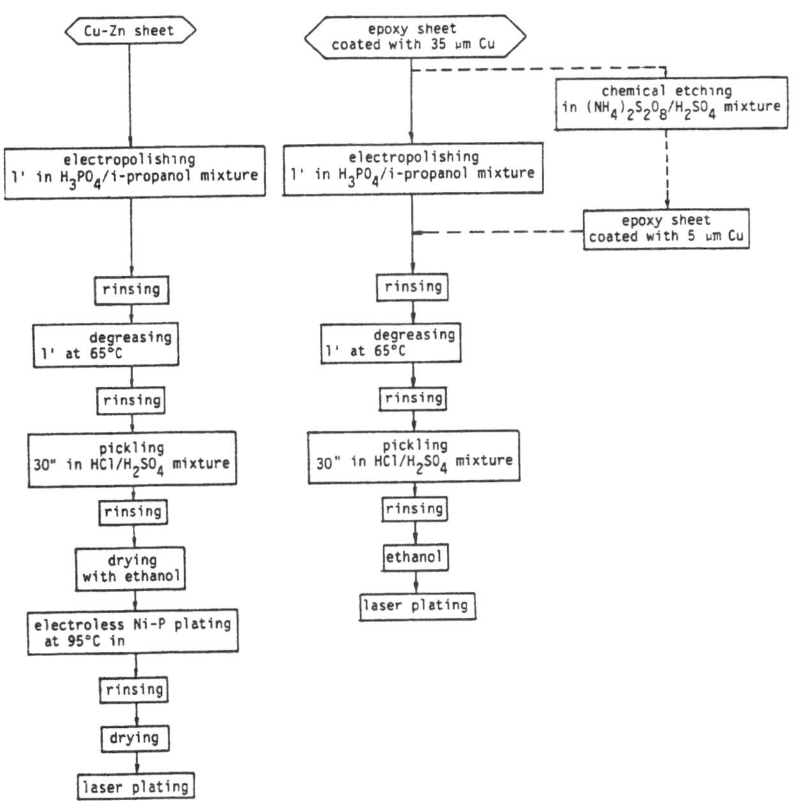

energy loss is demonstrated by a set of SEM pictures of cathode areas taken after irradiation either in the presence or absence of electrolyte in the plating cell. In the absence of electrolyte, the laser beam irradiation causes the formation of a hole through a gold-plated brass plate (see Fig. 6a,b). From Fig. 6b it can be concluded that the heat-affected zone is very limited since the original lenticular structure of the gold is visible close to the laser bore. In the presence of electrolyte the radial expansion of the heat-affected zone along the substrate surface is much larger. No drilling is noticed, but a local melting and recasting of the gold coating occurs at some distance away from the laser-irradiated zone (see Fig. 7a,b). The root of this expansion probably lies in the formation of bubbles at the cathode surface due to a local overheating of the electrolyte. These bubbles also inevitably deflect the laser beam.

The effect of the duration of laser irradiation on the size of the gold-enhanced deposit is shown in Fig. 8. For comparison, the thickness

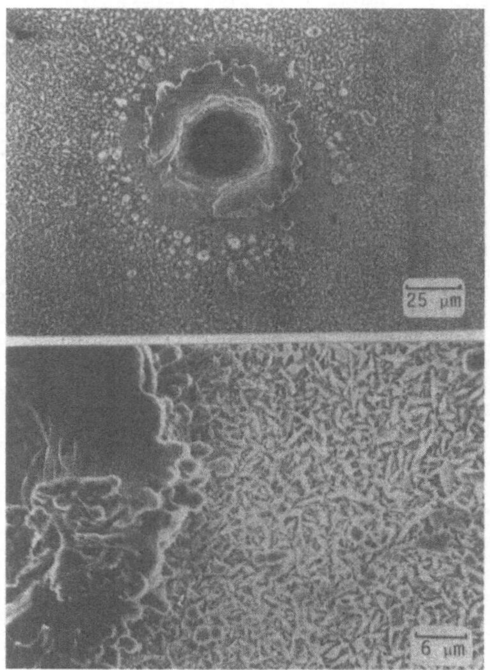

FIGURE 6. Effect of laser irradiation (Nd:YAG : 30 A, 1 kHz, 1') on a gold-plated brass plate in absence of an electrolyte.

of the galvanostatically deposited gold background is also plotted in Fig. 8. It seems that on a 35 µm Cu-plated epoxy sheet the width and height of the gold spot increase linearly with time. The rate of deposition perpendicular to the cathode surface enhances by a factor of 50x, independent of the duration of laser irradiation. This rather low enhancement in comparison to values reported in the literature (13) has certainly to be related to the non-optimal laser beam conditions used. However, since the experimental conditions used in the present work have been chosen based on a possible industrial practice in reel-to-reel plating, the data obtained are certainly realistic. On the other hand, the time of irradiation is too long due to the low duty cycle inherent to lasers operating in the pulsed mode. The typical nodular morphology of a gold laser-enhanced spot is shown in Fig. 9.

Since the frequency of the laser beam largely influences the peak power density (cfr. Table 1), it is also important to be aware of the effect of frequency on spot size. In Fig. 10 such results are given for two types of cathode material, namely, epoxy coated with a 35 µm or a 5 µm copper layer. For the epoxy + 35 µm copper it seems that an optimum is reached at 2 kHz. This optimum results from a compromise between a sufficient power density to enhance the electrolytic deposition and a maximum off time to avoid too large heat losses between two successive

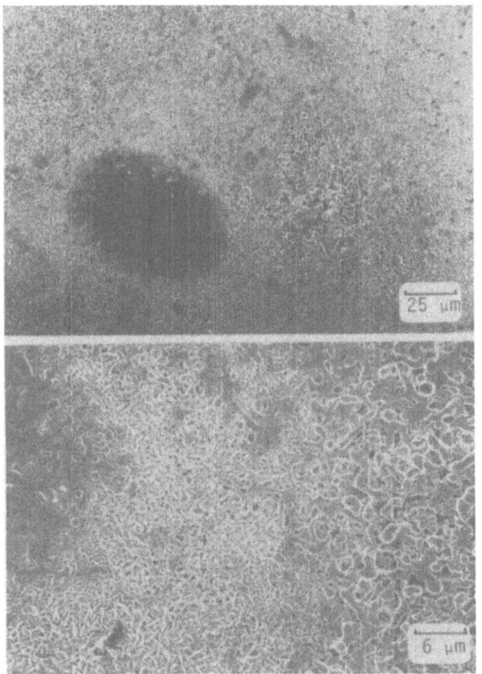

FIGURE 7. Effect of laser irradiation (Nd:YAG : 35 A, 1 kHz, 5') on a gold-plated brass plate in presence of a cobalt-containing gold cyanide electrolyte.

pulses. The importance of a correct selection of cathode material becomes evident when one compares results obtained with a 35 µm or 5 µm Cu-coated epoxy sheet (Fig. 10). For the 5 µm Cu-coated epoxy material, a dome-like gold deposit is obtained over the entire frequency range of the Q-switched Nd:YAG laser. The explanation for this is probably the fact that in a thin copper layer the heat diffusion is more restricted than in a thick one. These findings agree well with those of Al-Sulfi (19). On the Ni-P coated brass, dome-shaped deposits could only be obtained up to 1 kHz. Enhanced laser deposition results from an interrelationship between an induced raise of temperature and modified electrochemical conditions.

4. MECHANISMS OF LASER-ENHANCED PLATING

Looking back on the possible interaction between laser beam irradiation and electrochemical processes induced or enhanced during electrolysis, electroless or immersion plating, one can put forward:

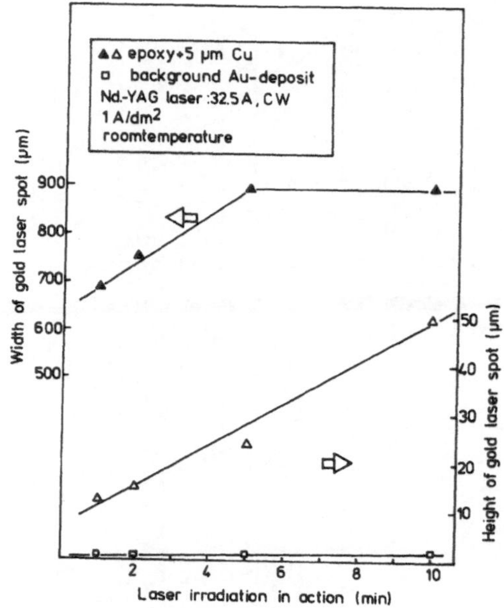

FIGURE 8. Size of laser-enhanced gold spots vs. duration of laser irradiation.

- Models based on a modification of the temperature along the electrolyte-cathode interface induced by an energy transfer from the laser beam to the irradiated material,
- Models based on a modification of the electrochemical deposition conditions induced by these temperature variations.

For relatively low laser intensities the temperature of the solid-liquid interface in the irradiated zone will remain below the boiling temperature of the solution. An increase of the plating rate will in that case only occur as far as the rate of the electrode reaction is temperature dependent. Below boiling only a very modest contribution from convection can be expected. Once boiling starts, a considerable enhancement of the convective transport towards the cathode occurs due to bubble explosion and/or ejection. Kuiken et al. (24) demonstrated both experimentally and theoretically that the application of a thin layer of a relatively poor heat-conducting material on a good heat-conducting substrate material may lead to a considerable local temperature increase. The dimensionless parameter determining this effect is, according to them, given by the product of the ratio of the thermal conductivities of substrate (k_2) and top layer (k_1) material and that of the layer thickness (d) and laser-spot diameter (a):

$$F = \left\{\frac{k_2}{k_1}\right\} \left\{\frac{d}{a}\right\}$$

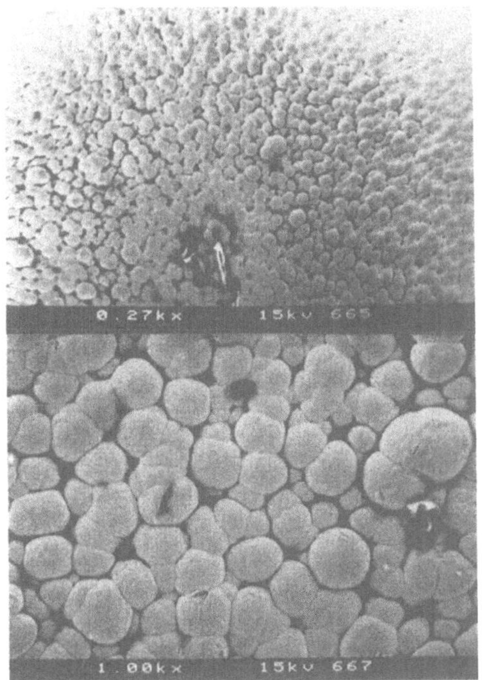

FIGURE 9. SEM micrographs of the morphology of a laser-enhanced gold spot on an epoxy + 5 μm Cu layer. Laser irradiation (Nd:YAG : 32.5 A, 5 kHz, 10') was performed during gold electrolysis at 1 A/dm^2.

The higher the F value, the larger the temperature enhancement will be, and the higher the conductivity of the plated material, the wider the spot will grow.

Considering now electrochemical processes, different formulae can be used to discriminate possible mechanisms affected by temperature variations:

(1) The Nernst equation, giving the rest potential (E) for the reaction OX + ne = RED

$$E = E^\circ + \frac{RT}{nF} \log \frac{[OX]}{[RED]}$$

(2) The Butler-Volmer equation giving the current density (i) at low overpotentials ($\eta = E' - E$)

$$i = i_o \left\{ \exp[\frac{\alpha\eta F}{RT}] - \exp[\frac{-\beta\eta F}{RT}] \right\}$$

with i_o the exchange current density.

(3) The limiting current density based on a limited mass transport

$$i_{lim} = \frac{FDC_o}{\delta}$$

with D the diffusion coefficient, δ the thickness of the diffusion double layer, C_o the bulk concentration of metal ions.

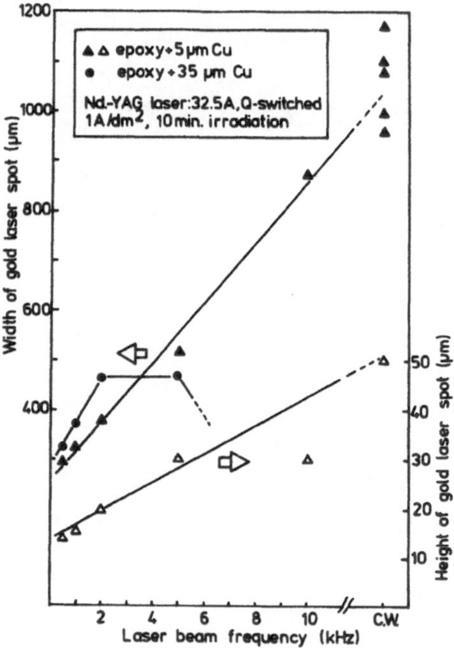

FIGURE 10. Size of laser-enhanced gold spots vs. laser beam frequency.

As can be seen from these formulae, the rest potential as well as the current density and the limiting current density are all temperature dependent. Experimental work done by Puippe (15) demonstrated indeed that the rest potentials for Cu/Cu^{++} and Au/Au^{+} shift towards more positive values with increasing temperature. Due to this positive shift of the rest potential at the hotter part of the cathode, it is possible to plate locally on a large cathode with no background plating and even without the use of an electrical circuit. The effects of agitation and increased temperature have been schematized by Romankiw (25) and are shown in Fig. 11. The relative importance of both parameters is, however, far from being well understood.

Finally, it should be mentioned that based on experiments performed by von Gutfeld (13), showing that back illumination of a thin cathode led to the same enhancement as that for front illumination (13), Puippe (15) excluded a significant contribution of a photocatalytic effect.

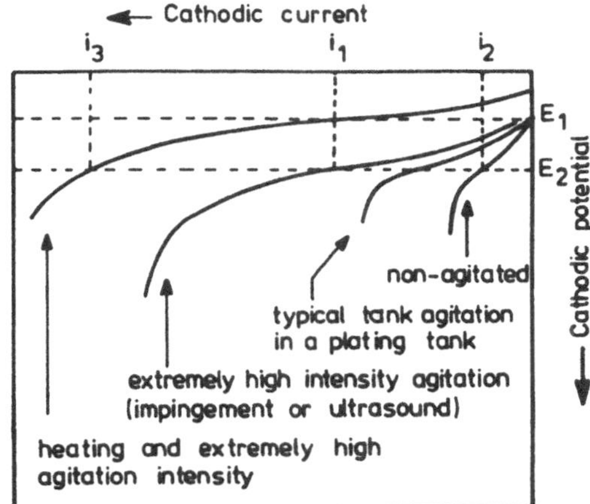

FIGURE 11. Shift in the current potential curve due to high substrate heating and accompanying intense local agitation (25).

Recently Zahavi (23), on the contrary, concluded that laser-induced gold deposition on GaAs substrates took place primarily through a photoelectrochemical deposition. From this controversy it is evident that the mechanism of laser-induced and -enhanced plating has still to be clarified.

ACKNOWLEDGMENTS

The authors would like to acknowledge the use of the facilities of Siemens, N.V., Oostkamp (Belgium). We gratefully thank Dr. J. Vanhumbeeck and ir. A. Mattelin from Siemens, N.V., for their contribution to this investigation.

REFERENCES

1. W. M. Steen and J. Powell, Mat. Eng. 2, 157-162 (1981).
2. K. Mukherjee and J. Mazumder, "Lasers in Metallurgy," Proc. 110th AIME Annual Meeting, Chicago (Feb. 22-26, 1981).
3. M. Bertolotti, Physical Processes in Laser-Materials Interactions (Plenum Press, 1983), ISBN 0-306-41107-5.
4. W. W. Duley, Laser Processing and Analysis of Materials (Plenum Press, 1982), ISBN 0-306-41067-2.
5. R. B. Diegle, "Glassy Alloys - New Class of Corrosion-Resistant Coatings," SAMPE-Quarterly 13, 26-31 (1982).
6. C. W. Draper, J. of Metals 34, 24-32 (1982).
7. A. Berlmondo and M. Castagna, Thin Solid Films 64, 294-256 (1979).
8. J. D. Ayers, R. J. Schaefer, and W. P. Robey, J. of Metals 33, 19-23 (1981).
9. H. Bhat, H. Heman, and R. J. Coyle, "Laser-Treated Plasma-Sprayed Ni-Base Alloy Coatings, Proc. 112th AIME Annual Meeting, Atlanta (March 7-10, 1983).

10. L. Baufay, D. Dispa, A. Pigeolet, and L. D. Laude, J. Cryst. Growth 54, 143-147 (1982).
11. D. J. Ehrlich, R. M. Osgood, and T. F. Devisch, IEEE J. Quantum Electron. 16, 1233-1243 (1980).
12. D. J. Ehrlich, R. M. Osgood, and T. F. Deutsch, J. Electrochem. Soc. 128, 2039-2041 (1981).
13. R. J. von Gutfeld, E. E. Tynan, R. L. Melcher, and S. E. Blum, Appl. Phys. Lett. 35, 651-653 (1979).
14. R. J. von Gutfeld, R. E. Acosta, and L. T. Romankiw, "Laser-Enhanced Plating and Etching; Mechanisms and Applications," IBM J. Res. Develop. 26, 136-144 (1982).
15. J. C. Puippe, R. E. Acosta, and R. J. von Gutfeld, J. Electrochem. Soc. 128, 2539-2545 (1981).
16. R. J. von Gutfeld, M. H. Gelchinski, and L. T. Romankiw, J. Electrochem. Soc. 130, 1840-1844 (1983).
17. R. J. von Gutfeld and L. T. Romankiw, "Laser-Enhanced Plating," Gold Bulletin 15, 120-123 (1983).
18. News and Update, J. of Metals 36, 8 (1984).
19. A. K. Al-Sufi, H. J. Eichler, and J. Salk, J. Appl. Phys. 54, 3629-3631 (1983).
20. R. F. Karlicek, K. M. Donnelly, and G. J. Collins, J. Appl. Phys. 53, 1084-1090 (1982).
21. A. Auerbach, J. Electrochem. Soc. 132, 130-132 (1985).
22. J. Zahavi and S. Tamir, "Laser-Induced Gold Deposition on a Silicon Substrate," Proc. Int. Conf. on Laser Processing and Diagnostics, Linz (July 15-19, 1984).
23. J. Zahavi and M. Halliwell, "Laser Beam Inducing Selective Plating Processes on GaAs Semiconductor Substrates, Proc. Interfinish '84, Jerusalem (Oct. 21-26 1984).
24. H. K. Kuiken, F. E. P. Mikkers, and P. E. Wierenga, J. Electrochem. Soc. 130, 554-558 (1983).
25. L. Romankiw, Invited Paper, 60 Jahrestag Forschungsinstituts für Edelmetalle und Metallchemie, Schwäbisch Gmünd, Germany (Sept. 26, 1983).

EDITED QUESTIONS - CHAPTER 7

J. TARDIEU de MALEISSYE

Q. In the case of pulsed irradiation, can you have higher pressures at greater power density and still have truly selective excitation via multiphoton coherent interaction?
A. True, selective excitation requires in this case an extremely low reactant pressure.

Q. Do you observe any fluorocarbons?
A. No, only ethylene and transparent hydrocarbons.

Q. Can you increase the yield by focusing tighter?
A. No, in fact, because when you increase the energy density by focusing, you decrease the irradiated volume and the number of molecules in the beam.

Q. Since interaction is multiphoton in nature, there should be a power law dependence between beam intensity and yield, so tightening the focus should increase the yield.
A. Under our experimental conditions there are no multiphoton processes as under pulsed irradiation and low pressure.

Q. What physical differences between C_2H_6 and C_4H_{10} cause the difference in the decomposition behavior?
A. If physical properties are concerned, it is both thermal conductivity and heat capacity which can cause such a difference in decomposition.

Q. Have you observed convection as well as diffusion and have you any way of observing this?
A. The presence of convection during irradiation may be qualitatively observed by the carbon deposit on the walls.

Q. Do you envisage any competition from this technique to the arc and plasma techniques used in the chemical engineering industry for the producton of "strange hydrocarbons"?
A. It is doubtful that "strange hydrocarbons" should be produced in this way. Its eventual concurrence with arc and plasma depends on the reaction of chemical reagents.

T. JERVIS (comment)
At Los Alamos, arc and plasma techniques create a wide size range of powders of this type; the laser technique forms a much narrower distribution and finer powders. So, although cheaper than the laser technique, the powders are not as suitable for very high strength ceramics, though the total volume produced by the laser technique is much smaller.

T. JERVIS

Q. How would you compare this process to classical photolithography?
A. The idea is not to create complete circuits by this technique, rather to make interconnections between larger circuits. As yet, only simple circuits such as small amplifiers have been made.

Q. Have you carried out any stress measurements on the films?
A. No.

Q. Was the sample horizontal or vertical to the beam?
A. It is vertical.

Q. Does the beam impinge on the surface?
A. No, it is going across the substrate. The plasma created by the beam at the pressures used is typically 2 mm diameter and its length depends on the nature of the beam and the focal length of the lens, and it is more than that distance above the substrate. The substrate received some shock wave and an ultra-violet pulse, but we don't think these phenomena have any significant effect.

Q. What was the pulse length used?
A. The laser is a CO_2 TEA laser, so the pulse length of the spike is about 50 ns.

Q. How many pulses per second do you achieve? How many nanometers per shot are deposited? How long to deposit one micrometer?
A. Typically 1-2 nm per shot. We use 1 Hz, so the system relaxes between shots; typically it takes 10 to 15 minutes to get one micrometer.

Q. Is there any specific direction that your group is interested in?
A. We are interested in all amorphous material work and solid-state reactions.

Q. Would it be possible to preionize the plasma in order to gain better control of the process?
A. It may be, there are many modifications we could make.

Q. You have used Auger analysis extensively. Could you comment on the accuracy of this technique?
A. On the whole, it is better than 10% with trace elements, but with a stronger signal it is much more accurate.

J. P. CELIS

Q. Does the laser irradiation increase the rate of other reactions, like, for example, hydrogen evolution?
A. Yes, in some instances H_2 evolution can even be seen with no potential applied.

A. GREELY

Q. What is the minimum concentration of an element that can be analyzed by this technique?
A. On the order of 1 ppm.

Q. In the transient nucleation model can you take superheating into consideration?
A. Yes we can.

Q. Is there any auxiliary ionization used on the mass spectrometer.
A. No.

CHAPTER 8 - LASER ANNEALING OF SILICON

CHAPTER INTRODUCTION

J. M. POATE, P. S. PEERCY, AND S. U. CAMPISANO

The observation in the latter part of the 1970s that laser irradiation of ion-implanted Si could remove the ion-implantation damage gave rise to the field that came to be known as laser annealing. The field has grown at an enormous rate; less than a decade later it remains an active area of research and has also spawned related fields that potentially have considerable technological importance. The background and developments of this field are reviewed in the articles by Poate and Peercy in this chapter.

This field has led to significant advances in several areas of solid-state physics and materials science. The ability to rapidly heat and melt surfaces with well-defined geometries to give known and controllable quenching rates up to 10^{12} K/sec, for example, has allowed, for the first time, amorphous Si to be quenched from the melt. At such high quench rates novel supersaturated Si solutions have been formed. Transient reflectance and conductance techniques have been developed to probe the melt duration at the surface at these ultra-rapid velocities as discussed in the article by Peercy. These rapid heating and diagnostic techniques have allowed us to address, for the first time, fundamental thermodynamic and kinetic properties of amorphous and crystalline Si as discussed in the article by Poate. The first-order phase transition of the melting of a-Si has been unambiguously observed and the melting point established. The liquid produced in these transient regimes can be undercooled considerably, thus leading to the formation of amorphous Si from the melt. The interfacial velocity and undercooling at which this transition takes place has been measured. The behavior of dopants at the liquid-solid interface results in novel segregation and supersaturation phenomena. Indeed, velocity-dependent segregation coefficients have been measured for the first time. The ability to measure directly the resulting liquid-solid or amorphous-crystalline interface velocity has allowed the first microscopic probing of interface kinetics that control these phenomena. The application of these dynamic techniques, in conjunction with ion beam analysis, electron microscopy and related techniques, has permitted detailed analysis of the solidification dynamics and resulting microstructures. Our current understanding of the segregation phenomena at these rapidly moving interfaces, and some of the open questions in this area, are addressed in the articles by Campisano and Aziz in this chapter.

A major driving force behind the initial development of this field was to use lasers to anneal ion-implantation damage in semiconductors. Although it was demonstrated that laser annealing can remove damage from ion-implanted semiconductors and restore electrical activity, it now appears that simpler heating schemes will be used. However, the concept of heating for times and temperatures different from those used in conventional semiconductor processing furnaces came directly from laser annealing. For example, the technique of rapid thermal annealing (RTA) is becoming very important in the processing of semiconductors. Similarly, the growth of novel structures and lateral epitaxial Si on insulators by scanned lasers gave birth to the silicon on insulator (SOI) field. This field now ranges from laser to strip heater crystallization and from buried insulators produced by ion implantation to epitaxial fluoride structures. The subject of SOI is one of the most active areas of Si crystal growth.

This NATO ASI has addressed the subject of Laser Treatment of Metals. As discussed in this chapter, many of the most powerful real-time and analytical techniques developed for the study of laser-silicon interactions are now being applied to the study of laser treatment of metals. For example, as discussed in the chapter by Spaepen and Peercy, picosecond lasers are extending the known compositional ranges for amorphous metallic alloys. Similarly, the transient techniques developed in the work on Si are permitting real-time measurements of melt kinetics in metals.

LASER ANNEALING OF SILICON

J. M. POATE
AT&T Bell Laboratories, Murray Hill, NJ

Key Words: laser annealing, amorphous Si, epitaxy

1. INTRODUCTION

Silicon is one of the most studied and best understood of all materials because of its importance to the integrated circuit industry. The emergence of laser annealing (1,2) in the last ten years has brought about new insight into some of its basic properties and new ways of processing. A quick look at the way integrated circuits are made reveals the reasons for the interest in laser annealing. To make integrated circuits, manufacturers slice very pure crystals of Si into thin wafers. Then they use complex fabrication techniques to produce electrically doped regions close to the surface of the Si and to produce insulating and conducting films that overlay the surface. These doped regions and films can be as thin as a few hundred atomic layers.

Dopants can be introduced by diffusion, which requires heating the wafer to about 1000°C for half an hour. Ion implantation is an alternative method of introducing dopants, but this also requires high-temperature heating to remove damage caused by the implantation process. Other currently practiced processing steps also entail heating the whole wafer for extended periods. Heating the entire wafer is not ideal because it limits the range of surface structures that one can produce. Focusable sources such as lasers, electron beams and even ion beams are attractive alternatives because they permit heating and modification of only the regions of interest (3).

The first demonstration of the utility of directed energy processing came from the initial Russian studies which showed that pulsed or continuous wave laser radiation removes ion-implantation damage in semiconductors. Thus the term "laser annealing" was coined. It is something of a misnomer, as most of the annealing mechanisms result from liquid or solid-phase recrystallization. What laser annealing offers to basic Si crystal growth studies is the ability to heat and quench well-defined surface layers in novel temperature and time regimes. This article will firstly concentrate on some of these aspects of crystal growth. Significant discoveries have been made concerning the kinetic and thermodynamic properties of crystalline, amorphous and liquid Si and these will be reviewed. Laser annealing has already spawned several technological offshoots and these will also be reviewed.

2. EPITAXY AND KINETICS

Figure 1 shows schematically the solidification or crystallization processes that result in epitaxial crystallization. The upper part shows solid-phase epitaxy. Amorphous Si is thermodynamically unstable in contact with crystalline Si and furnace heating will cause the amorphous layer to recrystallize. If the interface is clean, epitaxial

VERTICAL EPITAXY

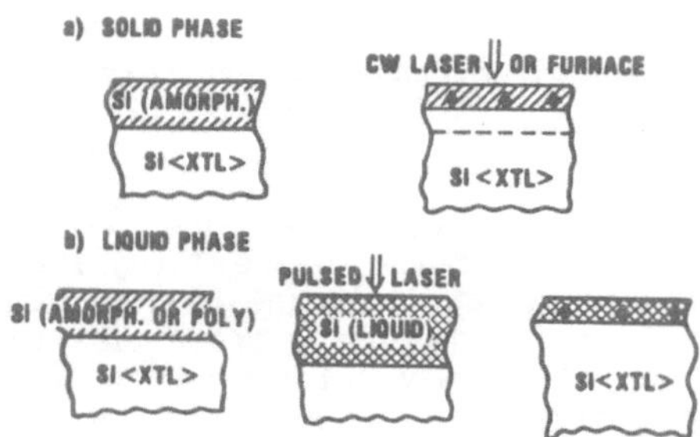

FIGURE 1. Schematic of vertical epitaxy. The regrowing interface, in both the solid and liquid phases, moves in a planar fashion to the surface.

growth will ensue. Implantation, for example, can produce amorphous layers with defective but clean interfaces. The lower part of the figure shows liquid-phase epitaxy.

The solid-phase epitaxial growth process is clearly illustrated by the series of transmission electron microscope (TEM) micrographs in Figure 2. Annealing for various times at 525°C results in regrowth of the amorphous layer produced by the implantation of 200 keV Sb^+ at $4.4 \times 10^{15}/cm^2$ into (100) Si. The epitaxial regrowth rates are about 0.15 nm/min for these annealing conditions. The dark band of

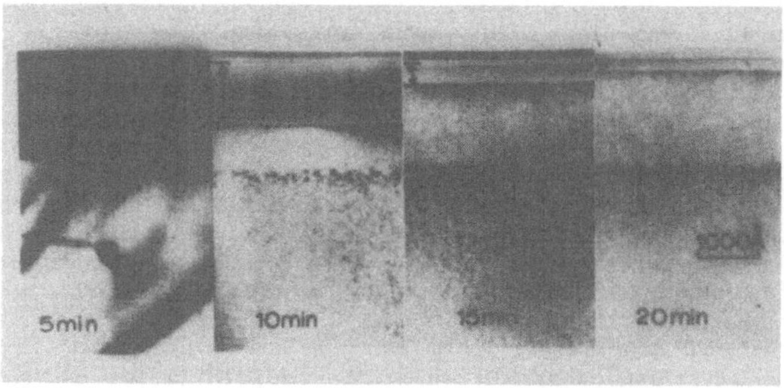

FIGURE 2. Transmission electron microscope cross-sectional micrograph for 200 keV Sb^+ ($6.0 \times 10^{15}/cm^2$) implants in Si annealed at 525°C. From J. Fletcher, J. Narayan, and O. N. Holland, Inst. Phys. Conf. Se. 60, 295 (1981).

interstitial defects at ~ 160 nm below the surface corresponds to incompletely annealed end-of-range damage resulting from beam heating.

The series of cross-section micrographs in Figure 3 provides an excellent illustration of amorphization and liquid-phase-crystallization processes in Si. Figure 3a shows an amorphous surface layer and a deeper band of isolated interstitial defects produced by implantation with As^+ ions. Irradiation with a 30-nsec ruby laser produces the following effects. Figures 3b and 3c illustrate that, at low-energy

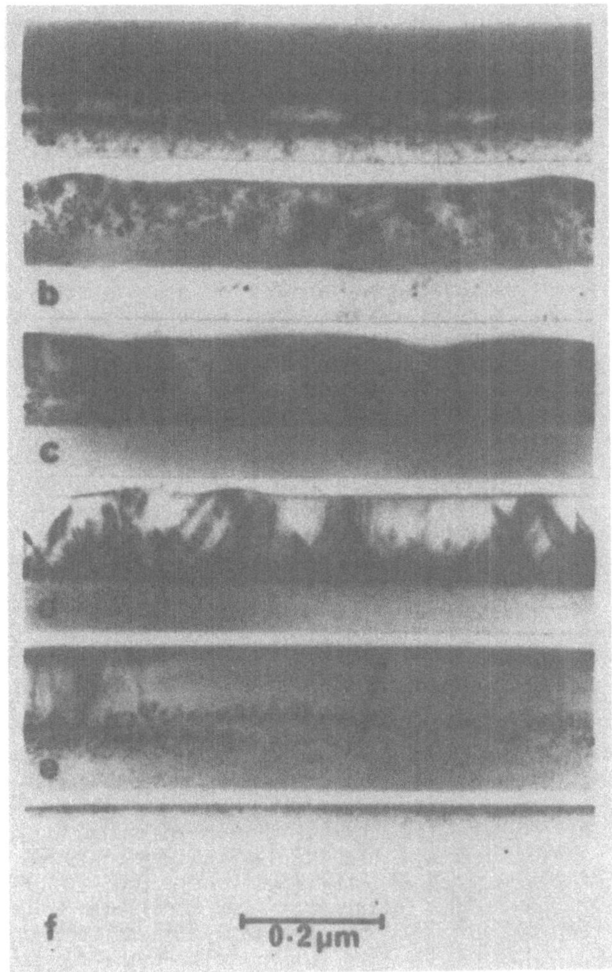

FIGURE 3. TEM cross-sectional images of (001) Si implanted with 150-keV As^+ ions ($4 \times 10^{15}/cm^2$). (a) As-implanted, (b) 0.20 J/cm^2, (c) 0.35 J/cm^2, (d) 0.85 J/cm^2, (e) 1.00 J/cm^2, (f) 1.20 J/cm^2. From A. G. Cullis, H. C. Webber, and N. G. Chew, Appl. Phys. Lett. 36, 547 (1980).

irradiation, an amorphous-to-polycrystalline transition occurs in the outer regions of the amorphous layer. This can be attributed to localized near-surface melting, in which the melt front did not extend into the underlying crystal. As there is no seed for epitaxy, solidification produces polycrystalline Si. Results such as these shown in Figures 3b and 3c presented an interesting puzzle at low irradiation energies because the melt depths (i.e., polycrystalline thickness) were much greater than expected from simple heat flow arguments. This puzzle has only been resolved in the past two years. It has been discovered, as discussed by Peercy in this chapter, that low-energy irradiation produces an explosive crystallization front which propagates through the amorphous layer. Figures 3d and 3e show an amorphous-to-single crystal transition in which the melt has just penetrated into the underlying crystal during the laser irradiation and then resolidified from the bulk seed crystal towards the surface. But the single crystal epitaxy is defective because not all the end-of-range defects have been removed. Irradiation at a higher energy density (Figure 3f), which induces melting beyond the region of isolated defects, produces an extended defect-free single crystal via liquid-phase epitaxial growth. The entire melting and recrystallization process occurs in a time of less than 100 nsec with solidification velocities of approximately 2 m/sec. One of the intriguing features of the first experiments on laser annealing was the fact that high-quality single-crystal Si could be grown when amorphous, implanted layers were melted with Q-switched ruby laser irradiation and solidified with such high velocities. The reason for this behavior lies in the high-yield strength of Si. Metals will usually slip when quenched at such rates.

A parameter of crucial importance in epitaxy is the velocity at which the crystallizing interface advances. Although amorphous Si is thermodynamically unstable in the presence of crystalline Si, it does not crystallize at room temperature because of kinetic barriers to atomic motion. However, at quite modest temperatures the amorphous layer crystallizes epitaxially. Figure 4 shows the exponential rate at which the velocity of the crystallizing interface increases with temperature. The continuous line is an extrapolation of furnace measurements of crystallization rates in the temperature range 500-600°C. At temperatures of about 1100°C, a crystalline layer 100 nm thick will grow from the amorphous material in about 1 msec. It is not possible to heat for such short times in conventional furnaces.

An elegant technique has been developed by Olson and co-workers (4) for the monitoring of solid-phase epitaxy of elevated temperatures. They heat the surface with a single, long pulse from a continous-wave argon laser and observe the crystal growth directly by monitoring the reflectivity of light from a probing laser. Interference between light reflected from the surface and light reflected from the amorphous crystal interface causes the reflectivity to oscillate as a function of time. Thus they measure directly the time for the interface to travel one wavelength. Figure 5 shows these solid-phase epitaxy rates (4). These measurements indicate solid-phase regrowth of amorphous Si to within 50°C of the 1423°C melting temperature of crystalline Si, as shown in Figure 4. However, the curve above 1100°C is dashed because there are predictions that amorphous Si melts at temperatures considerably beneath the crystalline melting temperature. The thermodynamics of Si will be discussed later.

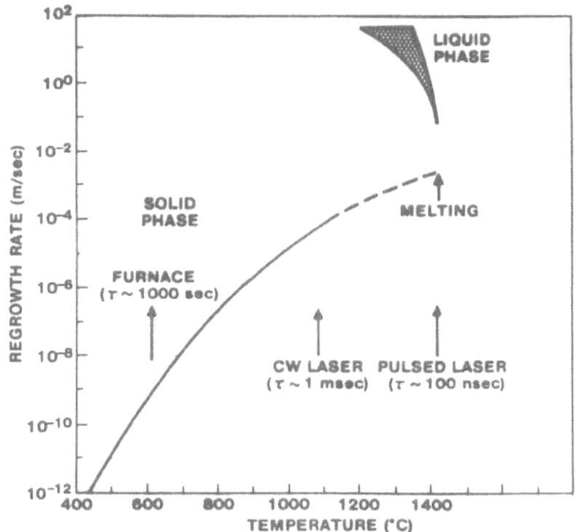

FIGURE 4. Schematic of Si crystallization rates (in meters per second) versus temperature. The solid-phase data come from measurements of the regrowth of amorphous Si on Si. The liquid-phase data come from calculations of the velocity of the liquid-solid interface in laser-induced surface melting.

The interface velocities are clearly higher when thin surface layers are melted using pulsed laser irradiation. As Figure 4 shows, there is a sharp jump in the crystallization velocity above the solid-phase values because of the much greater mobility of atoms in the liquid and because of the very high temperature gradients present in pulsed laser melting. The hatched region shows the velocities that are experimentally attainable using pulsed irradiation. The velocity depends on the rate at which the latent heat of crystallization is extracted from the interface; it therefore depends on the thermal conductivity of crystalline Si and the temperature gradient in the solid. Calculations of interface velocities agree well with direct velocity measurements by the transient conductance technique as discussed by Peercy in this chapter. At velocities of about 3 m/sec the melt crystallizes with a high degree of epitaxial perfection. This type of crystal growth should be contrasted with conventional growth from the liquid phase, where the growth rates are typically 10^{-5} m/sec. What ultimately determines the velocity of crystallization is the degree of supercooling, or undercooling, of the growing interface with respect to the melting temperature. The greater the undercooling the greater the velocity. At present there is only one good estimate of the relationship of undercooling to interface velocity in Si as will be discussed later. The hatched region just indicates plausible values of velocities and undercooling.

The upper limit to the recrystallization velocity occurs when solidification is so fast that an amorphous layer forms instead of a crystalline one, because the atoms do not have time to find equilibrium

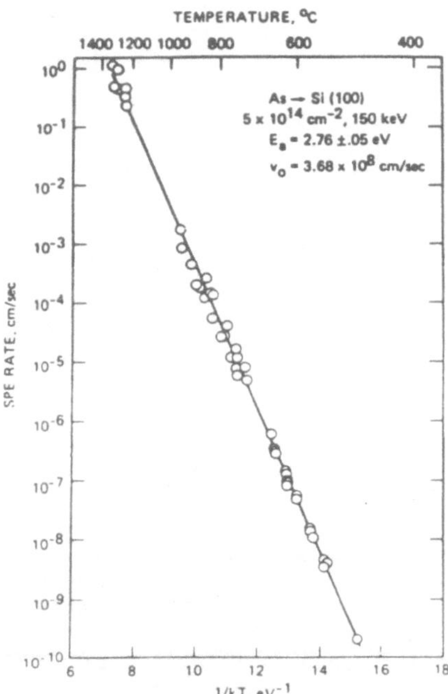

FIGURE 5. Dependence of solid-phase epitaxy rate on temperature in As-implanted (150 keV, $5 \times 10^{14}/cm^2$) Si (100) samples. All rates measured by time-resolved reflectivity; temperatures less than 645°C measured with thermocouple in thermal equilibrium with sample; temperatures greater than 645°C measured by time-resolved reflectivity. From Olson (4).

locations at the moving interface. Figure 4 shows that the range of crystallization velocities, from the amorphous solid and the liquid phases, is quite remarkable - one can vary them experimentally over 14 orders of magnitude.

One of the most striking manifestations of the rapidly moving liquid-solid interface is the incorporation, or trapping, of dopants in the solid at concentrations in excess of equilibrium solubilities. Dopants are implanted in crystalline Si, folowed by pulsed laser melting of the resulting implanted amorphous layer and part of the underlying crystalline Si. Rutherford backscattering and ion-channeling techniques are used to observe the depth distribution and lattice-site location of the impurities in the recrystallized surface layer. The impurity depth distributions are fitted to theory by using known Si liquid-state diffusivities and by assuming a unique interfacial segregation coefficient. This subject is reviewed by Campisano in this chapter.

3. THERMODYNAMICS AND AMORPHOUS Si

The condensed phases that take part in these rapid-heating transformations are amorphous, crystalline and liquid Si. The thermodynamic relationships of the liquid and crystal phases are well established, but there is some uncertainty regarding the amorphous phase. The fact, however, that amorphous Ge and Si are in a higher free energy state than the crystalline state led Bagley and Chen (5) and Spaepen and Turnbull (6) to propose that the amorphous phase melts at a discrete temperature (T_{al}) which is lower than the crystalline melting temperature (T_{cl}). Figure 6 shows the calculation of Donovan et al. (7) of the Gibbs free energy of liquid and amorphous Si referenced to crystalline Si. These calculations were based on calorimetric measurements (7) of the heat of crystallization (ΔH_{ac}) of amorphous Si. The two curves of the amorphous free energies give upper and lower limits. The intersection of the amorphous and liquid free energy curves gives, by definition, the amorphous melting temperature (T_{al}). The hatched region, therefore, in the curves gives an idea of the uncertainty in T_{al}. We see that $T_{al} \approx 0.8\ T_{cl}$ or $T_{cl} - T_{al} \approx 250°C$, a remarkable difference in melting temperatures for two solid phases of the same element.

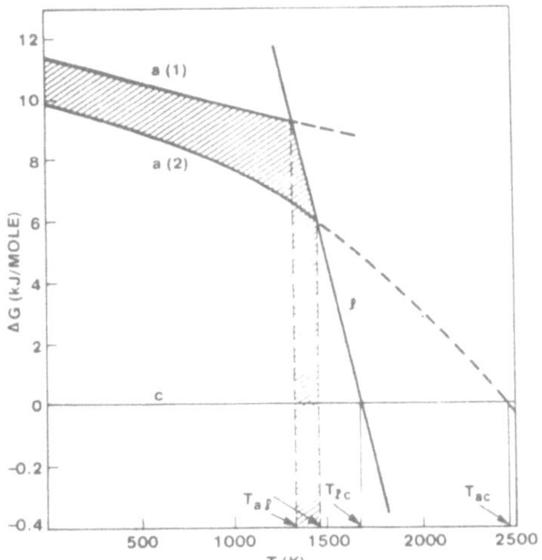

FIGURE 6. Gibbs free energy differences for Si crystal (c), metallic liquid (l), and amorphous (a). The different estimates for the amorphous melting temperature T_{al} correspond to the two estimates of the heat capacity. From Donovan et al. (7).

The argument regarding this large depression in melting temperature is based on the premise that the phase transition from the amorphous to liquid phase is discontinuous and first order. The physical reasoning behind this premise is plausible when it is realized that the transition involves a fundamental change in bonding from the covalent, amorphous phase with fourfold coordination to the metallic liquid with 11- to 12-fold coordination. Clearly, this transition will only occur in very rapid heating measurements; otherwise, the amorphous phase will recrystallize directly in the solid phase as observed in furnace heating measurements, for example. We have directly observed (8) this transition using the transient conductance technique (Peercy, this chapter) and indeed measure $T_{cl} - T_{al} \approx 250°C$. The evidence for this first-order transition therefore looks pretty solid. There is a puzzle, however, in the data of Olson (4), where solid-phase epitaxy is observed at temperatures within 50°C of T_{cl}. It is important to resolve this dilemma.

The amorphous-liquid transition should be reversible so that undercooling or supercooling the melt beneath T_{al} should lead to growth of amorphous Si in the melt. When ultrafast laser heating is used, it is possible to quench amorphous Si from the melt. This effect was originally demonstrated by Liu et al. (9) and Tsu et al. (10) and was the first time that amorphous Si had been quenched from the melt. We have determined (11) by the transient conductance technique that amorphous Si is formed when the liquid-solid interface velocity exceeds 15 m/sec. At such a velocity, therefore, the liquid must have a greater undercooling than 250°C. Amorphization conditions are usually quoted in quench rates, in this case 10^{12}°C/sec, but interfacial velocities are more meaningful physically. Laser annealing affords the opportunity of measuring such interfacial parameters.

Fundamental to melting-solidification theory is the relationship between undercooling and crystal growth and superheating and melting. Figure 7 from Spaepen and Turnbull (12) shows the various regimes for crystal growth or melting of Si. The constant f case refers to growth or melting away from the [111] direction. The curves for dislocation

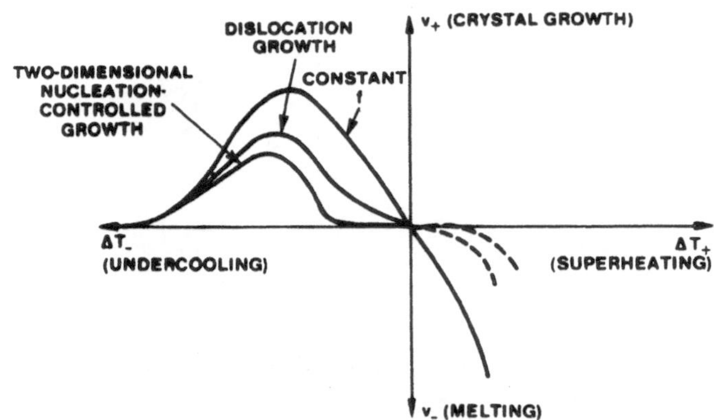

FIGURE 7. Schematic diagram of the crystal growth (v_+) or melting (v_-) velocities in various regimes for a Si crystal surrounded by its melt. The dashed lines represent melting of a thin layer on a flat Si crystal. From Spaepen and Turnbull (12).

and two-dimensional nucleation apply to regrowth of Si in the [111] direction. Although Si is such an important material, data on velocities versus growth or melting are remarkably sparse or non-existent. In fact, the only data we are aware of come from laser annealing and transient conductance experiments (see Peercy, this chapter), where the undercooling at an interface velocity of 6 m/sec has been deduced to be 90°K. This corresponds to an undercooling rate of 15°K/m/sec. This number is consistent with the laser amorphization experiments where the undercooling at 15 m/sec must be greater than 250°K (i.e., the freezing point depression of amorphous Si).

Unusual solidification scenarios can result when amorphous Si is melted using very short laser pulses. We have investigated the melting of thin (100 nm) amorphous layers formed by the implantation of such dopants as As, Bi and In. Amorphous Si can be solidified from the melt if very short heating pulse lengths are employed (typically 2 nsec ruby) to melt only partially through the amorphous thickness. Calculations show that the solidification velocity is substantially less than 15 m/sec, which is the velocity needed to form amorphous Si at the liquid-crystal interface. It is obviously easier to propagate an amorphous solid from an amorphous interface than from an ordered, crystalline interface. The temperature of the liquid, however, must be depressed beneath T_{al} for the solidification of amorphous Si.

The dopants can be segregated in a novel fashion by these amorphous-liquid interfaces. Figure 8 shows cross-section transmission electron microscope images of the In- and As-implanted layers following laser irradiation. The In sample shows a band of segregated In which is buried some 40 nm beneath the surface of the amorphous Si. This band is only some 1.5 nm wide. The fact that the In layer in the present experiment is buried and not zone refined to the surface can be explained by a very unusual solidification scenario. Solidification of the amorphous phase starts at the liquid-amorphous interface. This interface moves toward the surface with concomitant segregation of In. The remaining liquid is so undercooled, however, that solidification can proceed from the surface after possible nucleation at residual surface impurities. The buried In layer, therefore, represents the location at which these two interfaces collide. The complete dopant profiles have been measured by Rutherford backscattering and interfacial segregation coefficients have been estimated. These are the first measurements of segregation coefficients at the amorphous-liquid interface. The In segregation coefficients are very similar to those measuered for the crystal-liquid interface at the same velocity. No buried bands are observed for As because the segregation coefficients are effectively unity.

4. APPLICATIONS

Extensive research over the past six years has indicated that pulsed lasers probably will not find widespread use as heating sources for removing Si implantation damage. Rapid melting and solidification do not appear to be compatible with maintaining structural integrity on Si wafers that have already been patterned with metal and dielectric films. Nevertheless, pulsed lasers, or other pulsed sources, may find applications in contacting metal films to Si and compound semiconductors.

Laser annealing has led to two important technological developments in semiconductor processing. One is almost trivial. All the research on novel heating schemes demonstrated to the semiconductor engineers

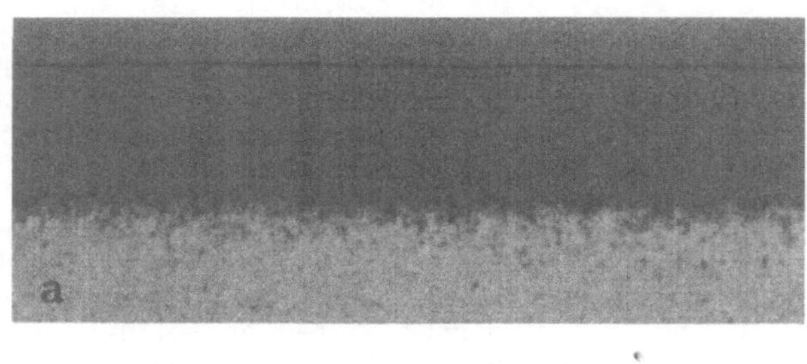

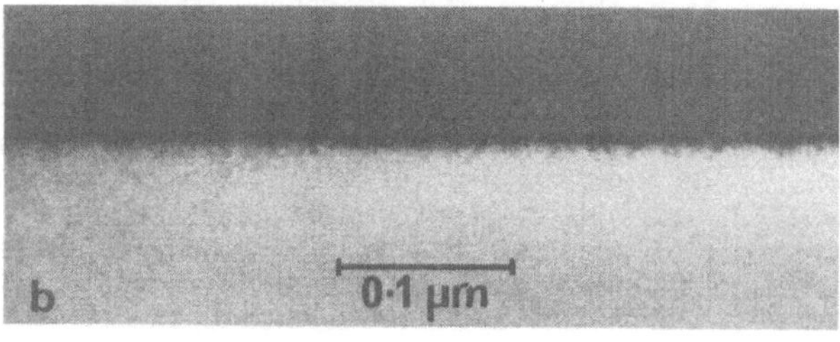

FIGURE 8. Cross-sectional TEM images of amorphous ion-implanted and laser-annealed layers: (a) In^+ at 0.25 J/cm^2, note buried band of segregated In; (b) As^+ at 0.25 J/cm^2. From S. U. Campisano, D. C. Jacobson, J. M. Poate, A. G. Cullis, and N. G. Chew, Appl. Phys. Lett. 46, 846 (1985).

that Si wafers do not necessarily have to be annealed at the canonical conditions of 1000°C for 30 minutes. In fact, a 100 nm amorphous layer will recrystallize epitaxially (see Figures 4 and 5) in 10^{-2} sec at such temperatures. Annealing for 30 minutes therefore represents a considerable degree of overkill. New transient heating schemes have been developed using, for example, arc lamps as the heating source. Wafers can be heated at temperatures of approximately 1000°C for times of approximately 1 sec. This is rapid thermal annealing (RTA). One of its advantages is that implantation damage can be annealed without significant dopant diffusion. The technique also looks particularly promising for the annealing of compound semiconductors.

One of the most important offshoots of laser annealing research is the technology for forming crystalline Si on amorphous, insulating substrates. Manufacturers have produced small-grain polycrystalline Si on amorphous SiO_2 for many years by methods involving chemical vapor deposition. However, the resulting material has an exceedingly fine grain size of about 50 nm, so that while it is useful for making electrical interconnections, its electrical transport properties are much poorer than single-crystal Si and it is uninteresting as a material in which to fabricate active devices. The situation is very different if single-crystal Si can be grown on insulators. Silicon-on-insulator

(SOI) technology offers many exciting device implications such as [3D] circuits, increased speed due to the dielectric isolation and radiation hardness.

The many possibilities of laser melting of Si using continuous wave lasers led to the concept of lateral epitaxy, illustrated schematically in Figure 9. Polycrystalline or amorphous Si is melted and the melt puddle scanned over the dielectric SiO_2. If the initial melt takes place over a Si seed, very large grains of single-crystal Si can be produced on SiO_2. This Si quality compares favorably with the best known SOI material, epitaxial silicon-on-sapphire. Because of its localized heating, this laser-scanning technique is finding application in producing the first [3D] Si circuits.

LATERAL EPITAXY

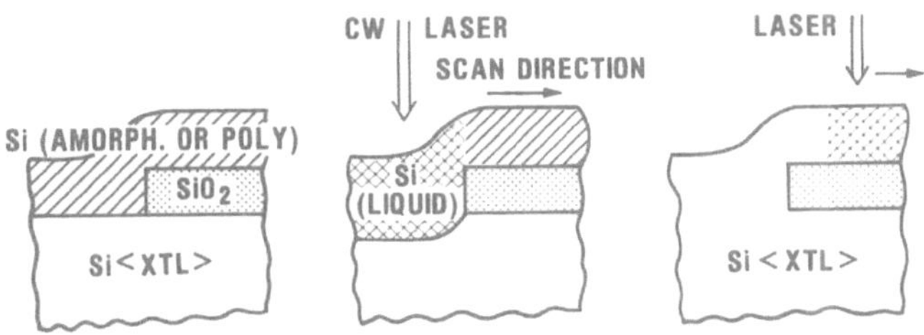

FIGURE 9. Schematic of lateral epitaxy. The melt puddle formed by a cw laser is scanned. Lateral epitaxy thus occurs at the trailing edge of the melt puddle.

A laser is not the only means of producing a moving molten zone for lateral crystal growth on amorphous substrates. Fan and his co-workers (13) used graphite-strip heaters to melt a layer of Si on SiO_2. A schematic of this apparatus is shown in Figure 10. It is quite simple in concept and very successful in application. One of the heaters is narrow and defines the molten zone. It moves parallel to the surface of the film at a speed of about 5 mm/sec. Such a strip heater is shown schematically in Figure 10. The Si is encapsulated between two layers of SiO_2. Pfeiffer and co-workers (14) have been able to recrystallize 4" wafers using this technique.

The success of laser annealing in demonstrating lateral epitaxy has led not only to strip heater technology but also to other SOI technologies. For example, buried oxide layers can be formed by oxygen implantation in Si. Following implantation, the surface Si layer is highly disordered but not amorphous. High-temperature ($\approx 1200°C$) annealing will restore the crystallinity of the upper Si layer. The whole field of SOI research is one of the most active areas of Si crystal growth.

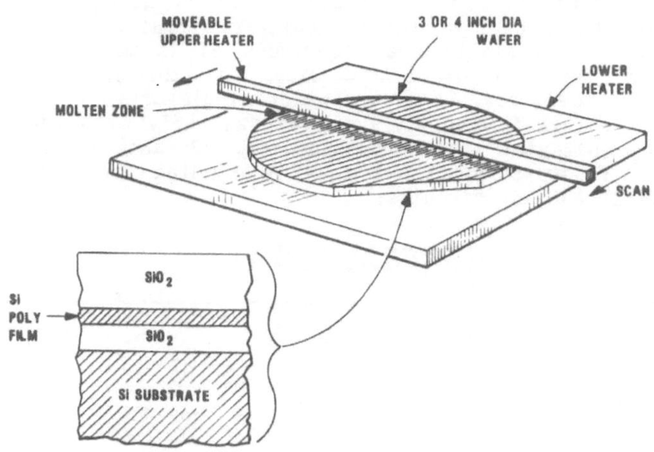

FIGURE 10. Schematic of a carbon strip heater and SOI structure.

REFERENCES

The progress of the field is nicely detailed in eight Materials Research Society annual symposia from 1978 to 1984; references 1 and 2 give much of the background.

1. Laser-Solid Interaction and Laser Processing-1978, edited by S. D. Ferris, H. J. Leamy, and J. M. Poate, AIP Conference Proceedings No. 50 (AIP, New York, 1979).
2. Laser and Electron Beam Processing of Materials, edited by C. W. White and P. S. Peercy (Academic Press, New York, 1980).
3. Laser Annealing of Semiconductors, edited by J. M. Poate and J. W. Mayer (Academic Press, New York, 1982).
4. G. L. Olson, Materials Research Society Symposium Proceedings (Materials Research Society, 1984), Vol. 35, p. 25.
5. B. G. Bagley and H. S. Chen, Ref. 1, p. 97.
6. F. Spaepen and D. Turnbull, Ref. 1, p. 93.
7. E. P. Donovan, F. Spaepen, D. Turnbull, M. J. Poate, and D. C. Jacobson, J. Appl. Phys 57, 1795 (1985).
8. M. O. Thompson, G. J. Galvin, J. W. Mayer, P. S. Peercy, J. M. Poate, D. C. Jacobson, A. G. Cullis, and N. G. Chew, Phys. Rev. Lett. 52, 2360 (1984).
9. P. L. Liu, R. Yen, N. Bloembergen, and R. T. Hodgson, Appl. Phys. Lett. 34, 864 (1979).
10. R. Tsu, R. T. Hodgson, T. Y. Tan, and J. E. E. Baglin, Phys. Rev. Lett. 42, 1356 (1979).
11. M. O. Thompson, J. W. Mayer, A. G. Cullus, H. C. Webber, N. G. Chew, J. M. Poate, and D. C. Jacobson, Phys. Rev. Lett. 50, 896 (1983).
12. F. Spaepen and D. Turnbull, Chapter 2 in Ref. 3.
13. J. C. C. Fan, M. W. Geis, and B.-Y. Tsaur, Appl. Phys. Lett. 38, 365 (1981).
14. L. N. Pfeiffer, K. W. West, S. Paine, and D. C. Joy, Materials Research Society Symposium Proceedings (Materials Research Society, 1984), Vol. 35, p. 583. This MRS proceedings gives a good review of the SOI field.

MEASUREMENT OF MELT AND SOLIDIFICATION DYNAMICS DURING PULSED LASER IRRADIATION

P. S. PEERCY
Sandia National Laboratories, Albuquerque, New Mexico 87185

Key Words: laser annealing, transient conductance, solidification velocity

1. INTRODUCTION

When an absorbing solid is irradiated with a short pulse from a Q-switched or mode-locked laser, the temperature of the near surface region can be increased to values in excess of the melting temperature. Under these conditions, surface melting, followed by rapid solidification, can occur (1). Under normal conditions, melt initiates at the irradiated surface and propagates in to some maximum depth. After reaching this maximum depth, the liquid-solid interface returns to the surface as the molten region resolidifies. The well-defined and precisely-controlled temperature gradients afforded by surface melting permit melt and solidification to be investigated over an unprecedented range of solidification velocities (2). Real-time measurements of crystallization under rapid solidification conditions are providing unique insights into the thermodynamic and kinetic parameters which control the solidification process. Furthermore, the steep temperature gradients associated with pulsed surface melting can lead to the formation of novel non-equilibrium systems, including metastable phases and supersaturated solutions (3).

Studies of laser-induced surface melting, popularly known as "laser annealing" when applied to semiconductors because it removes implantation damage in Si and introduces implanted dopants onto electrically active lattice sites, are significantly expanding our understanding of the thermodynamics and kinetics of metastable and nonequilibrium phase formation. Most of the studies of "laser-annealed" materials have relied on post-annealed examinations, such as ion channeling and electron microscopy, to deduce information about the annealing process. These experiments do not yield direct information on the dynamics of the annealing process. In those studies the dynamics of melting and solidification must be inferred from numerical model calculations. The quantity that is perhaps most important in determining the resulting phases and microstructures is the solidification velocity. While it is well recognized that the velocity is of central importance to rapid solidification processing, there were no techniques available to measure the liquid-solid interface velocities under the rapid melt and solidification conditions associated with pulsed laser-induced surface melting before the development of the transient conductance technique (4). As will be demonstrated, direct measurement of this interface velocity provides a wealth of information about the thermodynamics and kinetics of the processes that control rapid solidification and the resulting microstructures.

Draper, C.W. and Mazzoldi, P. (eds.), Laser Surface Treatment of Metals. ISBN 90-247-3405-3.

The recently developed transient conductance technique permits real-time measurements of the molten layer thickness and solidification velocity for liquid-solid interface velocities up to 10^{11} nm/sec. The transient conductance measurements were first used to demonstrate that annealing proceeds by surface melting followed by rapid solidification (4,5-7) and that the annealing phenomena are well described by purely thermal processes governed by the energy absorption and heat transport (7-9). Applications of these techniques, in conjunction with transient reflectance techniques to measure the melt duration at the irradiated surface, have been reported for Si (4,5-7) Si on sapphire (SOS) (10) and compound semiconductors (11). As noted above, the usual scenario is for melt to nucleate at the irradiated surface and for a single liquid-solid interface to propagate into the sample during melting and subsequently return to the surface during the solidification. However, simultaneous measurements of the transient conductance and surface reflectance (12) have demonstrated the existence of such novel phenomena as propagating molten layers (13), surface nucleation of solid on top of molten layers (14), and internal nucleation of melt (15).

In studies of amorphous Si (a-Si), these measurements of the melt dynamics were used to determine the melting temperature of the amorphous phase (14) and the mechanism by which explosive crystallization occurs. These measurements reveal that the origin of the unique microstructure (16,17) that consists of a layer of coarse-grained polycrystalline Si on top of a layer of fine-grained polycrystalline Si is the result of explosive crystallization (13,14).

The above conclusions were verified by measurements of Si-Ge alloys (14,18) with a composition that had a melting temperature similar to that of a-Si. In addition, measurements in Si which contains impurities (14,15) were used to determine the effects of impurities on the solidification velocity. The velocity changes were then used to determine the metastable alloy phase diagram.

2. EXPERIMENTAL DETAILS

The concept behind the transient conductance measurements is that, for many solids, the electrical conductivity changes discontinuously at phase changes. Indeed, many semiconductors become metallic upon melting; for example, molten Si is metallic, and the conductivity increases by a factor of ~ 30 upon melting (19). As a result, if the conductance of sample with a well-defined geometry is measured in real time, the change in conductance with melting permits direct determination of the melt depth as a function of time. The experimental arrangement for such transient conductance measurements is illustrated schematically in Fig. 1. The samples are irradiated with a Q-switched ruby laser at either the fundamental ($\lambda = 0.694\ \mu m$) or frequency-doubled wavelength ($\lambda = 0.347\ \mu m$) at selected pulse widths between 2 and 70 nsec. The laser beam was incident through a fused silica beam homogenizer (20) to assure uniform ($\pm$ 5%) irradiation across the active region. In this configuration, the entire sample, including the contacts, was irradiated.

The earliest transient conductance measurements were made with a bias voltage, supplied by a battery and fast capacitor network, applied across a bar of bulk Si (4). While this arrangement was adequate for relatively long (> 25 nsec) laser pulses, a system with a greater bandwidth was necessary for measurements with shorter pulse lengths. A charge line configuration was therefore developed to provide a larger bandwidth for the study of very fast phenomena (21). In this

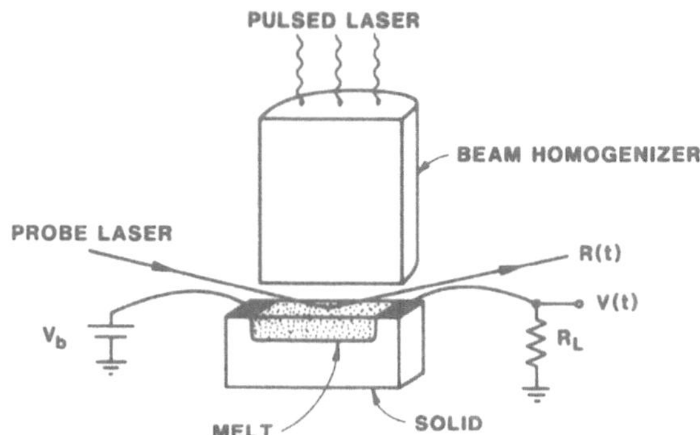

FIGURE 1. Schematic illustration of the experimental arrangement for simultaneous measurement of the transient conductance and surface reflectance for real-time measurements of melt and solidification dynamics (Ref. 5).

configuration, typical bias voltages of 20 to 40 V were applied, and the time-dependent voltage across the load resistor was monitored using a Tektronix 7912AD transient digitizer. The overall system bandwidth was >400 MHz. As noted above, molten Si is metallic, and the 30-fold increase in σ is used in the transient conductance technique to obtain direct measurements of the liquid thickness. Under conditions in which thermal and photo-induced contributions to the conductivity can be neglected, the current flowing through the load resistor is determined by the thickness of the liquid layer. In the charge line configuration, the transient voltage V(t) measured by the transient digitizer can be converted to an equivalent molten layer thickness d(t) by

$$d(t) = \frac{\rho}{R_L} \frac{L}{W} (V_b/V(t) - 2)^{-1} \tag{1}$$

where ρ is the resistivity of molten Si (80 $\mu\Omega$-cm), V_b is the applied bias voltage, R_L is the impedance of the charge lines (50 Ω) and L/W is the length-to-width ratio of the sample. For data taken in this configuration, measurements were made on SOS that was photolithographically patterned to yield L/W = 55.5, giving high depth sensitivity. A related, but slightly different equation converts the measured V(t) to d(t) for the original configuration noted above. After the raw data are illustrated in Fig. 2, the remaining transient conductance data will be presented after conversion to d(t).

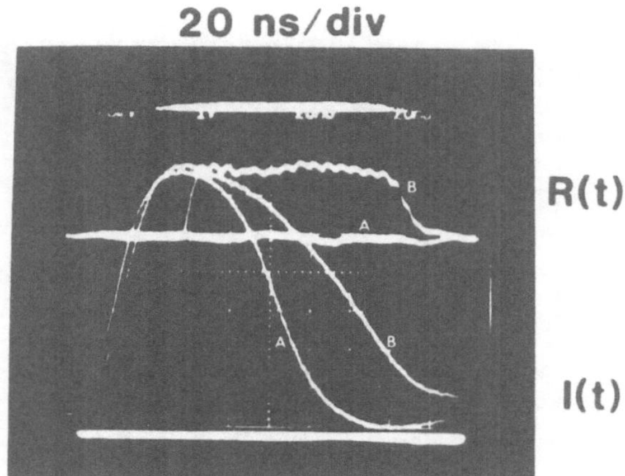

FIGURE 2. Photograph of scope traces showing the simultaneous transient conductance I(t) and reflectance R(t) for two laser energy densities on bulk Si. Curves A were taken at an incident energy density of 0.75 J/cm, just below the melt threshold energy density of 0.80 J/cm, whereas curves B were taken at 1.45 J/cm (Ref. 5).

The time-dependent reflectance R(t) was monitored simultaneously with the transient conductance. The R(t) measurements were used to determine the time during the laser pulse at which melt initiated and the melt duration at the surface. Since this technique is sensitive only to changes in the reflectivity within the absorption depth of the probe beam ($\sim$ 20 nm), these simultaneous measurements were especially valuable in the study of buried molten layers.

Except for the initial studies in bulk Si, samples consisted of either 0.5 or 1.0 μm SOS. For the studies of the thermodynamic properties of a-Si, amorphous layers were produced by implantation of Si at various energies. For the studies of As, Sn and In impurities, these species were implanted into 0.5 μm SOS at the necessary energy to yield the desired depth distribution. The Ge-Si alloys were formed by electron beam evaporation from Ge-Si mixtures, and the resulting alloy composition was measured by Rutherford backscattering. The dependence of the melting temperature of Ge-Si alloys on composition has previously been measured (22). The temperature T at which the free energies of the solid and liquid are equal was calculated as a function of alloy composition and found to vary approximately linearly with composition between the melting temperatures of Ge and Si.

3. RESULTS AND DISCUSSION

3.1. Bulk Silicon

Results from simultaneous measurements of the transient voltage V(t) and reflectance R(t) measured in bulk Si are shown in Fig. 2. The transient conductance data were taken with a bias voltage of 40 V to overcome any non-ohmic features in the contact resistance. Data are shown for two incident laser energy densities E: one at E = 0.75 J/cm^2, below the melt threshold energy density E_m of 0.8 J/cm^2 for 30 nsec pulses at 0.694 um, and the other at E = 1.45 J/cm^2, above E_m. For E = 0.75 J/cm^2 (curves A) the transient conductance signal is produced by the photoconductivity of Si, which is consistent with the observation that there is no significant change in R(t) for this energy density. For $E > E_m$, however (curves B), R(t) increases at the onset of melting and remains high throughout the ~ 120 nsec melt duration. Correspondingly, there is an increase in V(t) at times after the photoresponse has decayed to zero. This increase is caused by the conductance through the molten Si layer and decays as the layer resolidifies. These data demonstrate the presence of melting in bulk Si. Although the photoconductive response obscures the melt-in region of the data, data such as these can be used to evaluate theoretical models for the solidification velocity following pulsed melting.

Detailed numerical calculations, similar to those of Baeri et al. (8) and Wood et al. (9), were performed to obtain the melt depth versus time to compare with these data. These initial calculations used a simple heat flow model for the solidification, in which the latent heat liberated at the advancing liquid-solid interface is balanced by heat conduction into the substrate under steady-state conditions. For the case of pulsed laser melting, the temperatures of gradients are initially established by the energy absorption profile of the incident laser pulse and evolve in time through thermal diffusion. The numerical calculations include temperature-dependent values of the thermal conductivity, heat

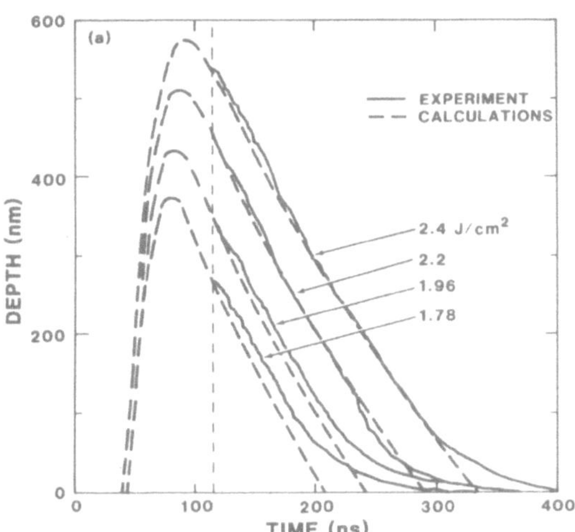

FIGURE 3. Calculated melt depth versus time compared to the melt depth measured by the transient conductance technique; because of the large photoresponse, only the steady-state solidification region can be compared to the calculations (Ref. 7).

capacity, and electrical conductivity. Finally, the measured values of the absorption coefficient in the solid and liquid phases (23) were used to determine accurately the fraction of the incident energy that was absorbed. Comparison of the measured and calculated melt depth versus time for bulk Si are given in Fig. 3 for various incident laser energy densities. The dashed curves are the measured d(t) values and the solid lines are the d(t) values calculated as described above. Even with Au doping to reduce the carrier lifetime, bulk Si exhibits appreciable photoconductivity. Because of the large photoconductivity response, d(t) was not determined during melt-in or for short times after the maximum melt depth. This constraint limits comparison between theory and experiment for bulk Si to the solidification regime. In this regime, examination of the calculated and measured d(t) curves in Fig. 3 reveals good agreement, indicating that the steady-state solidificaton regime is accurately described by a purely thermal treatment for melt and resolidification.

Numerical calculations such as those described above also give the total melt duration at the surface. This duration can be readily measured as a function of the incident laser energy density E, as shown by the data in Fig. 4. These data were taken with a 30 nsec pulse from a ruby laser, and the melt duration was measured using the 0.488 μm line from an argon laser as the probe beam. The measured melt duration is compared with the calculated duration in Fig. 5. As in the case of the solidification velocity, agreement between the measured and calculated values is excellent.

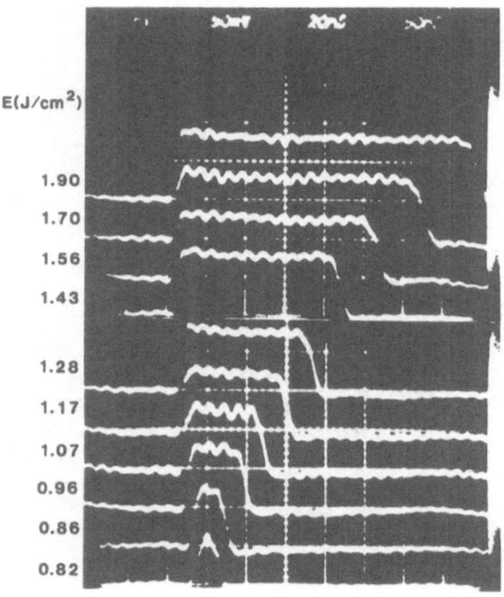

FIGURE 4. Transient reflectance measured using the 488 nm line of an Ar laser for various incident annealing energy densities.

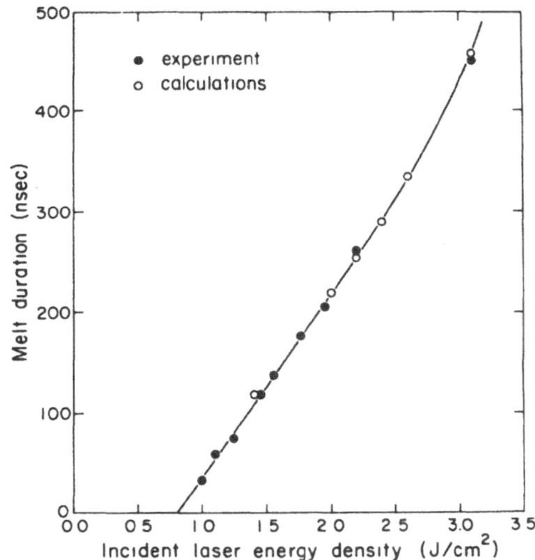

FIGURE 5. Melt duration as a function of incident laser energy density obtained from transient reflectance (solid circles) compared to the calculated duration (open circles) (Ref. 7).

Measurements such as those summarized above illustrate that the melt and solidification process in bulk Si is controlled by heat transport in the longer time regimes discussed above and can be quantitiatively understood on the basis of numerical heat flow calculations. As will be discussed below, however, detailed studies of the approach to equilibrium provide important information on the interfacial kinetics during solidification.

3.2. Silicon on Sapphire (SOS)

As noted in the introduction, the short carrier lifetime in SOS leads to a significantly smaller photoconductive response than that observed in bulk Si. This small photoresponse of SOS permits one to use the transient conductance technique for detailed studies of both the melt and solidification dynamics. Furthermore, because of this low photoresponse, the melt dynamics in the very fast time regime accessed by 2 nsec pulses at either 0.694 or 0.347 μm can be examined. As a result, most of the recent measurements of melt and solidification dynamics in Si have been performed in 0.5 or 1.0 μm thick SOS. A typical melt depth transient converted to d(t) via Eq.(1) is shown in Fig. 6 for the sample formed on 0.5 μm SOS. Also shown is the transient reflectance R(t) and the 1.35 J/cm^2 30 nsec annealing pulse at 0.694 μm. The small peak in the d(t) which occurs at the peak of the laser pulse is produced by the photoconductive response of the SOS; as can be seen, this photoresponse is small compared to that of bulk Si, and for convenience it was converted to an equivalent melt depth. The reflectance and the melt-induced contribution to the transient conductance increase simultaneously, indicating that melt initiates at the irradiated (free)

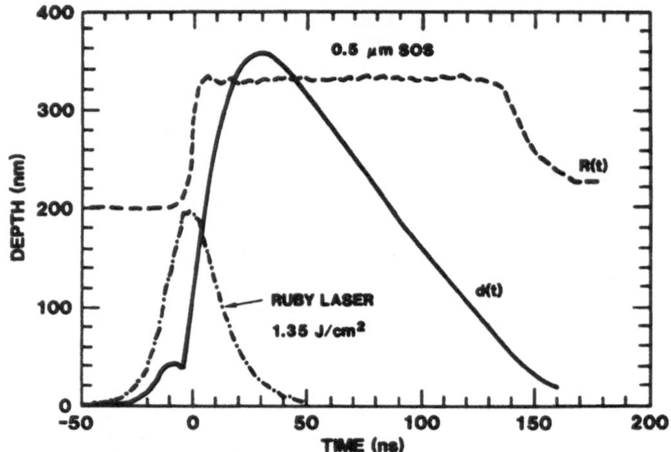

FIGURE 6. Typical surface reflectance R(t) and melt depth d(t) versus time measured from transient conductance for SOS (Ref. 14).

surface. The derivative of d(t) gives the instantaneous velocity so that data such as these can be used to study both the solidification velocity, as discussed above, and because the photoresponse corresponds only to an equivalent depth of ~ 30 nm, to measure the melt velocity throughout most of the melt depth. (In the studies of amorphous Si discussed below, the equivalent depth from the photoconductive response is even less than for crystalline SOS, permitting a more detailed study of the melt velocity.)

The d(t) behavior measured for 0.5 μm SOS irradiated at a variety of incident energy densities is shown in Fig. 7. As can be seen from those data, the melt depth versus time can be measured with a minimum of uncertainty in SOS throughout the total melt duration. These data illustrate that the melt threshold energy density E_m for 0.5 μm SOS is ~ 0.5 J/cm^2. As the incident laser energy density E is increased, the maximum melt depth increases until the melt extends through the entire 0.5 μm Si film at $E \geq 1.5$ J/cm^2. As in the case of bulk Si, the steady-state solidification velocity can be accurately calculated under the above assumptions. As will be discussed below, however, the approach to steady state near the turnaround of the solid-liquid interface contains important information on the solidification kinetics and interfacial dynamics under rapid solidification conditions. This region of the d(t) curve will be discussed in more detail in Section 3.5

3.3. Amorphous Silicon (a-Si)

Measurements of the free energy of a-Si (24) indicate that the amorphous phase should melt at a temperature substantially below the melting temperature of crystalline silicon (c-Si). (A detailed description of the thermodynamic properties of a-Si is given in the paper by Poate

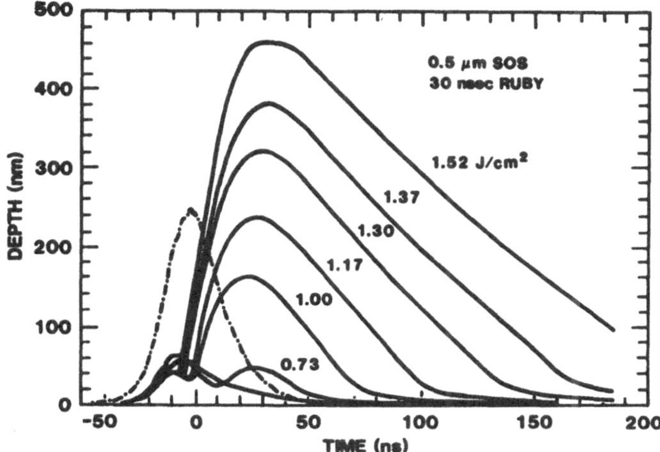

FIGURE 7. A series of current transients, converted to depth versus time, to show the time-dependent melt depth in 0.5 μm SOS at various incident energy densities.

elsewhere in this chapter.) Because a-Si transforms rapidly to c-Si by a solid phase process at temperatures in excess of 600°C, this melting temperature difference cannot be measured by conventional techniques, and attempts to determine the melting temperature difference have yielded estimates ranging from $T_a = T_c \pm 10$ to $T_a = T_c - 550$ (25,26). In addition to the uncertainty over the values of such fundamental thermodynamic parameters as the melting temperature, pulsed laser melting of a-Si has raised fundamental questions concerning the thermodynamics and kinetics that control the melt and resolidification process. For example, at incident laser energy densities insufficient to melt completely through the amorphous layer to yield epitaxial regrowth, part of the a-Si film can be transformed to polycrystalline Si. However, the thickness of this polycrystalline layer does not increase linearly with incident laser energy density. Furthermore, detailed examination of the microstructure of the transformed material reveals two distinct microstructures: a fine-grained (< 10 nm) layer beneath a coarse-grained surface layer. Prior to the measurements of the melt and resolidification dynamics, it was assumed that, as in the case of melts on single crystals, the melt front propagated to the full extent of the resulting polycrystalline layer. This assumption led to various interpretations of the kinetics of the process, ranging from small, but highly temperature dependent, thermal conductivity (16) to bulk nucleation and "slush zones" (27-29). However, direct measurements of the melt dynamics demonstrate that the melting temperature of a-Si is ~225 K below the melting temperature or c-Si and that the extent of the fine-grained polycrystalline Si does not represent the direct laser-induced melt depth; rather, the fine-grained polycrystalline Si is produced by explosive crystallization (13).

First, consider the melting temperature of a-Si. Melt depths as a function of time, determined from the transient conductance measurements, are shown in Fig. 8 for a series of laser energy densities incident on a-Si layers 330 nm thick (produced by Si implantation) on 0.51 μm SOS. The thickness of the implantation-produced amorphous layer

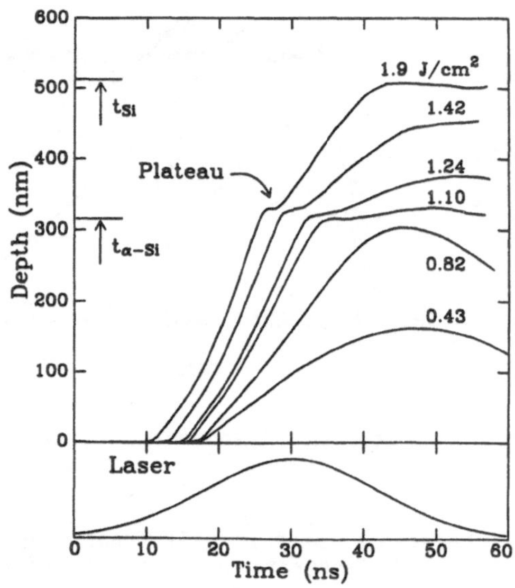

FIGURE 8. Melt depth versus time for ~ 210 nm a-Si films on SOS irradiated with various laser energy densities (Ref. 13).

and the SOS thickness were measured by Rutherford backscattering. Transient reflectance measurements demonstrated that melt originated at the irradiated surface before the peak of the laser pulse. As the melt reached the amorphous-crystalline interface, a plateau with an incident energy density dependent duration between 2 and 6 nsec, was observed. To confirm that this plateau is indeed produced by differences in the thermodynamic properties between a-Si and c-Si, similar measurements were performed on samples with 215 and 400 nm a-Si thicknesses. The results, shown in Fig. 9, demonstrate similar plateaus when the melt front reaches the amorphous-crystalline interface.

The plateau observed in the traces in Figs. 8 and 9 is consistent with a first-order phase transition of a-Si to metallic liquid at a melting temperature that is reduced from the melting temperature of c-Si. Specifically, the data are interpreted as follows. Melt initiates at the irradiated surface when the temperature exceeds the melting temperature T_m^a of a-Si. The melt propagates into the a-Si film at this reduced temperature until it encounters the a-Si/c-Si interface. Because the temperature of the molten liquid is below the melting temperature of c-Si, the melt front must pause at this interface until enough energy is absorbed from the laser to raise the liquid temperature to T_m^c. At that time, the melt front can propagate into the

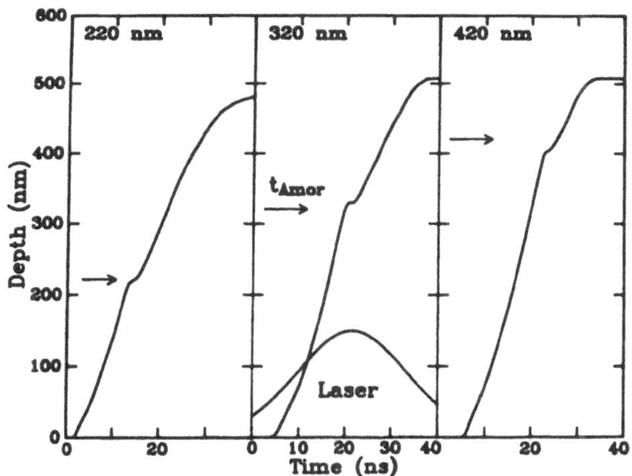

FIGURE 9. Melt depths versus time for various thicknesses of a-Si (Ref. 14).

underlying c-Si. It should also be noted that the melt velocity (slope of the melt depth versus time) differs in a- and c-Si, reflecting the different latent heats and thermal conductivities of the two phases.

The absolute temperature difference between the melting temperature of a-Si and c-Si can be determined from the plateau width (Δt) and the incident laser intensity I(t) by

$$c_p d\Delta T + \kappa \frac{\partial T}{\partial x} = (1 - R_\ell) \int_{\Delta t} I(t)dt \qquad (2)$$

where C_p is the specific heat of the liquid, d is the thickness of the molten layer, κ is the thermal conductivity of the crystalline phase, $\partial T/\partial x$ is the temperature gradient at the interface and R_ℓ is the reflectivity of the liquid at the laser wavelength. As noted above, thermodynamic parameters of a-Si cannot be readily measured at high temperature. Lack of high-temperature knowledge of the thermal conductivity of a-Si introduces an uncertainty in $\partial T/\partial x$. Upper and lower limits can be determined for ΔT, however, by assuming $\kappa_a << \kappa_c$ and $\kappa_a = \kappa_c$, the thermal conductivity of c-Si. This procedure yields a melting temperature reduction of $\Delta T = 225 \pm 50$ K, in reasonable agreement with the estimate of Donovan et al. (24).

If similar a-Si samples are irradiated at laser energy densities only slightly above the threshold for surface melting, markedly different behavior is observed from that for high-energy irradiation of c-Si. Shown in Fig. 10 are d(t) and R(t) for an incident energy density of 0.20 J/cm^2, slightly above the melt threshold energy density of

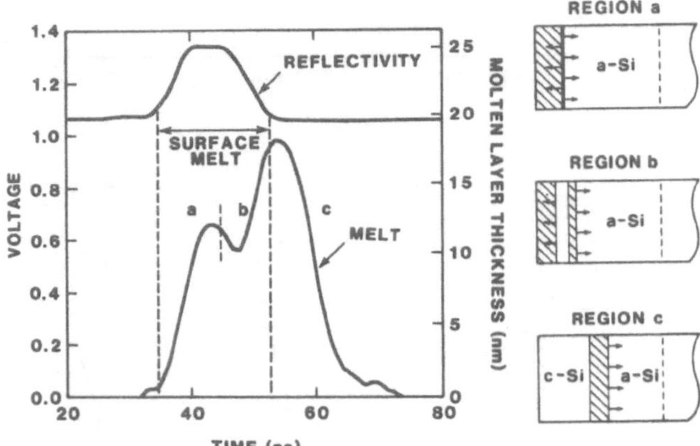

FIGURE 10. Transient conductance measurements of molten layer thickness and simultaneous surface reflectance for a 0.20 J/cm^2 pulse incident of a 320 nm thick a-Si film. The schematic diagrams at the right illustrate the various regions described in the text for the explosive crystallization process (Ref. 13).

~ 0.14 J/cm^2. Of particular interest is the double-peaked structure observed in d(t) and the fact that R(t) returns to its solid phase value before the molten layer completely disappears. These data are interpreted as follows: Melt initiates at the irradiated surface, as demonstrated by comparison of d(t) and R(t), and propagates into a depth of ~12 nm, whereupon this primary melt begins to solidify. This region is denoted as region a and is illustrated schematically in the upper part of Fig. 10b. Associated with the solidification of the primary melt, the latent heat of crystallization $\Delta H_{\ell c}$ is released and heats the underlying a-Si to its reduced melting temperature. The underlying a-Si then melts to create a buried molten layer. While the interface from the primary melt returns to the surface, the buried molten layer propagates into the sample, as illustrated schematically in the center trace in Fig. 10b. At later times, the interface from the original melt has returned to the surface, leaving a buried molten layer in the sample beneath a solid surface. This region is indicated as region c and is illustrated in the lower schematic of Fig. 10b. Explosive crystallization thus becomes a self-sustaining process, mediated by a buried molten layer. The energy released by crystallization at the rear interface of the buried molten layer is sufficient to raise the temperature of the a-Si at the front interface to the melting temperature of a-Si and to supply the latent heat ΔH_{al} between amorphous and liquid Si. Because the melting temperature of a-Si is less than that of c-Si, the melt is severely undercooled. The rapid nucleation at the crystal-liquid interface in this undercooled melt is presumed to result in the fine-grained polycrystalline Si observed after the explosive crystallization.

Further evidence for this interpretation is obtained by comparison of the microstructure measured by cross-section TEM at various laser energy densities. An example of the microstructure, which shows the coarse-grained polycrystalline Si on fine-grained polycrystalline Si on the underlying crystalline Si is given in the inset of Fig. 11. Also shown in Fig. 11 is the primary melt depth, defined as the initial depth melted by the energy absorbed from the incident laser beam, and the total transformed polycrystalline thickness versus incident laser energy density. Once the incident laser energy density exceeds the melt

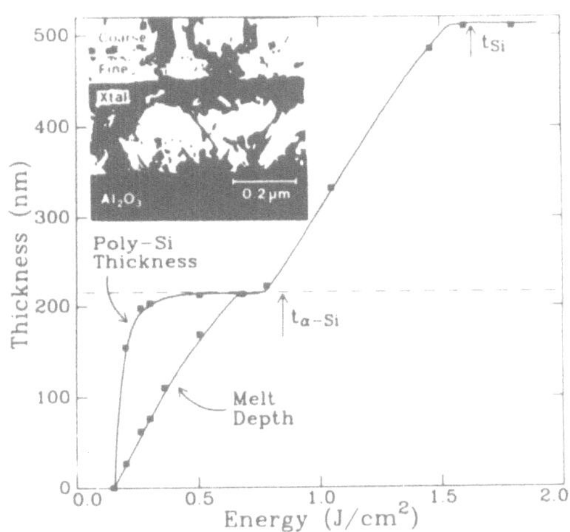

FIGURE 11. Thickness of the primary melt and total poly-Si versus incident energy density on a 215 nm a-Si film. The inset shows a TEM cross section, illustrating the coarse- and fine-grained poly-Si (Ref. 13).

threshold energy density, essentially the entire amorphous thickness is transformed to crystalline Si for a 30 nsec laser pulse at 694 nm. Furthermore, there is a plateau in the transformed thickness versus incident energy density that occurs when the total amorphous layer has been transformed. This plateau in melt depth versus energy density is a result of the reduced melting temperature of a-Si compared to that of c-Si.

One of the ramifications of explosive crystallization, mediated by a rapidly propagating buried molten layer, is that unusual impurity redistribution can be expected. For example, explosively transformed silicon which contains impurities with a low solubility in the solid phase can be expected to show impurity segregation ahead of the solidifying interface. Evidence for such internal impurity segregation has been observed by Narayan et al. (30) and by Sinke and Saris (31).

3.4. Si-Ge Alloys: A Model System

Although significant progress has been made in the qualitative understanding of the melt and solidification dynamics in c-Si, quantitative studies of the effects of undercooling and overheating on interface dynamics require a model system with known and easily altered thermodynamic properties. As illustrated in the measurements reported below, alloys of Si and Ge provide such a model system (18). These alloys form a continuous solid solution (32) with well-known thermodynamic parameters (22). The melting temperature (T_m) can be varied continuously from the 1210 K melting point of pure Ge to the 1685 K melting point of pure Si. These parameters are summarized in Table 1. Furthermore, since the thermal conductivities of Ge-Si alloys are reduced by almost an order of magnitude from the crystalline value of elemental silicon (33), the alloy system can be used to directly model the melting of a-Si.

Alloys of Si-Ge with the desired composition $Si_{100-x}Ge_x$ were electron beam deposited onto 0.5 μm SOS. The Si-Ge alloys were annealed at 800°C for 1 hour to produce large-grained polycrystalline films. Thicknesses and compositions of the deposited layers were measured by Rutherford backscattering analysis (RBS).

TABLE 1. Melting temperature T_m and latent heat ΔH for Si, Ge and $Si_{100-x}Ge_x$ alloys.

Si	Ge	T_m	T_m	ΔH
100%	0%	1685 K	0 K	50.55 kJ/mole
75%	25%	1566 K	119 K	47.1 kJ/mole
50%	50%	1447 K	238 K	43.7 kJ/mole
0%	100%	1210 K	475 K	36.94 kJ/mole

The melting temperature of the $Si_{50}Ge_{50}$ alloy composition is comparable to the measured value for a-Si. A typical depth versus time trace for a 150 nm $Si_{50}Ge_{50}$ alloy layer irradiated at ~1 J/cm^2 is shown in Fig. 12b. During melting, a ledge is observed at ~160 nm. The depth at which the ledge occurs corresponds to the thickness of the alloy layer. For comparison, similar data for a-Si on c-Si are shown in Fig. 12a. The similarity between the melt depth versus time for this $Si_{50}Ge_{50}$/c-Si structure and for a-Si/c-Si structures is readily evident.

As in the case for a-Si on c-Si, the occurrence of the ledge in the melt depth versus time is interpreted in terms of the reduced melting temperature of the surface alloy as follows: Melting initiates from the surface at the melting temperature of the surface alloy. Since this temperature is less than the melting temperature of c-Si, when the liquid-solid interface reaches the c-Si/alloy interface, the temperature of the liquid is insufficient to melt c-Si. The ledge results as the melt front pauses at the alloy/c-Si interface while the laser deposits sufficient energy to raise the liquid layer from the alloy melting temperature to the c-Si melting temperature. This temperature difference is ~230 K and results in a ~2.4 ns ledge.

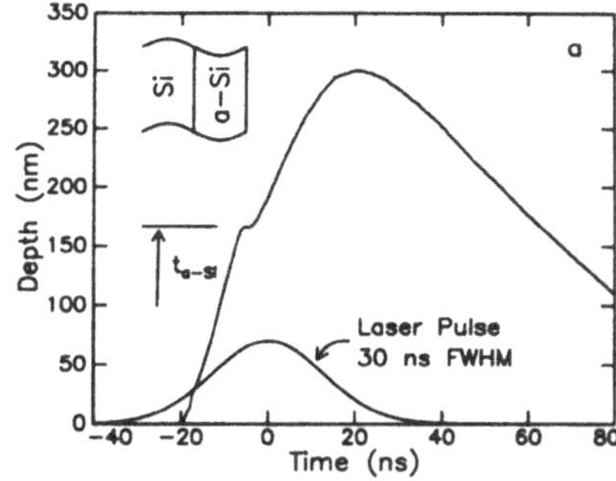

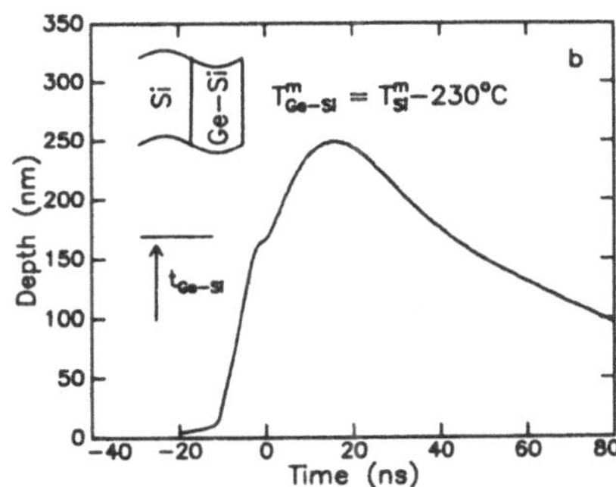

FIGURE 12. Melt depth versus time for $Si_{50}Ge_{50}$ alloys on Si, illustrating the plateau that reflects the melting temperature difference between the alloy and crystalline Si (lower curve) compared to the melt depth versus time for a-Si on c-Si (upper curve) (Ref. 18).

As noted earlier, Ge-Si alloys allow the melting temperature to be continuously changed from 1210 to 1685 K. As a result, structures can be fabricated which permit the effect of overheating and undercooling to be measured directly. These measurements will not be discussed here; for further information the reader is referred to Refs. 14 and 18.

3.5. Velocity-Undercooling Relationship

When a liquid is in contact with its own solid, solidification occurs if the temperature of the liquid at the interface is decreased below the melting temperature. The driving force for solidification is the free energy difference ΔG between the liquid and the solid. Several theoretical models have been developed to relate this driving force for solidification to the interfacial velocity and thereby derive a relationship between undercooling and v (34-37). In general, the velocity of a planar liquid-solid interface can be expressed in terms of the free energy change upon solidification as

$$v = \lambda \omega f e^{-\Delta Q/RT}[1 - \exp(-\Delta G/RT_i)] \quad (3)$$

where ω is an attempt frequency to overcome a barrier of height ΔQ, λ is the jump distance, f is the sticking coefficient and T_i is the interface temperature. While Eq.(3) provides a general form for the velocity versus undercooling, there are a variety of theoretical views as to what the prefactor $\lambda \omega f e^{-\Delta Q/RT}$ should be; however, prior to the transient conductance technique, there were no reliable techniques for measuring the solidification velocity in elemental systems to test these theories.

Since the prefactor is unknown, Eq.(3) is expanded about the melt temperature T_m for small values of the undercooling $\Delta T = [T_m - T_i]$, assuming a constant prefactor. Under this assumption, Eq.(3) reduces to

$$v \simeq \beta[T_m - T_i] = \beta\Delta T \tag{4}$$

where β is a measure of the slope of the velocity versus undercooling curve. As will be discussed below, detailed measurements of the transitional region between melt and solidification permit estimates of β in this velocity-undercooling relationship.

The melt depth versus time is shown in Fig. 13 for a SOS sample melted with a 3.5 nsec laser pulse. The numerical derivative of d(t) to give the velocity versus time after the melt front has reached its maximum depth and the sample starts to solidify is shown, along with the laser pulse. The important feature of these data for our consideration

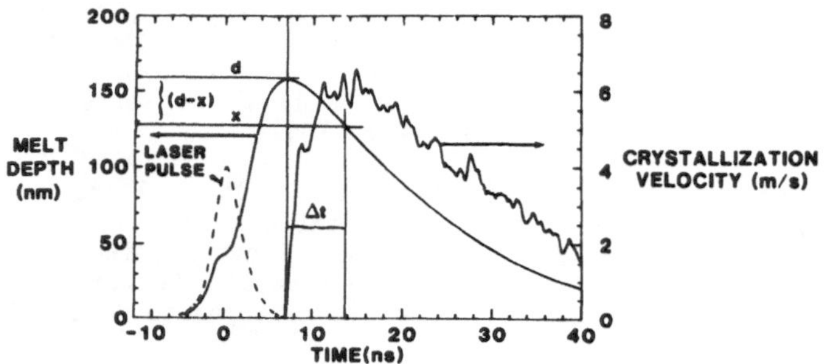

FIGURE 13. Melt depth versus time for SOS irradiated with a 3.5 nsec pulse from a ruby laser and the solidification velocity obtained by taking the numerical derivative of d(t). Also shown is the laser pulse (dashed line). The maximum melt depth $d = x_{max}$ and the melt depth x at v_m, which occurs at time Δt after $v = 0$ the maximum melt depth, are also indicated (Ref. 30).

is the time Δt required for the velocity to increase from $v = 0$ (at the peak melt depth d) to its maximum value v_m. At all times conservation of energy at the liquid-solid interface requires

$$J_\ell + v\Delta H = J_s \tag{5}$$

where J_s is the heat flux transported into the solid, $v\Delta H$ is the heat released by solidification and is the heat flux J_ℓ that flows from the liquid to the interface. In general, J_ℓ will be comprised of two terms: the energy deposited by the laser and carried by thermal conductivity into the solid and the energy released by the liquid as it undercools. These contributions can be evaluated numerically using the computer-based heat transport formalisms to determine precisely the undercooling (38); however, in the case of very short laser pulses which deposit negligible energy after the peak melt depth, $v = 0$, approximate analytical solutions, which yield physical insight into the important processes, can be used to estimate the undercooling (39).

To illustrate these solutions, consider the total heat transported into the solid in the time Δt between time $t = 0$, when $v = 0$, and $t = t_m$ when $v = v_m$. This can be determined by integrating Eq.(5) over the time Δt from t to t_m:

$$\int_{\Delta t} J_\ell dt + \int_{\Delta t} v \Delta H dt = \int_{\Delta t} \kappa \frac{\partial T}{\partial x} dt \tag{6}$$

If one assumes that the thermal conductivity of the molten Si is high and that no laser energy is deposited after the time $t = 0$, then the integral over J_ℓ will be simply given by

$$\int_{\Delta t} J_\ell = 0.5\ C_p (x + x_{max})\ \Delta T \tag{7}$$

where C_p is the heat capacity of molten Si, x_{max} is the maximum melt depth d, x is the melt depth at t_m and ΔT is the undercooling. Similarly, the integral of the latent heat released is $\Delta H(x_{max} - x)$. The most difficult term to evaluate is the integral of J_s -- i.e., the integral over $\kappa(\partial T/\partial x)$. This term is normally evaluated numerically in heat flow calculations; however, for the short times (~5 nsec) under consideration in the present case, we will assume that $\kappa \partial T/\partial x$ can be approximated as constant. In that case, $J_\ell \approx v_m \Delta H$ from steady-state considerations so that the integral over $\kappa \partial T/\partial x$ is $\approx v_m \Delta H \Delta t$. Under these approximations, the relationship between the velocity and the undercooling becomes

$$v_m \Delta H \Delta t \simeq 0.5\ C_p (x + x_{max}) \Delta T + (x_{max} - x) \Delta H \tag{8}$$

Application of Eq.(8) to the data of Fig. 13 yields an undercooling $T \simeq 90$ K at the interface velocity of 6 m/sec. Assuming that the velocity is linearly proportional to the undercooling yields $v = 0.07 (T_m - T_i)$ (m/sec)/K. This analysis thus demonstrates that these measurements can be used to determine the relationship between undercooling and interfacial velocity directly. Because of the importance of this relationship for rapid solidification processing, and because of the uniqueness and simplicity of this technique for such measurements, it is anticipated that it will be widely applied to determine undercooling-velocity relationships.

3.6. As in Si

It is well established that impurity or solute atoms can be incorporated at concentrations substantially in excess of the equilibrium solid solubility (3,40) during the rapid solidification that follows surface melting with a pulsed laser. Several theoretical treatments have been given for the kinetics that control the formation of such supersaturated solutions (36,41). In general, these treatments include a velocity-dependent interfacial segregation coefficient; however, because of the lack of direct measurements of the solidification velocity v, theoretical treatments to date have assumed that v is independent of the impurity content of the solid. To determine if impurities do alter v and thus evaluate the limits of validity of the treatments noted above, the transient conductance technique has been used to measure impurity-related effects on v.

First, consider the case of As, which is a common dopant in Si. As will be discussed below, As directly affects v and can lead to such novel effects as buried molten layers and internal nucleation of melt. Although impurity-induced buried molten layer formation has been proposed to explain anomalous impurity distributions after pulsed laser melting (42,43), the d(t) and R(t) measurements permit direct observation of surface nucleation of solid and buried nucleation of melt necessary to yield the buried molten layers.

Measurements were performed on 0.5 μm SOS implanted with various fluences of As at 250 or 275 keV. The As depth distributions before and after melting were determined by ion backscattering/channeling analysis. For the 275 keV implant energy, the measured As distribution peaked at 160 nm with a full width at half maximum (FWHM) of 100 nm.

Measurements of d(t) are shown in Fig. 14 for a sample implanted with 5×10^{16} As/cm^2 to give a peak As content of 7 at.%. Since As is quenched into electrically active sites, the contribution to the electrical conductivity in the solid phase from As donors can be significant. That contribution accounts for the value of d(t) at long

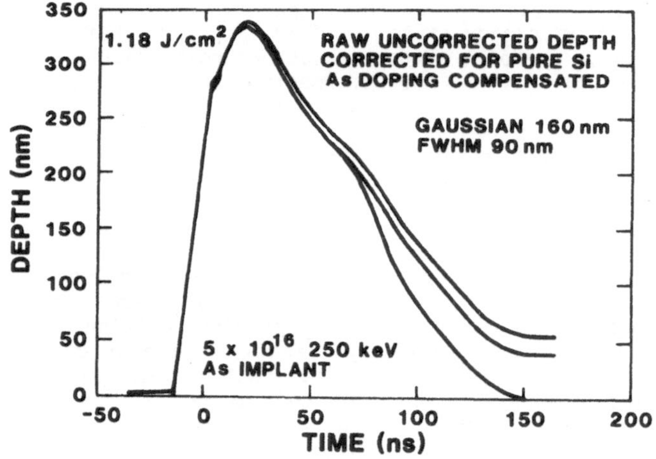

FIGURE 14. Melt depth versus time for Si implanted with 5×10^{16} As/cm^2. The upper curve shows the data before correction for either As doping or thermal contributions to the conductivity; the center curve shows thermal corrections, whereas the bottom curve shows d(t) corrected for both thermal and doping contributions (Ref. 15).

times after the melt has solidified. The magnitude of the contribution from As doping is compared to that from thermally generated carriers in the center curve. To obtain the liquid thickness, the contribution to σ from the As doping was deconvoluted. The deconvolution assumed that the conductance due to As doping was linear with the As concentration measured after irradiation. The actual d(t) after this deconvolution is given by the bottom curve.

The deconvoluted d(t) is compared in Fig. 15 for samples implanted with 1.6×10^{16} and 5×10^{16} As/cm^2. The effect of the increased As doping can be seen in the regrowth at a depth $\sim$160 nm near the peak of the As impurities. These deviations are more pronounced in the solidification velocity versus depth traces shown in Fig. 15b. The dotted curve is v for undoped SOS and shows the velocity decreasing with time as the heat is conducted into the substrate. For both the 1.7 and 7 at.% samples, the interface velocity is depressed as the interface approaches the peak As concentration at 160 nm. Once the interface passes through the As peak, the velocity is enhanced above the solidification velocity for undoped Si melted under similar conditions. The interpretation of these velocity changes is given below.

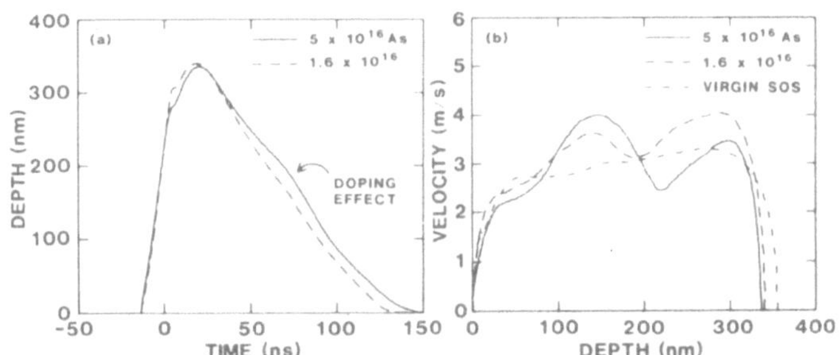

FIGURE 15. (a) Deconvoluted d(t) data for Si implanted with 1.6 and 5×10^{16} As/cm^2. (b) Velocities obtained by numerical differentiation of the curves in part a; also shown for comparison is the velocity for unimplanted SOS (Ref. 15).

Under steady-state conditions, energy released by the advancing liquid-solid interface must be balanced by thermal conduction of heat into the substrate.

$$v\Delta H = \kappa(\partial T/\partial x) \tag{9}$$

The incorporation of As into the solidifying SOS can modify the kinetics by several effects: (1) changes in the latent heat, (2) changes in the equilibrium melting temperature, and (3) modifications in the kinetic undercooling-velocity relationship. As discussed below, changes in the melting temperature dominate the observed changes in v in this rapid quench regime.

The melt depth extends beyond the As profile for the traces in Fig. 15. The samples thus begin solidifying in undoped Si where the undercooling necessary to satisfy Eq.(9) is established. As the interface approaches the As impurities, the melting temperature is reduced, which reduces the undercooling and thus v. With Equation 9 no longer satisfied, the excess heat flowing into the substrate cools the liquid layer until steady-state conditions are reestablished. Once the interface passes the peak As concentration, the melting temperature increases and the inverse process occurs. The additional heat now released at the liquid-solid interface raises the liquid temperature, again reestablishing steady-state conditions.

In the approximation that quasi-steady-state conditions are maintained throughout the process, Eq.(9) can be modified to include the effect of the changing liquid temperature. The energy balance equation now includes an additional term at the interface resulting from the heat capacity of the liquid layer. The heat release from the liquid is given by $C_p d(t)(\partial T_m/\partial t)$ where C_p is the specific heat of the liquid layer. The thermal conductivity of molten Si is assumed to be sufficiently large that temperature gradients in the liquid can be ignored. The time derivative can be replaced by the convective derivative $-v(dT_m/dx)$ and Eq.(9) becomes:

$$x(dT/dx) = v_n \Delta H = vdH - vC_p d(t)(dT_m/dx) \tag{10}$$

or

$$(dT_m/dx) = (1 - v_n/v)\Delta H/C_p/d(t) \tag{11}$$

where v_n is the normal velocity for an undoped sample. Equation 11 shows that the velocity from the impurities should vary as the derivative of the impurity concentration, and thus be antisymmetric as seen in Fig. 15. Equation 11 conceptually provides a direct means of determining the melting temperature as a function of the As concentration, and estimates for the data in Fig. 15b indicate melting temperature reductions of 40 K for the 1.6×10^{16} As/cm^2 implants and 150 K for the 5×10^{16} As/cm^2.

If the interpretation that the velocity decrease in the As-Si alloy is produced by the reduction in T_m is correct, then effects due to this reduced T_m should appear in other experiments. For example, the high thermal conductivity of molten Si requires that the surface temperature follow the interface temperature and thus it is possible to cool the surface sufficiently to observe solid nucleation. This temperature reduction can be achieved in two manners, increasing the As concentration further or reducing the laser pulse width to increase the interface velocity and thus the undercooling. The results of two experiments designed to test the hypothesis are shown in Fig. 16. Figure 16b shows a 5×10^{16} As/cm^2 implant irradiated with a 3.5 ns FWHM pulse while Fig. 20b shows an 8×10^{16} As/cm^2 implant irradiated with a 28 ns FWHM pulse. Correction for the As doping in the conductance has not been made; thus the data represent an apparent melt depth only. Simultaneous transient conductance and surface reflectance measurements indicate that surface nucleation of solid occurred in both cases. Consider the data shown in Fig. 16a for 3.5 ns FWHM irradiation. Within experimental uncertainty, the reflectivity increases at

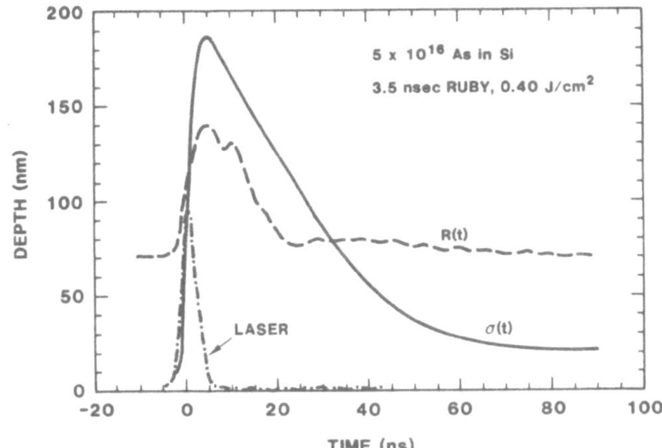

FIGURE 16. (a) Transient conductance and reflectance for Si implanted with 5×10^{16} As/cm^2 and irradiated with a 3.5 nsec pulse, illustrating surface nucleation of solidification.

the same time as the transient conductance, indicating that melt initiates at the free surface. However, it is evident that surface solidification begins when the liquid-solid interface is still ~ 160 nm below

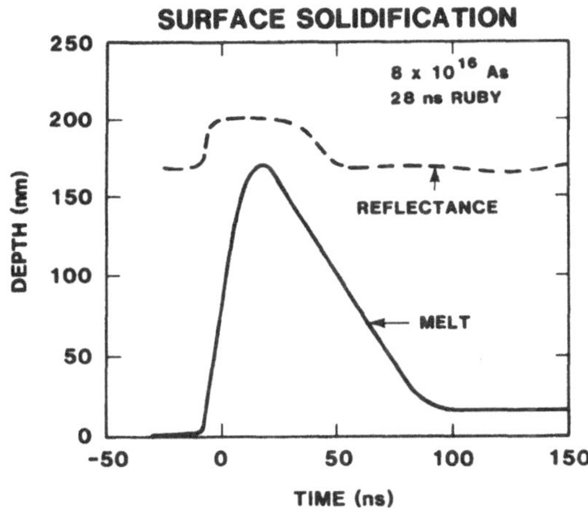

FIGURE 16. (b) Data similar to those in (a) for a 30 nsec pulse incident on an 8×10^{16} implant (Ref. 15).

the surface, i.e., near the maximum of the As profile. After solidification initiates, a buried molten layer results and the transient conductance measurement no longer yields a simple melt depth but rather the thickness of the buried layer. Similar conclusions are obtained from the 3.5 nsec data in Fig. 16b.

Further support for the reduced melting temperature in the Si-As alloy system is given by similar measurements at higher As concentrations using 28 ns pulses. Transient conductance and surface reflectance measurements on a 1.2×10^{17} As/cm^2 implant are shown in Fig. 17. At this concentration, the surface reflectivity shows the surface remaining solid while a buried molten layer 150 nm thick is produced.

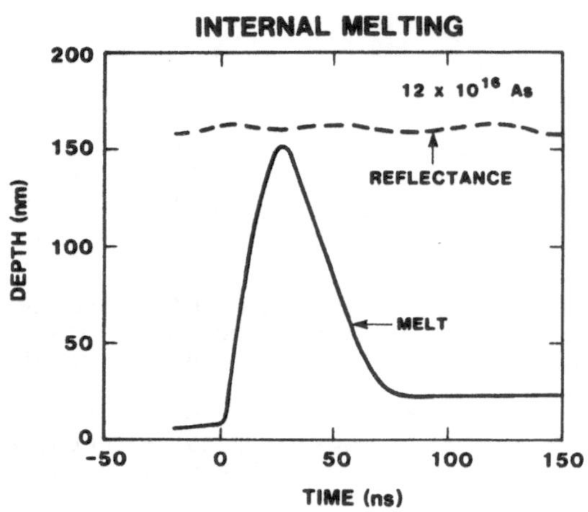

FIGURE 17. Transient conductance and reflectance measurements for a 1.2×10^{17} implant showing internal nucleation of melt due to the As-induced decrease in the melting temperature (Ref. 15).

We interpret this result to indicate interior nucleation of melt due to the extreme reduction in the melting temperature at the peak of the As profile. While changes in the interface velocity and the surface nucleation can be explained through kinetic arguments, nucleation of the internal melt provides evidence for a significantly reduced melting temperature at these As concentrations.

3.7. Metals

There has recently been significant growth in the study of new alloy structures that can be formed by the rapid solidification that results when alloys are rapidly quenched from the melt. The most common so-called Rapid Solidification Processing (RSP) techniques are melt-spinning or splat cooling at quench rates 10^5-10^7 K/sec; however, because the heat transfer rate is not well known and geometries are complex, it is difficult to estimate the quench rates accurately. Furthermore, perhaps the most important parameter in determining the resulting phase and microstructure is the solidification velocity, which cannot be measured in these conventional RSP. In very recent measurements of Al, Tsao and co-workers (44) have shown that the transient conductance technique permits direct measurement of this velocity in metals.

The resistance of Al decreased discontinuously by a factor of ~ 2.2 upon melting. This change in ρ is smaller than the factor of ~ 30 change for Si. Therefore, it is necessary that the measurements be performed on thin films of Al; otherwise, conductivity through the unmelted Al will dominate the measured response. Al films ~ 30 nm thick were e-beam evaporated through a mask onto oxidized Si to form samples with L/w of 65. Since the thickness of the Al was small compared to the thermal diffusion distance in the time of the laser pulse, the temperature was approximately uniform throughout the Al film, which greatly simplifies the data analysis.

The resistance change versus time for various irradiation energy densities is shown in Fig. 18. Note that, in contrast to Si, the conductance decreases (resistance increases) under pulsed laser irradiation.

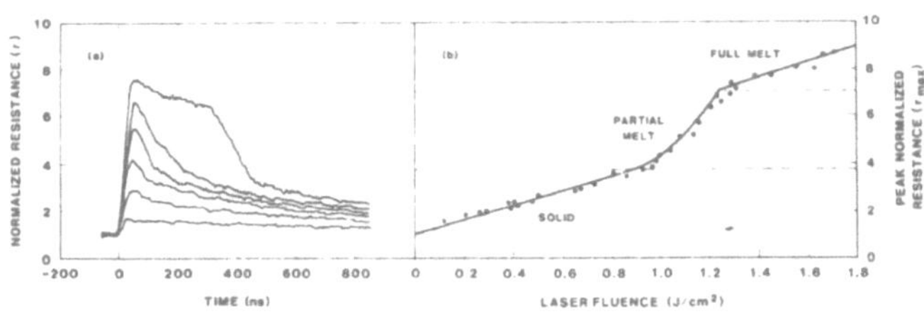

FIGURE 18. Time-resolved resistances normalized to room temperature resitances for Al films irradiated with various incident energy densities. (b) Peak normalized resistance versus incident laser energy density compared to numerical heat flow calculations (solid line). The horizontal dashed lines indicate the onset of melt and complete melting of the film (Ref. 44).

This resistance increase reflects the increase in resistance with increasing temperature, followed by a further increase upon melting. Because of the simple geometry chosen for the experiment, the resistance change can be quantitatively evaluated to determine the sample temperature as a function of time.

The peak resistance, normalized to the room temperature resistance to remove any uncertainties from film inhomogeneities, is plotted in Fig. 18b. The breaks in the slope of the curve, indicated by the horizontal dashed lines, are taken to be the onset of melting and complete melting of the film. The calculated resistance change at the melt threshold agrees within experimental uncertainty with previous measurements of the temperature dependence of the resistivity of Al; however, the calculated value at the point identified as complete melting is ~ 20% higher than the observed value. The reason for this difference is not yet known. The solid line through the data is the peak normalized resistance calculated using a simple heat flow model for heating, melt and solidification of the film; details are given in Ref. 44.

The measured resistance versus time can be converted into a melt depth versus time, similar to the case for Si. Results of this conversion are given in Fig. 19. The upper curve in the figure is the measured resistance versus time and the center trace shows the measured transient reflectance versus time, using the techniques described above for Si. The discontinuous change in the reflectivity upon melting, even though small, permits the melt duration at the surface to be measured. The melt depth versus time determined from the transient conductance is given in the bottom trace. Comparison of the melt depth and reflectance traces shows that melt initiates at the irradiated surface and propagates to some depth, whereupon the liquid-solid interface motion reverses and the interface returns to the surface. Numerical derivatives of the melt depth with respect to time yield a peak melt-in velocity of 16 m/sec and a maximum solidification velocity of 3 m/sec for Al on 0.75 μm SiO_2 films, in agreement with values expected from heat-flow calculations.

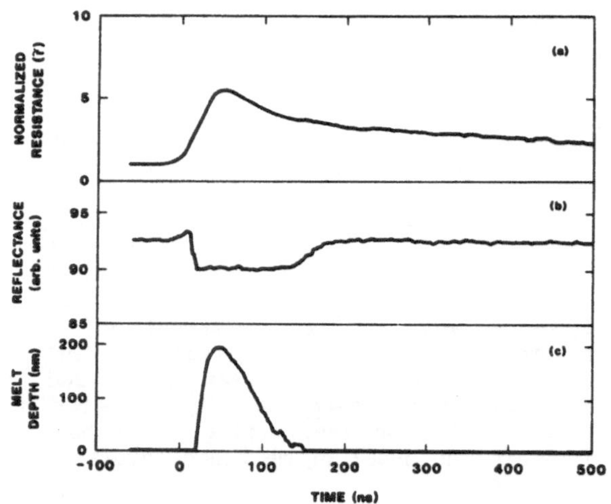

FIGURE 19. (a) Time-resolved resistance and (b) transient reflectance during pulsed laser iradiation with 1.14 J/cm^2. (c) Inferred melt depth versus time from the data in (a) (Ref. 44).

These initial transient conductance studies in Al provide the first measurement of the liquid-solid interface versus time in metals. This ability to measure d(t), and therefore v(t), should prove extremely valuable in the study of RSP in metals. Control of the interface velocity by control of the laser pulse width or the thermal conductivity of the substrate permits the velocity to be varied over wide ranges of interest to RSP. In addition, direct measurement of the velocity will permit fundamental studies of such phenomena as interfacial instability at high solute concentrations to determine the important kinetic parameters that govern the resulting microstructures.

5. SUMMARY

In summary, real-time measurement of the melt depth versus time and simultaneous measurement of the melt duration at the surface provide unique information about the melt and solidification dynamics resulting from pulsed laser irradiation. These measurements have permitted determination of the fundamental properties of metastable phases, such as the melting temperature of a-Si, and the study of such novel melt and solidification scenarios as buried molten layers. These buried molten layers mediate the explosive transformation that occurs to transform a-Si to c-Si; they also occur in ion-implanted materials that have a very non-uniform melting temperature versus depth. This effect was demonstrated by the measurement of Si(As) at high As concentrations.

Although measurements after pulsed irradiation with such techniques as ion beam analysis and electron microscopy provide invaluable information on the resulting microstructures, the transient conductance and reflectance techniques are the only techniques available at present for dynamic measurements of the melt and solidification process. In addition to the studies of Si discussed above, these transient techniques have proven to be generally applicable to semiconductors. In a recent important advance, they have also been extended to metals, and it is anticipated that future studies in metals will provide new information about the rapid solidification processes of importance for technological applications that are discussed in other chapters of this volume.

ACKNOWLEDGMENT

This work was performed at Sandia National Laboratories supported by the U.S. Department of Energy under contract number DE-AC04-76DP00789.

REFERENCES

1. See, e.g., N. Bloembergen, in Laser-Solid Interactions and Laser Processing, edited by S. D. Ferris, H. J. Leamy, and J. M. Poate, AIP Conference Proceedings No. 50 (AIP, New York, 1979), p. 1.
2. J. M. Poate and J. W. Mayer, in Laser Annealing of Semiconductors, edited by J. M. Poate and J. W. Mayer (Academic Press, New York, 1982), Chap. 1.
3. See, e.g., C. W. White, B. R. Appleton, and S. R. Wilson, in Ref. 2, Chap. 5.
4. G. J. Galvin, M. O. Thompson, J. W. Mayer, R. B. Hammond, N. Paulter, and P. S. Peercy, Phys. Rev. Lett. 48, 33 (1982).
5. P. S. Peercy, G. J. Galvin, M. O. Thompson, J. W. Mayer, and R. B. Hammond, Physica B 116, 558 (1983).
6. M. O. Thompson, G. J. Galvin, J. W. Mayer, R. B. Hammond, N. Paulter, and P. S. Peercy, in Laser and Electron Beam Interactions with Solids, edited by B. R. Appleton and G. R. Celler (North Holland, New York, 1983), p. 209.
7. G. J. Galvin, M. O. Thompson, J. W. Mayer, P. S. Peercy, R. B. Hammond, and N. Paulter, Phys. Rev. B 27, 1079 (1983).
8. P. Baeri, S. U. Campisano, G. Foti, and E. Rimini, J. Appl. Phys. 50, 788 (1979).
9. R. F. Wood and G. E. Giles, Phys. Rev. B 23, 2923 (1981).
10. M. O. Thompson, G. J. Galvin, J. W. Mayer, P. S. Peercy, and R. B. Hammond, Appl. Phys. Lett. 42, 445 (1983).
11. G. J. Galvin, M. O. Thompson, J. W. Mayer, P. S. Peercy, and R. B. Hammond, in Laser Processing of Semiconductor Devices, edited by C. C. Tang, Proc. SPIE, 385, 38 (1983).
12. D. H. Auston, C. M. Surko, T. N. C. Venkatesan, R. E. Slusher, and J. A. Golovchenko, Appl. Phys. Lett. 33, 437 (1978).
13. M. O. Thompson, G. J. Galvin, J. W. Mayer, P. S. Peercy, J. M. Poate, D. C. Jacobson, A. G. Cullis, and N. G. Chew, Phys. Rev. Lett. 52, 2360 (1984).
14. P. S. Peercy and M. O. Thompson, in Energy Beam-Solid Interactions and Transient Thermal Processing 1984, edited by D. K. Biegelsen, G. A. Rozgonyi, and C. V. Shank, Materials Research Society Symposium Proceedings (Materials Research Society, Pittsburgh, 1985), Vol. 35, p. 53.
15. P. S. Peercy, M. O. Thompson, and J. Y. Tsao, Appl. Phys. Lett. 47, 244 (1985).
16. H. C. Weber, A. G. Cullis, and N. G. Chew, Appl. Phys. Lett. 43, 669 (1983).
17. J. Narayan and C. W. White, Appl. Phys. Lett. 44, 35 (1984).
18. M. O. Thompson, P. S. Peercy, J. Y. Tsao, and M. J. Aziz, Appl. Phys. Lett. (to be published).
19. Liquid Semiconductors, edited by V. M. Glazov, S. N. Chizkovskaga, and N. N. Glagoleva (Plenum Press, New York, 1969).
20. A. G. Cullis, H. C. Weber, and P. Bailey, J. Phys. E 12, 688 (1979).
21. M. O. Thompson, Ph.D. Thesis, Cornell University, 1984.
22. J. P. Dismukes and L. Ekstrom, Trans. Metall. Soc. 233, 672 (1965).
23. P. S. Peercy and W. R. Wampler, Appl. Phys. Lett. 40, 768 (1982).
24. E. P. Donovan, F. Spaepen, D. Turnbull, J. M. Poate, and D. C. Jacobson, Appl. Phys. Lett. 42, 698 (1983).

25. S. A. Kokorowski, G. L. Olson, J. A. Roth, and L. D. Hess, Phys. Rev. Lett. 48, 498 (1982).
26. P. Baeri, G. Foti, J. M. Poate, and A. G. Cullis, Phys. Rev. Lett. 45, 2036 (1980).
27. R. F. Wood, D. H. Lowndes, and J. Narayan, Appl. Phys. Lett. 44, 770 (1984).
28. D. H. Lowndes, R. F. Wood, C. W. White, and J. Narayan, in Energy Beam-Solid Interactions and Transient Thermal Processing, edited by J. C. C. Fan and N. M. Johnson (North Holland, New York, 1984), p. 99.
29. D. H. Lowndes, R. F. Wood, and J. Narayan, Phys. Rev. Lett. 52, 5621 (1984).
30. J. Narayan, C. W. White, O. W. Holland, and M. J. Aziz, J. Appl. Phys. 56, 1821 (1984).
31. W. Sinke and F. W. Saris, Phys. Rev. Lett. 53, 2121 (1984).
32. M. Hansen and K. Anderko, Constitution of Binary Alloys, 2nd ed. (McGraw-Hill, New York, 1958).
33. B. Abeles, P. S. Beers, G. D. Cody, and J. P. Dismukes, Phys. Rev. 125, 44 (1962).
34. J. W. Cahn, W. B. Hillig, and G. W. Sears. Acta Metall. 12, 1421 (1964).
35. F. Spaepen and D. Turnbull, in Laser Annealing of Semiconductors, edited by J. M. Poate and J. W. Mayer (Academic Press, New York, 1982), Chap. 2.
36. K. A. Jackson, in Surface Modification and Alloying by Laser, Ion and Electron Beams, edited by J. M. Poate, G. Foti, and D. C. Jacobson (Plenum Press, New York, 1983), Chap. 3.
37. J. Q. Broughton, G. H. Gilmer, and K. A. Jackson, Phys. Rev. Lett. 49, 1496 (1982).
38. M. O. Thompson, P. H. Bucksbaum, and J. Bokor, in Energy Beam-Solid Interactions and Transient Thermal Processing - 1984, edited by D. K. Biegelsen, G. A. Rozgonyi, and C. V. Shank, Materials Research Society Symposium Proceedings (Materials Research Society, Pittsburgh, 1985), Vol. 35, p. 181.
39. G. J. Galvin, J. W. Mayer, and P. S. Peercy, Appl. Phys. Lett. 46, 644 (1985).
40. J. M. Poate, in Laser and Electron Beam Interactions with Solids, edited by B. R. Appleton and G. K. Celler (North Holland, New York, 1981), p. 121.
41. M. J. Aziz, J. Appl. Phys. 53, 1158 (1982).
42. S. U. Campisano, J. M. Poate, D. C. Jacobson, A. G. Cullis, and N. G. Chew, in Energy Beam-Solid Interactions and Transient Thermal Processing, edited by J. C. C. Fan and N. M. Johnson (North Holland, New York, 1984), p. 189.
43. S. U. Campisano, D. C. Jacobson, J. M. Poate, A. G. Cullis, and N. G. Chew, Appl. Phys. Lett. 46, 846 (1985).
44. J. Y. Tsao, S. T. Picraux, P. S. Peercy, and M. O. Thompson, Appl. Phys. Lett. (to be published).

IMPURITY SEGREGATION, SUPERSATURATION AND INTERFACE STABILITY

S. U. CAMPISANO
Dipartimento di Fisica dell'Universita, corso Italia 57, 95129, Catania, Italy

Key Words: laser annealing, dopant distribution, diffusion

The presence of an interface separating two media, one ordered (crystal) and one disordered (either amorphous or liquid), has a profound influence on dopant depth distribution and lattice location. The differences in dopant behavior between crystallization at the liquid-solid and amorphous-solid interfaces are illustrated by the following example. The implantation of Te in Si produces an amorphous layer which can be crystallized in the liquid or solid phase by laser or furnace annealing, respectively. Figure 1 shows (1) the depth profiles of Te implanted in silicon after pulsed laser annealing and solid-phase regrowth, respectively. In both cases the low aligned yields indicate that almost 100% of the Te atoms which are retained inside the crystal are located on substitutional lattice sites. The concentration of the substitutional Te is about 10^5 times the maximum equilibrium solubility. Supersaturated solid solutions, therefore, result from both liquid-phase and solid-phase crystallization processes. There is, however, a marked difference in the depth profiles of Te after laser or furnace annealing: In the process involving the liquid phase, part of the dopant is rejected to the sample surface, while after the low-temperature furnace annealing no profile modification is observed.

The profile modification after laser irradiation has been accounted for (2,3) by the normal freezing approach. As the dopant has different solubilities in the solid and the liquid layer, the advancing solid front will reject it to the high-solubility phase, i.e., into the liquid. Because the surface region is the last to solidify, the dopant will be accumulated at the surface. These concepts have been well known for many decades and are commonly used for zone refining during crystal growth processes from the liquid phase. The main difference between conventional crystal growth and laser annealing is the growth velocity: from 10^{-7} m/s for conventional growth to about 10 m/s for laser annealing.

The dopant profile after directional solidification is uniquely determined by the following parameters: the starting profile, the diffusivity in the liquid phase, the solidification velocity and the interfacial distribution coefficient. This last parameter is defined as $k' = C_s/C_l$ where C_s and C_l are the isothermal solubility in the solid and liquid phase measured at the interface. For usual crystal growth conditions k' coincides with the equilibrium segregation coefficient k_0. For the case of a dilute alloy undergoing directional solidification, the impurity redistribution at the liquid-solid interface is shown schematically in Figure 2. The two cases refer to a negligible and to a finite value of the solidification velocity. Under equilibrium conditions the concentration ratio in the solid and liquid can be determined by means of the phase diagram.

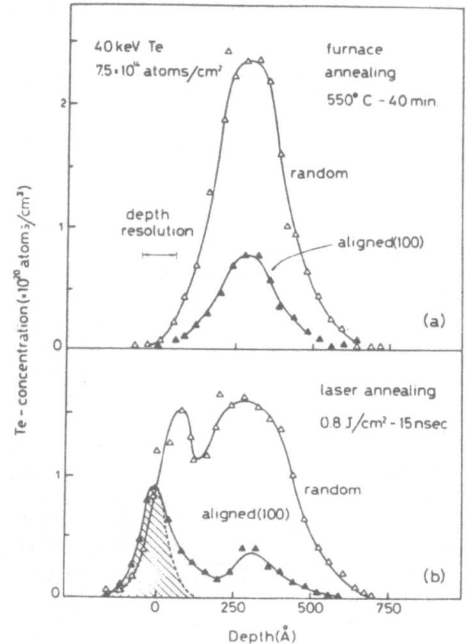

FIGURE 1. Rutherford backscattering and channeling depth profiles of Te atoms implanted in silicon after thermal and laser treatments. The ratio of the aligned (100) and random yield gives the measure of substitutionality of the Te. A ratio of 5%, for example, indicates that 100% of the Te is substitutional.

Estimates of the parameters that determine the final dopant profile can be obtained from the literature (e.g., dopant diffusion in the liquid) and from measurement (e.g., interface velocity). It is then possible to determine the nonequilibrium interfacial distribution coefficient from a comparison with the experimental results and the calculated profile where the k' value is the only fitting parameter. An example of the dopant distribution in the two media for a Gaussian initial profile for a segregation coefficient of 0.1 and a solidification velocity of 2 m/s is reported in Figure 3 at different times during the solidification process. Results of such a comparison are shown in Figure 4 for the case of Bi in silicon. The comparison has been extended to a wide velocity range and for different crystal orientations (4) and the results are summarized in Figure 5. The interfacial distribution coefficients, k', are much larger than the equilibrium k_o

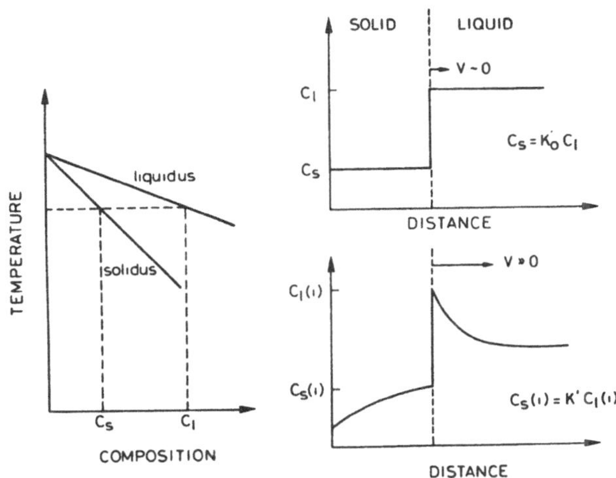

FIGURE 2. Distribution of dopant in the solid and in the liquid phases at negligible and at finite solidification velocity.

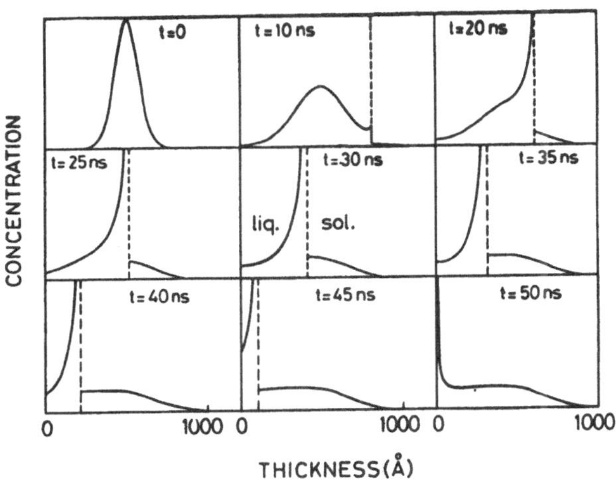

FIGURE 3. Numerical simulation of diffusion and segregation at a fast-moving liquid-solid interface for an initial Gaussian distribution of the dopant.

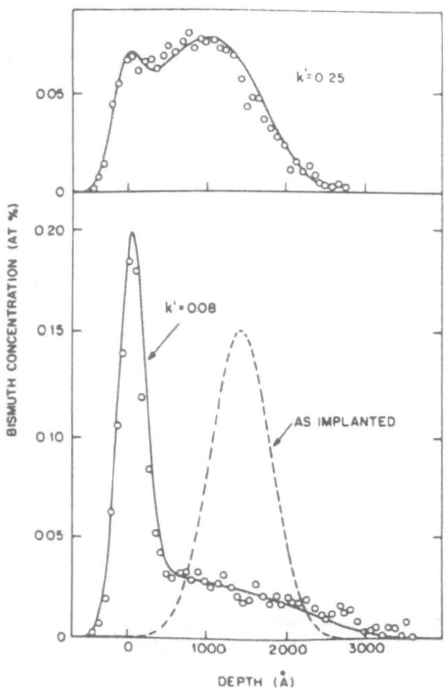

FIGURE 4. Depth profiles of Bi implanted in Si after laser recrystallization. The full lines are calculated by using the numerical fitting procedure.

figure and they depend upon velocity and crystallographic orientation of the substrate. The k' values have been measured for a large variety of dopants as a function of the solidification velocity, and a summary of experimental results is reported in Figure 6. The measured interfacial segregation coefficient increases with solidification velocity and reaches a value close to unity. It should be noted that in the following article Aziz presents somewhat different values for Bi segregation coefficients than those presented here. The reason for this discrepancy lies in different assignments of interfacial velocities either from calculation or measurement.

Dopants in silicon can be separated into two general classes: slow substitutional diffusers and fast interstitial diffusers. For slow diffusers the general trend is that of enhanced trapping. For fast diffusers no evidence of enhanced trapping has been observed: They are generally rejected at the sample surface as if the process occurred under equilibrium conditions. The enhanced trapping of substitutional impurities has been modeled theoretically using different approaches (5,8). There is, however, a simple picture which gives an understanding of the trapping process. The enhanced trapping is due to the competition between impurity diffusion in the liquid phase away from the

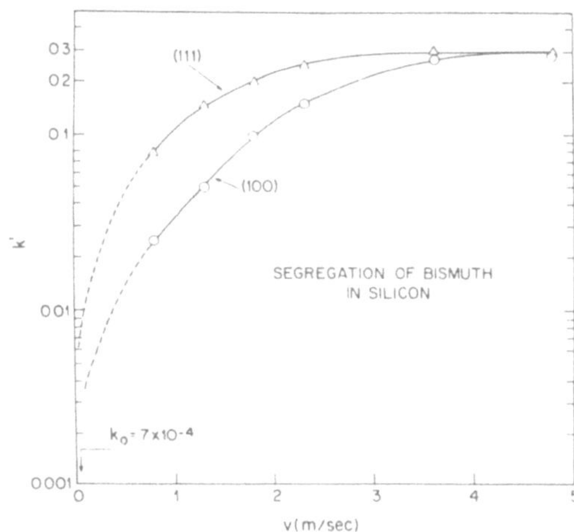

FIGURE 5. Values of the interfacial segregation coefficient for Bi in silicon as a function of the solidification velocity and for two crystal orientations.

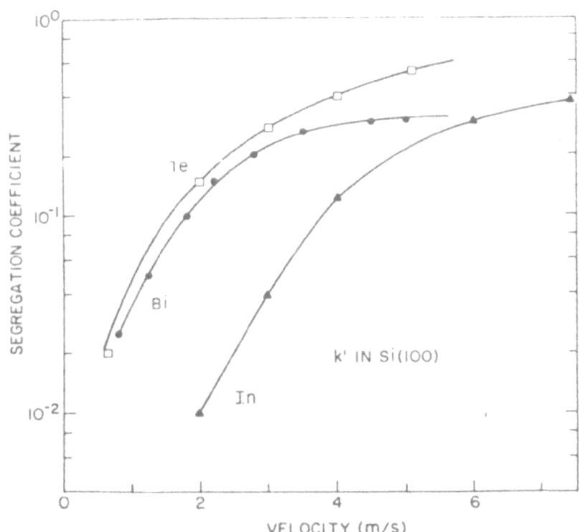

FIGURE 6. Values of the interfacial segregation coefficient for Te, Bi and In in Si (100) as a function of the solidification velocity.

advancing interface and trapping at the interface solid. There are two characteristic time intervals: the time required to regrow one monolayer of thickness $x, t_g = x/v$, and the time required to diffuse through one monolayer $t_D = x^2/D_i$, where D_i is the diffusivity in the near interface region. If $t_D < t_g$, the dopant can escape from the advancing solid front and will be rejected into the high-solubility phase, i.e., into the liquid. On the other hand, if $t_D > t_g$, the dopant is trapped by the fast interface and will occupy a local minimum in the free energy curve, i.e., a substitutional position. For a quantitative estimate of the critical velocity separating these two regimes $v = D_i/x$, an evaluation of D_i is necessary. Because the diffusion coefficient of impurities in silicon can change greatly on going from the solid to the liquid phase, it has been proposed (8) that an average value should be employed for D_i where: $D_i = (D_s D_l)^{1/2}$, with D_s and D_l the diffusion coefficients in the solid and in the liquid at the melting temperature, respectively. D_l is typically of the order of 10^{-4}-10^{-5} cm^2/sec while Ds can range from 10^{-13} to 10^{-5} cm^2/sec for slow and fast diffusers, respectively. Di will vary, accordingly, from 10^{-9} to 10^{-5} cm^2/s for slow and fast diffusion, respectively. The critical velocities, assuming $x \sim 10^{-8}$ cm, are therefore 0.1 and 10 m/sec, respectively, for slow and fast diffusers. For all pulsed laser annealing experiments interface velocities are on the order of a few meters per second, and substitutional diffusers will be trapped while interstitial diffusers will be rejected in the liquid phase.

To test this simple model, an experiment has been performed to compare segregation effects in silicon and germanium substrates. Si and Ge both have a diamond-like structure and similar lattice parameters: fast and slow diffusers in Si will behave in a similar manner in Ge. One exception is Zn: It is fast in Si and slow in Ge. The experimental results obtained by laser iradiation of Zn-implanted Si and Ge are reported in Figs. 7 and 8. The Zn is completely rejected to the Si surface, while it is retained in excess of the maximum solubility limit in Ge.

The same concept may be applied to explain enhanced impurity trapping during solid-phase regrowth (9). In this last case, the interface separates two media, crystal and amorphous, which are both solid. In a first approximation, we may assume that the diffusion coefficient in the amorphous phase is comparable to that in the crystalline one. The interfacial diffusivity will thus be $D_i = D_s$, where D_s is the diffusion coefficient at the annealing temperature. D_i can vary from 10^{-20} to 10^{-5} cm^2/sec for slow and fast diffusers, respectively. The corresponding critical velocities for enhanced trapping will be 10^{-12} and 10^3 cm/sec, respectively. The typical regrowth velocity is 10^{-9} cm/sec at T = 500°C. Slow diffusers will thus be trapped in substitutional lattice sites. Fast diffusers can migrate in the amorphous region, giving rise to small precipitates which can enhance the nucleation of polycrystalline silicon from the amorphous phase, thus inhibiting the solid-phase regrowth.

The experiments on impurity segregation show the formation of supersaturated solid solutions following laser annealing. The excess of solubility ranges from a factor of about 5 for those elements characterized by a large equilibrium solubility such as B and As to a factor of 1000 or more for those elements characterized by small solubilities such as Bi, Te, etc. During fast solidification processes we may consider

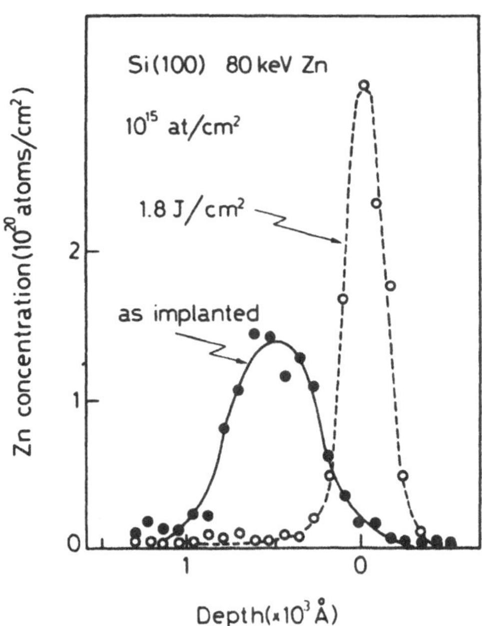

FIGURE 7. Backscattering depth profiles of Zn in Si after laser irradiation.

two different cases: dopants which are characterized by an interfacial distribution coefficient equal to unity and dopants which have a k' value smaller than unity. In the first case, such as As or B in silicon at several m/s, the maximum amount of dopant that can be retained on lattice sites is limited by the thermodynamic limit defined by the concentration at which the solidus and the liquidus free energy curves cross (10), as illustrated in Figure 9. In the case of boron, moreover, due to the difference in covalent radii between B and Si, the amount of strain due to B incorporation is so large that substrate cracking is the limiting factor. Many of the dopants, however, have a k' value different from unity. For these dopants the maximum concentration that can be retained on substitutional lattice sites is limited by morphological instabilities (11,12) at the liquid-solid interface. The large build-up of impurities rejected in the liquid phase by the advancing solid front causes a lowering of the freezing temperature of such a layer. If the actual temperature in the near interface region is higher than that determined by the dopant concentration, interfacial instabilities develop (13). The process is schematically illustrated in Figure 10. It has been shown (12) that to fulfill these constitutional supercooling

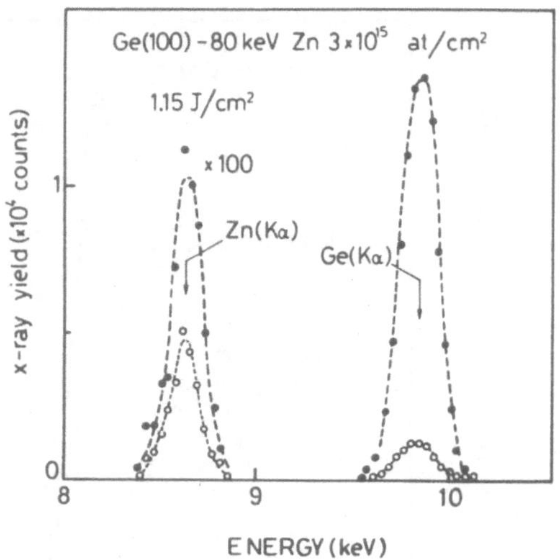

FIGURE 8. X-rays induced by 2.0 MeV He from a laser-irradiated Zn-implanted Ge sample.

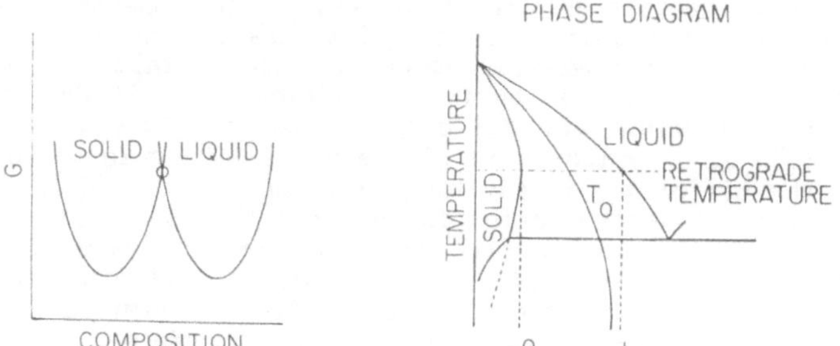

FIGURE 9. Schematic representation of the "thermodynamic limit" to nonequilibrium dopant incorporation.

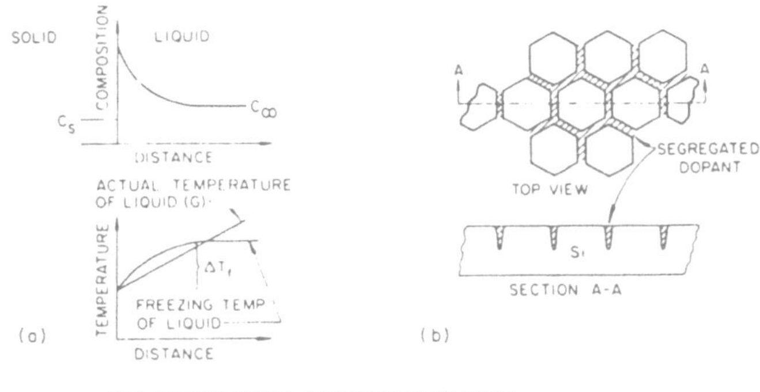

FIGURE 10. Schematic representation of the conditions giving rise to constitutional supercooling instabilities.

conditions, under laser annealing solidification regime, we must exceed a concentration:

$$C(s) = k'/(1 - k') \times \Delta H/2\kappa \times D_\ell/m \times 1/s \qquad (1)$$

where s is the tabulated stability function of Sekerka (13), ΔH is the enthalpy of melting, κ is the thermal conductivity of the solid close to the melting point, D_ℓ is the liquid-phase diffusivity and m is the slope of the liquidus curve.

The maximum substitutional concentration (12) calculated according to the previous expression is reported in Figure 11 for a wide velocity range. It must be noted that for these calculations we used the experimental values of $k'(v)$, which were determined at a low dopant concentration, i.e., when no interface instability occurs. The k' values are reported in the same figure, together with the measured values of the maximum substitutional concentration. There is quite good agreement between experiments and calculations. In fact, the concentration calculated through the above equation is the one at which the onset of interfacial instability should occur. There is no a priori reason to assume that such a concentration is the maximum value that can be incorporated on lattice sites. It will be interesting to investigate this point further. It is important to point out then that in the presence of a precipitate structure, such as that observed after constitutional supercooling, it is not possible to determine the k' value by fitting the profile of retained dopants.

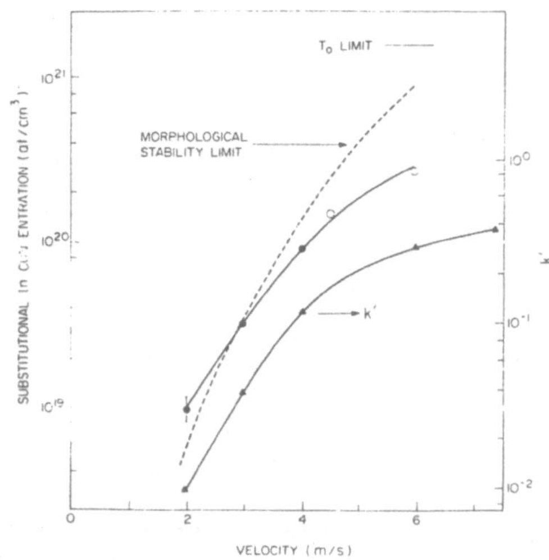

FIGURE 11. Measured value of the maximum substitutional concentration for In in silicon as a function of the solidification velocity. In the same figure are reported the values calculated according to the stability theory and the k' values adopted in these calculations.

REFERENCES

1. S. U. Campisano, E. Rimini, P. Baeri, and G. Foti, Appl. Phys. Lett. 37, 170 (1980).
2. P. Baeri and S. U. Campisano, in Laser Annealing of Semiconductors, edited by J. P. Poate and J. W. Mayer (Academic press, New York, 1982), Chap. 4.
3. S. U. Campisano, Appl. Phys., A 30, 195 (1983).
4. P. Baeri, G. Foti, J. M. Poate, S. U. Campisano, and A. G. Cullis, Appl. Phys. Lett. 38, 800 (1981).
5. K. A. Jackson, in Surface Modification and Alloying, edited by J. M. Poate, G. Foti, and D. C. Jacobson (Plenum Press, New York, 1983), Chap. 3.
6. K. A. Jackson, G. H. Gilmer, and H. J. Leamy, in Laser and Electron Beam Processing of Materials, edited by C. W. White and P. S. Peercy (Academic press, New York, 1980), p. 104.
7. M. A. Aziz, J. Appl. Phys. 53, 1158 (1982).
8. S. U. Campisano and P. Baeri, Appl. Phys. Lett. 42, 1023 (1983).
9. S. U. Campisano, P. Baeri, M. G. Gimaldi, G. Foti, and E. Rimini, Appl. Phys. Lett. 37, 719 (1980).
10. G. J. Baker and J. W. Cahn, Acta Metall. 17, 575 (1969).
11. E. Rimini and S. U. Campisano, in Chemical Instabilities, edited by G. Nicolis and F. Baras (Riedel Publ. Co., Amsterdam, 1984), p. 367.
12. S. U. Campisano and J. M. Poate, Appl. Phys. Lett. 47, 485 (1985).
13. R. F. Sekerka, J. Cryst. Growth 61, 499 (1983).

MODELING AND MEASUREMENTS OF SOLUTE TRAPPING*

M. J. AZIZ
Solid State Division, Oak Ridge National Laboratory, Oak Ridge, TN 37831

Key Words: laser annealing, diffusion, segregation coefficients

ABSTRACT

The fraction of impurity atoms in the liquid at the solid-liquid interface that joins the crystal, known as the segregation coefficient k, during rapid crystal growth is known to deviate away from the equilibrium value towards unity as the interface speed v increases. Several plausible models have been proposed that account qualitatively for this behavior with different functional forms of $k(v)$. Measurements are reported here of the segregation behavior during rapid solidification following pulsed laser melting of Bi-implanted Si. The time-evolution of the melt depth has been measured by the transient conductance technique. The as-implanted and final Bi depth profiles have been measured by Rutherford backscattering. The velocity dependence of the segregation coefficient of Bi in (100) Si has thus been determined to sufficient accuracy to allow us to distinguish between models. Implications for the mechanism of solute trapping are discussed. The effect of solute trapping on the crystal growth velocity is discussed.

1. INTRODUCTION

Pulsed laser melting experiments have reached a crystal growth regime where deviations from local equilibrium are obvious and interface motion is no longer heat-flow limited. These experiments offer the opportunity to study the interface kinetics in high-mobility systems for the first time. The first part of this paper describes a simple model, applicable to both metals and semiconductors, for the kinetics of the fundamental atomic processes occurring at the interface during rapid solidification of binary alloys. The result is a pair of "interface response functons" which predict (a) how much impurity should be incorporated into the solid, and (b) how fast the interface should move in terms of the local conditions at the interface, namely, temperature and composition. Some recent experiments that so far have been possible only in semiconductors are then described; the results support the model and rule out others. Finally, the consequences are discussed for a metallic alloy system of interest.

Consider what happens upon cooling of a liquid in an alloy system such as that shown in Fig. 1. The phase diagram contains all of the information needed to determine what will happen upon extremely slow cooling of a liquid as shown in Fig. 1a. The system would be under

---

* Research sponsored by the Division of Materials Sciences, U.S. Department of Energy, under Contract DE-AC05-84OR21400 with Martin Marietta Energy Systems, Inc.

conditions of metastable global equilibrium if there exists a time regime where nucleation of the α phase is prevented but the system is cooled slowly enough so that bulk diffusion continuously establishes compositional equilibrium throughout the liquid and the solid β phase. In this case, the composition of the bulk of the two phases in equilibrium would trace a path down the liquidus and solidus, along their metastable extensions below the eutectic temperature if necessary, until the relative amount of liquid, given by the "lever rule," vanished. In practice, this scenario virtually never happens in thermal processing of materials. Long-range diffusion through the bulk of a solid phase, and often transport through the liquid, is too slow to maintain compositional equilibrium throughout the bulk of the materials under conventional processing conditions. In this case, however, short-range diffusion across the solid-liquid interface may still be sufficiently rapid to effect interequilibration of the atoms in the liquid monolayer and the solid monolayer adjacent to the interface. Such is the model of local equilibrium: The compositional relationship between the two phases is the equilibrium relationship across the interface; this provides a boundary condition for macroscopic mass transport equations that determine the compositions far from the interface. Local equilibrium implies that given a composition in the liquid at the interface, the solid will grow (a) at the equilibrium liquidus temperature, and (b) with the equilibrium solidus composition (1) as shown in Fig. 1b.

In a rapid quenching process such as splat cooling of molten alloys or regrowth from laser-induced melting, the interface temperature is often unknown. Knowledge of the initial and final temperatures and compositions may be insufficient to determine whether local equilibrium existed at the interface. As shown in Fig. 1c, local equilibrium can only hold if the interface temperature during the quench corresponds to point "B," i.e., the composition of the growing solid must correspond to the solidus curve.

Baker and Cahn proved that local equilibrium is <u>not</u> maintained during splat quenching of Zn-Cd alloys (2), as shown in Fig. 1d. The solidus of Cd in β-Zn is characterized by a maximum Cd concentration at solid compositions above which solidification under local equilibrium conditions cannot occur. The formation of solids with Cd concentrations greater than this maximum demonstrated that the solid composition at the interface was far from the solidus curve, inspiring efforts to model the deviations from local equilibrium.

Pulsed laser melting experiments on doped semiconductors provided planar liquid-solid interfaces and a one-dimensional experimental geometry. Heat-flow calculations and post-irradiation analysis of dopant distributions (34) showed that: (a) maximum equilibrium solubilities could be exceeded by several orders of magnitude, and (b) the partition coefficient k, defined by the ratio of the impurity concentration in the growing solid to that in the liquid at the interface, departs from its equilibrium value and approaches unity. In such a case, it can often be shown that the impurity has actually undergone an increase in chemical potential upon solidification, termed "solute trapping" (1,2).

A number of physically plausible models have been proposed (5-13) to explain how the host atoms persuade the impurity atoms to increase their chemical potential and join the crystal. They are in qualitative agreement with the existing data, which show the partition coefficient

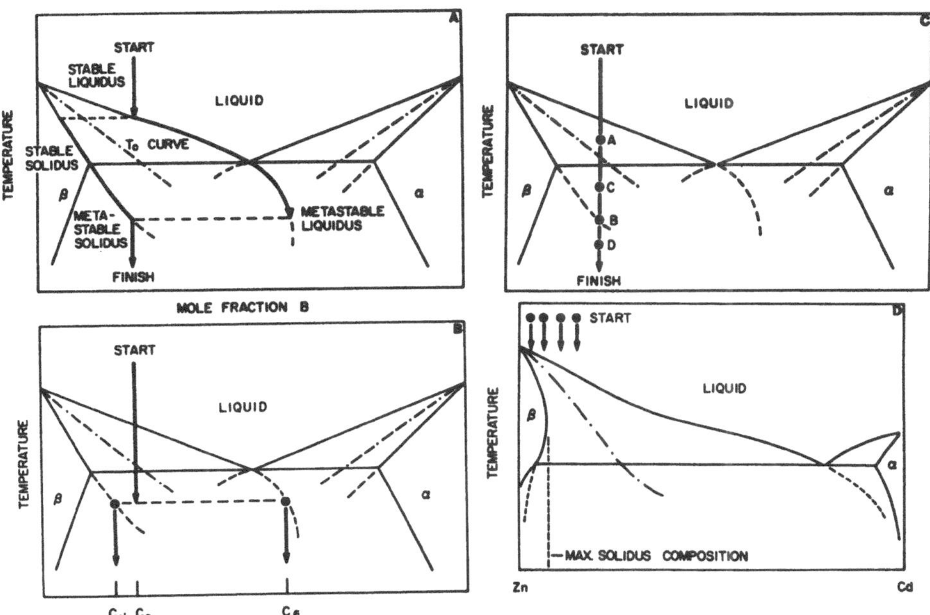

FIGURE 1. (a) Paths taken by liquid and solid phases during cooling sufficiently slow to establish stable for metastable global equilibrium. (b) State of solid and liquid at interface during solidification under conditions of local equilibrium. Given a composition of the liquid at the interface, the solid grows at the equilibrium temperature, with the equilibrium composition. (c) Possible states of solid at interface during rapid quench that produced solid of same composition as original bulk liquid. A: thermodynamically forbidden; B: local equilibrium condition; C,D: thermodynamically allowed by no local equilibrium. (d) Splat-quenching experiments that trapped Cd in Zn, proving local disequilibrium.

monotonically increasing from its equilibrium value k_e and toward unity as the interface speed v increases.

The basis for the model described here is the relatively new idea that crystallization and interdiffusion at the interface involve processes that are fundamentally different. Conventional modeling of interface kinetics (10) uses the same atomic motions to describe crystallization as those to describe interdiffusion in the liquid. In such a case, the growth speed can never exceed the maximum diffusive speed, which is typically on the order of 1-10 meters per second, given by $v_D = D_i/\lambda$, where D_i is the coefficient for interdiffusion across (not along) the interface and λ is the interatomic distance. However, the collision-limited growth model developed by Turnbull and co-workers (14-21), which has received recent support from the molecular dynamics work of Broughton et al. (22), indicates that for metallic and other simple molecular systems, such a scaling is invalid and that v_s, the speed of sound, should be the only limit to the crystal growth rate. Consequently, the growth speed can very much exceed the diffusive speed, and when it does so in alloys, we expect suppressed segregation and a diffusionless transformation.

The reason that crystal growth in metals should not scale with diffusion is illustrated in Fig. 2. A crystallization event consists of an atom shifting its position a small distance to move from a potential well in the liquid structure to a well on the crystal lattice. Since no bonds must be broken, the activation barrier for this reaction ought to be quite small. A diffusive jump, on the other hand, is a different atomic process requiring the cooperation of the neighboring atoms in this system. Position shifts of a fraction of an interatomic distance do not accomplish the solute-solvent redistribution which is necessary to avoid solute incorporation into the crystal. A solute atom must accomplish three things to avoid crystallization: It must escape from its potential well, as shown by the dashed arrow in Fig. 2, as the energy of the well increases and the well moves to the lattice site; it must push solvent atoms out of the way; and it must be replaced by a solvent atom on the lattice site or else it will be pushed right back to where it came from.

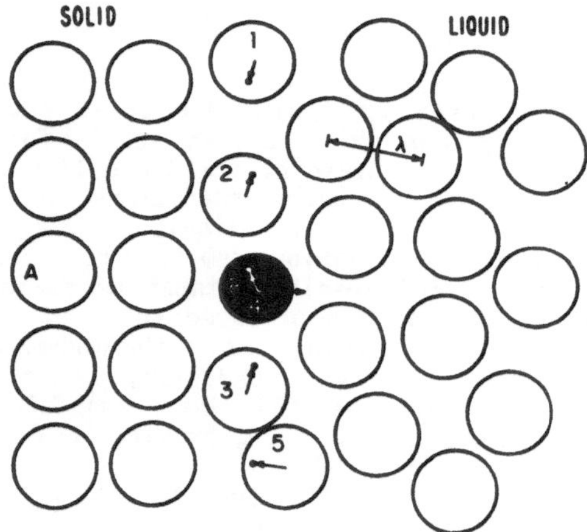

FIGURE 2. Choreography of Solute Trapping. In order to avoid incorporation into the crystal (solid arrow), the "B" atom must: (1) ESCAPE from its potential well (dashed arrow) as the well gains energy and moves to the lattice site (solid arrow), (2) PUSH "A" atoms out of the way, (3) BE REPLACED with an "A" atom on the lattice site.

Atoms in the interface region tend to interdiffuse in order to establish equilibrium compositions on either side of the interface. As the interface passes, solute-solvent redistribution only occurs during a limited time. Before the interface arrives, the driving force for redistribution is zero; afterwards, atomic mobilities are too low to permit significant interdiffusion. When $v << v_D$ there is plenty of time for the atoms at the interface to equilibrate. As the growth velocity becomes greater, solute and solvent atoms have less time while they are in the interface region to interdiffuse and maintain local equilibrium. When $v >> v_D$ the atoms have virtually no time to interdiffuse; the interface passes and locks the liquid composition into the bulk of the solid before the atoms have a chance to react.

If growth occurs by the rapid lateral passage of steps of height λ, then the average time between the passage of steps is $\tau = \lambda/v$. The time it takes solvent atoms to shift to their lattice positions is negligible when compared to τ, and the shifts can be treated as virtually instantaneous. On the other hand, if continuous solidification occurs, the impurity atom is being dragged toward its lattice site during a time period of order τ. In the former case, an analysis of solute diffusion back into the liquid (11) during the interval τ yields, for a dilute solution of B in A

$$k(v,T) = k_e(T) + [1 - k_e(T)] \exp(- v_D/v) \tag{1}$$

where T is the interface temperature, the equilibrium segregation coefficient $k_e(T)$ is the ratio of the solidus composition to the liquidus composition at the temperature T of the undercooled interface, and the diffusive speed v_D is the only fitting parameter in the model. This model should apply whenever the chemical potential of the solute atom is raised from its liquid value to its solid value during a time interval that is very short compared to τ. In the latter case, the limit of strict steady-state fluxes on a microscopic scale, the fluxes and concentrations become time-independent and a similar analysis (12) yields

$$k(v,T) = [(v/v_D) + k_e(T)]/[(v/v_D) + 1] \tag{2}$$

which shows the same qualitative features as in stepwise growth, a transition from equilibrium segregation ($k = k_e$) to complete solute trapping ($k \rightarrow 1$) as the interface speed surpasses the diffusive speed. In the continuous growth model, however, the transition is more gradual than in the stepwise growth model.

2. EXPERIMENTAL RESULTS

The most significant experimental progress has been made in the field of pulsed laser melting of semiconductors. Progress was rapid because defect-free plane-front solidification is routinely attained and because in many cases k_e is so small that when k approaches unity, tremendous changes are effected in the final impurity distribution.

The pioneering work of Baeri et al. (3) and of White et al. (23) showed that k can in fact increase several orders of magnitude above k_e at high interface speeds and demonstrated the velocity dependence of k by varying the laser parameters to cover a range of regrowth velocities during pulsed laser melting of ion-implanted Si. When compared in detail, the results of the two groups were seen to be somewhat different. Certain studies showed an effect termed "saturation," where $dk/dv \to 0$ at some value of $k < 1$. This effect was claimed to have been observed for Bi (24), In (25), and Sb (26) in Si. In a separate study of Bi in Si, the effect was not observed (23). This saturation phenomenon is intriguing because it cannot be explained by a simple model; it indicates, if correct, that more complicated solute trapping models (27) (8) (13) are necessary for understanding the phenomenon.

A study was recently undertaken (28) to see whether any of the existing models could yield quantitative agreement with the data and to examine the saturation phenomenon in detail. To obtain high precision data, we used the transient conductance technique for measuring the interface velocity for Bi-implanted Si (29), thereby eliminating errors that arose in the previous studies, which could only estimate v by the use of heat-flow calculations. The time evolution of the melt depth was measured by roughly 1 ns resolution with this technique. The initial and final Bi profiles were determined to high accuracy by Rutherford Backscattering Spectroscopy (RBS) carried out in glancing angle geometry.

The analysis was performed by numerical simulation with a finite-element solution of the diffusion equation, using the measured as-implanted profile and the measured melt depth as a functon of time for each sample. Diffusion was permitted in the liquid but not in the solid phase. During solidification a fraction k of the impurity in the liquid at the interface was incorporated into the crystal. The parameters allowed to vary were the bulk liquid-phase diffusivity D_L and the partition coefficient during solidification k. Comparison with the measured profiles yielded unique value for both D_L and k.

We show in Fig. 3 the results of analysis of several samples. The models discussed before for stepwise growth and for continuous growth are shown, as is the two-level Baker model (8,11,19), where the impurity is treated as if diffusing down a steep energy gradient in a continuum. For this model, k is given by $k = \{\beta + \ln k_e\}/\{\beta + [(1/k_e) \ln k_e \cdot \exp(-\beta)]\}$, where $\beta \equiv v/v_D$. The diffusive speed v_D is the only free parameter in all three models; it has been chosen in each case to yield the best fit to the data. Note that in all three equations, v only appears as the ratio v/v_D. Thus when a model is plotted as k versus $\log v$, as in Fig. 3, the only effect of varying the free parameter v_D is a rigid horizontal shift of the curve, with no change in the slope. We can therefore conclude that the stepwise growth model of Aziz and the two-level Baker model produce curves that rise too steeply to account for our data. The continuous growth model, on the other hand, fits our data quite well.

Data from the original work of Baeri et al. (24) and of White et al. (23) are also shown in Fig. 3. While sufficient to establish without a doubt that k increases far beyond k_e as v increases, we see here that their data are not accurate enough to allow any conclusions regarding appropriate models or the presence of the saturation effect discussed earlier. Note that there is no evidence in our data for such a saturation effect. Although it is possible that the disagreement between our results and theirs reflects a composition dependence or some other genuine difference in $k(v)$ between the experiments, we believe the disagreement is most likely due to errors in their calculations of the time evolution of the melt depth, which would feed back to produce errors in the apparent k.

There are other solute trapping models worthy of consideration. One model due to Jackson and co-workers (10) produces a $k(v)$ curve similar

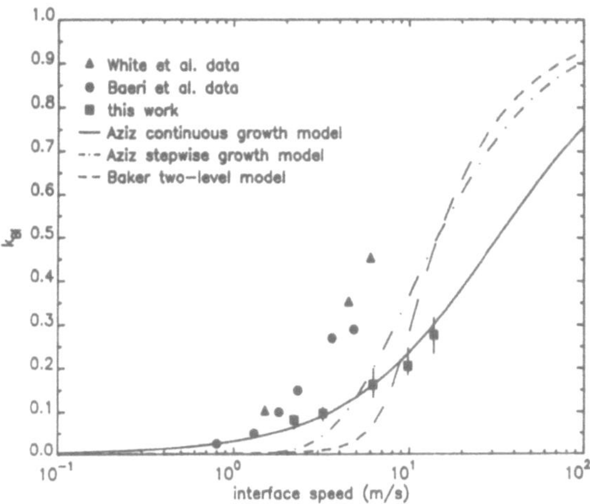

FIGURE 3. Dependence of partition coefficient on velocity. Triangles and circles: velocity estimated from heat-flow calculations. Squares: velocity measured by transient conductance. Continuous growth model: v_D = 32 m/s. Stepwise growth model: v_D = 10 m/s. Baker model: v_D = 1 m/s.

to that of the continuous growth model discussed here, but has been rejected because it cannot account for solute trapping on both ends of a phase diagram (28). We are unable to compare our results to the models of Hillert and Sundman (9) and of Gilmer (13) because they involve complex computer calculations that we cannot perform.

It is seen that nonequilibrium partition coefficients in semiconductors can be measured to significantly higher accuracy than has been done before by combining transient conductance and glancing angle RBS measurements, thereby eliminating errors resulting from heat-flow calculations. We see no evidence for saturation of the partition coefficient at values less than unity, for dilute solutions of Bi in Si (100). Our results for partitioning in this system at measured interface speeds between 2 and 14 m/s are consistent with a model where the potential of the impurity atom is raised gradually from its value in the liquid to that in the bulk of the solid over the same period in which it is trying to diffuse back into the liquid.

3. GROWTH VELOCITY

Onsager's reciprocity relations (30) imply that if crystal growth affects the amount of solute incorporation, then solute trapping will in turn affect the growth rate. The common asumption of heat-flow-limited growth is in many cases a useful one. It may, however, become unrealistic at high velocities and solute concentrations, where the interface reaction kinetics can come into play. The implications of equation (2) for crystal growth rate are decribed below.

For pure systems, the crystal growth process is understood as follows (31). In equilibrium, the rates at which atoms join and leave the crystal are equal. When there is a finite driving force for crystallization, the former exceeds the latter by a Boltzmann factor $\exp(\Delta\mu/RT)$; the growth velocity is given by their difference. The kinetics are manifested by an intrinsic growth-velocity limit, which is the speed of the forward reaction alone, $v_o(T)$. This is the speed with which the interface would propagate at infinite driving force (i.e., when the back reaction disappears). The growth velocity is then written as $v = v_o(T)[1 - \exp(\Delta\mu/RT)]$. This expression becomes the familiar $v = M\Delta G$ at small driving forces. Inverting the above expression, we have $\Delta\mu = RT \ln(1 - v/v_o)$. The left-hand side is the driving free energy; the right-hand side can be thought of as the free energy dissipated by the irreversible crystallization reaction at the interface. Thus the velocity-driving force relation can be written $\Delta G_{DF} = \Delta G_F$, where ΔG_{DF} is the driving energy, expressed as free energy per mole, and ΔG_F, the "interface friction energy" due to a finite interfacial mobility, is the free energy dissipated per mole of material solidified. The available driving force is dissipated by the irreversible processes at the interface. We can phrase this statement in an alternative way by dividing each side of the previous equation by the molar volume (32). We then say that the sum of the forces per unit area on an interface moving at constant velocity is zero.

For alloys, we can write $\Delta G_{DF} = \Sigma\Delta G_{DISS}$, where the $\Sigma\Delta G_{DISS}$ are the losses due to all of the simultaneous dissipative processes. In the steady state, the system does no work on the surroundings and so the driving free energy must be entirely dissipated by irreversible processes during the transformation. If we can calculate the dissipation and the driving force as functions of velocity, we have an equation that predicts the growth velocity. Ignoring heat conduction, the two dissipative processes at the interface are the crystallization and redistribution reactions. The dissipative terms associated with them are, respectively, the "interface friction energy" ΔG_F and the "solute drag energy" ΔG_D (32-34). By assuming interface friction to be the same for alloys as for pure systems, we can calculate these terms (12). The results are $\Delta G_F = RT \ln(1 - v/v_o)$ and, for the dilute solution continuous growth model, Eq.(2), $\Delta G_D = X_S RT[1 - k)/k] \ln[k/k_e(T)]$. The driving force is given by (34) $\Delta G_{DF} = X_S\Delta\mu_B + (1 - X_S)\Delta\mu_A$; the growth velocity equation becomes

$$\Delta G_{DF}(v) = \Delta G_F(v) + \Delta G_D(v) \tag{3}$$

It turns out that one of the dissipative terms is often negligible compared to the other; the transition occurs over a small velocity range. Consequently, the equation can be simplified away from the transition. For e-beam melting experiments on Ag(Cu), with interface velocities in the centimeter-per-second to meter-per-second range (35), ΔG_D dominates most of the time; for laser annealing of doped Si with meter-per-second velocities, ΔG_F almost always dominates. During a diffusionless transformation in any system, ΔG_D vanishes.

The dilute solution approximation is invalid when the mole fraction of solute is no longer negligible or when activity coefficients γ are no longer constants. When the appropriate corrections to the fluxes and driving forces in the continuous growth model are made (12), the results are

$$k_B = \frac{[(v/v_D) + \kappa_o]}{[(v/v_D) + 1 - (1 - \kappa_o)X_{li}]} \tag{4}$$

$$\Delta G_D = X_s[(1 - k)/k]\, RT \ln \frac{k}{k_A \kappa_o} \tag{5}$$

where $\kappa_o(X_s, X_{li}, T) \equiv \exp[-\Delta(\mu_B' - \mu_A')/RT]$, $\mu'(X,T) \equiv \mu(X,T) - RT \ln X = \mu°(T) + RT \ln \gamma(X,T)$, X_{li} is the mole fraction of B in the liquid at the interface, $k_A \equiv X_s^A/X_{li}^A$, γ is the activity coefficient, A = solute, B = solvent, and Δ = "solid minus liquid." The implicit assumption has been made that at the interface the transition state behaves in an ideal manner. In practice, temperature and composition dependence may show up in D_i. These equations predict that when the interface encounters a region of high impurity content during regrowth from pulsed laser melting, the interface slows down for two reasons. If $k_e < 1$ the driving force for solidification decreases with increasing solute content. In addition, the solute drag term, which always acts to hinder interface motion, increases with increasing solute content. Such an effect has been observed in silicon (36,37). Unfortunately, quantitative tests of the theory have not yet been possible due to problems modeling the thermodynamics of highly doped semiconductors.

Metals, on the other hand, are much better understood thermodynamically, enabling quantitative predictions to be made. Some predictions for the Ag-Cu system follow.

Equations 3, 4 and 5 were solved numerically. For the Ag-Cu system, the thermodynamic model of Murray (38) was used to obtain the chemical potential of Ag and of Cu across the phase diagram. The following parameters were used: $\lambda = 0.2$ nm, $v_o = 340{,}000$ cm/s, $D_i = 0.00122 \exp[-(10\ \text{kcal/mole})/RT]$ cm^2/s. The results are plotted as interface temperature and compositions on the phase diagram in Fig. 4; we see that for a given composition X_{li} in the liquid at the interface, the solid composition increases and the interface temperature drops as the velocity is increased. In a steady-state e-beam melting experiment, the solid composition is constrained to be equal to the bulk liquid composition. The velocity is independently controlled; the dependent variables are X_{li} and T. The way they behave is shown in Fig. 5. As the velocity is increased, the liquid composition at the interface decreases due to solute trapping, and the interface temperature actually rises, trying to follow the liquidus. When the T_o line is reached, a diffusionless transformation becomes thermodynamically possible. However, diffusionless solidification does not commence until some distance beyond the T_o line, when the velocity is great enough to suppress the redistribution reaction. Figure 6 illustrates that in the model for the Ag(Cu) system, two effects facilitate trapping at high

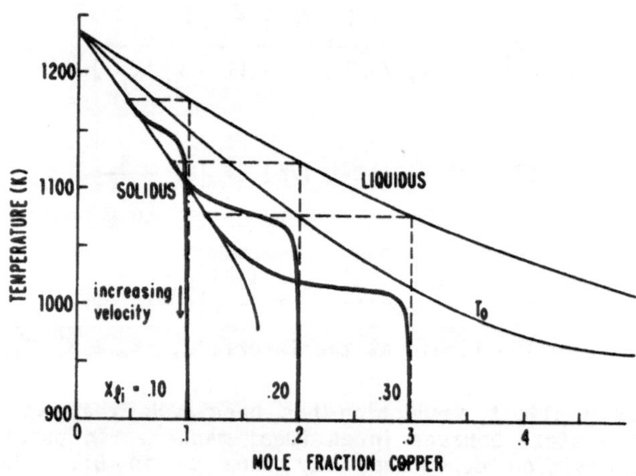

FIGURE 4. Interface temperature and solid composition for fixed X_{li} in Ag(Cu). For a given liquid composition X_{li} at the interface, the solid composition increases and the interface temperature drops as the velocity is increased.

concentrations. The interface diffusivity drops by a factor of two as we go from the melting point of silver to the eutectic temperature, thus making the redistributive reaction more difficult while not sensibly affecting the growth mobility. In addition, the driving force for redistribution is smaller at high concentrations.

The results of the e-beam melting experiments of Boettinger et al. (35) are consistent with Fig. 6. They find the onset of microsegregation-free solidification to occur at lower velocities as Cu is added to Ag. The magnitude of the effect is close to that in Fig. 6. It is hoped that recent experimental advances in metals (39) will allow a quantitative test of the theory.

ACKNOWLEDGMENTS

The experimental work was done in collaboration with J. Y. Tsao, M. O. Thompson, P. S. Peercy, and C. W. White. The computer calculations were done with the assistance of E. Nygren and K. F. Kelton.

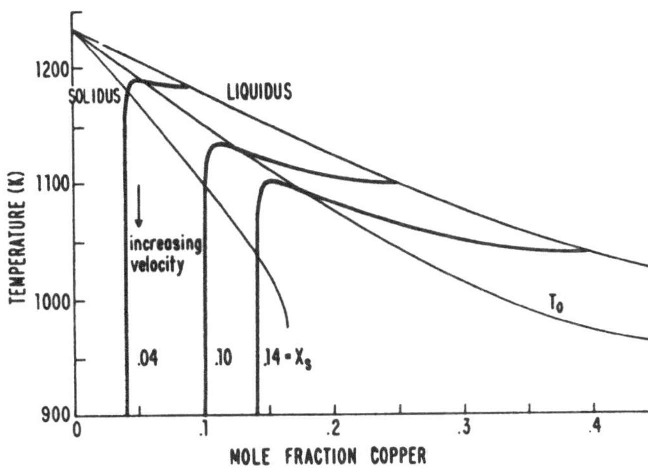

FIGURE 5. Interface temperature and liquid composition at interface for fixed X_S. when the T_0 line is crossed, the diffusionless transformation becomes thermodynamically possible, but it does not occur until some distance beyond.

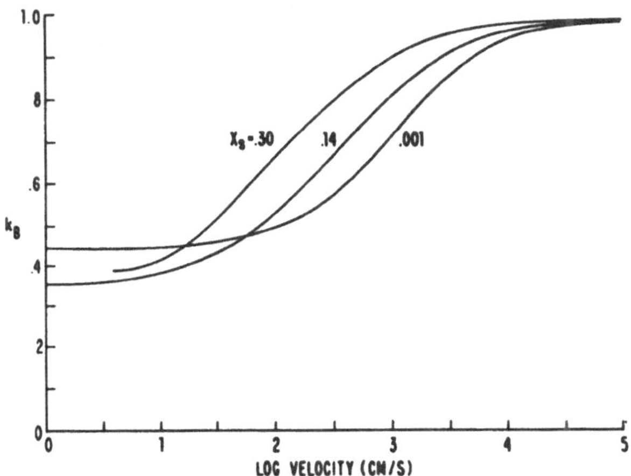

FIGURE 6. Segregation coefficient vs. velocity for dilute and concentration alloys of Cu in Ag. In this system, two effects facilitate trapping at higher concentrations. The interface diffusivity drops and the driving force for redistribution drops.

REFERENCES

1. J. C. Baker and J. W. Cahn, in Solidification (American Society for Metals, Metals Park, Ohio, 1970), pp. 23-58.
2. J. C. Baker and J. W. Cahn, Acta Metall. 17, 575 (1969).
3. C. W. White, S. R. Wilson, B. R. Appleton, and F. W. Young, Jr., J. Appl. Phys. 51, 738 (1980).
4. P. Baeri, J. M. Poate, S. U. Campisano, G. Foti, E. Rimini, and A. G. Cullis, Appl. Phys. Lett. 37, 912 (1980).
5. R. N. Hall, J. Phys. Chem. 57, 836 (1953).
6. A. A. Chernov, in Growth of Crystals, edited by A. V. Shubnikov and N. N. Sheftal (Consultants Bureau, New York, 1962), Vol. 3, p. 35.
7. J. C. Brice, The Growth of Crystals from the Melt, (North-Holland, Amsterdam, 1965).
8. J. W. Cahn, S. R. Coriell, and W. J. Boettinger, in Laser and Electron Beam Processing of Materials, edited by C. W. White and P. S. Peercy (Academic, New York, 1980), p. 89.
9. M. Hillert and B. Sundman, Acta Metall. 25, 11 (1977).
10. K. A. Jackson, in Surface Modification and Alloying by Laser, Ion and Electron Beams, edited by J. M. Poate, G. Foti, and D. C. Jacobson (Plenum, New York, 1983), p. 51.
11. M. J. Aziz, J. Appl. Phys. 53, 1158 (1982).
12. M. J. Aziz, Appl. Phys. Lett. 43, 552 (1983).
13. G. H. Gilmer, Mat. Res. Soc. Symp. Proc. 13, 249 (1983).
14. D. Turnbull, Contemp. Phys. 10, 473 (1969).
15. D. Turnbull, in Solidification (American Society for Metals, Metals Park, Ohio, 1970), pp. 1-22.
16. D. Turnbull, J. Phys. (Paris) Colloq. C-4 (1974).
17. D. Turnbull and B. G. Bagley, in Treatise on Solid State Chemistry, edited by N. B. Hannay (Plenum, New York, 1975), Vol. 5, pp. 513-54.
18. F. Spaepen and D. Turnbull, in Rapidly Quenched Metals, 2nd International Conference, edited by N. J. Grant and B. C. Giessen (MIT, Cambridge, MA, 1976), pp. 205-29.
19. F. Spaepen and D. Turnbull, in Laser Annealing of Semiconductors, edited by J. M. Poate and J. W. Mayer (Academic, New York, 1982), pp. 15-42.
20. D. Turnbull, Metall. Trans., A 12, 693 (1981).
21. S. R. Coriell and D. Turnbull, Acta Metall. 30, 2135 (1982).
22. J. Q. Broughton, G. H. Gilmer, and K. A. Jackson, Phys. Rev. Lett. 49, 1496 (1982).
23. C. W. White, B. R. Appleton, B. Stritzker, D. M. Zehner, and S. R. Wilson, Mat. Res. Soc. Symp. Proc. 1, 59 (1981).
24. P. Baeri, G. Foti, J. M. Poate, S. U. Campisano, and A. G. Cullis, Appl. Phys. Lett. 38, 800 (1981).
25. J. M. Poate, Mat. Res. Soc. Symp. Proc. 4, 121 (1982).
26. C. W. White, D. M. Zehner, S. U. Campisano, and A. G. Cullis, in Surface Modificiation and Alloying by Laser, Ion and Electron Beams, edited by J. M. Poate, G. Foti, and D. C. Jacobson (Plenum, New York, 1983), p. 94.
27. M. J. Aziz, Ph.D. Thesis, Harvard University, 1983, pp. 76-82.
28. M. J. Aziz, J. Y. Taso, M. O. Thompson, P. S. Peercy, and C. W. White, Mat. Res. Soc. Symp. Proc. 35, 153 (1985).
29. M. O. Thompson, G. J. Galvin, J. W. Mayer, P. S. Peercy, and R. B. Hammond, Appl. Phys. Lett. 42, 445 (1983).
30. L. Onsager, Phys. Rev. 37, 405 (1931); 38, 2265 (1931).

31. J. W. Christian, Theory of Transformations in Metals and Alloys, Part I, 2nd ed. (Pergamon, Oxford, 1975), p. 479.
32. M. Hillert and B. Sundman, Acta Metall. 24, 733 (1976).
33. J. W. Cahn, Acta Metall. 10, 789 (1962).
34. M. Hillert and B. Sundman, Acta Metall. 25, 11 (1977).
35. W. J. Boettinger, D. Shechtman, R. J. Schaefer, F. Biancaniello, Metall. Trans., A 15, 55 (1984).
36. G. J. Galvin, J. W. Mayer, and P. S. Peercy, Mat. Res. Soc. Symp. Proc. 23, 111 (1984).
37. P. S. Peercy and M. O. Thompson, Mat. Res. Soc. Symp. Proc. 35, 53 (1985).
38. J. A. Murray, Metall. Trans., A 15, 261 (1984).
39. P. S. Peercy, this volume.

EDITED QUESTIONS - CHAPTER 8

POATE, PEERCY, CAMPISANO, AZIZ

JOHN POATE

Q. Laser melting of Si - is it done in air or vacuum?
A. Most often it is done in air.

Q. Beam homogenizer - is it used for achieving spatial or temporal coherence?
A. Beam homogenizer rod is used to get spatial coherence so as to eliminate hot spots in the laser-annealed area.

Q. If this is the case, the sample has to be kept close to the homogenizer, so as to avoid beam divergence?
A. Yes. Indeed, the working distance is very close.

Q. In the case of cw laser regrowing of c-Si from a-Si, is it done in one pass?
A. No. A 6" wide layer to be treated with a 2.0 mm diameter beam would take hours. In fact, the state of the art is that we no longer use lasers.

Q. Comment on the future for laser processing of semiconductors?
A. Very bleak, unless you develop laser systems, which can heat up fairly large areas and hold them at about 1000°C for some time.

PAUL PEERCY

Q. In transient conductance measurements, why do you need to illuminate the contact areas?
A. When a sample is melted, the molten Si resistance will be dominated by the contact resistance. In order to suppress this, it is necessary to illuminate the contact area.

Q. How do you measure the energy density accurately?
A. Measure the beam energy after it comes out of the lightguide, using light-sensing diodes.

Q. What is the thermal conductivity of a-Si?
A. It is very low at room temperature and increases to a value 2/3 times lower than c-Si at the melting temperature.

Q. In case of explosive crystallization, is it possible to control the thickness of the second molten layer?
A. It varies with the substrate temperature. If the substrate is at room temperature, it could be up to 18 nm. It also depends on the interface temperature which in turn depends on the pulse length.

Q. The proportionality constant between regrowth velocity and the interfacial undercooling, ß - should it only be determined experimentally?
A. Yes.

Q. All the previous work described about As in Si and the transient conductance method - was that done using a-Si or c-Si?
A. a-Si. But it is possible to do it with c-Si as well.

UGO CAMPISANO

Q. How do you obtain the Zn segregation coefficient in Ge and Si?
A. K' is the only fitting parameter used to compare calculated with experimental profiles.

Q. Interfacial breakdown in case of implanted samples - how is the cell structure detected?
A. By microscopy - TEM.

MICHAEL AZIZ

Q. What is happening to White et al. data, as regards fitting on the solute trapping theory curve?
A. After repeated analysis, it was found that the composition analysis was wrong and is higher. In fact, reevaluation shows that is lower.

Q. In his paper regarding trapping becoming easier in Ag-Cu system as Cu content increases, Boettinger suggested that those bands existed just because you were moving towards the eutectic, and therefore for the given interface speed and undercooling, the absolute temperature and diffusive speeds were lower and this is the reason. Is it taken into account?
A. This is the value given. Diffusive speed is in there.

PARTICIPANTS LIST AND BRIEF PHOTO HISTORY

CLIFTON W. DRAPER, PAOLO MAZZOLDI AND LUIGI DONA

One of the thrusts of the ASI was to provide sufficient informal format so as to promote discussions across the "double jump" barriers. We did manage to schedule in some brief periods of physical exercise and mental relaxation. In some of the following figures and photos we share a few of these moments with you.

The highlight of week I was the national single elimination ping-pong tourney.

<u>Opening Round</u>

US vs. non-NATO,
UK vs. Portugal & Spain,
France vs. Germany,
Italy vs. Turkey et al.

<u>Semi's</u>

US vs. UK,
France vs. Turkey et al.

<u>Finals</u>

US vs. France

<u>Winner</u>

France

In the final matches the French team of Gerard Coquerelle and Thierry Manderscheid, coached by Monique Calvo, soundly defeated the US representatives: Elton Kaufman, Clif Draper, Mike Aziz and player-coach Paul Peercy.

The second week featured a football (soccer) match between native English-speaking and non-English-speaking countries. In other words, US, Canada, UK and Israel vs. all others. The onslaught ended after four periods: non-English - 8 goals, English - nil. The local <u>Italian</u> referee from Empoli called offsides on the only goal scored by the English-speaking squad, which preserved the shutout and embarrassment. Week II also featured the meeting's social dinner at which Paolo Mazzoldi and Luigi Dona made fun at the expense of the Materials Research Society (MRS). As one of the Institute's co-sponsors, the MRS was represented by its 1985 president, Elton Kaufmann. He and other MRS activists present at the ASI were the targets of most of the humor.

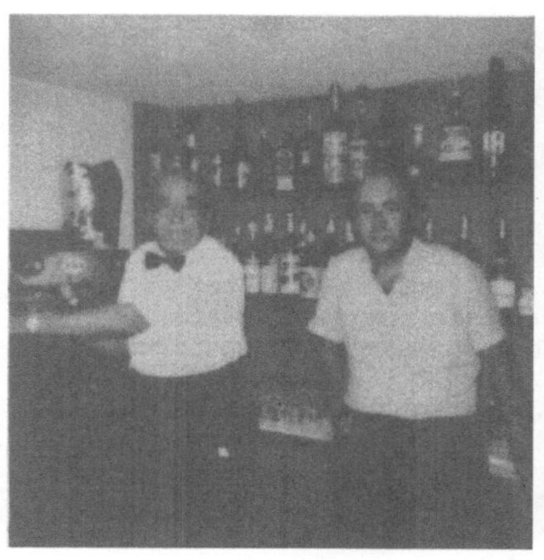

Vincenti Narciso and Professor Mazzoldi

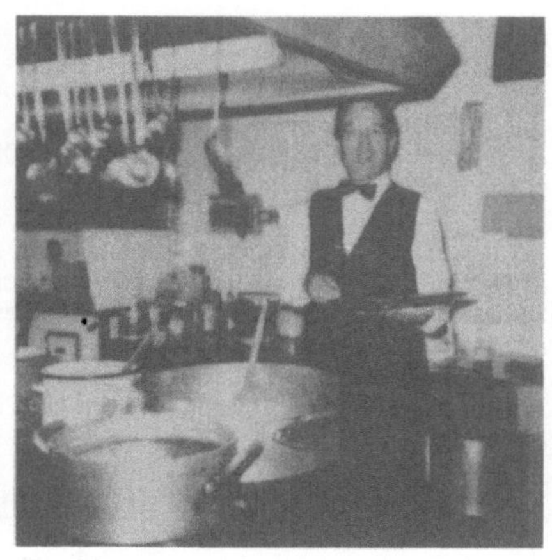

Moreno Nucci

Important to the success of our ASI: Our bartender Signore Narciso with Professor Mazzoldi. In charge of Capruccini's ristorante, Signore Moreno Nucci. The two most gracious conference secretaries, Signorina Carla Carbone and Signorina Maria Grazia Dogliotti.

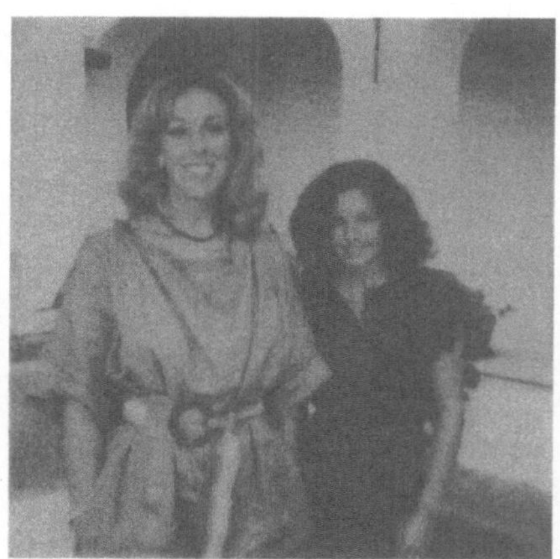

Carla Carbone and Maria Grazia Dogliotti

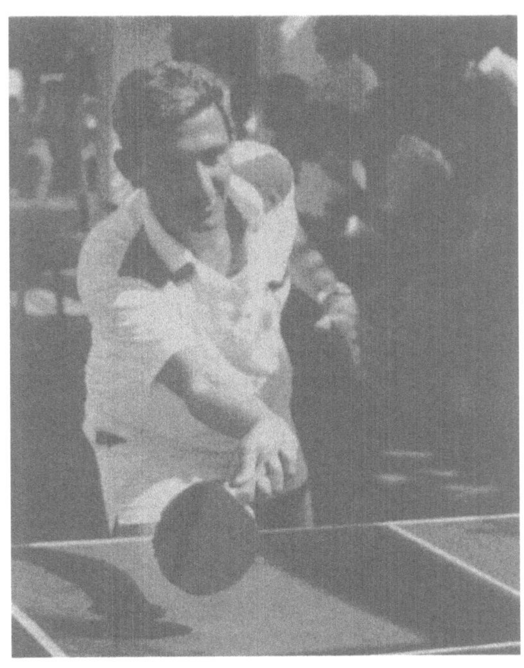

Dr. Gabriel Laufer, from Technion in Israel, delivers a forehand for the non-NATO team. His knowledge of laser surgery was more dangerous than his ping-pong.

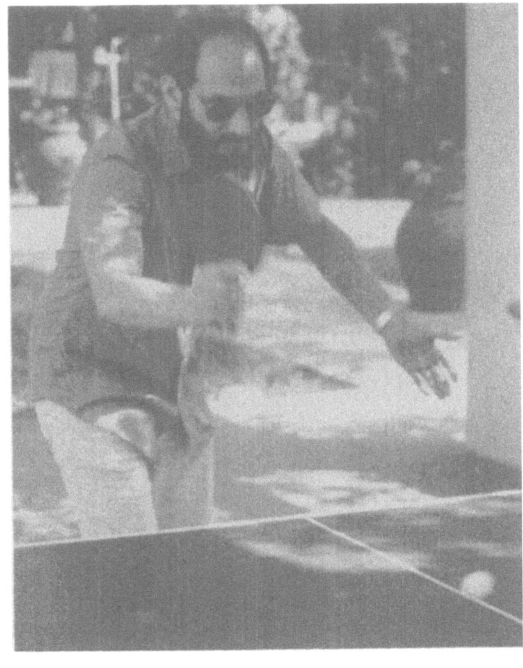

Dr. Elton Kaufmann, from Lawrence Livermore Laboratories, USA, and 1985 president of the Materials Research Society serves a high-velocity backhand with considerable angular momentum across to non-NATO first-round opponent.

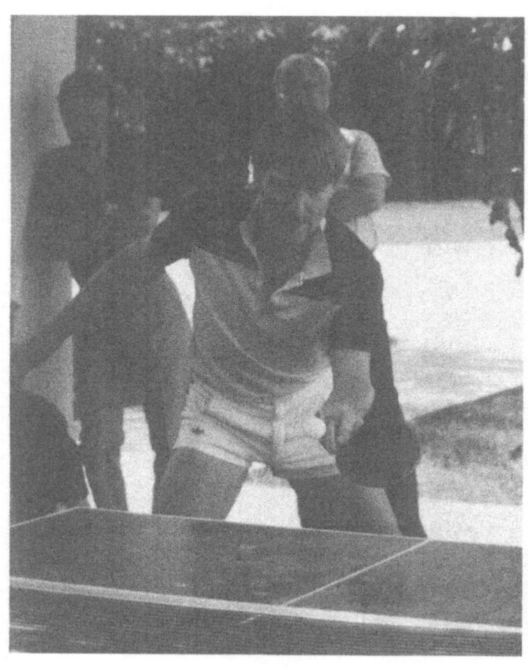

Mr. Thierry Manderscheid from CITROEN, France, proved to be too much for every opponent he faced. Much to the dismay of the English-speaking community, he was equally dangerous on the football (soccer) field.

Dr. Ir. Jean-Pierre Celis from Katholieke Universiteit, Belgium, uses a bit of body language to help the ball clear the net to the opponent's side.

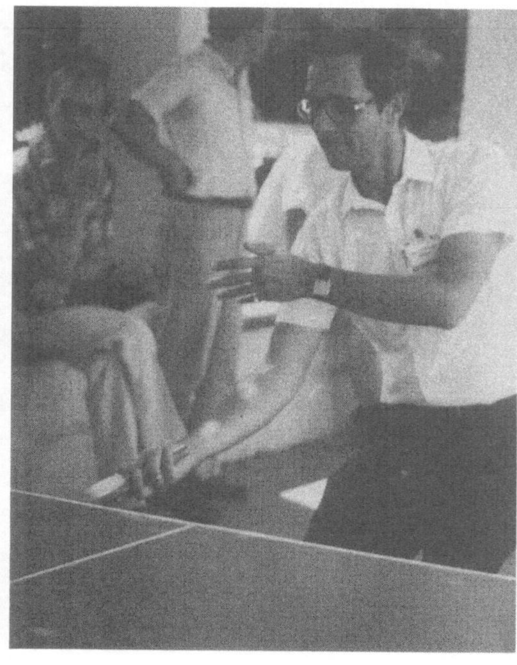

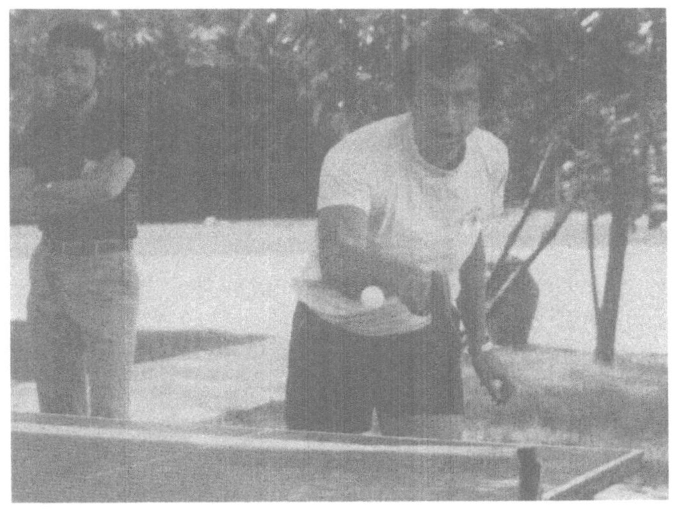

Dr. Bernd Stritzker from KFA, Germany, keeps his eye on the ball and calculates the incoming trajectory.

The grand champions - the French team of Gerard Coquerelle, Theirry Manderscheid and coach Monique Calvo.

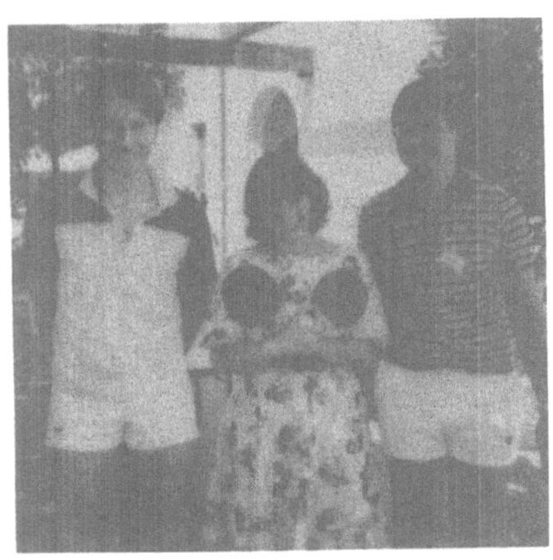

Ping-Pong Grand Champions
"The French"

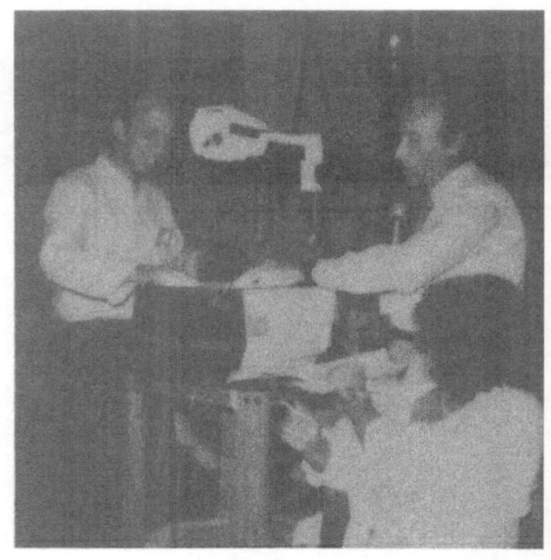

The Roots of Early
Materials Research

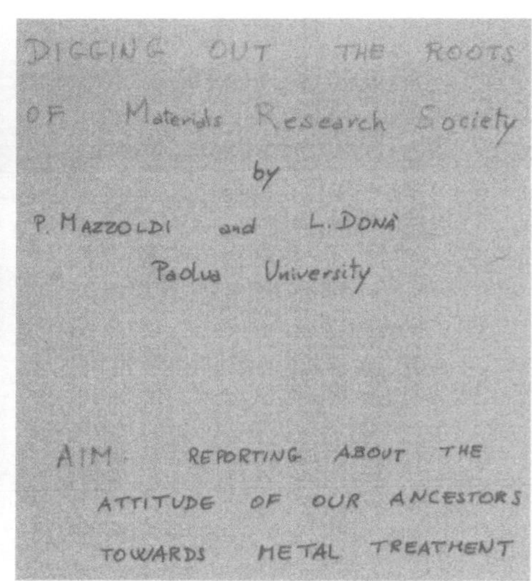

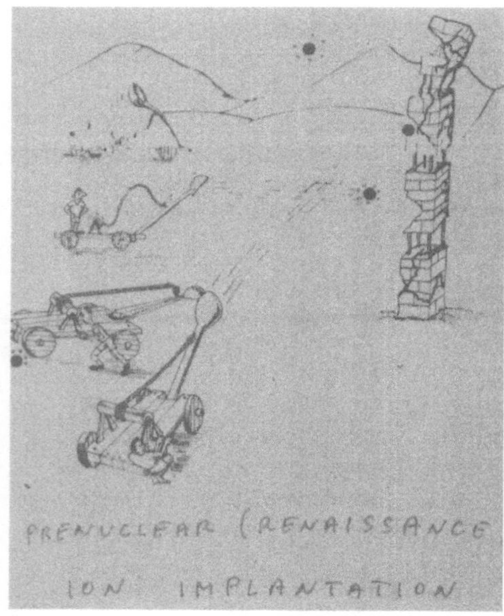

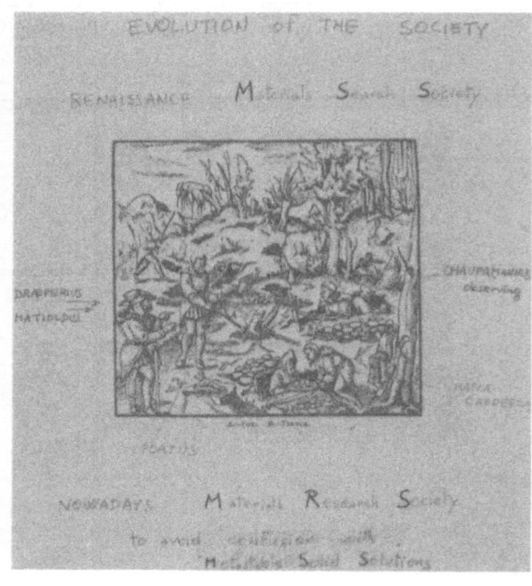

Paolo Mazzoldi and Luigi Dona entertain the participants at the social dinner at the expense of the Materials Research Society and our colleagues in the ion implantation community.

We close this book with reference to the meeting group photograph, its key and the complete listing of conference attendees. We thank all of you for your time and energy that resulted in such a successful meeting and, we are confident, useful book.

Key to Group Photograph

1. Ralf Koppmann, Germany
2. Todd Rockstroh, USA
3. Jean-Pierre Girardeau-Montaut, France
4. Paul Peercy, USA
5. Emmanuel Kerrand, France
6. Gerard Coquerelle, France
7. Pierre Magnin, Switzerland
8. Bernard Vannes, France
9. Thomas Jervis, USA
10. José Soares, Portugal

11. Jean Tardieu de Maleissye, France
12. Momcilo Tosic, Yugoslavia
13. Carolyn MacDonald, USA
14. Dale Jacobson, USA
15. Lindsay Greer, UK
16. Ed McCafferty, USA
17. Henri Van Dorssen, Netherlands
18. Vittoria Contini, Italy
19. Michael Aziz, USA
20. Marco Vittori, Italy

21. Fernanda da Silva, Portugal
22. Rui Vilar, Portugal
23. Satish Vitta, UK
24. Marcello Baricco, Italy
25. Bill Steen, UK
26. Etienne Petit, Belgium
27. Elton Kaufmann, USA
28. Margaret Steen, UK
29. Aubrey Helms, USA
30. Moreno Nucci, Italy

31. Malcolm Macintyre, UK
32. Monique Calvo, France
33. Nilgun Tezey, Turkey
34. Emmanuel Kerrand, France
35. Hans Bergmann, Germany
36. Barry Mordike, Germany
37. Clifton Draper, USA
38. Tassilo Keilmann, Germany
39. Pim Kool, Netherlands
40. Atilla Aydinli, Turkey

41. Luigi Dona dalle Rose, Italy
42. Fritz Keilmann, Germany
43. Jyotirmoy Mazumder, USA
44. Carla Carbone, Italy
45. Walter Duley, Canada
46. Russell J. Wallace, USA
47. Uberto Macchioni, Italy (taking pictures)
48. Aldo La Rocca, Italy
49. Maria Grazia Dogliotti, Italy
50. Thierry Manderscheid, France

51. Jean-Pierre Celis, Belgium
52. Claude Chabrol, France
53. Bernd Stritzker, Germany
54. Janet Folkies, UK
55. Marios Petropoulos, Belgium
56. Carmen Afonso, Spain
57. Charles Marsden, UK
58. Paolo Gay, Italy
59. Paolo Mazzoldi, Italy
60. Joachim Frölingsdorf, Germany

61. Andrew Bloyce, UK
62. Gabriel Laufer, Israel
63. Giancarlo Battaglin, Italy
64. Steve Williamson, USA
65. Dan Gnanamuthu, USA
66. Michael Berry, USA

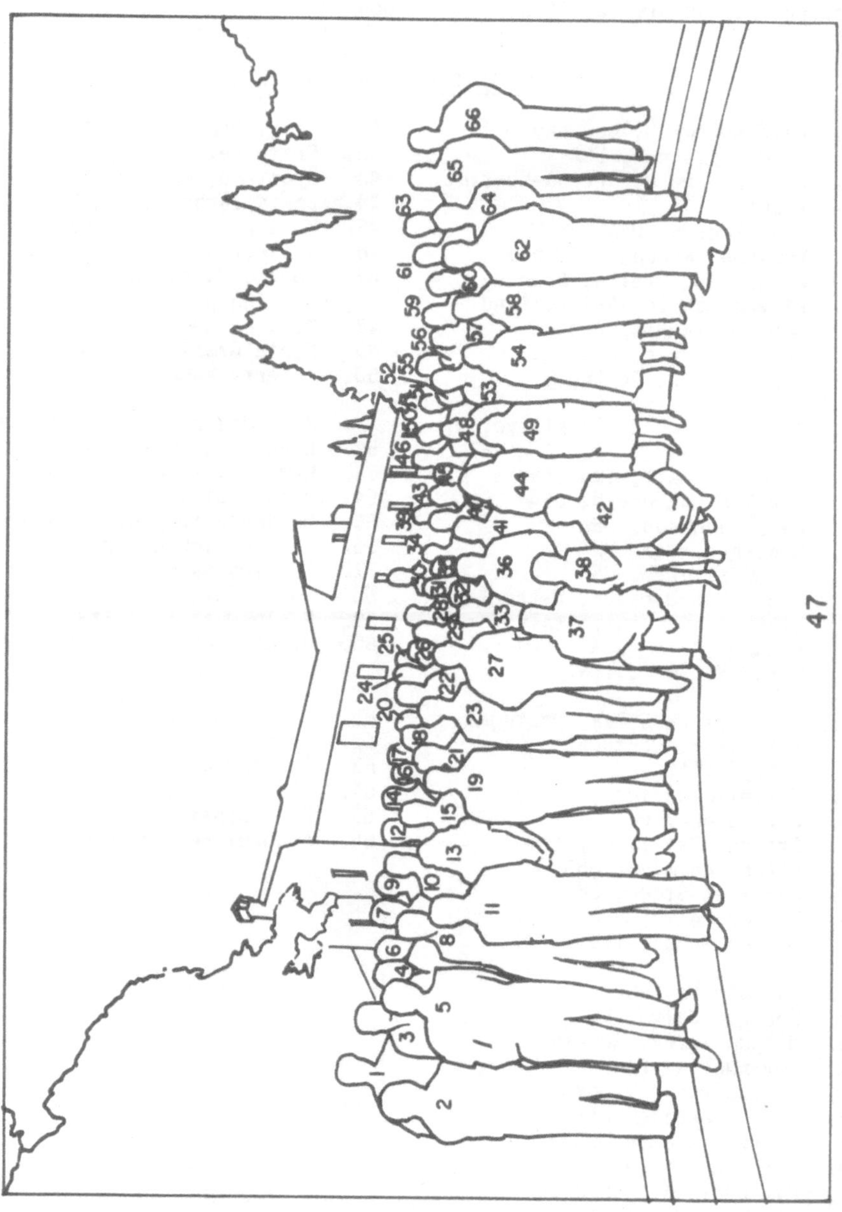

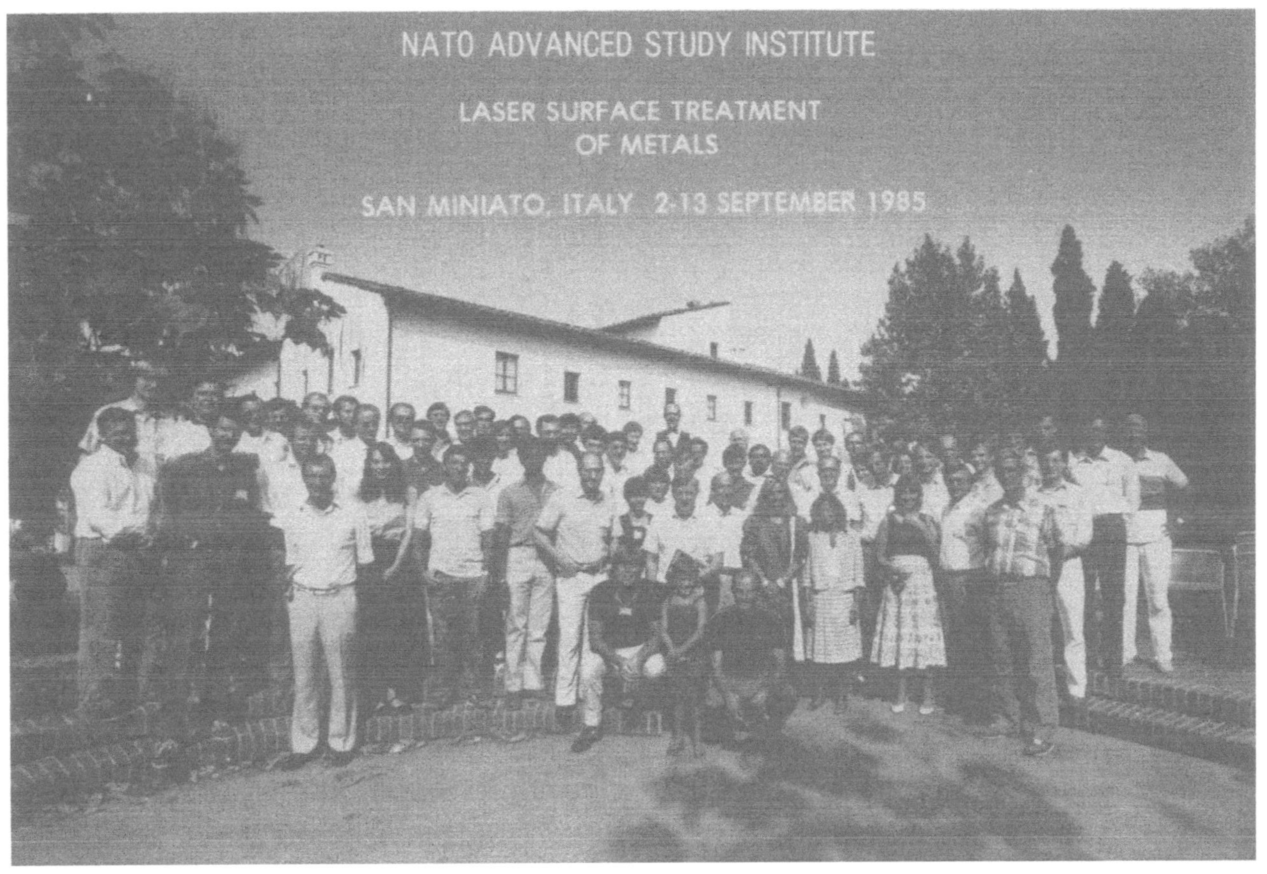
NATO ADVANCED STUDY INSTITUTE
LASER SURFACE TREATMENT
OF METALS
SAN MINIATO, ITALY 2-13 SEPTEMBER 1985

INVITED PARTICIPANTS AT NATO ASI.263/84

DIRECTORS AND COMMITTEE (also Lecturer*)

DR. CLIFTON W. DRAPER
AT&T Technologies
Engineering Research Center
P.O. Box 900
Princeton, NJ 08540

PROF. PAOLO MAZZOLDI
Dipartimento di Fisica
dell'Universita degli Studi
Via Marzolo, 8
35131 Padova, Italy

PROF. BARRY L. MORDIKE
Technische Universitat Clausthal
AgricolastraBe 2, D-3392
Clausthal-Zellerfeld, W. Germany

PROF. W. (BILL) M. STEEN*
Dept. of Metallurgy & Mat'l Sci.
Imperial College of Science & Tech.
London, S.W.7
United Kingdom

PROF. FRANS SPAEPEN*
Division of Applied Sciences
Harvard University
Cambridge, MA 02138

DR. A. BERNARD VANNES
Institut National des Sciences
Appliquees de Lyon
Villerubanne, France

LECTURERS (also International Organizations**)

MR. R. MALCOLM MACINTYRE
Rolls-Royce Limited
P.O. Box 3
Barnoldswick, Colne, Lancs
BB8 5RU England

PROF. HANS W. BERGMANN
Technische Universität Clausthal
Agricolastrasse 2, D-3392
Clausthal-Zellerfeld, W. Germany

DR. ALDO LA ROCCA
FIAT AUTO
Central Staff
Corso Orbanano, 637
10137 Torino, Italy

DR. ED MCCAFFERTY**
Naval Research Laboratory
Code 6314
Washington, DC 20375

PROF. WALTER W. DULEY
Dept. of Physics
York University
Downsview, Toronto
CANADA M3J 1P3

PROF. LUIGI F. DONA DALLE ROSE
Dipartimento di Fisica
Via Marzolo, 8
35131 Padova, Italy

DR. PAUL S. PEERCY
Sandia National Laboratories
P.O. Box 5800, Org. No. 1110
Albuquerque, NM 87185

DR. ELTON N. KAUFMANN**
P.O. Box 808 L-217
Lawrence Livermore National Lab.
Livermore, CA 94550

DR. BERND STRITZKER
KFA-IFF
D-5170 Julich Postfach 1913
West Germany

PROF. JEAN TARDIEU DE MALEISSYE
Universite' P. et M. Curie
4, Place Jussieu-Tour 55
75230 Paris Cedex 05
FRANCE

DR. JOHN M. POATE
AT&T Bell Labs
600 Mountain Ave.
Murray Hill, NJ 07974

PROF. S. UGO CAMPISANO
Universita di Catania
Istituto di Fisica
Corso Italia, 57
I 95129 Catania
Sicily, Italy

PARTICIPANTS

DR. CARMEN N. AFONSO
Instituto de Optica
C.S.I.C.
Serrano, 121
28006 Madrid, Spain

DR. ATILLA AYDINLI
Hacettepe University
Dept. of Physics Engineering
Beytepe-Ankara-Turkey

DR. MICHAEL J. AZIZ
Oak Ridge National Laboratory
Solid State Division, Bldg. 3003
Oak Ridge, TN 37831

MR. GIANCARLO BATTAGLIN
Dipartimento di Fisica
Via Marzolo 8
35131 Padova, Italy

PROF. MICHAEL BERRY
Department of Chemistry
Rice University
P.O. Box 1892
Houston, TX 77251

MR. TONY S. BRANSDEN
UKAFA Culham Laboratory
Abingdon Oxfordshire
OX14 3DB, United Kingdom

DR. BULGARELLI
Centro Informazioni Studi
Esperienze (CISE)
PO Box 12081
20100 Milan, Italy

DR. IR. JEAN-PIERRE CELIS
Katholieke Universitit Leuven
Metallurgy & Materials Eng.
de Croylaan 2
B-3030 Leuven, Belgium

DR. VITTORIA CONTINI
ENEA Cassaccia
Via Anguillarese Km. 1.300
C.P. 2400 - Roma, Italy

DR. GERARD COQUERELLE
ETCA
16 Bis, Ave Prieur de la Cote D'Or
94114 Arcueil Cedex, France

DR. DIEGO CRUCIANI
RTM
10080 Vico Canavese (Torino)
Italy

DR. M. FERNANDA DA SILVA
LNETI
Dept. of Physics
E. N. No. 10
2685 Sacaven, Portugal

MR. HENRI VAN DORSSEN
Martinus Nijhoff Publishers
Spuiboulevard 50
PO Box 163/3300 AD Dordrecht
The Netherlands

DR. RENATO FESTA
ENEA
C.R.E. CASACCIA-S.P. Anguillarese,
301 Casella Postale N.
2400-00100 Roma A.D., Italy

ING. PAOLO GAY
Centro Ricerche FIAT
Strada Torino 50
10043 Italy

PROF. JEAN-PIERRE GIRARDEAU-MONTAUT
Universite' Claude Bernard-Lyon I
Groupe de Physique des Interactions
Laser-Materiaux
UER de Physique-Bat. 205
43, Boulevard du 11 Novembre 1918
69622 Villeurbanne Cedex, France

MR. DANIEL S. GNANAMUTHU
Science Center
Rockwell International
1049 Camino Dos Rios
P.O. Box 1085
Thousand Oaks, CA 91360

DR. A. LINDSAY GREER
University of Cambridge
Dept. of Metallurgy & Mat. Sci.
Pembroke St.
Cambridge CB2 3QZ ENGLAND

DR. THOMAS JERVIS, MS E549
Los Alamos National Laboratory
P.O. Box 1663
Los Alamos, NM 87545

DR. FRITZ KEILMANN
Max-Planck-Institute
Solid State Research
Heisenberg Str. 1
D-7000 Stuttgart 80
West Germany

MR. EMMANUEL KERRAND
Laboratoires de Marcoussis
Centre de Recherches
de la Compagnie
Generale d'Electricite'
Route de Nozay
91460 Marcoussis FRANCE

PROF. W. H. (PIM) KOOL
Delft University of Technology
Department of Metals
Rotterdamseweg 137
2628 AL Delft
The Netherlands

DR. GABRIEL LAUFER
Faculty of Mechanical Engrg.
Technion
Technion City
Haifa 32000, Israel

DR. PIERRE MAGNIN
ECOLE POLYTECHNIQUE FEDERALE
DE LAUSANNE
Centre de traitement des
materiaux par laser
CH-1015 Lausanne, Switzerland

MR. THIERRY MANDERSCHEID
CITROEN
35 rue Grange Dame Rose
92360 Meudon La Foret
France

PROF. JYOTIRMOY MAZUMDER
University of Illinois at
Urbana-Champaign
1206 West Green St.
Urbana, IL 61801

PROF. EMILIO RAMOUS
Istituto Chimica Industriale
Via Marzolo 9
35131 Padova, Italy

DR. ING. GIUSEPPE RICCIARDI
RTM
10080 Vico Canavese (Torino)
Italy

DR. DAVID M. ROESSLER
Physics Dept.
General Motors Research Labs
Warren, MI 48090

DR. JOSE C. SOARES
Universidade de Lisboa
Centro De Fisica Nuclear
Av. Prof. Gamma Pinto, 2
1699 Lisboa Codex, Portugal

DR. M. NILGUN TEZEY
Bogazici University
App. Physics Dept.
Bebek-Istanbul
Turkey

PROF. MOMCILO M. TOSIC
"Boris Kidrich"
Institute of Nuclear Sciences
P.O. Box 522
11001 Belgrade
Yugoslavia

PROF. RUI VILAR
Universidade De Coimbra
Faculdade De Ciencias E Tecnologia
Seccao Autonoma
De Engenharia Mecania
3000 Coimbra-Portugal

DR. MARCO VITTORI
C.R.E. Casaccia
Div. Scienza Dei Materiali
Casella Postale N. 2400-00100
Rome, Italy

DR. RUSSELL J. WALLACE
Lawrence Livermore
National Laboratory
P.O. Box 808, L-370
Livermore, CA 94550

GRADUATE STUDENTS

MR. MARCELLO BARICCO
Universita di Torino
Instituto di Chimica Gen. ed Inorg.
via P. Giuria, 9
10125 Torino, Italy

MR. ANDREW BLOYCE
University of Birmingham
Dept. of Metallurgy
P.O. Box 363, Birmingham
B15 2TT, United Kingdom

MS. MONIQUE CALVO
Equipe Materiaux-Microstructure
du L.A. 251
I.S.M.R.A. Universite
14032 Caen Cedex France

MISS CLAUDE CHABROL
INSA-CALFETMAT
BAT. 303
69621 Villeurbanne Cedex
France

MS. JANET A. FOLKES
Metallurgy Department
Imperial College
London SW7 2BP

MR. JOACHIM FROHLINGSDORF
KFA Julich Gmbh, IFF
D-5170 Julich
P.O. Box 1913
West Germany

MR. AUBREY HELMS
Princeton University
Dept. of Chemistry
Princeton, NJ 08544

MR. DALE C. JACOBSON
AT&T Bell Laboratories
1E 256
600 Mountain Ave.
Murray Hill, NJ 07974

MR. RALF KOPPMANN
KFA Julich GmbH
Institut fur Plasmaphysik
Postfach 1913 D-5170 Julich
West Germany

MS. CAROLYN MACDONALD
502 Gordon McKay Laboratory
9 Oxford St.
Harvard University
Cambridge, MA 02138

MR. CHARLES F. MARSDEN
Imperial College
Metallurgy Dept.
London SW72BP
United Kingdom

MR. ETIENNE PETIT
Labo. ESCA
Facultes Universitaires Notre Dame
De La Paix
rue de Bruxelles, 61
B-5000 NAMUR, BELGIUM

MR. P. MARIOS PETROPOULOS
Faculte' des Sciences
Universite de L'Etat A Mons
Avenue Maistriau 23
7000 Mons Belgium

MR. TODD J. ROCKSTROH
Mechanical Engrg. Bldg.
1206 W. Green St.
Urbana, IL 61801

MR. SATISH VITTA
University of Cambridge
Dept. of Metallurgy & Mat. Sci.
Pembroke St., Cambridge
CB2 3QZ ENGLAND

MR. STEVE WILLIAMSON
University of Rochester
Laboratory for Laser Energetics
250 East River Road
Rochester, NY 14623

National Distribution of Participants

Nationality	Organizing Committee & Lecturers		Invited Participants		Graduate Students		Totals
Belgium	1		1		2		4
Canada	1						1
France	2		4		2		8
Federal Republic of Germany	3		1		2		6
Italy	4		9		1		14
Netherlands			2				2
Portugal			3				3
Spain			1				1
Turkey			2				2
United Kingdom	2		2		4		8
United States	3		7		5		15
Intern. Organizations	2**						2
Other			3				3
Totals	18	+	35	+	16	+	69

**President, Materials Research Society
Chairman, Corrosion Division, The Electrochemical Society

Index